W9-BHT-797

Understanding Pharmacology

Essentials for Medication Safety

evolve

ELSEVIER

YOU'VE JUST PURCHASED
MORE THAN
A TEXTBOOK!

Evolve Student Resources for *Workman: Understanding Pharmacology, 2nd edition*, include the following:

- Interactive Review Questions
- Answer Keys
- Essential Drug Patient Teaching Handouts
- Video Clips
- Drug Dosage Calculators
- Spanish/English Audio Glossary

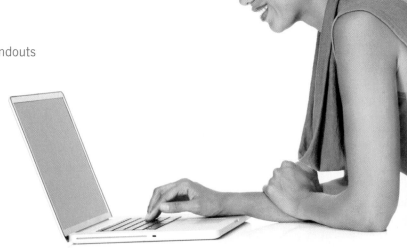

Activate the complete learning experience that comes with each textbook purchase by registering at

http://evolve.elsevier.com/Workman/pharmacology/

REGISTER TODAY!

You can now purchase Elsevier products on Evolve!
Go to evolve.elsevier.com/html/shop-promo.html to search and browse for products.

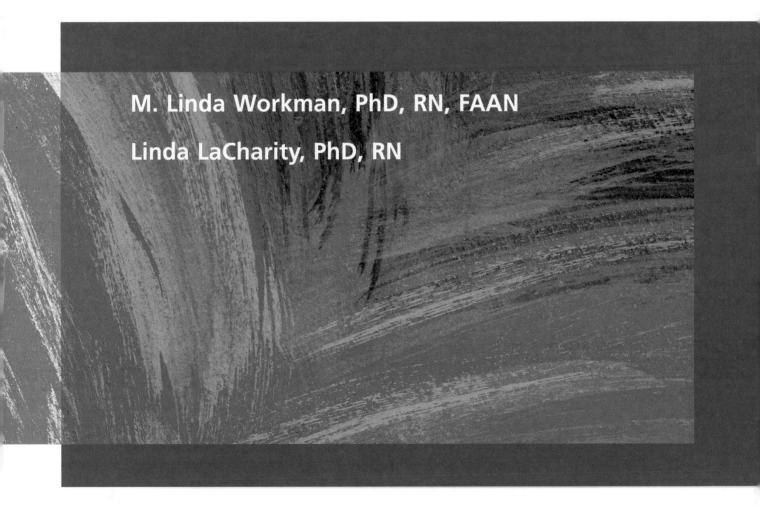

Understanding Pharmacology
Essentials for Medication Safety

2 EDITION

M. Linda Workman, PhD, RN, FAAN

Linda LaCharity, PhD, RN

ELSEVIER

ELSEVIER

3251 Riverport Lane
St. Louis, Missouri 63043

UNDERSTANDING PHARMACOLOGY: ESSENTIALS FOR
MEDICATION SAFETY, SECOND EDITION   ISBN: 978-1-4557-3976-9
Copyright © 2016, by Elsevier Inc. All rights reserved.

No part of this publication may be reproduced or transmitted in any form or by any means,
electronic or mechanical, including photocopying, recording, or any information storage and
retrieval system, without permission in writing from the publisher. Details on how to seek
permission, further information about the Publisher's permissions policies and our arrangements
with organizations such as the Copyright Clearance Center and the Copyright Licensing Agency,
can be found at our website: www.elsevier.com/permissions.

This book and the individual contributions contained in it are protected under copyright by the
Publisher (other than as may be noted herein).

Notices

Knowledge and best practice in this field are constantly changing. As new research and
experience broaden our understanding, changes in research methods, professional practices, or
medical treatment may become necessary.

Practitioners and researchers must always rely on their own experience and knowledge in
evaluating and using any information, methods, compounds, or experiments described herein.
In using such information or methods they should be mindful of their own safety and the safety
of others, including parties for whom they have a professional responsibility.

With respect to any drug or pharmaceutical products identified, readers are advised to check
the most current information provided (i) on procedures featured or (ii) by the manufacturer of
each product to be administered, to verify the recommended dose or formula, the method and
duration of administration, and contraindications. It is the responsibility of practitioners, relying
on their own experience and knowledge of their patients, to make diagnoses, to determine
dosages and the best treatment for each individual patient, and to take all appropriate safety
precautions.

To the fullest extent of the law, neither the Publisher nor the authors, contributors, or editors,
assume any liability for any injury and/or damage to persons or property as a matter of
products liability, negligence or otherwise, or from any use or operation of any methods,
products, instructions, or ideas contained in the material herein.

Previous edition copyrighted 2011.

International Standard Book Number: 978-1-4557-3976-9

Senior Content Strategist: Nancy O'Brien
Content Development Manager: Ellen Wurm-Cutter, Laurie Gower
Content Development Specialist: Heather Rippetoe, Laura Goodrich
Publishing Services Manager: Jeff Patterson
Senior Project Manager: Jodi M. Willard
Design Direction: Renee Duenow

Printed in Canada

Last digit is the print number: 9 8 7 6 5

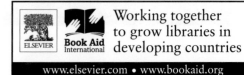

To David, Emmy, and Violet, who complete my rainbow.

M. Linda Workman

To my mother, the late Routh Annette Jenkins. An extraordinary woman and the inspiration for my research and the shaping of my career.

Linda LaCharity

About the Authors

M. Linda Workman, a native of Canada, received her BSN from the University of Cincinnati College of Nursing and Health. She later earned her MSN and a PhD in Developmental Biology from the University of Cincinnati. Linda's more than 30 years of academic experience include teaching at the diploma, associate degree, baccalaureate, and master's levels. Her areas of teaching expertise include medical-surgical nursing, pharmacology, physiology, and pathophysiology. Linda has been called the "Mr. Rogers" of nursing education for her ability to creatively present complex physiologic concepts in a manner that promotes student retention of the information. She has been recognized nationally for her teaching expertise and has received Excellence in Teaching awards from Raymond Walters College, the University of Cincinnati, and Case Western Reserve University. Currently she consults with a variety of nursing programs on teaching and curricular issues and co-authors a medical-surgical nursing textbook (Ignatavicius and Workman: *Medical-Surgical Nursing: Patient-Centered Collaborative Care*) and a genetics textbook.

Linda LaCharity received her BSN from Kent State University's College of Nursing. During her career in the U.S. Army Nurse Corps, she earned an MN from the University of Washington in Seattle. Linda earned her PhD from the University of Cincinnati. She worked as a staff nurse and nurse manager in adult medical-surgical and critical care settings supervising RNs, LPN/LVNs, and nursing assistant staff. Linda's academic experience includes teaching EMTs and critical care nurses for the military and across the curriculum at the University of Cincinnati (BSN, MSN, Accelerated BSN/MSN, and PhD). Her area of teaching expertise in both classroom and patient care settings is adult health. She was director of the Accelerated Program and an Assistant Professor in the College of Nursing at the University of Cincinnati in Cincinnati, Ohio. Retired in 2013, she continues to write textbooks.

Reviewers and Advisory Board

REVIEWERS

Chris Bridgers, PharmD
Saint Joseph's Hospital
Atlanta, Georgia

Andrew D. Case, BSN, MSN
Professor of Human Anatomy, Physiology, and
  Pharmacology
Southeast Community College
Lincoln, Nebraska

Diane K. Daddario, MSN, ACNS-BC, RN, BC, CMSRN
Clinical Nursing Instructor
Pennsylvania College of Technology
Williamsport, Pennsylvania

Michael Dorich, PhD, CST, CAHI
Program Director, Surgical Technology
Pittsburgh Technical Institute
Oakdale, Pennsylvania

Gail E. Dunham, MSN
Professor of Nursing
Mid Michigan Community College
Harrison, Michigan

Sally Flesch, RN, BSN, MA, EdS, PhD
Coordinator, Professor
Practical Nursing Program
Black Hawk College
Moline, Illinois

Cathy Maddry, MSN, MA, RN, Alumnus CCRN
Department Head
Heath Occupations
Northwest Louisiana Technical College
Minden Louisiana

Mary E. Stassi, RN-BC
Health Occupations Coordinator
St. Charles Community College
Cottleville, Missouri

Claudia Stoffel, MSN, RN, CNE
Practical Nursing Program Coordinator
West Kentucky Community and Technical College
Paducah, Kentucky

Audrey Tolouian, MSN, BSW, (EdD)
Clinical Instructor, School of Nursing
University of Texas
El Paso, Texas

Erin Yesenosky, MSN
Nursing Instructor
Greater Altoona Career & Technology Center
Altoona, Pennsylvania

ADVISORY BOARD

Nancy Bohnarczyk, MA
Adjunct Instructor
College of Mount St. Vincent
New York, New York

Sharyn P. Boyle, MSN, RN-BC
Instructor, Associate Degree Nursing
Passaic County Technical Institute
Wayne, New Jersey

Nicola Contreras, BN, RN
Faculty
Galen College
San Antonio, Texas

Dolores Cotton, MSN, RN
Practical Nursing Coordinator
Meridian Technology Center
Stillwater, Oklahoma

Sharon Gordon, MSN, RN, CNOR-E
Practical Nursing Faculty
Lehigh Carbon Community College
Schnecksville, Pennsylvania

Nancy Haughton, MSN, RN
Practical Nursing Program Faculty
Chester County Intermediate Unit
Downingtown, Pennsylvania

Shelly Hovis, MS, RN
Director, Practical Nursing
Kiamichi Technology Centers
Antlers, Oklahoma

Dawn Johnson, RN, MSN, Ed
Practical Nurse Program Director
Great Lakes Institute of Technology
Erie, Pennsylvania

Kristin Madigan, RN, MS
Nursing Faculty
Pine Technical and Community College
Pine City, Minnesota

Hana Malik, RN, MSN, FNP-BC
Academic Director
Illinois College of Nursing
Lombard, Illinois

Barb Ratliff, RN, MSN
Associate Director of Health Programs
Butler Technology and Career Development Schools
Hamilton, Ohio

Faye Silverman, RN, MSN/Ed, PHN, WOCN
Director of Professional Nursing
Kaplan College - North Hollywood Campus
North Hollywood, California

Russlyn A. St. John, RN, MSN
Professor and Coordinator, Practical Nursing
Practical Nursing Department
St. Charles Community College
Cottleville, Missouri

Fleur de Liza Tobias-Cuyco, BSC, CPhT
Dean, Director of Student Affairs, and Instructor
Preferred College of Nursing
Los Angeles, California

Preface

The authors of this text are nurses and educators with many decades of clinical and teaching experience. Our concept of what is needed in a pharmacology textbook is derived from the desire to create a book that will help students identify the most important content areas for safe drug administration and patient teaching. With this goal in mind, we developed a unique format based on four focus areas:

- Why specific drugs are prescribed as therapy for common health problems
- How different drugs work to induce their intended responses
- What critical actions and assessments to perform before and after administering drugs
- Which points are most important to teach patients about their drug therapy

Using these focus areas, we present pharmacology content in a framework that promotes in-depth learning versus rote memorization, which is truly essential in understanding the principles of pharmacology and safe drug administration. Interwoven within the textbook are areas that highlight specific safety issues with regard to medication administration. The impetus for this inclusion are the recommendations championed by the American Association of Colleges of Nursing, collectively known as the Quality and Safety Education for Nurses (QSEN) practice standards. Although this initiative is nursing based, the focus on safety must be a major directive for all health care professionals involved in the prescribing, preparing, dispensing, and administering aspects of drug therapy. Specific actions related to safety are noted with "QSEN" throughout the text.

CHAPTER ORGANIZATION

The textbook has been expanded to accommodate requested information in content areas not presented in the first edition. These areas now include immunizations and drugs affecting the immune system, drug therapy for adrenal gland problems, nutritional supplements, drug therapy for musculoskeletal problems, and drug therapy for common problems of the male and female reproductive systems. The text has been reorganized into 10 units totaling 32 chapters to streamline access to specific content areas. Unit I provides an overview of general content important for safe medication administration. Unit II provides essential mathematical concepts and practice for safe dosage calculation. Unit III focuses on content that has application to many body systems, such

as inflammation, infection, pain, and cancer. The remaining seven units are divided by the body system most closely associated with the specific drug therapy. For example, Unit V, Drug Therapy for Problems of the Circulatory and Cardiac Systems, is further divided into six chapters that include drug therapy affecting urine output, hypertension, heart failure, dysrhythmias, high blood lipids, and blood clotting. We believe this content arrangement synchronizes the information for students when they are studying specific health problems and issues. Although information regarding normal physiology and pathophysiology is still presented, this information has been streamlined to promote the pharmacology focus of the text.

Our presentation style for the content of this text is direct, active, and clear. Health care terms and related physiological mechanisms are explained in clear, straightforward, everyday language to promote better student understanding and application of the content in the clinical setting. Photographs and other illustrations have been selected and developed to better explain drug administration techniques, drug actions, and appropriate health care interventions.

Chapter **Objectives** presented at the beginning of each chapter focus the student on "need to know" information, clarifying which issues have the highest priority for safe drug administration. A list of **Key Terms** includes phonetic pronunciations, definitions, and page numbers where each term is first used.

The **mathematics review chapters** (Chapters 3, 4, and 5) are written in a self-paced, guided-study format and contain easy-to-understand explanations and examples. **Try This!** boxes provide more than 150 practice questions within these chapters, in addition to the end-of-chapter review material. Answers to these exercises are found at the end of the chapters.

In-text **drug tables** outline the most common drugs used to treat highlighted disorders and diseases. Generic and trade names and common dosage ranges for adults and children are included.

Discussion sections on **"What To Do Before," "What To Do After,"** and **"What to Teach Patients"** about each highlighted drug or drug category emphasize the important aspects of drug administration, monitoring, follow-up, and patient teaching.

Life Span Considerations sections receive particular attention in most chapters. Differences in actions, the risks for side effects, precautions, or dosing for pediatric patients, pregnant or breastfeeding patients, or older adults are presented as appropriate for each drug class.

A **Get Ready for Practice!** section at the end of each chapter features Key Points, Additional Learning Resources, Review Questions, and Critical Thinking Activities.

- **Key Points** emphasize selected need-to-know content from the chapter to help students study for tests and certification/licensure exams.
- **Additional Learning Resources** sections refer students to related review material in the accompanying Study Guide and on the Evolve website at http://evolve.elsevier.com/Workman/pharmacology/.
- **Review Questions** correspond item-by-item with the Objectives at the beginning of the chapter. Drug calculation questions are also included in this section. Answers to the Review Questions are located on the Evolve site. These review questions are divided by basic and advanced level concepts.
- **Critical Thinking Activities** are true-to-practice case studies that present issues and problems requiring clinical decision making related to individual patients receiving pharmacologic therapy. Answer guidelines to the questions are available on the secure Evolve instructor website at http://evolve.elsevier.com/Workman/pharmacology/.

LEARNER-FRIENDLY INSTRUCTIONAL DESIGN

One of the most innovative features of this text is its unique instructional design. A single column presents the narrative, and a wide margin is used to reinforce important concepts and prevent medication errors with special boxed features. This wide margin also allows generous space for note-taking. Special learning features found in the wide margin include the following:

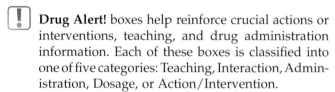

Drug Alert! boxes help reinforce crucial actions or interventions, teaching, and drug administration information. Each of these boxes is classified into one of five categories: Teaching, Interaction, Administration, Dosage, or Action/Intervention.

Memory Jogger boxes highlight and summarize essential information, including major categories of drugs and the diseases they are used to treat.

Clinical Pitfall boxes focus on information vital for safe practice and medication administration.

Common Side Effects boxes focus on individual drug groups and feature unique icons that promote rapid recognition.

Do Not Confuse boxes highlight look-alike/sound-alike drug names.

Did You Know? boxes help students link pharmacology content to the world around them.

Cultural Awareness boxes emphasize important cultural considerations related to pharmacology.

We believe you'll find that the authors and publisher have crafted a balance of these features to minimize wasted space and at the same time promote in-depth learning versus rote memorization.

TEACHING AND LEARNING PACKAGE

FOR STUDENTS

A companion **Study Guide,** available for purchase at elsevier.com, features a variety of engaging learning activities that complement those in the textbook. Clinically focused Medication Safety Practice questions and a Practice Quiz are provided in each chapter along with a variety of other Learning Activities that promote an understanding of pharmacology and safe drug administration.

The **Evolve website** at http://evolve.elsevier.com/Workman/pharmacology/ provides free student learning resources that include the following:

- Over 390 **Interactive Review Questions** in multiple-choice and alternate item formats, with rationales for correct and incorrect answers, help students review important chapter material.
- **Answer Keys** are provided for the in-text Review Questions, in-text Critical Thinking Activities, and Study Guide.
- **Video Clips** explain important concepts from anatomy and physiology to drug administration and are keyed to the text by distinctive icons.
- Twelve interactive **Drug Dosage Calculators** offer a quick way to calculate IV dosages, body surface area, oral doses, and more.
- An extensive **Spanish/English Audio Glossary** provides a vast array of health care–related terms and their definitions (with audio) in both English and Spanish.
- A collection of **Essential Drug Patient Teaching Handouts** can be used to provide patients with information on almost any available drug in both English and Spanish.

FOR INSTRUCTORS

The comprehensive *Evolve Resources with TEACH Instructor Resource* provides everything a new or seasoned instructor will need to teach the content, including the following:

- **TEACH Lesson Plans,** based on textbook Objectives, tie together the text and all other learning resources in ready-to-use, customizable lessons.

- A high-quality **Test Bank,** delivered in ExamView, RTF, and ParTest formats, as well as within the Assessment area of Evolve, contains more than 1200 test items created by the authors. Approximately 50% of these items are written at the Applying or higher cognitive level of Bloom's taxonomy. Each question includes the correct answer, rationale, and cognitive level, as well as corresponding textbook page numbers, where appropriate (page numbers are not appropriate for questions at the Applying level or above because they draw on multiple sources of information).
- A collection of **PowerPoint Lecture Slides** with **Audience Response System Questions** highlight key concepts and discussion in the text.

- An **Image Collection** contains every reproducible image from the text. Images are suitable for incorporation into classroom lectures, PowerPoint presentations, or distance-learning applications.

Understanding Pharmacology: Essentials for Medication Safety, together with its fully integrated multimedia ancillary package, provides the tools needed to fully understand pharmacology principles and how to apply them effectively and safely in today's health care environment. For more information on any of these innovative companion publications, or if you simply wish to provide us feedback, please contact your Elsevier sales representative, visit us at http://www.us.elsevierhealth.com/, or contact Elsevier Faculty Support at 1-800-222-9570 or sales.inquiry@elsevier.com.

Acknowledgments

Many talented people are needed to make any textbook a success. The authors wish to acknowledge the following individuals and groups for their guidance, dedication, hard work, constructive criticism, and creative input that were so important to this project: Nancy O'Brien, Heather Rippetoe, Laura Goodrich, Jodi Willard, all of the reviewers, and Yvonne LaCharity and Gregory Workman—our very own math experts. A special thank you to Teri Hines Burnham for her unflagging belief in this project.

Special Features

Understanding Pharmacology: Essentials for Medication Safety, 2nd edition, focuses on an *understanding* of pharmacology principles and safety of drug administration by using clear, everyday language. Full-color illustrations and a unique, user-friendly design accompany practical, understandable discussions of important drugs and drug classes.

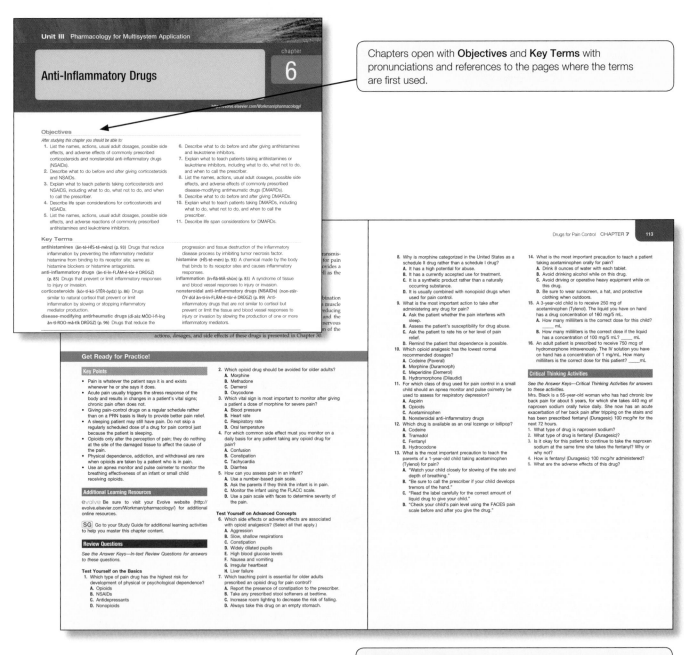

Chapters open with **Objectives** and **Key Terms** with pronunciations and references to the pages where the terms are first used.

Get Ready for Practice! sections include **Key Points**, **Critical Thinking Activities**, and **Review Questions** grouped by basic and advanced-level concepts.

Drug Alert! boxes highlight important tips for safe medication administration.

Video clips illustrate medication administration procedures.

Full-color illustrations explain key procedures, pathophysiology, and pharmacology concepts.

Try This! boxes in the math chapters let you practice math and dosage calculation concepts as you learn them. Answers are found at the end of the chapter.

Memory Jogger boxes summarize essential information, including major categories of drugs and the diseases they are used to treat.

Did You Know? boxes relate pharmacology content to everyday life.

Clinical Pitfall boxes highlight critically important clinical situations to avoid.

Drug tables provide generic drug names, brand names, and typical dosage ranges. Canadian and High-Alert drugs are noted with special icons.

Do Not Confuse boxes highlight look-alike/sound-alike drugs to help you avoid drug errors.

Common Side Effects boxes use memorable, easy-to-recognize icons to emphasize common side effects of drugs.

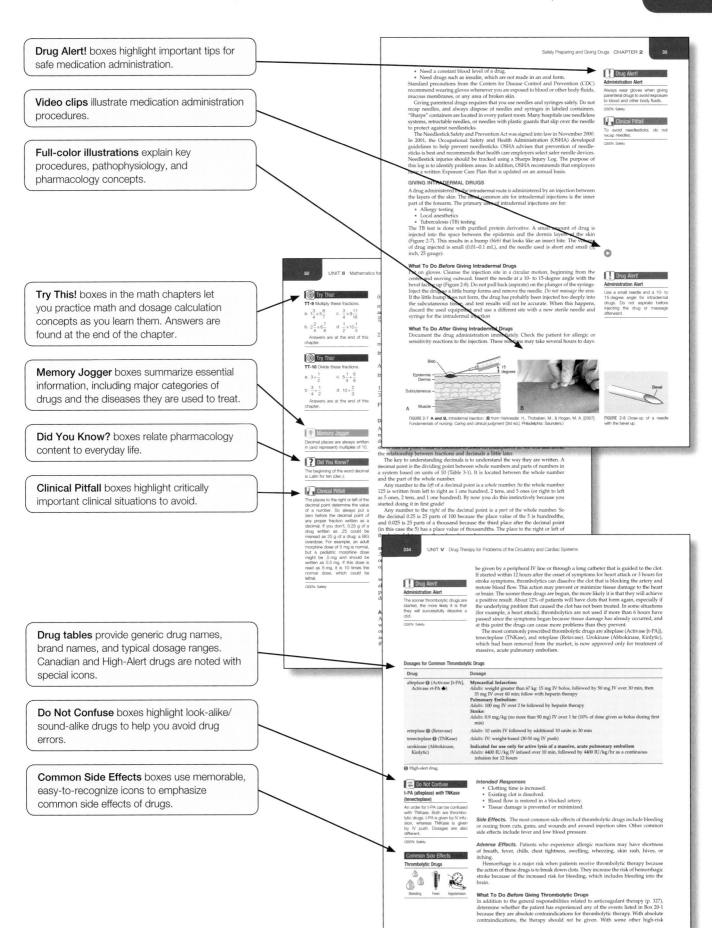

Contents

chapter

Drug Regulation, Actions, and Responses

1

http://evolve.elsevier.com/Workman/pharmacology/

Objectives

After studying this chapter you should be able to:

1. Define the common terms associated with drug therapy.
2. Explain the differences of a drug therapeutic effect (intended action), a drug side effect, and an adverse drug effect.
3. Compare the activity of a cell when an agonist drug binds to the receptor and when an antagonist drug binds to the receptor.
4. Explain the similarities and differences between allergic responses and personal responses to drugs.
5. Explain the purposes, advantages, and disadvantages of the different routes of drug administration.
6. Describe the processes and organs involved in drug metabolism and elimination.
7. Explain the influence of drug half-life, peak blood level, and trough of blood level on drug activity.
8. Describe the ways in which drug therapy for children differs from drug therapy for adults.
9. Describe two changes in older adults that make drug action, drug metabolism, and drug elimination different from that of younger adults.
10. Explain how pregnancy and breastfeeding should be taken into consideration with drug therapy.

Key Terms

absorption (ăb-SŌRP-shŭn) (p. 11) Movement of a drug from the outside of the body into the bloodstream.

adverse drug reaction (ADR) (ĂD-vŭrs DRŬG rē-ĂK-shŭn) (p. 8) Same as adverse effect.

adverse effect (ĂD-vŭrs ĕf-FĔKT) (p. 8) A drug effect that is more severe than expected and has the potential to damage tissue or cause serious health problems. It may also be called a toxic effect or toxicity and usually requires intervention by the prescriber.

agonist (ĂG-ŏn-ĭst) (p. 6) An extrinsic drug that activates the receptor site of a cell and mimics the actions of naturally occurring body substances (intrinsic drugs).

allergic response (ă-LŬR-jĭk rē-SPŎNS) (p. 9) Type of adverse effect in which the presence of the drug stimulates the release of histamine and other body chemicals that cause inflammatory reactions. The response may be as mild as a rash or as severe and life threatening as anaphylaxis.

antagonist (ăn-TĂG-ŏn-ĭst) (p. 7) An extrinsic drug that blocks the receptor site of a cell, preventing the naturally occurring body substance from binding to the receptor.

bioavailability (bī-ō-ă-vāl-ă-BĬL-ĭ-tē) (p. 11) The percentage of a drug dose that actually reaches the blood.

black box warning (BLĂK BŎKS WŌR-nĭng) (p. 9) A notice that a drug may produce serious or even life-threatening effects in some people in addition to its beneficial effects.

brand name (BRĂND NĀM) (p. 4) A manufacturer-owned name of a generic drug; also called "trade name" or "proprietary name."

contraindication (KŎN-tră-ĭn-dĭ-KĀ-shŭn) (p. 9) A personal or health-related reason for not administering a specific drug to a patient or group of patients.

cytotoxic (sī-tō-TŎKS-ĭk) (p. 8) Drug action that is intended to kill a cell or an organism.

distribution (dĭs-trĭ-BYŪ-shŭn) (p. 14) (drug distribution) The extent that a drug absorbed into the bloodstream spreads into the three body water compartments.

drug (DRŬG) (p. 2) Any small molecule that changes any body function by working at the chemical and cell levels.

drug therapy (DRŬG THĂR-ă-pē) (p. 3) The planned use of a drug to prevent or improve a health problem.

duration of action (dū-RĀ-shŭn of ĂK-shŭn) (p. 11) The length of time a drug is present in the blood at or above the level needed to produce an effect or response.

elimination (ē-lĭm-ĭ-NĀ-shŭn) (p. 15) The removal of drugs from the body accomplished by certain body systems.

enteral route (ĔN-tĕr-ŭl ROWT) (p. 11) Movement of drugs from the outside of the body to the inside using the gastrointestinal tract.

first-pass loss (FŬRST PĂS LŎS) (p. 15) Rapid inactivation or elimination of oral drugs as a result of liver metabolism.

generic name (jĕn-ĂR-ĭk NĀM) (p. 3) National and international public drug name created by the United States Adopted Names (USAN) Council to indicate the usual use or chemical composition of a drug.

half-life (HĂF LĪF) (p. 16) Time span needed for one half of a drug dose to be eliminated.

high-alert drug (HĪ ă-LŬRT DRŬG) (p. 4) A drug that has an increased risk for causing patient harm if it is used in error.

intended action (ĭn-TĔN-dĕd ĂK-shŭn) (p. 3) Desired effect (main effect) of a drug on specific body cells or tissues; same as therapeutic response.

loading dose (LŌ-dĭng DŌS) (p. 16) The first dose of a drug that is larger than all subsequent doses of the same drug; used when it takes more drug to reach steady state than it does to maintain it.

mechanism of action (MĔK-ă-nĭz-ŭm of ĂK-shŭn) (p. 6) Exactly how, at the cellular level, a drug changes the activity of a cell.

medication (mě-dĭ-KĀ-shŭn) (p. 2) Any small molecule that changes any body function by working at the chemical and cell levels (same as a drug).

metabolism (mě-TĂB-ō-lĭz-ĭm) (p. 14) (drug metabolism) Chemical reaction in the body that changes the chemical shape and content of a drug, preparing the drug for inactivation and elimination.

minimum effective concentration (MEC) (MĬN-ĭ-mŭm ĕf-FĔK-tĭv kŏn-sĕn-TRĀ-shŭn) (p. 10) The smallest amount of drug necessary in the blood or target tissue to result in a measurable intended action.

over-the-counter (OTC) (Ō-vŭr THĒ KOWN-tŭr) (p. 4) Drugs that are approved for purchase without a prescription.

parenteral route (pă-RĔN-tĕr-ăl ROWT) (p. 11) Movement of a drug from the outside of the body to the inside of the body by injection (intra-arterial, intravenous, intramuscular, subcutaneous, intradermal, intracavitary, intraosseous, intrathecal).

peak (PĒK) (p. 17) Maximum blood drug level.

percutaneous route (pĕr-kū-TĀN-ē-ŭs ROWT) (p. 11) Movement of a drug from the outside of the body to the inside through the skin or mucous membranes.

pharmacodynamics (făr-mă-kō-dĪ-NĂM-ĭks) (p. 5) Ways in which drugs work to change body function.

pharmacokinetics (făr-mă-kō-kĭn-ĔT-ĭks) (p. 10) How the body changes drugs; drug metabolism.

pharmacology (făr-mă-KŎL-ō-jē) (p. 3) The science and study of drugs and their actions on living animals.

physiologic effect (fĭ-zē-ō-LŌ-jĭk ĕf-FĔKT) (p. 8) The change in body function as an outcome of the mechanism of action of a drug.

potency (PŌ-tĕn-sē) (p. 11) The strength of the intended action produced at a given drug dose.

prescription (prē-SKRĬP-shŭn) (p. 4) An order written or dictated by a state-approved prescriber for a specific drug therapy for a specific patient.

prescription drugs (prē-SKRĬP-shŭn DRŬGZ) (p. 4) The legal status of any drug that is considered unsafe for self-medication or has a potential for addiction and is only available by a prescription written by a state-approved health care professional.

receptors (rē-SĔP-TŬRZ) (p. 6) Physical place on or in a cell where a drug can bind and interact.

side effects (SĪD ē-FĔKTS) (p. 3) Any minor effect of a drug on body cells or tissues that is not the intended action of a drug.

steady state (STĔD-ē STĀT) (p. 11) Point at which drug elimination is balanced with drug entry, resulting in a constant effective blood level of the drug.

target tissue (TĂR-gĕt TĬ-shū) (p. 6) The actual cells or tissues affected by the mechanism of action or intended actions of a specific drug.

transdermal (trănz-DŬR-mŭl) (p. 12) Type of percutaneous drug delivery in which the drug is applied to the skin, passes through the skin, and enters the bloodstream.

trough (TRŎF) (p. 17) The lowest or minimal blood drug level.

vaporized (VĀ-pŭr-īzd) (p. 15) Changing of a drug from a liquid form to a gas or mist that can be absorbed into the body by inhalation.

DRUG THERAPY

OVERVIEW

When used appropriately, drugs can help prevent, reduce, or correct a health problem. Some health problems are minor or temporary. Other health problems are complicated, serious, or chronic and require long-term treatment and monitoring. Drugs are often used to diagnose or treat health problems. A **drug** is any small molecule that changes a body function by working at the chemical and cell levels. So, many everyday substances are drugs, including caffeine, alcohol, and nicotine. Some drugs are manufactured from chemicals, others are taken from plants, and still others are taken from a person or animal to be used by another person. For example, insulin can be made in a laboratory, or it can be taken from the pancreas of a cow or pig and given to humans. (There are no plant sources of insulin.)

Some people use the term **medication** for substances that are used to treat health problems and the term *drug* for substances that are harmful or can be abused. However, these terms mean the same thing, and any drug or medication can be misused.

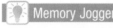 Memory Jogger

Any drug (medication) can be misused and harm a person.

When a plan to prevent or improve a health problem includes the use of drugs, it is called **drug therapy.** Drug therapy includes these factors:

- Identifying the specific health problem
- Determining what drug or drugs would best help the problem
- Deciding the best delivery method and schedule
- Ensuring that the proper amount of the drug is given
- Helping the patient become an active participant in his or her drug therapy

The prescriber's role in drug therapy is to select and order specific drugs. The authority to prescribe varies by state. State-approved prescribers may include physicians, dentists, podiatrists, advanced practice nurses, and physician's assistants. The pharmacist's role is to mix (compound) and dispense prescribed drugs. The pharmacy technician's role is to mix and dispense prescribed drugs under the direction of a registered pharmacist. The nurse's role is to administer prescribed drugs directly to the patient. In some states, medical assistants can administer drugs to patients under the direction of a prescriber or other licensed health professional. Because nurses often are the last checkpoint for safe drug therapy, they must know the purposes, actions, side effects, problems, delivery methods, and necessary follow-up care for different drugs. Along with prescribers and pharmacists, nurses teach patients about the drugs they have been prescribed.

It is important to understand the interactions and mechanisms by which various types of drugs influence body activity. Drugs are prescribed or used to improve some body condition or function. But the body actually makes some of its own drugs in the form of hormones, enzymes, growth factors, and other substances that change the activity of cells. The chemicals the body makes are called *intrinsic drugs*—the insulin made by the pancreas is one example of an intrinsic drug. Other drugs are made outside of the body and must be taken into the body to change cell, organ, or body action. These drugs are known as *extrinsic drugs* because the body does not make them. The study of drugs and how they work **(pharmacology)** is concerned mainly with extrinsic drugs. However, many effective extrinsic drugs are nearly identical to the drugs the body creates. For example, the body makes endorphin, which is very similar to the extrinsic drug morphine. Morphine is a very effective pain reliever because it has the same action as endorphin at the cell level.

Any drug affects some tissue or organ in the body. The reason a drug is prescribed is that it has at least one desired effect that improves body function; this is called the **intended action** or the *therapeutic response.* Think about a drug that widens (dilates) blood vessels and thereby lowers blood pressure. The therapeutic response of such a drug is to lower blood pressure; thus it is classified as an antihypertensive drug. In addition to its intended action or therapeutic response, there may be many minor changes in body function that occur when the drug is taken. These minor effects of a drug on body cells or tissues that are not the intended actions are known as **side effects.** Side effects can be helpful or may cause problems. For example, a drug to treat high blood pressure (hypertension) that widens blood vessels also may cause the side effects of dizziness and ankle swelling. All drugs have at least one intended action and at least one side effect. The safety of any drug is determined by balancing the seriousness of the side effects against the benefit of the therapeutic effect.

DRUG NAMES

Most drugs have more than one name, which can be confusing. There are three types of drug names: the chemical name, the generic name, and the brand name (trade name). The *chemical name* of a drug describes the exact chemical composition of atoms and molecules for the main ingredient of the drug. For example, the chemical name for Cozaar is: 2-butyl-4-chloro-1-[p-(O-1H-tetrazol-5 phenyl)benzyl] imidazole-5-methanol monopotassium salt. Chemical names are used only by the chemists who develop and manufacture the drug.

The **generic name** of a drug is a shorter, simpler name used by pharmacists, physicians, nurses, and other health care professionals. The generic name for Cozaar is losartan. The United States Adopted Names (USAN) Council creates the generic

Memory Jogger

Professionals who may prescribe drugs vary by state and may include physicians, advanced practice nurses, dentists, podiatrists, physician's assistants, and veterinarians.

Memory Jogger

Your body actually makes drugs. Drugs made by the body are called *intrinsic drugs.*

Memory Jogger

All drugs have at least one intended action and at least one side effect.

Did You Know?

The chemical name of a drug is not used by patients or health care providers.

names used for all drugs made in the United States. The rules used to name drugs help to ensure that the generic name is relatively short, gives some clue as to its use or chemical composition, and does not sound too much like any other known drug name. Often some part of all generic names for drugs of one class (also known as a "drug family") will be the same. For example, all the generic names for blood pressure control drugs that are angiotensin II receptor antagonists (also known as angiotensin receptor blockers [ARBs]) end in "-sartan," (such as eprosartan, losartan, telmisartan). Most beta-blockers end in "-olol" (such as atenolol, metoprolol, and propranolol). After the generic name is approved, it is public and not owned by any one drug company. When a generic drug name is written, the first letter is not capitalized.

Brand names are created by each drug company that makes and sells a specific drug. Other terms for "brand name" are *proprietary name* and *trade name.* Each company owns its brand names. For example, many drug companies make aspirin, and each one has its own recognized brand name for it. St. Joseph Aspirin is the aspirin made by the McNeil Company; Bufferin is the aspirin made by Bristol-Myers Squibb. The first letter of a brand name is always capitalized, and the name will often be followed by either the symbol ® (for registered trademark) or ™ (for trademark).

DRUG CATEGORIES

Any drug has the potential to harm a person if it is taken improperly or in large quantities. Some drugs have more powerful and dangerous effects than others. The U.S. government has classified drugs into two categories based on their potential for harm. These categories are over-the-counter drugs and prescription drugs.

Over-the-Counter Drugs

Drugs that are weaker and have less potential for harmful side effects are available for purchase without a prescription. These drugs are called **over-the-counter (OTC)** drugs. OTC drugs are considered safe for self-medication when the package directions for dosage and schedule are followed. Examples of OTC drug types include aspirin, antacids, vitamin supplements, and antihistamines. These drugs may be sold almost anywhere.

OTC drugs are convenient and allow you to control your own health care to some extent. However, some problems do exist with OTC drugs. Many patients do not consider them to be even slightly dangerous. All drugs, even vitamins, can be misused and cause harmful side effects when taken too often or in high doses. In addition, some people do not consider OTC drugs to be "real drugs" and may not mention them when they are asked what drugs they take on a daily basis. An OTC drug can cause health problems and may also interact with prescription drugs. Always ask specifically whether a patient takes any OTC drugs daily.

Prescription Drugs

Drugs that have a greater potential for harm, strong sedating effects, or a potential for addiction are considered too dangerous for self-medication. These drugs are classified as **prescription drugs** and are available only from a pharmacy with a drug order from a state-authorized prescriber. A **prescription** is an order written or dictated by a state-approved prescriber for a specific drug therapy for a specific patient.

High-Alert Drugs

Some prescription drugs have the designation of high-alert drugs. A **high-alert drug** has an increased risk for causing a patient harm if it is used in error. The error may be a dose that is too high, a dose that is too low, a dose given to a patient for whom it was *not* prescribed, and a dose *not* given to a patient for whom it was prescribed. One way to remember the more commonly prescribed high-alert drugs is with the term *PINCH.* In this term, *P* is for potassium, *I* is for insulin, *N* is for narcotics (more commonly called opioids), *C* is for cancer chemotherapy agents, and *H* is for heparin

Memory Jogger

The generic name of a drug often has some part that is the same for all drugs in that class or "family."

Memory Jogger

OTC drugs can be harmful when directions for dosage and schedule are not followed.

Drug Alert!

Interaction Alert

When taking a history, always ask what specific OTC drugs the patient uses daily.

QSEN: Safety

or any other drug that strongly affects blood clotting. Although calculating drug dosages and administering drugs always requires care and concentration, extra care is needed when calculating and administering high-alert drugs. When possible, always check the order for a high-alert drug with another licensed health care professional or pharmacist. Specific high-alert drugs are highlighted throughout the clinical chapters of this textbook.

Herbal Products

Herbals are natural products made from plants that cause a response in the body similar to that of a drug. Many herbal products, also called *botanicals*, have been used as drug therapy for centuries. This area of drug therapy is the least defined, least understood, and least regulated. Such products are available for sale almost everywhere, and individuals may even grow, collect, or make their own. Use of these products with or without the supervision of a prescriber is often termed *herbal therapy, homeopathic therapy, natural therapy,* or *alternative therapy.*

An even bigger problem is that most people who use herbal preparations consider them to be "natural" and therefore safe. However, herbal products do have cellular effects that can be harmful or interact with other drugs. For example, both white willow bark products and gingko biloba reduce blood clotting. If either of these is taken by a person who is also taking the prescription drug warfarin (Coumadin), the risk for a brain hemorrhage is high. When asked what drugs he or she is taking, a patient may not even mention herbal preparations that are taken on a daily basis, increasing the risk for an interaction with a prescribed drug.

Because many people consider herbal products to be safe, they may take large quantities of the products, believing that if one dose is good, five doses must be even better. For example, many people use the juice of the stinging nettle as a natural diuretic. It does increase urine output, but excessive doses cause dehydration and low blood potassium levels (*hypokalemia*).

Your responsibility with herbal therapy is to obtain correct information about what specific herbal products a patient is using and make sure that the prescriber is aware of this information. You also can help a patient understand the proper uses for and potential problems with specific herbal therapies.

DRUG REGULATION

The United States Pharmacopeia (USP) is a national group responsible for developing standards for drug manufacturing, including purity, strength, packaging, and labeling. The Food and Drug Administration (FDA) is the U.S. government agency that is responsible for enforcing the standards set by the USP. The FDA and the USP work together to ensure continuing public protection and drug safety.

Another drug regulating body is the U.S. Drug Enforcement Administration (DEA). All prescribers within the United States must register with the DEA and obtain a DEA number for full prescriptive authority. Additionally, the DEA is responsible for enforcing all drug laws with regard to controlled substances and illegal drugs. This administration has categorized drugs that have a potential for addiction or abuse as "controlled substances." These substances are further classified by the degree of their potential for addiction and abuse into one of five "schedules." See Table 7-1 in Chapter 7 for the definitions and classifications of the schedule system.

WAYS IN WHICH DRUGS AFFECT THE BODY (PHARMACODYNAMICS)

MECHANISMS OF ACTION

An important aspect of drug therapy is **pharmacodynamics,** or how the drug works to change body function. Think of this as what the drug does to the body. Drugs affect body function by changing the activity levels of individual cells. Remember that each body cell has at least one job that it must perform to make the whole body function correctly. The job that any cell performs can be slowed, stopped, or speeded up when that cell is exposed to a specific drug. Exactly how a drug changes the

 Memory Jogger

One way to remember the more commonly prescribed high-alert drugs is with the term PINCH: *Potassium, Insulin, Narcotics* (more commonly called opioids), *Cancer* chemotherapy agents, and *Heparin* or any other drug that strongly affects blood clotting.

 Drug Alert!

Administration Alert

Always check the order for a high-alert drug with another licensed health care professional or pharmacist.

QSEN: Safety

 Memory Jogger

Herbal preparations are not regulated for effectiveness, purity, or drug strength.

 Drug Alert!

Action/Intervention Alert

When taking a history, always be sure to ask what specific herbal products the patient uses on a daily basis, including the brand names and the amounts.

QSEN: Safety

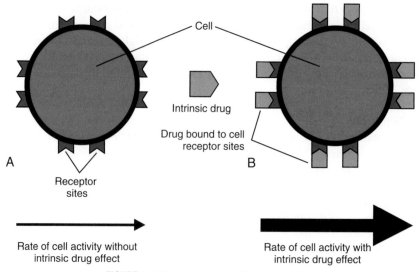

A

Receptor
sites

Rate of cell activity without
intrinsic drug effect

Cell

Intrinsic drug

Drug bound to cell
receptor sites

B

Rate of cell activity with
intrinsic drug effect

FIGURE 1-1 Receptors controlling cell activity.

 Memory Jogger

Receptors are physical places on or in cells that can bind with and respond to naturally occurring body chemicals. Their purpose is to control cell activity to meet the body's needs.

 Memory Jogger

A cell can respond to a drug by increasing its activity only when the drug fits into the receptor of the cell.

Cell with two different unbound
receptors and two different
free (loose) drugs

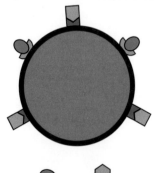

Receptor site
for drug A

Receptor site
for drug B

Cell with two different types of
drugs bound to their receptor sites

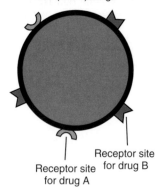

Drug A   Drug B

FIGURE 1-2 Cell with two types of receptors, unbound and bound.

activity of a cell is its **mechanism of action.** Most cells have receptors that control their activity. The actual cells or tissues affected by the mechanism of action or intended actions of a drug are known as the **target tissues.**

Receptors

Receptors are places on or in a cell where a drug can attach itself (bind) and control cell activity. In this way, the receptor acts as an ignition site for the cell's motor. When the right key (drug) is placed in the ignition (receptor) and turned, the cell motor starts, and the cell performs its special job better or faster. The right key for the ignition can be either an intrinsic drug such as the adrenaline made by the adrenal glands or an extrinsic drug such as epinephrine. (Chemically, epinephrine is almost identical to human adrenaline.) When the adrenal glands make and release adrenaline, it binds to adrenaline receptor sites on the heart muscle cells and makes those cells contract more strongly and rapidly. This action causes increased heart rate and higher blood pressure. When epinephrine is injected into a person, it binds to those same adrenaline receptor sites on the heart muscle cells and causes the same effects that adrenaline does. Figure 1-1 shows how cell receptors are used to control cell activity.

A cell can have more than one type of receptor; thus different drugs can affect the same cell in different ways. Figure 1-2 shows why a cell can respond to more than one drug. A cell can respond to a drug by changing its activity only when the proper drug fits into its receptor. If the wrong drug attempts to bind to a receptor, it will not activate that receptor—just as using the wrong key in a car ignition will not start the motor.

Many types of drugs work through cell receptors. These receptors can be on the surface of a cell or actually inside the cell. A cell with a receptor for a specific drug is known as the *target* for that drug. For example, the target of morphine is most brain cells (neurons) that perceive pain. Drug types that work by affecting cell receptors include opioid pain drugs, drugs for high blood pressure, diuretics, insulin, antihistamines, anti-inflammatory drugs, and antidiabetic drugs, to name only a few. For example, cells that are targets for antihistamines are those that have histamine receptors on their surfaces, such as mucous membrane cells, blood vessel cells, cells that line the airways, and stomach lining cells.

Receptor Agonists. When an extrinsic drug binds to the receptor of a cell and causes the same response that an intrinsic drug does, the extrinsic drug is called a receptor **agonist** because it is the right key to turn on that cell's ignition. Extrinsic drugs that are agonists have the same effects as the body's own hormones or natural

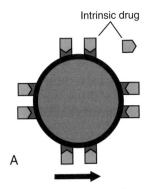

Intrinsic drug

A

Rate of cell activity when each specific receptor is bound with the naturally occurring substance (intrinsic drug).

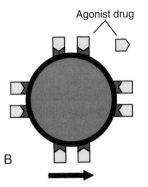

Agonist drug

B

Rate of cell activity when each specific receptor is bound with an extrinsic drug that is nearly identical to the naturally occurring substance (drug is an agonist).

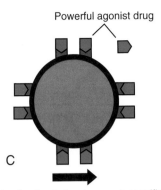

Powerful agonist drug

C

Rate of cell activity when each specific receptor is bound with an extrinsic drug that is even more powerful than the naturally occurring substance (drug is an agonist).

FIGURE 1-3 Comparison of cell activity when receptor sites are bound with different substances.

substances (intrinsic drugs) that activate or turn on a specific receptor type in or on a cell (Figure 1-3).

Agonist drugs must interact with the correct receptor for the drug to change the activity of the cell. Some agonist drugs change this activity to the same degree that intrinsic drugs do (see Figure 1-3, *B*). Other agonist drugs work but not quite as well as the intrinsic drug. Still other agonist drugs work more powerfully than intrinsic drugs (see Figure 1-3, *C*). Agonist drug strength is determined by how tightly the drug binds to the receptor and how long it stays bound. The more tightly bound a drug is to its receptor and the longer it stays attached, the stronger the effect of the drug on the activity of the cell. For example, hydromorphone (Dilaudid) is an opioid agonist that binds to the opioid receptor better than morphine does. As a result, hydromorphone provides longer pain relief at lower doses than morphine.

Receptor Antagonists. Sometimes the goal of drug therapy is to *slow* the activity of a cell. One way drugs can do this is by blocking the receptors of the cell so the intrinsic drug cannot bind with and activate the receptor. An extrinsic drug that works by blocking the receptor sites is called a receptor **antagonist**. An antagonist drug must be similar enough in shape to the intrinsic drug so it will bind with the receptor but not tightly enough or correctly enough to activate it. Antagonist action is like taking the key from one Chevrolet Impala and trying to start the motor of a different Chevrolet Impala. The key may fit into the ignition slot, but it will not turn on the motor. Instead, as long as the wrong key is in the ignition slot, the correct key cannot be placed in the slot, and the car does not run. The antagonist competes with the intrinsic drug for the receptor sites, blocking the receptors and slowing or stopping the activity of the cell. Antagonists have effects that are opposite of agonists. Figure 1-4 shows how antagonist drugs exert their effects on cells.

Receptors are the sites of direct action for many drugs. The final cell action when a drug binds to its receptor depends on both the nature of the drug (agonist or antagonist) and the nature of the receptor. Some drugs can act as agonists for certain cells and as antagonists for other cells. For example, epinephrine acts like an agonist when it binds to its receptors on heart muscle cells, making them contract more strongly and quickly. However, when epinephrine binds to muscle cells in the airways, it acts like an antagonist, causing these cells to relax rather than contract. Thus sometimes the same drug speeds up the activity of some cells and at the same time slows the activity of other cells. This is why you need to know the mechanism of action for each drug to understand both its intended actions and side effects. For example, when a person uses an epinephrine inhaler to widen the lung airways and breathe more easily, this is the intended action of the drug. The side effects are a more rapid heart rate and higher blood pressure.

 Memory Jogger

The effectiveness of an agonist drug depends on how tightly and how long it binds to its receptor.

 Memory Jogger

Agonists are drugs that act like naturally occurring drugs and "turn on" receptors when they bind, speeding up cell action. Antagonists bind to receptors but "block" them, slowing cell action.

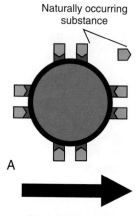

Naturally occurring substance

A

Rate of cell activity when each specific receptor is bound with the naturally occurring substance (intrinsic drug).

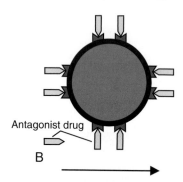

Antagonist drug

B

Rate of cell activity when each specific receptor is bound with an antagonist drug.

FIGURE 1-4 Comparison of cell activity when receptor sites are bound with the naturally occurring substance (intrinsic drug) **(A)** and with an extrinsic drug that is an antagonist **(B)** (blocks the receptor site, preventing the naturally occurring substance from binding).

 Memory Jogger

Drug side effects are expected, are mild, and may not occur in all patients.

Nonreceptor Actions

Some drugs exert their effects in a manner different from doing so through a receptor. Examples of drug types that do not use cell receptors to exert their effects include antibacterial drugs, cancer chemotherapy drugs, and most drugs that reduce blood clotting. The exact mechanism of action varies for each drug type that does not use receptors. For example, the targets of antibacterial drugs are bacteria. These drugs are either deadly (**cytotoxic**) to these organisms or prevent them from reproducing.

PHYSIOLOGIC EFFECTS

The outcome of the mechanism of action of a drug is its **physiologic effect**. Usually this effect can be felt by the patient or measured or observed by another person. For example, a drug that binds to airway receptors and dilates the airways has the physiologic effect of improving airflow in the airways. The improved airflow leads to better gas exchange. The patient notices easier breathing and you can observe improved oxygen saturation (SpO_2).

Both expected and unexpected patient responses are part of physiologic effects. These include intended actions, side effects, and adverse effects. Two specific types of adverse effects are allergic responses and personal (idiosyncratic) responses.

Intended Actions

The intended actions or therapeutic responses of a drug are the desired effect that improves body function and are the reason a drug is prescribed. All approved drugs have at least one expected intended action, and many have more than one.

Side Effects

Drug side effects are one or more effects on body cells or tissues that are **not** the intended action of drug therapy. All drugs have side effects. Generally side effects are the most common *mild* changes that occur in at least 10% of patients receiving a drug. *These effects are expected but do not occur in all patients.* Many are related to the mechanism of action of the drug and are temporary, resolving when the drug is discontinued. For example, people who take an oral penicillin for more than 5 days often develop diarrhea. This problem usually stops within 2 to 3 days after the drug is no longer taken. Although some side effects may be uncomfortable and may cause the patient to avoid a specific drug, they usually are not harmful. Examples of common side effects include:

- Constipation with the use of opioid analgesics
- Sexual disinterest or impotency with the use of certain antidepressants
- Diarrhea with the use of penicillin and other antibacterial drugs
- Drowsiness with the use of certain antihistamines
- Decreased blood clotting with the use of aspirin

Some drug side effects may even become a therapeutic effect. For example, aspirin has several therapeutic effects involved with pain relief, fever reduction, and reduction of inflammation. One of its side effects, decreased blood clotting, is now an intended action for prevention of heart attack (*myocardial infarction*).

Adverse Effects

A drug **adverse effect** or an **adverse drug reaction (ADR)** is a harmful side effect that is more severe than expected and has the potential to damage tissue or cause serious health problems. It may also be called a *toxic effect* or a *toxicity*. Often these effects occur with higher drug doses and are rare when the patient is taking normal doses of a specific drug. For example, many patients have the side effect of diarrhea when taking an antibacterial drug for 10 to 14 days. A few may have such severe diarrhea that they become dehydrated. At higher doses, a very few patients may develop the adverse effect of *pseudomembranous colitis,* which is profound bloody diarrhea and infection that can lead to complications such as perforation of the colon.

Although adverse effects are not common, it is important to know what types of ADRs and their signs and symptoms may occur with a specific drug so any problems are identified and managed early. Examples of ADRs include:

- Muscle breakdown with the use of "statin-type" cholesterol-lowering drugs
- Lung fibrosis with the use of amiodarone (a drug to correct abnormal heart rhythms)
- Pseudomembranous colitis with the use of antibacterial drugs such as amoxicillin and vancomycin
- Stevens-Johnson syndrome, a rare and severe skin reaction (Figure 1-5)

Usually when a patient has an adverse effect to a drug, he or she is taken off the drug. However, at times the patient requires the intended action, and the drug cannot be discontinued. In such cases, other precautions then are taken to limit tissue and organ damage.

Stevens-Johnson syndrome may result in a variety of rashes and skin blistering. The patient may lose body fluid and become dehydrated. The skin can slough, and the patient may then require skin grafts to restore skin integrity. Although this adverse reaction is more common as a response to some classes of drugs, it can occur as a result of any drug therapy.

Some adverse effects occur so commonly with a specific drug that the drug is removed from the market. Other drugs may continue to be prescribed but carry a black box warning. A **black box warning** means that a drug may produce serious or even life-threatening effects in some people in addition to its beneficial effects. This warning is printed on the package insert sheet and is bordered in black. Prescribers are instructed to make certain that such drugs are prescribed only for patients who meet strict criteria and who understand the serious nature of the possible adverse effects.

Allergic Responses. An **allergic response** is a type of adverse effect in which the presence of the drug stimulates the release of histamine and other substances that cause inflammatory reactions. It may be as mild as a skin rash or as severe and life threatening as anaphylaxis. Anaphylaxis is a severe inflammatory response with these symptoms:

- Tightness in the chest
- Difficulty breathing
- Low blood pressure
- Hives on the skin
- Swelling of the face, mouth, and throat (angioedema)
- Weak, thready pulse
- A sense that something bad is happening

If not recognized and treated quickly, anaphylaxis can lead to vascular collapse, shock, and death. The patient who develops a skin rash, hives, or mild throat swelling within hours or days of taking a drug may develop a more severe response and anaphylaxis the next time he or she takes the same drug. Usually when the person has a true allergic response to a drug, that drug and any from the same drug family should not be prescribed for him or her. This is known as a **contraindication**, which is a personal or health-related reason for not administering a specific drug to a patient or group of patients. Not all contraindications are for allergies. For example, a drug known to cause birth defects is considered an absolute contraindication for anyone who is pregnant. Another example is when two drugs interact very badly; one may be contraindicated for the time a patient is prescribed to take the other drug.

Another allergic reaction that can occur after weeks, months, and even years of therapy with a specific drug is *angioedema.* Although angioedema can occur in any part of the body, it is most serious when it occurs in the face and neck. The tongue, lips, and lower face swell to the point that the person has a hard time talking and

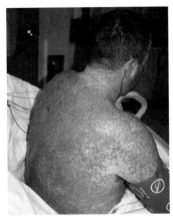

FIGURE 1-5 Steven's Johnson syndrome.

 Memory Jogger

An ADR is rare and serious and has the potential to damage organs (cause toxicities). Usually when a patient has an ADR, the drug is stopped.

 Memory Jogger

Drugs that carry a black box warning have more severe side effects and should only be used in patients for whom the potential benefits outweigh the possible drug risks.

 Memory Jogger

Anaphylaxis is the most severe type of allergic reaction to a drug and can lead to death if not treated quickly.

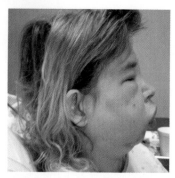

FIGURE 1-6 Angioedema of the face, lips, and mouth.

 Drug Alert!

Administration Alert

When a person has a true allergic response to a drug, do not administer that drug or any drug from the same drug family without additional precautions.

QSEN: Safety

 Drug Alert!

Action/Intervention Alert

Ask the patient about any adverse reactions, including allergic and personal reactions (idiosyncratic reactions), and record these in the patient's chart.

QSEN: Safety

 Memory Jogger

At the same time that a drug is having an effect on the body, the body is also having an effect on the drug.

may not be able to swallow (Figure 1-6). The swelling can extend to the throat, which is life threatening because the airway can become too narrow to breathe. Some of the more common drugs associated with angioedema include the angiotensin-converting enzyme inhibitors (ACE inhibitors) and some powerful antibiotics. People may not associate the problem with a drug they are taking because they may take the drug a long time before angioedema occurs. Patients experiencing angioedema should go to the nearest emergency department immediately and take all of their medications with them.

Personal/Idiosyncratic Responses. *Personal responses*, also known as *idiosyncratic responses*, are unexpected adverse effects that are unique to the patient and not related to the drug's mechanism of action. They are not true allergies but are related to the person's genetic differences in metabolism or immune function. For example, patients who have a deficiency of the enzyme glucose-6-phosphate dehydrogenase develop hemolytic anemia when they take the drug primaquine to prevent malaria.

Although the exact cause of personal responses is not always known, the effects can be severe and life threatening. For the purposes of prevention, they are documented in the patient's chart in the same way as severe drug allergies.

HOW THE BODY USES AND CHANGES DRUGS (PHARMACOKINETICS)

Most drugs must enter the body to produce their intended actions. Once a drug enters a living human body, the body exerts its effects on the drug. This process is known as **pharmacokinetics**. After absorption, the drug is affecting the body at the same time the body is affecting the drug. The body affects a drug by changing the structure of the drug so it can be inactivated and eliminated from the body. This "processing" of drugs by the body is why drugs must be taken repeatedly (for days and sometimes more than once each day) to continue to exert their intended actions. If drugs were never inactivated or eliminated, one dose would last for years and so would its intended actions and side effects.

A drug must enter the body and reach a high enough constant level in the blood or target tissue to produce the intended action. The lowest blood level needed to cause the intended action is known as the **minimum effective concentration (MEC)** (Figure 1-7). If the body eliminates the drug faster than it enters the body, the drug level at any given time will not be great enough to produce the intended action. If the body eliminates the drug more slowly than it enters the body, the drug level could become high enough to cause more side effects or adverse effects. For a drug

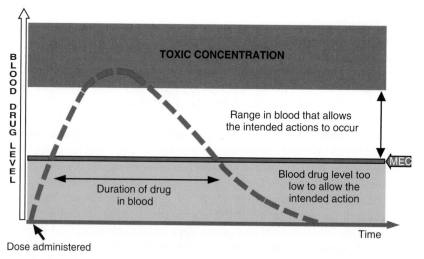

FIGURE 1-7 Minimum effective concentration *(MEC)* and blood level needed to allow the intended action to occur.

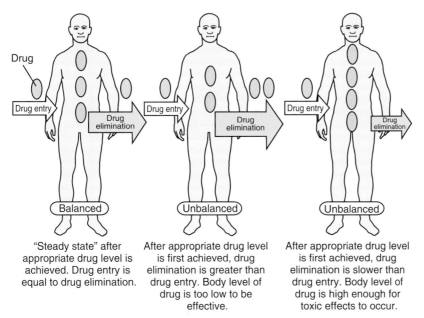

FIGURE 1-8 Comparison of body levels of drug when drug entry and elimination are balanced and unbalanced.

to do its job and produce the intended action without causing harm to the patient, its level in the blood has to be maintained by balancing drug entry with drug elimination. This balance, known as a **steady-state** drug level, keeps the amount of drug in the body high enough to produce the intended action continuously (Figure 1-8). The body processes drugs through the stages of absorption, distribution, metabolism, and elimination.

How long a drug remains in the blood at the MEC is its **duration of action**. The duration of action is one way to describe the **potency** of a drug. Drug potency is the strength of the intended action produced at a given dose. Drugs that have higher potency need lower doses to produce an intended action. Drugs that are less potent require higher doses to produce the same intended action. The longer a drug dose stays active in the body at or above the MEC, the more potent it is. In general, less potent drugs have fewer expected side effects but may need to be taken more often. A more potent drug may need to be taken only once or twice daily to achieve the intended action.

ABSORPTION

Drugs must come into contact with their target cells to cause a cell to change its activity. Extrinsic drugs must enter the body and get into the bloodstream to find their target cells. The movement of a drug from the outside of the body into the bloodstream is called **absorption**. The amount of a drug dose that actually reaches the blood is its **bioavailability.** If an entire drug dose reaches the bloodstream, its bioavailability is 100%. When only part of a drug dose gets into the blood, that drug is less than 100% bioavailable.

Drugs can enter the body in many ways:
- The **percutaneous route** means that the drug enters through the skin or mucous membranes.
- The **enteral route** refers to the gastrointestinal tract.
- The **parenteral route** means that the drug is injected into the body.

Table 1-1 lists the different routes of drug entry and their advantages and disadvantages. Chapter 2 describes how to administer drugs by these routes, along with any specific precautions needed.

Drugs are prepared differently by the manufacturer, depending on their intended routes. For example, drugs given by the parenteral route must be sterile, but those

 Memory Jogger

Drugs that have higher potency need lower doses to produce an intended action. Drugs that are less potent require higher doses to produce the same intended action.

 Memory Jogger

The three main drug entry routes are the percutaneous route, the enteral route, and the parenteral route.

Table 1-1   Advantages and Disadvantages of Drug Entry Routes

ROUTE	ADVANTAGES	DISADVANTAGES
Percutaneous	Convenient	Absorption dependent on circulation
Transdermal	Bypasses gastrointestinal tract Large selection of body areas	Absorption less predictable Can lead to skin breakdown
Sublingual	Less invasive Rapid absorption	Effect is reduced when patient eats or drinks
Buccal	Less invasive/obtrusive	Effect is reduced when patient eats or drinks
Rectal*	Usually painless	Embarrassing
Enteral	Convenient High patient acceptance Least expensive route because drugs need only to be clean, not sterile Large surface area for absorption	Can cause gastrointestinal disturbance First-pass loss Can bind to other substances in the tract and not get absorbed Absorption dependent on motility; has great individual variation
Parenteral	Speed 100% bioavailability Decreased first-pass loss	Speed Invasive administration Increased cost because drugs need to be sterile rather than just clean Discomfort

*Rectal drug delivery can be either percutaneous or enteral depending on how far into the rectum the drug is placed. Drugs placed within the lowest 1.5 inches are considered delivered by the percutaneous route. Those placed higher in the rectum are considered delivered by the enteral route.

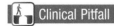

Clinical Pitfall

Do not give a drug that is prepared to be given by one route by any other route.

QSEN: Safety

given by the enteral route only need to be clean, not sterile. Some drugs prepared for the enteral route may have special coatings *(enteric coatings)* on them. These coatings either prevent the drugs from harming the stomach lining or prevent some of the enzymes and other substances in the digestive tract from destroying the drug before it can be absorbed.

Percutaneous Route

The percutaneous route of drug entry is the movement of the drug from the outside of the body to the inside through the skin or mucous membranes. Only lipid-soluble drugs—those that easily dissolve in lipids (fats) rather than water—can be absorbed percutaneously.

One method of the percutaneous route is **transdermal** delivery. In this method the drug is applied to the skin, passes through the skin, and enters the bloodstream to affect an internal organ. For example, nitroglycerin paste applied to the skin dissolves through the skin, then enters the bloodstream, and finally exerts its effect on blood vessels in the heart. Other drugs that are often given by this route using skin patches include certain types of pain medications and continuous hormone treatments.

Some drugs can be given through the mucous membranes of the mouth, nose, lungs, rectum, or vagina and have effects on deeper tissues. Mucous membranes have many blood vessels close to the surface, making movement of the drug through the membranes and into the bloodstream rapid and easy. Drugs given this way can be placed as tablets under the tongue or between the gum and the cheek, sprayed in the nose or under the tongue, inhaled through the nose or mouth, or placed as a liquid or a suppository in the rectum or vagina (see Figures 2-5, 2-16, and 2-17). Examples of drugs that can be given this way include hormones, pain medications, drugs for nausea and vomiting, and anesthetic agents.

Enteral Route

The enteral route of drug delivery is the movement of drugs from the outside of the body to the inside using the gastrointestinal (GI) tract. It is the most commonly used route of drug administration, and drugs are swallowed as liquids, tablets, or capsules. Most drugs that can be taken by mouth can also be placed directly into the stomach or intestines through a tube or into the rectum (when prescribed to do so). Once the drug is in the GI tract, it must dissolve and enter the bloodstream before it can exert its effects on target cells. Usually not all of a drug taken enterally enters the blood, and thus these drugs have *less* bioavailability than those given by the parenteral route. Enteral drugs are often given in higher doses than the same drug given parenterally just for this reason.

Absorption of oral drugs is affected by anything occurring in the stomach or intestines. Diarrhea can move drugs through the intestine so quickly that they are eliminated rather than absorbed. Food in the stomach or intestines slows or delays absorption. For this reason, some drugs such as the tetracycline antibiotics are not to be taken with food or milk. On the other hand, taking some oral drugs when the stomach is empty can cause such rapid absorption that the effects can occur too quickly and harm the patient.

Rectal drug delivery with drugs placed within the lowest 1.5 inches is considered delivered by the percutaneous route. Those placed higher in the rectum are considered delivered by the enteral route. The reason for this difference is the way venous blood leaves these areas. Venous blood from the last half of the mouth, the esophagus, the stomach, the intestines, and the higher part of the rectum drains into the liver before it returns to the heart as part of systemic circulation. This means that the liver has a chance to metabolize drugs from the gastrointestinal (GI) tract *before* they get to their target tissues. Blood from the lowest part of the rectum does *not* first enter the GI circulation, and drugs absorbed there do not get metabolized before they reach their target tissues.

Parenteral Route

The *parenteral route* involves giving drugs by injection, which bypasses the intestinal tract and other organs of digestion such as the liver, placing drugs more directly into the blood or target cells. Drugs can be injected into many structures:

- An artery, called an *intra-arterial injection* (administered by the prescriber)
- A vein, known as *intravenous injection*
- The skin, known as *intradermal injection*
- The fatty tissue below the skin, called a *subcutaneous injection*
- A muscle, or *intramuscular injection*
- A body cavity, known as *intracavitary injection* (administered by the prescriber)
- A joint, known as *intra-articular injection* (administered by the prescriber)
- A bone, or *intraosseous injection* (administered by the prescriber)
- The fluid of the brain or spinal cord, known as *intrathecal* (administered by the prescriber)
- Directly into specific tissues or organs (administered by the prescriber)

The parenteral route gets the drug into the bloodstream more quickly and more completely than other routes. For example, the dose of a drug given intravenously is entirely in the blood immediately after injection and then is 100% bioavailable. Not only do drugs work more quickly when given this way, but any problems the drugs may cause also occur more quickly. The parenteral route is more invasive and more dangerous to the patient than other routes. Give drugs parenterally only if they are made to be given by the parenteral route.

 Memory Jogger

Mucous membranes have many blood vessels close to the surface, making movement of the drug through the membranes and into the bloodstream rapid.

 Memory Jogger

Oral drugs have the least predictable absorption pattern.

 Memory Jogger

Drugs given by mouth usually require higher doses than the same drugs when given intravenously.

 Memory Jogger

The most rapid drug entry routes are intra-arterial and intravenous.

 Clinical Pitfall

Drugs prepared for the enteral route should never be given by the parenteral route.

QSEN: Safety

DISTRIBUTION

Once drugs are in the blood, they must be distributed to their target tissues, where the intended action is supposed to occur. Most drugs do not exert their mechanisms of action while in the blood. The bloodstream is just the "roadway" used by the body to get the drug to its target cells. Drugs can be distributed or spread to different body areas. **Distribution** of a drug is the extent that a drug spreads into three specific compartments. The *bloodstream* or *blood volume* (sometimes called the plasma volume) is the first drug compartment. This area is made up of the spaces in all the arteries, veins, and capillaries. The second drug compartment includes both the blood volume and the watery spaces between all body cells, also known as the *interstitial space.* The third drug compartment is the largest, including the blood volume, the watery spaces between the cells, and the space inside the cells (*intracellular space).*

How well a drug is distributed is determined by the size and chemical nature of the drug. Small drugs may have only a few molecules or parts. Smaller drugs are able to fit through cell channels and have a wide distribution into tissues and cells. Large drugs may be composed of many molecules and do not fit easily through cell pores or channels. Thus larger drugs have a more limited distribution within the body.

Some large drugs bind to proteins in the blood. These drugs do not touch or enter other cells; they can exert their effects only on cells in the blood. An example of this type of drug is an antibiotic that stays in the blood and affects only the microorganisms that are also in the blood. Drugs that distribute only to the blood volume are eliminated more rapidly than those that are distributed more widely. Thus drugs that distribute only to the blood volume may need to be taken three or four times a day to keep the drug level high enough to be effective.

Very small drugs and those that easily dissolve in fats can cross cell membranes and enter cells. Drugs that dissolve easily in fats are known as *lipid-soluble* drugs. These drugs are distributed the most widely, staying in the body longer and affecting more tissues and organs.

Some places in the body are more difficult for drugs to enter (such as the brain, eye [actually inside the eye], sinuses, and prostate gland). In addition, some body conditions can reduce drug distribution (such as when the patient is *dehydrated* [when he or she has too little body water] or has low blood pressure [*hypotension*]). If a person is taking more than one drug, the drugs can interact (meaning that the presence of one drug can change the distribution of another drug). This issue is a type of drug interaction and must be considered whenever the patient is taking more than one drug.

Another issue related to drug distribution is the "trapping" of drugs in certain tissues. This is called *sequestration.* Drugs that are more easily dissolved in fat often enter body fat cells and are sequestered there, with the drug being slowly released over time. Completely eliminating these drugs may take a long time. So the effects of sequestered drugs may be present for weeks or longer after the person has stopped taking the drug.

METABOLISM

Because any drug that enters the body is considered a "foreign" substance, the body takes steps to inactivate and eliminate it. Before most drugs can be eliminated, they must first be metabolized. **Metabolism** is a chemical reaction in the body that changes the chemical shape and content of the drug. Usually the changing of a drug by the body inactivates the drug and makes it easier to eliminate. A few drugs are actually activated by body metabolism before they can exert their effects and then are remetabolized or reprocessed for elimination.

A comparison of the use of the opioid drugs morphine and codeine is a clinical example of how metabolism works for drug elimination and drug activation. When a patient receives morphine for pain management, it is distributed throughout the

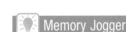

Memory Jogger

Drug distribution and activity are reduced in a patient who is dehydrated or has a very low blood pressure.

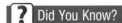

? Did You Know?

Body fat is a "time-release" capsule for drugs that have a fat base, retaining them for weeks to months.

body, including the brain. In the brain, it binds to opioid receptor sites to reduce the patient's perception of pain. At the same time, the liver inactivates the morphine through metabolism and readies it for elimination. This is why the effects of morphine wear off in a few hours and another dose of the drug then needs to be given for the patient to remain comfortable. Codeine is another opioid drug given for pain. However, when codeine is first taken into the body, it is not active and does not bind to the opioid receptor sites in the brain. It must be activated by metabolism and converted to morphine before it can relieve pain. Once this conversion takes place, codeine (now morphine) binds to receptor sites in the brain and reduces pain perception. When the metabolized codeine (now morphine) is remetabolized, it is ready to be eliminated from the body. The fact that codeine first has to be activated by metabolism before it can work as a pain reliever explains why morphine relieves pain faster than codeine.

Drugs can be metabolized to different degrees by different body tissues. The organs and cells most involved in drug metabolism are the liver, kidneys, lungs, and white blood cells. All these tissues contain special enzymes that break down and change the chemicals in the drugs.

Some factors that determine how fast and how well drugs are metabolized include genetic differences between people, whether the person has been exposed to that specific drug or similar drugs before, and the health of the liver and kidneys. Some people have genetic differences that allow them to make more of the enzymes used in drug metabolism. These people may need higher-than-average doses of drugs for the drugs to work well and may also need to take the drugs more often to keep a steady-state level. Other people have genetic differences that reduce the amount of enzymes they make for drug metabolism. These people need lower doses for the same effect compared with the "average" person.

The liver and kidneys are the most important organs for drug metabolism (Figure 1-9). If a patient has a problem with either the liver or the kidneys, drugs may be metabolized slowly and remain active longer. In this situation, high levels of a drug can quickly build up in the patient, often leading to toxic side effects.

ELIMINATION

Elimination is the removal of drugs from the body accomplished by certain body systems. Although many body systems eliminate drugs to some degree, the most active routes for drug elimination are the intestinal tract, the kidneys, and the lungs (see Figure 1-9). Drugs leave the body in the feces, urine, exhaled air, sweat, tears, saliva, and breast milk.

Drugs metabolized by the liver are sent to either the intestinal tract or the blood and then to the kidney for elimination. Even drugs given parenterally can be eliminated through the intestinal tract. When a drug is given orally, some of the drug is metabolized quickly by the liver and rapidly eliminated from the body. This rapid inactivation and elimination of oral (enteral) drugs is called **first-pass loss**. This is the reason an enteral drug is less bioavailable and the dosage is higher compared with the same drug given intravenously.

Drugs that are dissolved in the blood may leave the body in the urine. The drugs may change the color or smell of the urine. (This is why urine tests can determine whether a person is using certain illegal drugs.)

A few types of drugs are metabolized and eliminated through the lungs and leave the body in the exhaled air. Drugs that are small and easily turned into gases (**vaporized**) are eliminated by the lungs. This is why a Breathalyzer test can measure blood alcohol levels.

Just as for metabolism, the liver and kidneys are the most important organs for drug elimination. The liver metabolizes the drug to make it ready for elimination, which often is performed by the kidney. If a patient has a problem with either the liver or the kidneys, drugs may take a longer time to be eliminated from the body and can build up to toxic levels quickly. Liver damage is called *hepatotoxicity,* and kidney damage is called *nephrotoxicity.* Drugs that can cause liver damage are called

Memory Jogger

Metabolism changes the chemical structure of drugs; it can activate drugs, inactivate them, and prepare them for elimination.

Memory Jogger

Codeine must be metabolized to morphine before it can relieve pain.

Drug Alert!

Action/Intervention Alert

Anyone who has either liver or kidney problems must have the dosage and timing of drugs adjusted by the prescriber. Watch these patients carefully for signs of drug overdose.

QSEN: Safety

Did You Know?

Drugs administered intravenously can be eliminated through the intestinal tract.

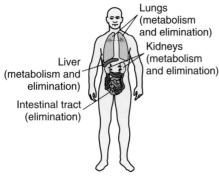

FIGURE 1-9 Major sites of drug metabolism and elimination.

Table 1-2	Time Needed to Completely Eliminate a Single-Dose Drug with a Half-Life of 6 Hours
TIME PASSED (HR)	**AMOUNT OF DRUG REMAINING IN THE BODY**
0 (time of drug administration)	500 mg
6	250 mg
12	125 mg
18	62.5 mg
24	31.25 mg
30	15.625 mg
36	7.813 mg
42	3.906 mg
48	1.953 mg
54	0.976 mg
60	0.488 mg

liver toxic or *hepatotoxic*. Drugs that can cause kidney damage are called *kidney toxic, renal toxic,* or *nephrotoxic.*

Half-Life

The **half-life** of a drug is the time span needed for one half of a single drug dose given to be eliminated. When multiple doses are given over time, the half-life for the total dosage also can be calculated. For example, the anti-inflammatory drug Aleve (naproxen) has a half-life of 12 hours. Suppose the first dose of the drug was 220 mg. Twelve hours after the drug was given, 110 mg of the drug remains in the body. Half of the remaining 110 mg is eliminated in the next 12 hours so that, 24 hours after the first dose, 55 mg of the drug remains in the patient's body. Thus if you received only a single 220-mg dose of a drug that has a half-life of 12 hours, it would take almost 48 hours for you to completely eliminate the drug (Table 1-2). The drug is considered eliminated when less than 10% of the drug remains, which would be between 36 and 48 hours for this example. For most drugs, at least five half-lives after the last dose are needed to eliminate a drug.

The half-life of a drug is related to how fast it is eliminated. Drugs that are eliminated rapidly have a short half-life; drugs eliminated slowly have a long half-life. The half-life of any drug is calculated based on research. The half-life is used to determine how much drug should be prescribed and how often it should be taken to get to and stay at a steady-state level (that is, a point at which drug elimination is balanced with drug entry). This steady-state level must be maintained at or above the minimum effective concentration (MEC). However, calculation of the MEC is based on the "average" response of the drug when it was given to a large number of test subjects. The same drug may have a different half-life in some patients because of differences in the patients' age, size, gender, race/ethnicity, metabolism, genetic heritage, and health and the presence of other drugs. Drugs with a short half-life are often prescribed to be taken more than once per day to get to and keep a steady-state level long enough to make the drug effective (produce its therapeutic effect). Drugs with a long half-life may be prescribed so the first dose is larger than the rest of the prescribed doses. This larger first dose is known as a **loading dose.** It is used to get the blood level up to the MEC as fast as possible. Once the MEC is achieved, all other doses can be smaller and still maintain the MEC because the drug has a long half-life and is eliminated slowly. One example of a drug that is usually prescribed with a higher loading dose than a maintenance dose is amikacin (Amikin), an antibiotic with a long half-life that is prescribed for serious life-threatening infections.

Memory Jogger

A drug with a half-life of 4 hours is *not* eliminated in 8 hours. Each portion *remaining* after a half-life time has passed is eliminated one half at a time.

Memory Jogger

Loading doses are often used for drugs that have a long half-life.

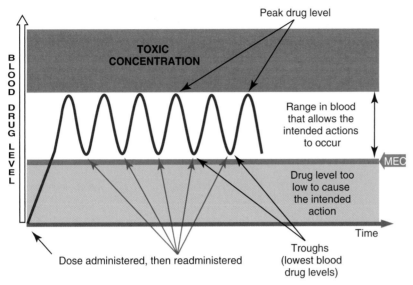

FIGURE 1-10 Peaks and troughs of blood drug levels. *MEC*, Minimum effective concentration.

Peaks and Troughs

Peaks and troughs describe the relationship between the actual dose of drug given and the blood drug level over time (Figure 1-10). The **peak** is the maximum blood drug level (like the top of a mountain), and the **trough** is the lowest or minimal blood drug level (like the bottom of a water trough for animals).

When patients have no severe health problems or unusual reactions to a drug and its metabolism, the peaks and troughs of a specific drug are already known (they have been worked out for the average person).

LIFE SPAN CONSIDERATIONS

SIZE

Children are smaller than most adults. Most drugs are given in smaller doses in proportion to the child's size, especially weight. Some drugs are prescribed in milligrams (mg) per kilogram (kg). Some prescribed drug doses are based on *body surface area (BSA)*—that is, they are calculated in milligrams per kilogram of body weight or milligrams per square meter (m^2). Either calculation must be made carefully and accurately because a math error of even one decimal place results in tremendous overdosing or underdosing.

Correctly calculating drug dosages for children is critical for preventing drug overdose. Follow these rules for pediatric drug administration:

- Always compare the drug dose prescribed for an infant or child with the recommended dose for the child's size.
- Question any drug prescription for a child in which the prescribed dose is greater or less than the recommended dose.
- Double check your drug dose calculation for an infant or child with a colleague or a pharmacist.

Drugs that have a specific type of effect or response on adults may have the opposite effect on children (these effects are called *paradoxical*). For example, the drug methylphenidate (Ritalin) stimulates the central nervous system of an adult and causes an overall increase in excitability and activity. This same drug reduces excitability and activity in children. Some drugs that cause drowsiness in adults may cause hyperactive behavior in children.

Other drug side effects that occur in children but not in adults can be related to the growth and maturity of specific tissues. For example, when teeth are developing, the antibiotic tetracycline changes the density of the tooth enamel and can result in tooth darkening. After teeth are mature, they are no longer at risk for this side effect.

 Memory Jogger

One kilogram is equal to 2.2 pounds. Therefore a person always weighs fewer kilograms than pounds.

| Table 1-3 | Laboratory Values for Liver Function |

TEST	NORMAL VALUES	SIGNIFICANCE OF ABNORMAL VALUES
Albumin	3.5-5.0 g/dL	Decreased values indicate possible liver disease.
Alanine aminotransferase (ALT)	4-36 IU/L	Increased values indicate possible liver disease.
Aspartate aminotransferase (AST)	10-35 units/L (higher in children)	Increased values indicate possible liver disease.
Lactate dehydrogenase (LDH)	100-190 IU/L (slightly lower in children)	Increased values indicate possible liver disease.
Alkaline phosphatase	30-120 units/L (higher in children)	Increased values indicate possible liver disease.
Bilirubin total serum	0.3-1.0 mg/dL	Increased values indicate possible liver disease.
Ammonia	10-80 mcg/dL	Increased values indicate possible liver disease.

From Pagana, K., & Pagana, T. (2014). *Mosby's manual of diagnostic and laboratory tests* (5th ed.). St. Louis: Mosby. *IU,* International units.

 Memory Jogger

Children may have completely different responses to a drug than an adult would have to the same drug.

As a result, the drug tetracycline is rarely used for pregnant women (when the first teeth are forming) or in children under the age of 12 years (when the permanent teeth are forming). Another example of a drug affecting development is the quinolone type of antibiotics. These drugs damage bone growth in children and are not prescribed for them unless an infection is life threatening and the organism responds only to a quinolone.

ORGAN HEALTH

The health of the organs most involved in drug distribution, metabolism, and elimination affect drug actions, especially the liver and kidneys. Along with physical immaturity and age-related changes in organ function, diseases can have an effect on organ function.

Liver Health

A healthy liver is important for good drug metabolism and elimination. The liver health status of any person should be known before drug therapy is started. Table 1-3 lists the normal values for tests of liver function.

Pediatric Considerations. Drug metabolism in children varies depending on age and organ maturity. A premature infant or newborn may have a slower rate of metabolism than an adult because the enzyme systems of the liver may not yet be fully active. Toddlers, preschool children, school-age children, and adolescents usually have *higher* rates of metabolism than do adults. A child may receive a much lower dose of a drug than an adult, but the dose may need to be given more often because it is metabolized and eliminated more rapidly.

Considerations for Older Adults. Many older adults have serious damage to the liver, making drug metabolism and elimination slower. Even older adults in good health have reduced liver function as a result of the aging process. Thus all older adults metabolize and eliminate drugs more slowly than younger adults, although this problem is greater in adults who have actual organ damage. Slow metabolism and elimination increase the half-life of a drug and make it easier to develop toxic drug levels in older adults.

Additionally, often an older adult may be prescribed many different drugs to take every day. New drugs may be prescribed and old ones may be discontinued. An

Table 1-4	Laboratory Tests Assessing Kidney Function
SUBSTANCE	**NORMAL VALUES**
Blood urea nitrogen (BUN)	10-20 mg/dL
Creatinine	*Males:* 0.6-1.3 mg/dL *Females:* 0.5-1 mg/dL
Sodium	136-145 mEq/L
Potassium	3.5-5 mEq/L
Calcium	9.0-10.5 mg/dL
Chloride	98-106 mEq/L
Magnesium	1.3-2.1 mEq/L
Bicarbonate	21-28 mEq/L

From Pagana, K., & Pagana, T. (2014). *Mosby's manual of diagnostic and laboratory tests* (5th ed.). St. Louis: Mosby.

important consideration to ensure that any patient is receiving the correct drugs at the correct dosages in any setting is the issue of *medication reconciliation*. It is the responsibility of the prescriber and the health care professional administering the drugs, especially nurses, to ensure that all of a patient's active drugs are properly listed in the patient record. More information on medication reconciliation is discussed in Chapter 2.

Kidney Health

Some drugs are metabolized and eliminated by the kidney. Others are metabolized elsewhere and just eliminated by the kidney. Thus a healthy kidney is important for drug elimination and prevention of toxic drug levels. The kidney (renal) health status of any person should be known before drug therapy is started. Table 1-4 lists the normal values for tests of kidney function.

Pediatric Considerations. An infant's kidneys do not concentrate fluids well. In addition, infants have a greater proportion of total body water than older children or adults. This means that drugs easily dissolved in water spread through proportionally more water, and drugs are lost by the kidney route more rapidly. Thus an infant may need a higher dose in terms of milligrams per kilogram than would a toddler or an older child. Water-soluble drugs are eliminated more rapidly in infants and young children than they are in adults.

Considerations for Older Adults. About two thirds of all adults over age 60 have reduced kidney size and kidney function. Because the kidney is important in eliminating drugs from the body, reduced kidney function in the older adult increases drug half-life. This means that one dose of a drug stays in the body longer and continues to have intended actions, as well as side effects in an older adult than in a younger adult.

Cardiopulmonary Health

The cardiovascular system ensures that drugs reach their target sites of action and sites for metabolism and elimination. The lungs and pulmonary system help metabolize and eliminate some drugs. Red blood cells (RBCs) carry oxygen, and white blood cells (WBCs) are sites of drug metabolism. Together the heart, blood, and lungs promote the health of all organs by ensuring adequate oxygenation. Thus a healthy heart, adequate blood pressure, and good oxygenation are needed for optimal drug therapy. Table 1-5 lists normal values for tests of cardiac, blood, and lung function.

Considerations for Older Adults. Many adults over age 70 years have some degree of heart failure and poor blood flow to the liver and other body areas. This reduced

 Memory Jogger

Older adults may need a lower drug dosage than younger adults because of reduced kidney or liver function, and they are at a higher risk for dosage-related side effects.

Table 1-5 Laboratory Tests Assessing Cardiovascular Function and Oxygenation

TEST	RANGE
BLOOD CELLS	
Red blood cells	
Women	4.2-5.4 million per cubic millimeter (mm^3) of blood
Men	4.7-6.1 million/mm^3 of blood
Platelets	150,000-400,000/mm^3 of blood
White blood cells, total	5000-10,000/mm^3 of blood
OXYGENATION	
Hematocrit	
Women	37%-47%
Men	42%-45%
Newborn to 6 months	44%-64%
Over 6 months	30%-44%
Hemoglobin	
Women	12-16 g/dL
Men	14-18 g/dL
Newborn to 6 months	10-17 g/dL
Over 6 months	10-15.5 g/dL
Oxygen saturation (SpO_2)	95%-100%
Arterial oxygen (PaO_2)	80-100 mm Hg
Arterial carbon dioxide ($PaCO_2$)	35-45 mm Hg
CARDIAC FUNCTION	
Brain natriuretic peptide (BNP)	Less than 100 pg/mL
Creatine kinase (CK)	
Women	30-135 units/L
Men	55-170 units/L
Newborns	68-580 units/L
Children	Same as adults
Creatine kinase-MM	100%
Creatine kinase-MB	0%
Creatine kinase-BB	0%

From Pagana, K., & Pagana, T. (2014). *Mosby's manual of diagnostic and laboratory tests* (5th ed.). St. Louis: Mosby.

blood flow both decreases drug effectiveness and limits how well drugs are distributed, metabolized, and eliminated.

The respiratory changes that occur with aging reduce lung volume and function to some degree in all older patients. These effects are made worse by a lifetime of exposure to inhaled irritants such as cigarette smoke, bacteria, air pollutants, and industrial fumes. These changes reduce lung metabolism and elimination of some drugs. Lung problems may reduce the effectiveness of drugs taken by inhalation.

Older adults often have fewer RBCs and WBCs than younger adults. These changes reduce oxygenation of all organs and limit drug metabolism.

SPECIAL POPULATIONS

Pregnancy

Pregnancy is the time for development of a new human being. Nearly every organ forms in the 9 months before birth. During pregnancy the mother's bloodstream is separated from the unborn baby's bloodstream by the placenta. However, the placenta is not a perfect barrier. Some drugs can cross the placenta and may affect the unborn baby, although not all drugs taken during pregnancy have harmful effects on the fetus. Regardless of the presumed safety of a drug, no prescribed or OTC drug should be taken during pregnancy unless it is clearly needed and its benefits outweigh any risks to the fetus.

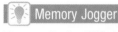 Memory Jogger

No prescribed or OTC drug is considered to be *completely* safe to take during pregnancy.

Drugs that can cause birth defects are *teratogenic* or *teratogens.* Some drugs are more teratogenic than others, and even one dose can cause a severe birth defect. Other drugs are less teratogenic and require either many doses or very high doses to cause even a minor birth defect. Not all pregnant women who take a teratogenic drug during pregnancy have a child with birth defects, but the *risk* for birth defects is higher. Usually drugs are avoided during pregnancy; however, certain health problems may need to be managed with drug therapy.

Drugs have the same effects on the fetus as on the mother but can cause more problems. For example, when a pregnant woman takes the anticoagulant warfarin, the unborn baby's blood is also less able to clot, and the fetus can bleed to death. Drugs that lower blood pressure can lower the fetus's blood pressure so much that the brain does not receive enough oxygen, and brain damage results.

The FDA has developed new guidelines for the "information for prescribers" section of the drug package inserts under the changed Physician Labeling Rule. The changes for the "Use in Special Populations" section include the eventual complete removal of the old pregnancy categories A, B, C, D, and X, in which the risk for birth defects or adverse pregnancy outcomes moved from no apparent increased risk (category A) through increasing risks to greatly increased risk (category X). Under the new guidelines, which are effective for some drugs as of June 2015, the subsections of "pregnancy" (including labor and deliver), "lactation" (breastfeeding), and "females and males of reproductive potential," replace the old categories. The package inserts must contain all appropriate information regarding when and how a drug may affect these special populations. This information is presented as a risk summary when a drug is known to be absorbed systemically (enter the bloodstream), and risk is classified in the following manner:

- Not predicted to increase risk
- Low likelihood of increasing risk
- Moderate likelihood of increasing risk
- High likelihood of increasing risk
- Insufficient data to assess the likelihood of increasing risk

This classification is used for risk to the fetus, risk to the pregnant woman (for problems when taking the drug, as well as problems that could occur from not taking the drug), risk for affecting the production of milk, risk for affecting the health of the nursing infant, and risk for affecting the fertility of females and males. It is the responsibility of the prescriber to know this information and to ensure that patients for whom the drugs are prescribed understand the risks versus the benefits of the prescribed therapy.

Lactation

Some drugs taken by a breastfeeding woman cross into the milk and are ingested by the infant. The effects of the drugs on the baby are the same as on the mother. For example, lipid-lowering drugs taken by a breastfeeding woman will lower her infant's blood lipid levels. Although the mother may need to lower her blood lipid levels, the infant does not. Low lipid levels in an infant may cause poor brain development and mental retardation.

When a breastfeeding woman has an infection, usually the infant does not; however, the antibiotic the mother takes can enter the breast milk and affect the infant. Some antibiotics such as penicillin may not cause a problem. Other antibiotics such as the quinolones, even taken for a short time, can disrupt bone development.

Before a drug is selected and prescribed for a breastfeeding woman, the effects on the infant must be considered. The mother's prescriber, the infant's health care provider, and the mother must discuss the issues together.

Breastfeeding is not recommended for mothers with chronic disorders that require daily drug therapy (e.g., seizures, hypertension, and hypercholesterol). For short-term health problems that require less than 2 weeks of drug therapy (e.g., infection),

Drug Alert!

Action/Intervention Alert

Before administering any newly prescribed drug, ask any female patient between the ages of 10 to 60 years if she is pregnant, likely to become pregnant, or breastfeeding.

QSEN: Safety

Box 1-1   Recommended Methods of Reducing Infant Exposure to Drugs During Breastfeeding

- For drugs that should not be given to infants:
  - Switch the infant to formula feeding temporarily or to breast milk obtained when you were not taking the drug.
  - Maintain your milk supply by pumping your breasts on a regular schedule, and discard the pumped milk.
  - When you are no longer taking the drug and it has been eliminated, resume breastfeeding.
- For drugs that do not have to be avoided but should have levels reduced:
  - Nurse your baby right before taking the next dose of the drug.
  - Drink plenty of liquids to dilute the amount of drug in the breast milk.
  - Take the drug just before the baby's longest sleep period.

 Drug Alert!

Action/Intervention Alert

If a woman is breastfeeding, urge her to discuss any drugs that she may be taking with her pediatrician.

QSEN: Safety

Drug Alert!

Teaching Alert

Warn patients taking prescribed drugs to check with the prescriber before starting any OTC drugs, vitamins, or herbal supplements.

QSEN: Safety

---

the breastfeeding woman can make adjustments to reduce the infant's exposure to the drug (Box 1-1).

Females and Males with Reproductive Potential

This special population refers to teenagers and adults who are capable of becoming pregnant (females) or are capable of causing a pregnancy (males). Some drugs reduce fertility temporarily and others can reduce it permanently. Other types of drugs can increase fertility. Any person who is prescribed to take a drug that can affect fertility should have full knowledge about such effects.

DRUG INTERACTIONS

Drugs can interact with other drugs, food, vitamins, and herbal compounds. These interactions can change the way a drug works or the timing of its action. Some interactions actually increase the activity of the drug, whereas others decrease it. Some drugs and herbal compounds are not compatible with each other and can lead to adverse effects. Always ask patients who are being prescribed a new drug what other drugs (prescribed or OTC), vitamins, and herbal supplements they are taking currently. Because the number of possible problem interactions is huge, always check with the pharmacy or a drug handbook for potential drug interactions.

Examples of interactions between drugs and between drugs and other common agents follow:

- Cimetidine (Tagamet) enhances the action of quinidine (Quinadure, Quinidex), increasing the risk for adverse effects.
- Ciprofloxacin (Cipro) increases the blood concentration of warfarin (Coumadin), increasing the risk for bleeding.
- Ibuprofen (Advil) and naproxen (Aleve) reduce the effectiveness of some antihypertensives such as captopril (Capoten) and lisinopril (Zestril), increasing the risk for heart failure and strokes.
- Grapefruit juice greatly increases the activity of many drugs, including felodipine (Plendil), midazolam (Versed), and lovastatin (Mevacor), increasing the risks for overdose and adverse effects. It can also decrease the activity of other drugs.
- St. John's wort, an herbal preparation, reduces the effectiveness of many drugs, including digoxin (Lanoxin), warfarin (Coumadin), and oral contraceptives (birth control pills). Reducing the effectiveness of digoxin may worsen heart failure; reducing the effectiveness of warfarin increases the risk for clot formation, strokes, and pulmonary embolism; reducing the effectiveness of oral contraceptives may lead to unplanned pregnancies.

Get Ready for Practice!

Key Points

- The prescriber's role in drug therapy is to select and order specific drugs. Prescribers may include physicians, dentists, podiatrists, advanced practice nurses, and physician's assistants.
- The health care professionals most responsible for teaching patients about their drugs include the prescriber, the pharmacist, and the nurse.
- Generic drug names are spelled with all lowercase letters; brand names (trade names) have the first letter capitalized.
- When possible, always check the order and dosage calculation of a high-alert drug with a licensed health care professional or pharmacist.
- Herbal products can cause problems if taken too often or with prescribed drug therapy.
- Drugs often work in the same way that body hormones, enzymes, and other proteins do.
- For a drug to work on body cells, it must enter the body.
- Most drugs exert their effects by binding to a cell receptor.
- Although some drug side effects may be uncomfortable and may cause the patient to avoid a specific drug, they usually are not harmful and do not cause extensive tissue or organ damage.
- True allergic drug reactions result when the presence of the drug stimulates the release of histamine and other body chemicals that cause inflammatory reactions.
- Anaphylaxis is the most severe type of allergic reaction to a drug and can lead to death if not treated quickly.
- At the same time that a drug is changing body activity, the body is processing the drug for elimination.
- Drugs have to reach a high enough level in the blood to exert their effects.
- The three main drug entry routes are percutaneous, enteral, and parenteral.
- A drug prepared to be given by one route should not be given by any other route.
- Any problem with the gastrointestinal tract can interfere with how fast a drug is absorbed.
- Never give by injection any drug made to be given by the enteral route.
- The side effects of a drug given intravenously can occur very rapidly.
- Drugs may take a longer time to work when a patient is dehydrated or has very low blood pressure.
- Taking more than one drug at the same time can change the effectiveness of both drugs.
- The most important organs for drug metabolism and elimination are the liver and kidneys.
- Drugs that have a long half-life stay in the body longer and are more likely to build up to toxic levels more quickly.
- Although the expected actions and patient responses are known for all approved drugs, some patients may react differently than expected. Whenever a patient receives the first dose of a drug, be alert to the possibility of unique responses.
- An infant may need a higher drug dose (in terms of milligrams per kilogram) than toddlers or older children because infants have a greater proportion of total body water.
- Unless a serious health problem exists in the pregnant woman, all types of drugs should be avoided (except for prenatal vitamins and iron supplements).
- When a female patient is prescribed to take a drug that is known to cause birth defects, be sure that she understands the risks, that her pregnancy test is negative, and that she is using one or more reliable methods of birth control (or completely abstains from sex) during treatment.
- Urge breastfeeding women to consult with their infant's health care provider before taking any prescribed or OTC drug.
- Always ask patients who are being prescribed a new drug what other drugs (prescribed or OTC), vitamins, and herbal supplements they are taking currently.
- Check with the pharmacy or a drug handbook for potential drug interactions.
- Warn patients taking prescribed drugs to check with the prescriber before starting any OTC drugs, vitamins, or herbal supplements.

Additional Learning Resources

evolve Be sure to visit your Evolve website (http://evolve.elsevier.com/Workman/pharmacology/) for additional online resources.

SG Go to your Study Guide for additional learning activities to help you master this chapter content.

Review Questions

See the Answer Keys—In-text Review Questions for answers to these questions.

Test Yourself on the Basics

1. Which function is primarily the role of the pharmacist in drug therapy?
   - A. Administering a prescribed drug directly to the patient
   - B. Teaching a patient the possible side effects of a prescribed drug
   - C. Changing the dose of a prescribed drug based on a patient's response
   - D. Dispensing a drug according to the instructions written in the prescription
2. What action or condition is a major disadvantage of the oral drug delivery route?
   - A. First-pass loss of drug is extensive.
   - B. Drug must be sterile rather than clean.
   - C. Only lipid-soluble drugs can be absorbed.
   - D. Adverse effects occur more rapidly than with other routes.

3. What major consideration allows a drug to be available over-the-counter (OTC) rather than by prescription?
   A. The drug has absolutely no side effects or intended responses.
   B. The cost of the drug must be lower than prescription drugs.
   C. The drug has not undergone any federally regulated safety testing.
   D. The drug is safe when the directions for dosage and scheduling are followed.

4. How much does a child who weighs 34 lb weigh in kilograms (kg)?
   A. 15 kg
   B. 34 kg
   C. 68 kg
   D. 74.8 kg

5. What is the minimal effective concentration (MEC)?
   A. The movement of drug from outside the body to the inside of the body without the use of needles or syringes.
   B. The way in which drugs work to change body function and the way in which the body changes drug composition.
   C. The smallest amount of drug necessary in the blood or target tissue to result in a measurable intended response.
   D. The smallest amount of drug lost as a result of liver metabolism and elimination before the drug reaches its target tissue.

6. Which statement about drug side effects is true?
   A. All drugs have at least one side effect.
   B. Side effects usually cause tissue damage.
   C. Side effects change pharmacokinetics and reduce a drug's main effect.
   D. Once a patient experiences a side effect, he or she cannot be prescribed that drug again.

7. What is the meaning of the word *contraindication* in relation to drug therapy?
   A. The reason a person should be given a drug by the parenteral route when most people take the drug by the enteral route.
   B. The type of reaction to a drug a patient experiences that is exactly the opposite of the drug's usual intended response.
   C. The trapping of a drug in the body's fat cells so that the drug is released slowly over time.
   D. A personal or health-related reason why a drug should NOT be given to a patient.

8. What route of drug administration is the most commonly used for drug therapy?
   A. Enteral
   B. Parenteral
   C. Inhalation
   D. Transdermal

9. Which organ is most heavily involved in drug metabolism?
   A. Stomach
   B. Rectum
   C. Spleen
   D. Liver

10. Which statement about drug half-life is true?
    A. A drug with a half-life of 2 hours is totally eliminated from the body in 4 hours.
    B. Drugs with a short half-life are more likely to be sequestered.
    C. Most drugs with a long half-life require less frequent dosing.
    D. Half-life is extended when the drug is taken with a full glass of water.

Test Yourself on Advanced Concepts

11. Which patient response indicates a drug's intended action or therapeutic response?
    A. Ankle swelling
    B. Bone strengthening
    C. Constipation
    D. Dizziness

12. Which condition would be considered a contraindication for a specific drug?
    A. The patient has loose stools when he takes an antibiotic for 2 weeks.
    B. The patient who is prescribed to take penicillin is 7 months pregnant.
    C. The patient prescribed to take lisinopril (Prinivil) has had swelling of the lips, face, and tongue when taking another drug from the same drug class (family).
    D. The patient prescribed to take diphenhydramine (Benadryl) for an allergic reaction usually gets sleepy after taking this drug.

13. What is an advantage of a drug with a long half-life?
    A. The drug is taken fewer times daily.
    B. The drug does not have to be metabolized before it is eliminated.
    C. Usually, a drug with a long half-life has fewer side effects than a drug with a short half-life.
    D. Most drugs with a long half-life are less expensive than are drugs with a shorter half-life.

14. Which patient response is a personal (idiosyncratic) adverse response to a drug rather than a true allergic reaction or general side effect?
    A. Prolonged hiccoughing while taking a drug to reduce nausea and vomiting
    B. A change in urine color to reddish orange while taking a bladder anesthetic for 3 days
    C. Development of a vaginal yeast infection while taking a tetracycline antibiotic for the past 10 days
    D. Swelling of the lips, tongue, and lower face while taking an angiotensin-converting enzyme inhibitor type of antihypertensive for 2 weeks

15. What type of reaction is a child having when he or she becomes more alert and excited when taking an antihistamine that usually makes people sleepy?
    A. Adverse reaction
    B. Allergic reaction
    C. Intended reaction
    D. Paradoxical reaction

16. Which condition represents the "steady-state" phase of drug metabolism?
    A. The drug is excreted at the same rate that it is absorbed, resulting in an even blood-drug concentration.
    B. The drug is excreted at a more rapid rate than it is absorbed, resulting in a lower blood-drug concentration.
    C. The drug is excreted at a slower rate than it is absorbed, resulting in a high blood-drug concentration.
    D. The drug is activated rather than inactivated by metabolic processing, resulting in the excretion of an active compound.

17. A patient who is breastfeeding her 6-week-old infant is prescribed to take montelukast sodium (Singulair) 10 mg orally daily (at 9:00 AM) for control of asthma. Which action should you teach her to reduce the infant's exposure to this drug?
    A. Breastfeed the infant no sooner than 1 hour after taking the drug.
    B. Avoid drinking fluids for 6 hours after taking the drug.
    C. Breastfeed the infant right before taking the drug.
    D. Take the drug on an empty stomach.

18. A drug is prescribed at 220 mg orally every 8 hours. How many total milligrams are given in a 24-hour period?
    A. 440
    B. 660
    C. 880
    D. 1100

19. A patient receives 250 mg of an oral drug at noon, 6 PM, and midnight. The drug has a half-life of 6 hours. How much of the drug remains in the patient at 6 AM the next day?
    A. 437.75 mg
    B. 375 mg
    C. 218.75 mg
    D. 187.5 mg

20. What is the weight in kilograms for a man who weighs 192 lb? _____ kg

Critical Thinking Activities

See the Answer Keys—Critical Thinking Activities for answers to these activities.

The patient is a 78-year-old woman who has only 20% kidney function. She also has diabetes and is prescribed insulin, which is eliminated by kidney action.

1. What type of dosage adjustment would you expect for this patient?
2. What problems could occur if the drug dosages are not adjusted?
3. Would this change in needed drug dosage be considered an idiosyncratic reaction? Why or why not?

Safely Preparing and Giving Drugs

http://evolve.elsevier.com/Workman/pharmacology/

Objectives

After studying this chapter you should be able to:

1. List the eight "rights" of giving drugs.
2. Identify four types of drug orders.
3. Explain ways to prevent drug errors.
4. List important principles related to preparing and giving drugs.
5. Describe responsibilities related to giving enteral drugs.
6. Describe responsibilities related to giving parenteral drugs.
7. Describe responsibilities related to giving drugs through the skin and mucous membranes.
8. Describe responsibilities related to giving drugs through the ears and eyes.
9. List responsibilities before and after a drug has been given.

Key Terms

buccal route (BŬK-ŭl ROWT) (p. 39) Application of a drug within the cheek or the cavity of the mouth.

drug error (DRŬG ĂR-ŭr) (p. 29) Any preventable event that may cause inappropriate drug use or patient harm while the drug is in the control of the health care professional or the patient. A drug error may cause a patient to receive the wrong drug, the right drug in the wrong dose, the wrong route, or at the wrong time.

enteral route See Chapters 1 and 24.

intradermal route (ĭn-tră-DŬR-mŭl ROWT) (p. 35) Injection of drugs within or between the layers of the skin.

intramuscular (IM) route (ĭn-tră-MŬS-kyū-lŭr ROWT) (p. 36) Injection of drugs into a muscle.

intravenous (IV) route See Chapter 1.

medication reconciliation (mĕ-dĭ-KĀ-shŭn rĕ-kŭn-sĭl-ē-ā-shŭn) (p. 30) The process of identifying the most accurate list of all medications that the patient is taking, including name, dosage, frequency, and route, by comparing the medical record to an external list of medications obtained from a patient, hospital, or other provider.

onset of action (ŎN-sĕt ŭv ĂK-shŭn) (p. 32) The length of time it takes for a drug to start to work.

oral route (ŌR-ŭl) (p. 32) Administration of drugs by way of the mouth.

parenteral route See Chapter 1.

percutaneous route See Chapter 1.

per os (PO) (PŬR ŎS) (p. 32) Giving drugs by way of the mouth.

PRN order (p. 29) An order written to administer a drug to a patient as needed.

rectal route (RĔK-tŭl ROWT) (p. 34) Movement of a drug from outside of the body to the inside of the body through the rectum.

single-dose order (SĬN-gŭl DŌS ŌR-dŭr) (p. 29) An order written to administer a drug one time only.

standing order (STĂN-dĭng) (p. 29) An order written when a patient is to receive a drug on a regular basis. Also called a routine order.

STAT order (STĂT) (p. 29) An order written to administer a drug once and immediately.

subcutaneous route (sŭb-kū-TĀN-ē-ŭs ROWT) (p. 36) Injection of drugs into the tissues between the skin and muscle.

sublingual (SL) route (sŭb-LĬN-gwŭl ROWT) (p. 39) Administration of drugs by placing them underneath the tongue.

suppository (sŭ-PŎZ-ĭ-tōr-ē) (p. 34) A small medication plug designed to melt at body temperature within a body cavity other than the mouth.

topical route (TŎP-ĭ-kŭl ROWT) (p. 39) Application of drugs directly to the skin.

transdermal route (trănz-DŬR-mŭl ROWT) (p. 39) A type of percutaneous drug delivery in which the drug is applied to the skin, passes through the skin, and enters the bloodstream.

unit-dose drugs (YŪ-nĭt DŌS) (p. 30) Drugs that are dispensed to fill each patient's drug orders for a 24-hour time period.

OVERVIEW

A major role of the health care professional administering medications is to give the drugs safely. Although other health care professionals also have major roles in the drug therapy process, you are responsible for providing competent and safe patient care.

You, along with prescribers and pharmacists, must teach patients about the drug or drugs that have been prescribed.

Administering drugs is one of the your most important responsibilities. But your responsibilities do not end with "giving" the drug to the patient. Every health care professional should be familiar with the professional practice act for the state in which he or she works.

To give drugs safely, you must understand the basic principles of drug administration. Check the expiration date to be sure that the drug is not outdated. Look carefully at intravenous (IV) drugs for any sediment or discoloration that may indicate that the drug is unstable and should not be used. Be sure to wash your hands and follow the eight "rights" of drug administration.

After giving a drug, you must check the patient for the expected results and for any side effects or adverse effects. You also have a duty to teach patients and their families about drugs, including the desired action, side effects, and when to call the prescriber.

THE EIGHT RIGHTS OF SAFE DRUG ADMINISTRATION

When preparing and giving drugs to patients safely, follow the eight "rights" for drug administration:
1. Right patient
2. Right drug
3. Right dose
4. Right route
5. Right time
6. Right documentation
7. Right diagnosis
8. Right response

Some sources cite an additional right to follow when giving drugs: the patient's right to refuse a drug.

THE RIGHT PATIENT

To make sure that the right patient is receiving any drug that has been prescribed, The Joint Commission (TJC) recommends checking two unique patient identifiers (name and birth date) before medication administration. An alert and oriented patient can be asked directly. If the patient is confused, hard of hearing, unconscious, or otherwise unable to reply, wash your hands first and then check the name, birth date, and identification number on his or her wristband. Some long-term care facilities such as nursing homes use pictures of patients to ensure that the correct patient receives the correct drugs. If a patient does not have an identification wristband, have one made and place it on his or her wrist. As an added safety measure, be sure to check the medication administration record (MAR) and the label on the patient's medication box with the wristband.

THE RIGHT DRUG

Each drug that is prescribed has a particular intended action. You must be sure that the drug being given is correct. Carefully compare the drug you are about to administer with the drug order. Be sure to give the drug in the form ordered by the prescriber (e.g., pill, capsule, liquid). Thousands of drugs are available today, and many of their names are so similar that they can be confusing. Be aware of these easily confused drug names. For more information about them, see "Confusing Drug Name Lists" later in this chapter.

 Memory Jogger

Safe drug administration requires that the person administering the drug be knowledgeable about these drug features:
- Purpose(s)
- Actions
- Side effects
- Abnormal reactions
- Delivery methods
- Necessary follow-up care

 Memory Jogger

Be sure to review the professional practice act (e.g., nurse practice act) for your state on the state board website.

 Memory Jogger

Remember to use the eight "rights" every time you prepare and administer drugs.

QSEN: Safety

 Drug Alert!

Action Alert

Be sure to always check two unique identifiers (e.g., name and birth date) to ensure that you are giving the right drug to the right patient.

QSEN: Safety

Memory Jogger

Minimum information required by the U.S. government for a written prescription:
- Date
- Patient's name
- Name and address of the prescriber
- Generic or brand name of the drug
- Strength of the drug
- Number of times per day that the drug is to be taken
- Any specific instructions for use
- Number of doses to be dispensed
- Number of refills allowed
- Prescriber's signature

THE RIGHT DOSE, ROUTE, AND TIME

A prescriber's drug order should be in written form and include all the minimum information required by the U.S. government. Verbal orders should be accepted only in emergency situations. As soon as the emergency has been resolved, verbal orders must be written and signed. Contact the prescriber whenever a drug order seems unclear or if a drug dosage is higher or lower than expected. For safety, when you contact the prescriber by telephone or follow a verbal order, be sure to write the order, read it back, and ask for confirmation that what you wrote is correct before administering any drug. Be sure to document that you read back the order to the prescriber.

THE RIGHT DOCUMENTATION

When you give a drug, record the action immediately. This is essential for all drugs, but it is especially important for drugs given on an as-needed (PRN) basis. Many pain-relieving drugs are prescribed to be given as needed. These drugs often require 20 to 30 minutes to take effect. If you fail to document giving one of these drugs, a patient may request and receive a second dose from another health care professional. When a patient is receiving a narcotic (opioid) pain drug, a second dose can cause complications such as a decreased respiratory rate. Documenting that a drug has been given may prevent another health care professional from mistakenly repeating the dose.

THE RIGHT DIAGNOSIS

Before giving a drug, you must be familiar with the patient's medical diagnosis. The diagnosis should match the purpose of the drug. If the diagnosis does not match its purpose, question the prescription.

You should also check any related laboratory tests before giving a drug. For example, if a patient's diagnosis is digitalis toxicity, be sure to check the digitalis level before giving this drug. If the drug you are giving may cause adverse effects on a major body organ, be sure to check laboratory values related to that organ. For example, before giving an aminoglycoside drug such as gentamicin, you should be sure to check kidney function test results such as creatinine and blood urea nitrogen (BUN).

Many drugs affect blood pressure, heart rate, or respiratory rate. Be sure to check a patient's vital signs before giving these drugs. If the patient's vital signs are outside of the normal limits, you should hold the drug and notify the prescriber. Be sure to check the patient's vital signs again after giving the drug.

THE RIGHT RESPONSE

After you give a drug, check the patient to make sure that the drug has the desired effect. For example, check the blood pressure for improvement after giving an antihypertensive drug. Be sure to document what you monitored and any other appropriate interventions.

THE RIGHT TO REFUSE

A patient has the right to refuse any drug. Be sure that he or she understands why the drug has been prescribed and the consequences of refusing to take it. When a patient refuses to take a drug, document the refusal, including the fact that the patient understands what may happen if the drug is not taken.

TYPES AND INTERPRETATION OF DRUG ORDERS

READING AND INTERPRETING DRUG LABELS

Knowing how to read and interpret drug labels for prescription or over-the-counter drugs is essential for ensuring that any medication is used correctly. Health care professionals must learn this skill to administer drugs and teach patients how to care for and use medications.

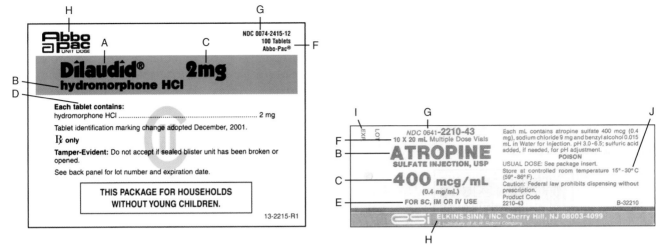

FIGURE 2-1 Drug labels. *A*, Trade name; *B*, generic name; *C*, drug strength; *D*, drug form; *E*, route of administration; *F*, total amount of medication in container; *G*, national drug code; *H*, manufacturer's name; *I*, expiration date; *J*, storage temperature. (From Fulcher, E. M., Fulcher, R. M., Soto, C. D. [2012]. *Pharmacology: Principles and applications* [3rd ed.]. St. Louis: Saunders.)

Drug labels provide important information (Figure 2-1) including:
- Trade (brand) name
- Generic name
- Drug strength (e.g., milligrams, micrograms, milliequivalents)
- Drug form (e.g., tablet, capsule, powder, solution, cream, suppository)
- Route of administration (e.g., subcutaneous, intramuscular, intravenous)
- Total amount of medication in the container (e.g., number of tablets)
- Directions for reconstitution (if needed before administration)
- National drug code (number assigned to identify the manufacturer, product, and size of container)
- Manufacturer's name
- Expiration date
- Controlled drug symbol (warning that drug may be habit forming) if needed

Labels may also include abbreviations that indicate modification of drug forms such as SR (slow release), CR (controlled release), LA or XL (long acting), DS (double strength), TR (time released), and XR or ER (extended release).

TYPES OF DRUG ORDERS

Remember, a drug order from a qualified prescriber is needed before any drug may be administered to a patient. Drug orders may be written by different types of health care providers, including physicians, dentists, and some advanced practice nurses. Common types of drug orders include standing (routine) orders, PRN orders, single-dose orders, and immediate (STAT) orders.

A **standing (routine) order** is written when a patient is receiving a drug on a regular basis. These drugs are prescribed for a specific number of days or until discontinued by the prescriber. Certain drugs such as narcotics (opioids) can be prescribed as standing orders only for a certain number of days. If the patient is to continue taking the drug after that number of days, the prescription must be renewed.

A **single-dose order** is an order to give a drug once only. A **PRN order** is given to the patient as needed. Prescribers usually designate a time interval between doses of these drugs. **STAT orders** are given one time immediately.

DRUG ERRORS

A **drug error** is defined as a preventable event that leads to inappropriate drug use or patient harm. A drug error can occur while the drug is in the control of health care professionals (e.g., in the hospital, pharmacy, or prescriber's office) or the patient.

 Memory Jogger

There are four common types of drug orders: standing (routine), single-dose, PRN, and STAT.

 Memory Jogger

Eight categories of drug errors include:
- Omission
- Wrong patient
- Wrong dose
- Wrong route
- Wrong rate
- Wrong dosage form
- Wrong time
- Error in preparation of dose

Memory Jogger

Because nurses administer most drugs to patients, they are the final defense for detecting and preventing drug errors.

QSEN: Safety

 Memory Jogger

The five steps of the medication reconciliation process are:
1. Develop a list of current medications
2. Develop a list of medications being prescribed
3. Compare the medications on the two lists
4. Make clinical decisions based on the comparison
5. Communicate the new list to appropriate caregivers and the patient

 Drug Alert!

Administration Alert

Most drug errors are made while giving drugs. Common errors include giving the wrong drug or giving the wrong dose. Follow the eight "rights" to prevent drug errors.

QSEN: Safety

 Did You Know?

You can find lists of confused drug names on the Internet at the website for the Institute for Safe Medication Practices (ISMP) (www.ismp.org).

Drug errors are a leading cause of death and injury. Medication errors cause at least one death every day and injure as many as 1.3 million people annually in the United States. Errors can occur when the prescriber writes the drug order, when the pharmacist dispenses the drug, or when the nurse or other health care professional administers the drug. *Because nurses give most drugs to patients, they are the final defense for detecting and preventing drug errors.*

PREVENTING DRUG ERRORS

To prevent medication errors, the five-step process of **medication reconciliation** has been developed. Medication reconciliation is the process of identifying the most accurate list of all medications that a patient is taking, including name, dosage, frequency, and route, by comparing the medical record to an external list of medications obtained from a patient, hospital, or other provider. When a patient visits a health care provider, is admitted to the hospital, or is transferred from unit to unit in the hospital, it is common to receive new prescriptions or to have changes made in currently prescribed drugs. The process of medication reconciliation is used during these transitions of patient care to avoid drug errors such as omissions, duplications, dosing errors, and drug interactions.

The medication reconciliation process consists of five steps:
1. Develop a list of current medications
2. Develop a list of medications being prescribed
3. Compare the medications on the two lists
4. Make clinical decisions based on the comparison
5. Communicate the new list to appropriate caregivers and the patient

When administering drugs, always follow the eight "rights." Many drug errors occur because one or more of the "rights" are not followed. If a drug prescription does not make sense, contact the prescriber to ensure that the order is correct. Always check drug dosage calculations with a coworker. Listen to the patient's questions about a drug or a drug dose. Administer drugs only after the patient's questions have been researched and answered appropriately. While giving drugs, concentrate on the task at hand. Often drug errors result from distractions or interruptions.

Bar-Code Systems

Currently many facilities use computerized charting. Computers are located in physician's offices, patient rooms, and nursing stations for ease in documentation of patient care. Facility computer systems are integrated to include various departments (e.g., pharmacy, radiology, dietary) and patient care units. As more hospitals are using bar-code systems, bar codes are added to each patient's identification wristband on admission. **Unit-dose drugs** (drugs dispensed to fill a patient's drug orders for a 24-hour period) and IV fluids are all bar coded. A bar-code scanner is used to ensure that each patient receives the right drug doses at the right time. Take the scanner to each patient's bedside to scan the identification band and the drugs that are given (Figure 2-2). Scanning automatically documents the drugs that have been given into the facility's computer system. Standing order, one-time, PRN, and STAT drugs are scanned. Research shows that bar-code systems dramatically decrease the number of drug errors.

Confusing Drug Name Lists

Lists of drug names that have been confused and involved in drug errors are published by organizations such as the Institute for Safe Medication Practices (ISMP). A partial list is provided in Box 2-1. As you read through this text, be sure to check the "Do Not Confuse" boxes for additional hints on how to avoid confusing drug names.

REPORTING DRUG ERRORS

When a drug error is made, report it immediately. Carefully watch the patient for any signs of an adverse reaction. Drug errors may result in life-threatening

| Box **2-1** | Examples of Easily Confused Drug Names |

FOSAMAX (alendronate) for osteoporosis
FLOMAX (tamsulosin) for enlarged prostate

LAMICTAL (lamotrigine) for epilepsy
LAMISIL (terbinafine) for fingernail fungus

OXYCONTIN (oxycodone) for pain
Ditropan (**OXYBUTYNIN**) for urinary
   incontinence

SINGULAIR (montelukast) for asthma
SINEQUAN (doxepin) for depression and
   anxiety

XANAX (alprazolam) for anxiety
ZANTAC (ranitidine) for heartburn and
   ulcers

complications such as coma or death. Most patient care facilities have a form and standard procedure that are used to report a drug error. The patient's prescriber must also be notified.

PRINCIPLES OF ADMINISTERING DRUGS

You must know the drug that you are administering, including its uses, actions, common adverse reactions, and any special precautions. You will probably become familiar with the drugs given most often in your institution. However, many drugs are not given on a daily basis, and new drugs are constantly being developed. Before giving a drug with which you are not familiar, seek out information from dependable sources such as pharmacists, drug inserts, and manufacturers' websites. In addition, *know the patient's drug history, allergies, previous adverse reactions, pertinent laboratory values, and any important changes in his or her condition before administering a drug.*

Often prescribers put limitations on when a drug should be given. For example, the prescriber may order that the drug be given only if the patient's blood pressure is greater or less than a particular value. Similar limitations may be based on heart rate, respiratory rate, or pain level. Be aware of the prescribed limitations and check them before giving the drug. If the patient's condition or vital signs are outside of the set limits, you must hold the drug and document the reason for your action.

When giving drugs, listen to your patient. Patient comments give clues to adverse reactions such as nausea, dizziness, unsteady walking, and ringing in the ears. These comments indicate that the patient may be having an adverse reaction, and you should hold the drug while you notify the prescriber.

GETTING READY TO GIVE DRUGS

There are several important guidelines to follow before preparing to give any drug:
- Always follow the eight "rights."
- Always check the written order.
- Check the patient's identification wristband and ask the patient's name and birthdate.
- Limit interruptions and distractions.
- Wash your hands and wear clean gloves when needed (e.g., parenteral, rectal routes).
- Keep drugs in their containers or wrappers until at the patient's bedside.
- Avoid touching pills or capsules.
- Never give drugs prepared by someone else.
- Follow sterile technique when handling syringes and needles.
- Remain alert to drug names that sound or look alike. Giving the wrong drug can have serious adverse effects.

Some pills and capsules are prepared for slow absorption. These drugs are often labeled enteric-coated, time release, or slow release. If chewed, crushed, or opened, these drugs may be absorbed too rapidly. This can irritate the gastrointestinal (GI) system or cause symptoms of overdose. If a patient cannot take pills or capsules, a liquid form of the drug may be a better option. A prescriber's order is needed to change the drug form.

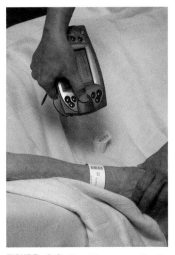

FIGURE 2-2 Checking a patient's wristband with a bar-code scanner. (From deWit, S. C., O'Neill, P. [2013]. *Fundamental concepts and skills for nursing* [4th ed.]. St. Louis: Saunders.)

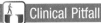 **Drug Alert!**

Action/Intervention Alert

Always report drug errors *immediately* so appropriate actions can be taken to counteract possible adverse reactions to the drug.

QSEN: Safety

Drug Alert!

Safety Alert

Know the patient's drug history, allergies, previous adverse reactions, pertinent laboratory values, and any important changes in his or her condition before administering any drug.

QSEN: Safety

Drug Alert!

Action/Intervention Alert

Always listen to patients when giving drugs because their actions and comments can be clues to adverse or side effects of drugs.

QSEN: Safety

Clinical Pitfall

Never crush tablets or open capsules without first checking with the drug guide or pharmacist.

QSEN: Safety

Giving drugs to children can be challenging and difficult. Tips that may help you give drugs to children are listed in Box 2-2.

GIVING ENTERAL DRUGS

A drug given by the **enteral route** is delivered from the outside of the body to the inside of the body using the GI tract. Enteral drugs enter the body in one of three ways: through the mouth (oral), by feeding tube (e.g., nasogastric tube or percutaneous endoscopic gastrostomy), or through the rectum.

ORAL DRUGS

Drugs are most commonly given by mouth or the **oral route**, also known as the enteral route. Orders for oral drugs are written as "PO," which means *per os* or "by mouth." Most drugs are available in one or more oral forms: tablets, capsules, and liquids. Oral drugs are easy to give as long as the patient can swallow. A major advantage of PO drugs is that if a patient receives too much, the drug can be removed by pumping the stomach or causing the patient to vomit. Oral drugs do not work well for patients suffering from nausea and vomiting. **Onset of action** for these drugs is slow because they must be absorbed through the GI tract.

What To Do *Before* Giving Oral Drugs

Be sure that the patient can swallow. Sit the patient upright and have a full glass of water ready. Tell him or her what drugs you will be giving and answer any questions asked. Tell the patient if there are any special instructions related to the drugs (e.g., getting up slowly from bed after new antihypertensive drugs are given). Ask him or her to place the tablets or capsules in the back of the mouth, take a few sips of water, and swallow the drugs. Unless the patient is on a fluid restriction, have him or her drink the entire glass of water because oral drugs dissolve better and cause less GI discomfort when they are given with enough water. Stay at the bedside until the drugs are swallowed. Do not leave drugs at the patient's bedside to be taken later. An exception may be made for antacids or nitroglycerin tablets *if* there is an order permitting this. You are responsible for documenting that drugs have been taken and must witness that this has occurred.

If the oral drug is in suspension form, be sure to shake it well. When giving oral liquid drugs, be sure to use a calibrated device to measure the correct dose (Figure 2-3) because household devices such as spoons or cups vary widely in size and their use can result in giving inaccurate doses. Always hold a calibrated medicine cup at eye level to measure the dose (Figure 2-4).

What To Do *After* Giving Oral Drugs

Document that the drug was given. If a drug was refused or not given, document the reason. Be sure to check the patient later for side effects, adverse effects, and the desired effect. For example, check the patient taking antihypertensive drugs for decreased blood pressure. Document your findings.

ORAL DRUGS GIVEN BY FEEDING TUBE

Oral drugs may be given by feeding tubes. Patients who are unable to swallow may be given oral drugs by a nasogastric tube. A nasogastric (NG) tube delivers drugs by a tube inserted through the nostrils to the stomach. A percutaneous endoscopic gastrostomy (PEG) tube is a feeding tube that is surgically implanted through the abdomen into the stomach.

What To Do *Before* Giving Drugs by NG or PEG Tube

As with all oral drugs, check the drug orders, which may be written as PO or by feeding tube. Check your drug book or with the pharmacist before crushing tablets or opening capsules. Wash your hands and place the patient upright. Check to make sure that the tube is located in the stomach by withdrawing (*aspirating*) stomach

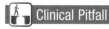

Clinical Pitfall

Never leave drugs at the bedside for the patient to take at a later time or ask someone else to administer drugs that you have prepared.

QSEN: Safety

Box 2-2 │ Tips for Administering Drugs to Children

DO'S

- Keep drugs in their original containers and never in dishes, cups, bottles, or other household containers.
- When dosage calculations are needed, have another nurse, prescriber, or pharmacist also perform the calculation to ensure accuracy.
- Check with a drug guide for information on dosage by milligrams per kilogram and ensure that the calculated dosage is within the guidelines.
- Question any order in which the prescribed dosage does not match the recommended dosage for body weight or size.
- Use appropriate measuring devices (see Figure 2-3) to ensure accurate doses of liquid drugs.
- Work with the pharmacist to ensure that a liquid oral drug or a crushed oral tablet is mixed with a small amount of pleasant, delicious-tasting liquid.
- Keep all drugs out of reach of children.
- Before crushing a tablet, check with the pharmacist or drug resource book to determine whether it should be crushed.
- Apply transdermal patch drugs to a child's back between the shoulder blades.
- Use two identifiers, including the child's name band, to identify him or her before administering any drug (this can include asking a parent the child's full name and date of birth).
- Position children in a sitting or semi-sitting position when administering an oral drug (to avoid aspiration or choking).
- Help a child rinse his or her mouth after taking an oral liquid drug.
- Watch an infant or child closely (at least every 15 minutes) for the first 2 hours after giving the first dose of a newly prescribed drug for expected and unexpected or unusual responses to the drug.
- Offer creative choices for the child who is old enough to understand such as:
  - Which drug to take first if more than one drug will be administered at the same time
  - Which type of drink the child would like as a follow-up after a drug is administered
  - Which leg or arm (when appropriate) the child would prefer be used for an injection
  - Which toy to hold during an injection
- When an infant or child is prescribed to take a drug at home, demonstrate to the parents exactly how to measure and give the drug. Have the parents demonstrate these acts.
- Obtain the assistance of another adult when administering a parenteral drug, drops or ointment to the eye, or drops to the ear of an infant or child.
- Select the smallest gauge and shortest needle that will safely deliver the injection.
- If possible, change needles after injecting the drug into the syringe (prevents any irritating drug residue from contacting the child's tissues).
- Follow agency policy for site selection of injectable drugs for a child.
- Use diversion during an injection.
- Try to avoid having the child see the needle or the actual injection.

DON'TS

- Don't refer to drugs as "candy."
- Don't place liquid drugs in a large bottle of formula (unless the child drinks the entire amount, he or she will not receive the correct dose).
- Don't place crushed drugs into the child's *favorite* food or snack (he or she may never eat that food again).
- Don't threaten a child with an injection in place of an oral drug.
- Don't lie to a child.

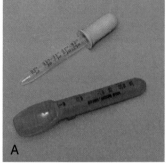

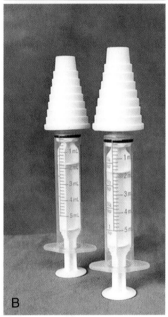

FIGURE 2-3 Calibrated devices for delivery of liquid oral drugs. **A,** Calibrated dropper and calibrated spoon. **B,** Calibrated oral syringes. (**A** from Hockenberry, M. J., & Wilson, D. [2006]. *Wong's nursing care of infants and children* [8th ed.]. St. Louis: Mosby. **B** courtesy Paul Vincent Kuntz, Texas Children's Hospital, Houston.)

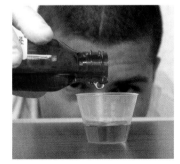

FIGURE 2-4 Checking the drug dose in a medicine cup. (From Perry, A. G., & Potter, P. [2009]. *Clinical nursing skills and techniques* [7th ed.]. St. Louis: Mosby.)

contents with a syringe, or you can attach an end-tidal carbon dioxide (CO_2) detector to the feeding tube. The presence of carbon dioxide indicates that the tube is in the trachea rather than the stomach.

If the patient is receiving a tube feeding, check the amount of tube feeding remaining in the stomach *(residual)*. Some drugs are not well absorbed when food is in the stomach (e.g., phenytoin [Dilantin]), and the tube feeding must be stopped for a period before and after administration. Liquid drugs should be diluted and flushed

Clinical Pitfall

Do *not* give a drug by NG tube if CO_2 is present when the tube is tested with an end-tidal CO_2 detector.

QSEN: Safety

 Drug Alert!

Administration Alert

Always check for correct placement of a feeding tube before giving drugs by this route to ensure that the drugs do not go into the lungs.

QSEN: Safety

Memory Jogger

Vasovagal reactions are a common cause of fainting from a decrease in heart rate and blood pressure.

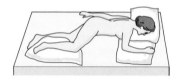

FIGURE 2-5 Sims' left position. For this position, the patient lies on one side with the knee and thigh drawn upward toward the chest.

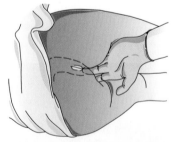

FIGURE 2-6 To administer a rectal suppository, push the suppository into the rectum about 1 inch.

through the tube. Crushed tablets and the contents of opened capsules are first dissolved in water before being given through the tube. To give the drugs, attach a large syringe to the tube, pour the liquid or dissolved drug into the syringe, and let it run in by gravity.

What To Do *After* Giving Drugs by NG or PEG Tube

After giving drugs by this route, flush the tube well to make sure it is clear. Use at least 50 mL of water to prevent the tube from becoming clogged. If the patient's NG tube is connected to suction, the tube should be clamped for at least 30 minutes after administering drugs before reattaching it to suction. This allows time for the drugs to be absorbed from the GI system. As with oral drugs, document what has been given and watch the patient for side effects, adverse effects, and the desired effects. Document your findings.

GIVING RECTAL DRUGS

Patients who are unable to swallow or have severe nausea and vomiting may need to have drugs given by the **rectal route** (movement of a drug from outside the body to inside the body through the rectum). These drugs may come as suppositories or in the form of an enema. A **suppository** is a small drug plug designed to melt at body temperature when placed within the rectum or vagina. With drugs given by this route, absorption is not as dependable or predictable as when drugs are given orally. The patient with diarrhea cannot hold them long enough for absorption to take place. The rate of absorption is also affected by the amount of stool present.

What To Do *Before* Giving Rectal Drugs

Ask whether the patient has any health problems such as diarrhea that may make using this route undesirable. Other reasons for not giving a rectal drug include recent rectal surgery or trauma and a history of *vasovagal reactions* (slowed heart rate and dilation of blood vessels, which can lead to fainting, sometimes called *syncope*).

Bring the drug, some lubricant, and a pair of disposable gloves to the bedside. Assist the patient to turn to the side with one leg bent over the other (Sims' position) (Figure 2-5). The left Sims' position is best for giving rectal suppositories.

Protect the patient's privacy by closing doors or drapes and keeping as much of the patient covered as possible. Explain what you will be doing and be sure to include any special instructions such as how long the drug must be held inside the rectum. Put on your gloves. Take the wrapper off the suppository and coat the pointed end with a small amount of water-soluble lubricant. Also apply a small amount of lubricant to the finger that you will be using to insert the drug. Hold the suppository next to the anal sphincter and explain that you are ready to insert the drug. Ask the patient to take a deep breath and bear down a little. With the pointed end first, push the suppository into the rectum about 1 inch (Figure 2-6).

What To Do *After* Giving Rectal Drugs

Remind the patient to remain on his or her side for about 20 minutes. Clean the patient's anal area and cover the patient. Remove gloves and wash your hands. Immediately document that the drug was given. Check the patient for any expected or unexpected responses and chart these. For example, if the patient was given a suppository to relieve constipation, be sure to note whether the patient later had a bowel movement.

GIVING PARENTERAL DRUGS

Drugs given by the **parenteral route** are injected through the skin. They may be injected intradermally, subcutaneously, intramuscularly, or intravenously. There are four primary reasons for giving drugs parenterally. The patient may:
- Be unable to take oral drugs.
- Need a drug that acts rapidly.

- Need a constant blood level of a drug.
- Need drugs such as insulin, which are not made in an oral form.

Standard precautions from the Centers for Disease Control and Prevention (CDC) recommend wearing gloves whenever you are exposed to blood or other body fluids, mucous membranes, or any area of broken skin.

Giving parenteral drugs requires that you use needles and syringes safely. Do not recap needles, and always dispose of needles and syringes in labeled containers. "Sharps" containers are located in every patient room. Many hospitals use needleless systems, retractable needles, or needles with plastic guards that slip over the needle to protect against needlesticks.

The Needlestick Safety and Prevention Act was signed into law in November 2000. In 2001, the Occupational Safety and Health Administration (OSHA) developed guidelines to help prevent needlesticks. OSHA advises that prevention of needlesticks is best and recommends that health care employers select safer needle devices. Needlestick injuries should be tracked using a Sharps Injury Log. The purpose of this log is to identify problem areas. In addition, OSHA recommends that employers have a written Exposure Care Plan that is updated on an annual basis.

GIVING INTRADERMAL DRUGS

A drug administered by the **intradermal route** is administered by an injection between the layers of the skin. The most common site for intradermal injections is the inner part of the forearm. The primary uses of intradermal injections are for:

- Allergy testing
- Local anesthetics
- Tuberculosis (TB) testing

The TB test is done with purified protein derivative. A small amount of drug is injected into the space between the epidermis and the dermis layers of the skin (Figure 2-7). This results in a bump *(bleb)* that looks like an insect bite. The volume of drug injected is small (0.01–0.1 mL), and the needle used is short and small ($\frac{3}{8}$ inch, 25 gauge).

What To Do *Before* Giving Intradermal Drugs

Put on gloves. Cleanse the injection site in a circular motion, beginning from the center and moving outward. Insert the needle at a 10- to 15-degree angle with the bevel facing up (Figure 2-8). Do not pull back (aspirate) on the plunger of the syringe. Inject the drug so a little bump forms and remove the needle. *Do not massage the area.* If the little bump does not form, the drug has probably been injected too deeply into the subcutaneous tissue, and test results will not be accurate. When this happens, discard the used equipment and use a different site with a new sterile needle and syringe for the intradermal injection

What To Do *After* Giving Intradermal Drugs

Document the drug administration immediately. Check the patient for allergic or sensitivity reactions to the injection. These reactions may take several hours to days.

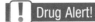
Drug Alert!

Administration Alert

Always wear gloves when giving parenteral drugs to avoid exposure to blood and other body fluids.

QSEN: Safety

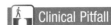
Clinical Pitfall

To avoid needlesticks, do not recap needles.

QSEN: Safety

Drug Alert!

Administration Alert

Use a small needle and a 10- to 15-degree angle for intradermal drugs. Do not aspirate before injecting the drug or massage afterward.

QSEN: Safety

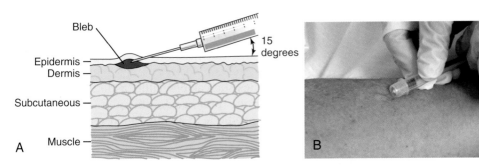

FIGURE 2-7 A and B, Intradermal injection. (**B** from Harkreader, H., Thobaben, M., & Hogan, M. A. [2007]. *Fundamentals of nursing: Caring and clinical judgment* [3rd ed.]. Philadelphia: Saunders.)

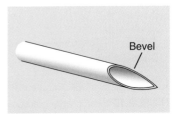

FIGURE 2-8 Close-up of a needle with the bevel up.

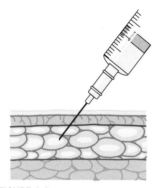

FIGURE 2-9 Subcutaneous injection.

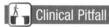

Clinical Pitfall

Be sure *not* to aspirate when giving subcutaneous heparin. Aspirating causes a vacuum and can lead to tissue damage and bruising when the heparin is injected.

QSEN: Safety

Drug Alert!

Administration Alert

IM injections of more than 3 mL are rare. To ensure that the drug dose is correct, carefully calculate and check it with another health care professional.

QSEN: Safety

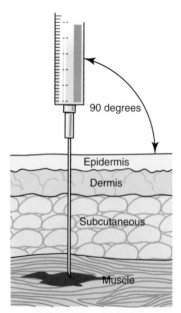

FIGURE 2-10 Intramuscular injection.

Making a circle around the injection site with a pen may help to accurately check the site. Document any reactions and notify the prescriber. TB tests must be checked and read 2 to 3 days (48 to 72 hours) after the injection.

GIVING SUBCUTANEOUS DRUGS

A drug given by the **subcutaneous route** is injected into tissues between the skin and muscle (Figure 2-9). Although several drugs are given by this route, two drugs commonly given subcutaneously are insulin and heparin. Subcutaneous drugs are absorbed more slowly than intramuscular drugs. Typically these injections are from 0.5 to 1 mL. When a larger volume of drug is ordered, give the injection in two different sites with different syringes and needles. Small, short needles are used (⅜ inch, 25 to 27 gauge). Sites for subcutaneous injections include the upper arms, the abdomen, and the upper back. Some sources also recommend use of the anterolateral thigh. Rotate the sites for the injections to avoid damage to the patient's tissues.

What To Do *Before* Giving Subcutaneous Drugs

Insert the needle at a 45-degree angle for most patients. If the patient is obese, you may need to use a 90-degree angle. If the patient is thin, you may need an angle that is less than 45 degrees. Before giving any subcutaneous injection, do *not* aspirate (pull back on the plunger of the syringe). Inject the drug and remove the needle.

What To Do *After* Giving Subcutaneous Drugs

Apply pressure to prevent bleeding. If a patient has a bleeding disorder or is receiving anticoagulation therapy, you may need to apply pressure longer until the bleeding has stopped. Document giving the drug immediately, including the site used for injection. Check the patient for side effects, adverse effects, and expected effects. Document your findings.

GIVING INTRAMUSCULAR DRUGS

A drug given by the **intramuscular (IM) route** is given by injection deep into a muscle (Figure 2-10). Because of the rich blood supply in the muscles, IM drugs are absorbed much faster than subcutaneous drugs. IM injections can also be much larger than subcutaneous injections (1 to 3 mL). Injections into an adult's arm should not be more than 2 mL. Infants and children usually do not receive more than 1 mL. If an injection order is for more than 3 mL, divide the dose and give two injections. Injections of more than 3 mL are not as well absorbed.

Needles for these injections are longer (1 to 1.5 inches) and larger (20 to 22 gauge). Sites for IM injections include the upper arm deltoid muscle, the thigh vastus lateralis muscles, and the ventrogluteal muscle in the hip (Figures 2-11 through 2-13). The dorsogluteal site is *not* favored because of the presence of nerves and major blood vessels. This site is avoided in obese patients because research has shown that injections do not reach the muscle. Be sure to rotate injection sites when multiple IM injections are prescribed. Table 2-1 describes the advantages and disadvantages of IM injection sites.

What To Do *Before* Giving Intramuscular Drugs

Help the patient into a comfortable position that is appropriate for the site you plan to use. Select the injection site by identifying the correct anatomic landmarks. Wash your hands and be sure to wear gloves. Cleanse the injection site. Using a 90-degree angle, insert the needle firmly into the muscle. *Aspiration is not recommended for IM injection of vaccines or immunizations.* For drugs such as penicillin, aspiration may be indicated. When indicated, aspirate the syringe (pull back on the plunger) to make sure that the needle is not in a vein. If the needle is in a vein, blood will appear in the syringe. Remove the needle and discard the drug if this happens. Get a new dose of the drug and a sterile needle and syringe and give the injection in another site. Once you have determined that the needle is not in a blood vessel, inject the drug and remove the needle.

Table **2-1**	Intramuscular Injection Site Advantages and Disadvantages	
INJECTION SITE	**ADVANTAGES**	**DISADVANTAGES**
Deltoid (upper arm)	Easily accessible Useful for vaccinations in adolescents and adults	Poorly developed in young children Only small amounts (0.5-1 mL) can be injected
Vastus lateralis (thigh)	Preferred site for infant injections Relatively free of large blood vessels and nerves Easily accessible	Intake or medication is slower than the arm but faster than buttocks
Ventrogluteal (hips)	Used for children age 7 or older and adults Less likely to be inadvertently injected subcutaneously	Patient anxiety due to unfamiliarity with site and visibility of site during injection

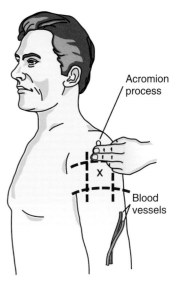

FIGURE 2-11 Deltoid (arm) intramuscular injection site landmarks.

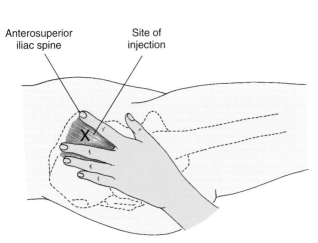

FIGURE 2-12 Ventrogluteal intramuscular injection site landmarks. (From Potter, P. A., & Perry, A. G. [2013]. *Fundamentals of nursing: Concepts, process, and practice* [8th ed.]. St. Louis: Mosby.)

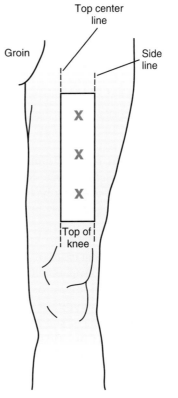

FIGURE 2-13 Vastus lateralis (thigh) intramuscular injection site landmarks.

Use the Z-track method of IM injection for drugs that are irritating to subcutaneous tissue or that may permanently stain the tissues (Figure 2-14). After drawing the drug into the syringe, draw in 0.1 to 0.2 mL of air. The air follows the drug into the muscle and stops it from oozing through the path of the needle. After you select and cleanse the site, pull the tissue laterally and hold it. Insert the needle into the muscle; inject the drug and release the tissue as you remove the needle. Releasing the tissue allows the skin to slide over the injection and seal the drug in the muscle.

[!] Drug Alert!

Administration Alert

With the Z-tract IM injection, draw up 0.1 to 0.2 mL of air after drawing up the drug. Injection of air keeps the drug in the muscle, and the drug does not ooze through the path of the needle.

QSEN: Safety

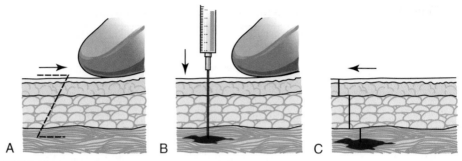

FIGURE 2-14 Z-track intramuscular injection. **A,** Displace the tissue downward, away from the injection site. **B,** Inject while holding the tissue away. **C,** Allow the displaced tissue to move back into place.

What To Do *After* Giving Intramuscular Drugs

Apply pressure after removing the needle to prevent bleeding. When charting the drug administration, be sure to include the injection site. Check the patient for adverse effects, side effects, and expected effects of the drug. Document your findings.

GIVING INTRAVENOUS DRUGS

A drug given by the **intravenous (IV) route** is injected directly into a vein (Figure 2-15). This route is selected when a drug needs to enter the bloodstream rapidly or when large doses of a drug must be given. The rates of absorption and action are rapid with this route. Emergency drugs may be given by a needle and syringe directly into a vein; however, most IV drugs are given slowly through a needle or catheter that has been inserted into a vein. The needle or catheter is attached to IV tubing with an injection port. IV drugs may be pushed slowly over 1 or more minutes, pushed rapidly over a few seconds, or given slowly by IV piggyback. They may be given through an IV line or a saline lock.

What To Do *Before* Giving Intravenous Drugs

Check the IV site to make sure that it is patent. Document the condition of the IV site. If the drug has been added to IV fluid, be sure to remove all air from the tubing. (This is called *priming* the IV tubing.) If the drug is to be administered in a continuous IV infusion or an IV piggyback, it should be placed on an infusion pump to control the rate.

In most cases, registered nurses (RNs) will give IV push and IV piggyback drugs. Be sure to check the scope of practice laws of your state. In some states, licensed practical nurses or licensed vocational nurses may administer IV drugs with additional training.

What To Do *After* Giving Intravenous Drugs

Document that the drug has been given, including the site and flow rate. Continue to check the IV site for signs of these conditions:

- Infection
- Escape of fluid from the vein into tissue (*extravasation*)
- Collection of fluid in the tissues (*infiltration*)

If fluid escapes or collects in the tissues, the IV catheter must be discontinued and replaced in a different vein. As with administration of any drug, check the patient for side effects, adverse effects, or expected effects of the drug. Document these effects. To learn more about IV fluids, see Chapter 5.

GIVING PERCUTANEOUS DRUGS

A drug given by the **percutaneous route** is applied to and absorbed through the skin and mucous membranes. Absorption of these drugs is affected by several factors:

- Size of area covered by the drug
- Concentration or strength of the drug

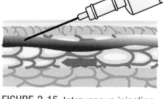

FIGURE 2-15 Intravenous injection.

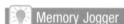
Memory Jogger

IV drugs may be given continuously or intermittently.

Drug Alert!

Administration Alert

Always check the IV site before administering IV drugs. If an IV line is not patent, the drug will go into the tissue instead of the vein and may cause tissue damage.

QSEN: Safety

- Time the drug remains in contact with the skin or mucous membranes
- Condition of the skin (breakdown, thickness, hydration, nutrition, and skin tone)

GIVING TOPICAL OR TRANSDERMAL DRUGS

A drug given by the **topical route** is applied directly to the skin for local effects. Topical drugs include creams, lotions, and ointments. They soften or lubricate the skin. Some are used to treat superficial infections of the skin. Topical drugs are applied in a thin, even layer over the affected area of skin.

A drug given by the **transdermal route** is applied to the skin, but it is absorbed and enters the bloodstream. The transdermal route allows the patient to maintain a steady blood level of the drug. For this reason, toxicity and adverse effects can usually be avoided. Examples of transdermal drugs are:

- Nitroglycerin to treat cardiac problems
- Scopolamine to treat dizziness and nausea
- Birth control
- Nicotine patches for smoking cessation
- Long-term pain drugs

They are applied as patches or ointments. Drug patches have a semipermeable membrane and an adhesive that attaches to the skin (Figure 2-16). Common sites of application include the chest, flank, back, and upper arms.

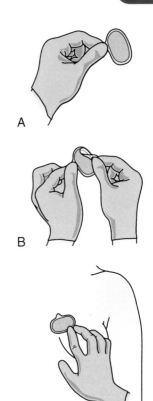

FIGURE 2-16 Applying a transdermal patch. **A,** Nitroglycerin patch. **B,** Remove plastic backing carefully, taking care not to touch the medication. **C,** Place the medication side of the patch on the patient's skin and press the adhesive to stay in place.

What To Do *Before* Giving Topical or Transdermal Drugs

Wash your hands and put on gloves. Clean the area of skin where the drug will be applied. Apply topical drugs in a smooth, thin layer, and cover the area. When administering transdermal drugs, remove old patches or doses of the drug. Be sure to remove all traces of the drug from the previous dosage site, and rotate sites to avoid skin irritation or breakdown.

Do not shave skin before applying topical or transdermal drugs. Shaving may cause skin irritation and change the absorption of the drug.

What To Do *After* Giving Topical or Transdermal Drugs

Document that the drug has been given, including the site where it was applied. Be sure to write the date, time, and your initials on the new patch. Check the patient for adverse effects or expected effects and document these. For example, headache and dizziness related to decreased blood pressure are common side effects of nitroglycerin ointment.

GIVING DRUGS THROUGH THE MUCOUS MEMBRANES

Drugs may be absorbed through the mucous membranes. The following are examples of drug forms used for the different mucous membranes found in the body:

- Buccal or sublingual drugs are used in the mouth.
- Drops and ointments are applied to the eyes, nose, or ears.
- Inhalation drugs are drawn into the lungs.
- Suppositories and creams are used in the vagina.

Drugs are usually well absorbed through these areas; however, the blood supply to mucous membranes varies. When you administer a drug through mucous membranes, be sure to use a sterile procedure before placing eye drops or ointments and a clean procedure before giving drugs into the ears, nose, mouth, or vagina.

What To Do *Before* Giving Drugs Through the Mucous Membranes

Always check the order and the patient's identity. Wash your hands and wear gloves. Follow the eight "rights."

Buccal and Sublingual Drugs. Drugs given by the **buccal route,** such as lozenges, are placed between the cheek and molar teeth of the upper jaw (Figure 2-17). A drug given by the **sublingual route,** such as nitroglycerin, is placed under the tongue

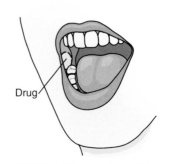

FIGURE 2-17 Giving buccal drugs.

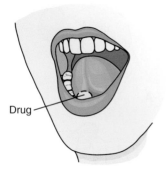

FIGURE 2-18 Giving sublingual drugs.

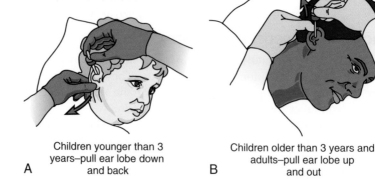

A   Children younger than 3 years–pull ear lobe down and back

B   Children older than 3 years and adults–pull ear lobe up and out

FIGURE 2-19 Giving ear drops. **A,** Children younger than 3 years: pull ear lobe down and back. **B,** Children older than 3 years and adults: pull ear lobe up and out.

> ⓘ **Drug Alert!**
>
> **Teaching Alert**
>
> Teach the patient to avoid swallowing any buccal or sublingual drugs.
>
> QSEN: Safety

> ⓘ **Drug Alert!**
>
> **Administration Alert**
>
> Before giving ear drops to children younger than 3 years, pull the ear lobe down and back to straighten the ear canal. Before giving ear drops to older children and adults, pull the ear lobe up and out to straighten the ear canal.
>
> QSEN: Safety

(Figure 2-18). The blood supply is very good in the mouth; therefore these drugs dissolve and are absorbed quickly. The patient should not eat or drink until the drug is completely dissolved. Teach the patient not to swallow or chew while the drug is in the mouth because these drugs are not effective if absorbed through the GI tract.

Ear Drops. Ear drops are drugs given to treat local infection or inflammation and should be kept at room temperature. Help the patient to lie on one side with the affected ear up. For children younger than 3 years, pull the ear lobe (*pinna*) down and back. For older children and adults, pull the ear lobe up and out (Figure 2-19). This straightens the ear canal. Do not let the ear dropper touch the ear. Have the patient stay in the same position for at least 5 minutes so the drug can coat the inner ear canal. Sometimes a cotton ball is ordered to be placed in the ear canal. Repeat this procedure for the other ear when both ears are affected.

Eye Drops and Ointments. Administration of eye drops and ointments is discussed in detail in Chapter 29.

Nose Drops. Nose drops or sprays are most often used to treat congestion or infection. To give nose drops, draw the drops into a dropper. Ask the patient to gently blow his or her nose and then lie down with the head hanging over the edge of the bed. Hold the dropper over a nostril and give the ordered number of nose drops. Do not let the dropper touch the nose. Repeat for the second nostril if needed.

To give nasal spray, position the patient sitting up with one nostril blocked by a finger. Place the tip of the spray in the other nostril. Ask the patient to take a deep breath. During the deep breath, squeeze a puff of spray into the nostril. Wipe the spray bottle tip if it is to be used with both nostrils. Nasal sprays are absorbed quickly from the nasal mucosa. Do not use the same spray container for any other patient.

Inhalers. Drugs may be inhaled through the respiratory tract. Different types of devices are used for delivery of inhaled drugs. Specific techniques for administering inhaled drugs are presented in Chapter 21.

Vaginal Drugs. Vaginal drugs are given to treat irritation or infection. Types of vaginal drugs include creams, jellies, tablets, foams, or suppositories. These drugs should be kept at room temperature. Ask the patient to empty her bladder then lie down. Be sure to put on gloves after washing your hands. Suppositories are lubricated and given in the same way as rectal suppositories. Creams, jellies, tablets, and foams are given with a special applicator that is placed in the vagina as far as possible. The plunger of the applicator is pushed to give the drug. Be sure to have the patient lie down for 10 to 15 minutes after receiving these drugs.

What To Do *After* Giving Drugs Through the Mucous Membranes

Always document that the drugs have been given, including the route. Check the patient for any expected or unexpected actions of the drug that you have given. Document these effects.

Get Ready for Practice!

Key Points

- Always follow the procedures of the eight "rights" when giving drugs (right patient, right drug, right dose, right route, right time, right documentation, right diagnosis, and right response).
- The four types of drug orders are standing (routine), single dose, PRN, and STAT.
- Most drug errors occur while giving drugs. Following the procedure of the eight "rights" helps prevent drug errors.
- Nurses give most drugs to patients, and they are the final defense for detecting and preventing drug errors.
- Medication reconciliation and bar-code systems for giving drugs have led to decreases in drug errors.
- Always report a drug error immediately so actions can be taken to counteract any possible adverse drug reactions.
- Always listen to patients for clues to adverse effects when giving drugs.
- Always check the written order and pertinent laboratory values and vital signs before giving a drug.
- Always check the patient for expected effects, side effects, and adverse effects after giving a drug.
- Never crush tablets or open capsules without checking with the pharmacist first.
- Check the patient's ability to swallow before giving oral drugs.
- Always wear gloves and use Standard Precautions to protect yourself from the risk of exposure to body fluids when giving drugs.
- To avoid needlesticks, do not recap needles.

Additional Learning Resources

evolve Be sure to visit your Evolve website (http://evolve.elsevier.com/Workman/pharmacology/) for additional online resources.

SG Go to your Study Guide for additional learning activities to help you master this chapter content.

Review Questions

See the Answer Keys—In-text Review Questions for answers to these questions.

Test Yourself on the Basics

1. Which of the eight rights should you apply immediately after you give a drug?
   - A. Right drug
   - B. Right patient
   - C. Right documentation
   - D. Right dosage

2. For which order do you administer a drug as the patient needs it?
   - A. Routine order
   - B. STAT order
   - C. One-time order
   - D. PRN order

3. Which process was developed to ensure that a patient receives the correct medications when transferred from the ICU to a medical patient care unit?
   - A. Medication reconciliation
   - B. Bar-code scanners
   - C. Online charting
   - D. Error reporting protocol

4. Which are parenteral routes? (Select all that apply.)
   - A. Sublingual
   - B. Intradermal
   - C. Buccal
   - D. Rectal
   - E. Subcutaneous
   - F. Intravenous

5. What must you do to protect yourself when giving a topical drug like nitroglycerin ointment?
   - A. Check the patient's blood pressure.
   - B. Put on clean gloves.
   - C. Spread the drug in a smooth layer.
   - D. Wear a disposable gown.

Test Yourself on Advanced Concepts

6. What is the best way to check that you are giving the drug to the right patient?
   - A. Ask the patient's name.
   - B. Look at the patient's bedside chart.
   - C. Check the patient's wristband.
   - D. Check two unique patient identifiers.

7. A patient receiving a daily dose of furosemide needs a daily dose of oral potassium. Which type of order does the prescriber use?
   - A. Standing/routine order
   - B. One-time order
   - C. PRN order
   - D. STAT order

8. Which intervention is the best way to prevent drug errors such as omissions, duplications, dosing errors, and drug interactions?
   - A. Double check the written drug order.
   - B. Follow the procedure of the eight "rights."
   - C. Use the process of medication reconciliation.
   - D. Check the patient's wristband for identification.

9. Before giving any drug that you are not familiar with to a patient, what do you need to know about the patient? (Select all that apply.)
   A. The patient's allergies
   B. Previous adverse reactions to drugs
   C. Pertinent laboratory values
   D. The patient's family history of illnesses
   E. Important changes in the patient's condition
   F. Any over-the-counter drugs that the patient is taking

10. Which priority assessment must you make before giving any patient an oral drug?
    A. Quiz the patient about the action of each drug.
    B. Make sure that the patient can swallow.
    C. Find out if the patient prefers cold or room temperature liquids.
    D. Ask the patient to repeat his or her name and birthdate.

11. Which actions are essential for safety when administering a parenteral drug to a patient? (Select all that apply.)
    A. Never recap needles.
    B. Clean the injection site in a circular motion from the outside to the inside.
    C. Use a 1-inch, 22-gauge needle and a 90-degree angle for injection.
    D. Place all used needles and syringes in a "Sharps" container.
    E. Wear gloves to avoid exposure to blood or body fluids.
    F. Always inject the drug in the same site.

12. You are teaching a patient about a prescribed transdermal drug. What will you be sure to tell the patient? (Select all that apply.)
    A. "This route will allow you to keep a steady blood level of the drug."
    B. "Be sure to apply the drug patch to your upper thigh."
    C. "Shave the hair from your skin before applying your transdermal patch."
    D. "Remove the old patch when you apply a new one."
    E. "Rotate the sites where you place the patch to avoid skin irritation or breakdown."
    F. "Remove any drug left on the old site."

13. You are to give ear drops to a 10-year-old child. Which technique will you use?
    A. Pull the ear lobe up and out.
    B. Pull the ear lobe down and back.
    C. Pull the ear lobe out and back.
    D. Pull the ear lobe up and back.

14. Your patient it to receive medications through an NG tube. What should you do when testing a patient's NG tube with an end-tidal CO_2 detector if CO_2 is present?
    A. Inject an air bolus to see if the tube is positioned in the stomach.
    B. Flush the tube with 20 mL of water.
    C. Hold the medication because the tube is in the trachea.
    D. Crush the pills and dilute them in water.

Mathematics Review and Introduction to Dosage Calculation

http://evolve.elsevier.com/Workman/pharmacology/

Objectives

After studying this chapter you should be able to:

1. Identify the numerator and denominator of a fraction.
2. Identify a proper and an improper fraction.
3. Change a whole number into a fraction.
4. Change a mixed number into a fraction.
5. Reduce a fraction to its lowest terms.
6. Calculate the lowest common denominator of a series of fractions.
7. Add two or more fractions and subtract two or more fractions.
8. Multiply two fractions and divide two fractions.
9. Identify the divisor and the dividend of a decimal problem.
10. Multiply two decimals and divide two decimals.
11. Change a fraction into a decimal and a decimal into a fraction.
12. Calculate a given percentage of a number.
13. Compare the dose on hand (what you have) with the dose that has been prescribed (what you want).
14. Calculate the number of tablets or amount of liquid drug needed to make the prescribed dose.
15. Convert a set of fractions into a proportion.
16. Solve for "*X*" (the unknown) in a math problem.

Key Terms

decimal (DĔS-ĭ-mŭl) (p. 50) The part of a whole number based on a system of units of 10 (for example, 0.5 is 5 tenths of 1).

decimal point (DĔS-ĭ-mŭl PŌYNT) (p. 50) The dividing point between whole numbers and parts of numbers in a system based on units of 10.

denominator (dē-NŎM-ĭn-ā-tŭr) (p. 46) The bottom number in a fraction, the dividing number (for example, in $\frac{3}{4}$ the denominator is 4); same as divisor.

dividend (DĬ-vĭ-dĕnd) (p. 52) The number to be divided in a division problem (for example, in $\frac{3}{4}$ the dividend is 3); same as numerator.

divisor (dĭ-VĬ-zŭr) (p. 52) The number the dividend is divided by (or that is divided into the dividend) (for example, in $\frac{3}{4}$ the divisor is 4); same as denominator.

fraction (FRĂK-shŭn) (p. 46) A part of a whole number obtained by dividing one number by a larger number.

improper fraction (ĭm-PRŎ-pŭr FRĂK-shŭn) (p. 47) A fraction that has a top number (numerator) that is larger than the bottom number (denominator). The final answer to an improper fraction is always greater than the number 1.

mixed-number fractions (MĬKST NŬM-bŭr FRĂK-shŭnz) (p. 47) Whole numbers with a fraction attached.

numerator (NŪ-mŭr-ā-tŭr) (p. 46) The top number in a fraction that is divided by the bottom number (denominator) (for example, in $\frac{3}{4}$ the numerator is 3; same as dividend).

percent (pŭr-SĔNT) (p. 53) The expression of how a number is related to 100; literally "for each hundred."

proper fraction (PRŎ-pŭr FRĂK-shŭn) (p. 47) A fraction in which the top number is smaller than the bottom number. The final answer to a proper fraction is always less than the number 1.

proportion (prō-PŌR-shŭn) (p. 56) An equal mathematic relationship between two sets of numbers.

quotient (KWŌ-shĕnt) (p. 52) The answer to a division problem.

reduced fractions (rē-DŪST FRĂK-shŭnz) (p. 47) Fractions that have been changed to their lowest common denominator (that is, both the numerator and the denominator of a fraction have been divided by the same number evenly).

scored tablet (SKŌRD TĂB-lĕt) (p. 55) A tablet that has a line etched into it, marking the exact midpoint. Cutting (or breaking) a tablet along this line gives you two halves with known dosages.

WHY DO HEALTH PROFESSIONALS NEED MATHEMATICS?

You have probably taken drugs at some time in your life, either over-the-counter or prescription drugs. As a nurse you will be responsible for giving drugs to others safely and accurately. As a pharmacy technician you will be responsible for preparing medications. As a medical assistant you may be responsible, under the direction of a health care provider, for giving drugs to others.

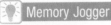
Memory Jogger

Use math correctly to calculate or check drug dosages, which is an important "right" of correct drug administration.

All drugs work better if they are given at the right dose. This is one of the eight rules for drug administration known as the *eight rights* (see Chapter 2). Understanding math helps to ensure that a drug is given at the right dose.

Drugs may not come from the pharmacy prepared in exactly the right dose to give to a patient. You may need to calculate *how much to give* from what you *have on hand* (available). Dosage calculations are performed in the same way whether the drug is a tablet, oral liquid, injectable liquid, or suppository.

This chapter and Chapters 4 and 5 contain all the basic skills and equivalencies needed to solve any drug dosage problem. Traditional math terms are used only when they help you to understand the dosage calculation concept. Basic math is logical, and you *can* understand it. If you already have a good working knowledge of the principles of basic math, check yourself by working the problems in the "MATH CHECK" section of this chapter.

MATH CHECK

The answers to these problems are located at the end of the chapter. If you work these problems correctly, you probably do not need to review the chapter. If you have a weakness in any specific area, review the content and principles for that area.

MATH CHECK PROBLEMS

MC-1: Change these mixed-number fractions into improper fractions.

a. $3\dfrac{5}{8}$

b. $7\dfrac{1}{3}$

MC-2: Reduce each of these fractions to their lowest common denominators.

a. $\dfrac{25}{75}$

b. $\dfrac{115}{130}$

MC-3: How many zeros can you chop and drop?

a. $\dfrac{180}{2200}$

b. $\dfrac{50,000}{100,000}$

MC-4: Which fraction represents the largest part of the whole for a and b? What is the lowest common denominator for each set of three fractions?

a. $\dfrac{1}{3}, \dfrac{10}{15},$ or $\dfrac{12}{24}$

b. $\dfrac{2}{4}, \dfrac{6}{8},$ or $\dfrac{3}{24}$

Which fraction represents the smallest part of the whole for c and d? What is the lowest common denominator for each set of three fractions?

c. $\dfrac{6}{8}, \dfrac{6}{12},$ or $\dfrac{2}{3}$

d. $\dfrac{8}{9}, \dfrac{1}{3},$ or $\dfrac{3}{27}$

MC-5: Add these fractions. If a sum is an improper fraction, convert it to either whole number or to a mixed-number fraction.

a. $\dfrac{1}{3}+\dfrac{2}{3}+\dfrac{3}{3}$

b. $\dfrac{9}{9}+\dfrac{5}{9}+\dfrac{7}{9}+\dfrac{4}{9}$

MC-6: Add these fractions. If the sum is an improper fraction, convert it to either a whole number or a mixed-number fraction. Reduce the answers to their lowest common denominators.

a. $\dfrac{2}{3}+\dfrac{6}{12}+\dfrac{6}{8}$

b. $\dfrac{1}{9}+\dfrac{3}{4}+\dfrac{2}{3}$

MC-7: Subtract these fractions. If a fraction is a mixed-number fraction, first convert it to an improper fraction. Reduce answers to their lowest common denominators.

a. $\dfrac{5}{6}-\dfrac{2}{6}$

b. $2\dfrac{5}{6}-1\dfrac{3}{6}$

MC-8: Subtract these fractions. If a fraction is a mixed-number fraction, first convert it to an improper fraction. Reduce answers to their lowest common denominators.

a. $\dfrac{7}{8} - \dfrac{2}{3}$

b. $6\dfrac{1}{3} - 2\dfrac{1}{2}$

MC-9: Multiply these fractions.

a. $1\dfrac{22}{24} \times \dfrac{1}{2}$

b. $4\dfrac{5}{8} \times \dfrac{2}{3}$

MC-10: Divide these fractions.

a. $\dfrac{7}{8} \div \dfrac{2}{3}$

b. $6\dfrac{3}{4} \div 2\dfrac{1}{3}$

MC-11: Decimals as parts of a whole:

a. 0.50 = How many parts of a whole?

b. 2.48 = How many whole numbers and how many parts of a whole?

MC-12: Multiply these decimals.

a. 16.5×0.5

b. 1.2×1.2

MC-13: Divide these decimals.

a. $52.8 \div 12$

b. $1.4 \div 1.4$

MC-14: Change the following fractions to decimals and decimals to fractions.

a. 0.065

b. $\dfrac{300}{650}$

MC-15: Work to three places and then round to two places.

a. $\dfrac{128.5}{80}$

b. $\dfrac{26.8}{13.4}$

MC-16: Convert the following percents into fractions.

a. $\frac{2}{3}\%$

b. 7%

MC-17: Find the percentages of the whole number.

a. 0.6% of 50

b. 20% of 120

MC-18: How many tablets should you give?

a. *Want* carvedilol 25 mg; *Have* carvedilol 6.25 mg

b. *Want* estrogen 0.0625 mg; *Have* estrogen 0.125 mg

MC-19: How many milliliters should you give?

a. *Want* diphenhydramine (Benadryl) 50 mg; *Have* diphenhydramine 25 mg/5 mL

b. *Want* chloral hydrate syrup 100 mg; *Have* chloral hydrate syrup 500 mg/5 mL

MC-20: How many milliliters should you give by injection?

a. *Want* penicillin 50,000 units; *Have* penicillin 1,000,000 units/50 mL

b. *Want* prochlorperazine (Compazine) 10 mg; *Have* prochlorperazine 5 mg/mL

MC-21: Express the following problems as a fractional proportion.

a. If one box of eggs has 18 eggs, then two boxes have 36 eggs.

b. If one chewable tablet of diphenhydramine contains 12.5 mg, then four chewable tablets have 50 mg.

MC-22: How many milliliters should you give?

a. *Want* carbamazepine (Tegretol) 75 mg oral suspension; *Have* carbamazepine 100 mg/5 mL

b. *Want* acetaminophen (Tylenol) 100 mg; *Have* acetaminophen 160 mg/5 mL

GETTING STARTED

Of course you can use a calculator to work all math problems, but beware! For a calculator to arrive at the correct answer, you must be sure to set the problem up correctly. This involves entering the numbers into the calculator in the right order. Entering the numbers into the calculator in the correct order is known as the *order of operation*. If you understand the math principle, you will be more likely to enter the numbers correctly. The location of the keys on a calculator can differ from one brand to another. So be sure to practice with your calculator before you use it at work to calculate drug dosages. *Practice makes perfect!*

Remember that math problems are punched into a calculator just like they are written or just like you would say them aloud. For example, 24 × 12 is punched in as 2, 4, ×, 1, 2 = *answer*. If you punch in any of the numbers backwards (for example, 4, 2, ×, 1, 2 or 2, 4, ×, 2, 1), the answer will be wrong.

Always use common sense whether you are using a calculator or a paper and pencil. Always ask yourself, *DOES IT MAKE SENSE?* Some people refer to this thinking as the "DIMS test." If the answer doesn't look right (for example, give 15 tablets), it probably isn't right! Think about it again and rework the problem.

Some types of drugs are *high-alert drugs* and are very dangerous if the dosage is miscalculated. These include *p*otassium, *i*nsulin, *n*arcotics, *c*hemotherapy and *c*ardiac drugs, and *h*eparin or other anticlotting drugs. Remember these dangerous drugs with the term *PINCH*. After you calculate one of these drug doses, always have another health care professional independently double check your calculation.

TALKING ABOUT NUMBERS: A WHOLE NUMBER VERSUS A PART OF A NUMBER

If you are comfortable with the difference between whole numbers and a part of a number, just skip to the next section. Let's review whole numbers versus fractions. A fraction is a part of a whole number obtained by dividing one number by a larger number. The simplest way to do this is to think about money. A \$1 bill represents the whole number one (1). A \$1.25 amount is both a whole dollar (1) and a part of another dollar. The 25 cents is a fraction of the second \$1. If you wrote it out, it would be 25 out of 100 cents, or $\frac{25}{100}$. The same amount written as a decimal would be \$0.25. Both express the exact same amount of money. So the dollar is a *whole number,* and the 25 cents is a *part* or *fraction* of another whole number. Figure 3-1 shows the relationship of a fraction (part of a whole number) to a whole number.

FRACTIONS

A **fraction** is a part of a whole number obtained by dividing one number by a larger number. Any fraction (for example, $\frac{25}{100}$) is actually a division problem. The fraction $\frac{25}{100}$ is the same as $100\overline{)25}$ or $25 \div 100$. So any number *over* another number is a fraction. The top number in a fraction, in this example 25, is called the **numerator.** Remember the numerator as being "numero uno," No. 1, the best! The number on the bottom in a fraction is the **denominator.** In the example $\frac{25}{100}$, the denominator is 100.

Any number can be expressed as a fraction, even a whole number. To make a whole number a fraction, simply make the denominator of the fraction 1. Thus the whole number 2 has the same value when written as the fraction $\frac{2}{1}$. When any whole number is written as a fraction, the whole number is always on top (numerator), and the denominator (1) is always on the bottom. Remembering this concept will help you solve drug dosage problems using fractions.

Different Types of Fractions

There are several types of fractions, including proper fractions, improper fractions, mixed-number fractions, and reduced fractions. The differences are simple, and you can do it!

 Drug Alert!

Administration Alert

Use the DIMS ("does it make sense") test when calculating a drug dose. If your answer requires more than four tablets or more than one syringe, it is probably wrong.

QSEN: Safety

 Memory Jogger

High-alert or PINCH drugs include potassium, insulin, narcotics (also known as opioids), chemotherapy and cardiac drugs, and heparin or other anticlotting drugs.

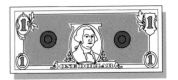

A one-dollar bill representing the whole number one

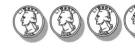

Four quarters, each representing 1/4 or 25% (0.25) of the whole one-dollar bill

FIGURE 3-1 Comparison of part of a number to a whole number.

 Memory Jogger

Remember the word NUDE. The top number in a fraction is the numerator (NU), and the bottom number is the denominator (DE): NU/DE

Memory Jogger

Whenever a whole number is written as a fraction, the whole number is on top, and the denominator is always 1.

Proper Fractions. A **proper fraction** is one in which the top number is smaller than the bottom number. So $\frac{25}{100}$ is a proper fraction. A proper fraction is the most common type of fraction. The value of a proper fraction is always less than the number 1. For example, the answer to $\frac{25}{100}$ (which is really $100\overline{)25}$ or $25 \div 100$) is **0.25,** a number less than 1.

Improper Fractions. Improper fractions didn't do anything wrong. They are just different from proper fractions, which represent only part of a whole number. A fraction can also have a top number (numerator) that is *bigger* than the bottom number (denominator) (for example, $\frac{125}{100}$). This number is still a fraction, but it represents *more* than the number 1. So an **improper fraction** is a fraction that has a top number (numerator) that is larger than the bottom number (denominator), meaning that the value is greater than 1. For example, $\frac{125}{100}$ is really $100\overline{)125}$ or $125 \div 100$, and the answer is **1.25.**

Mixed-Number Fractions. **Mixed-number fractions** are whole numbers with a fraction attached. For example, $1\frac{2}{4}$ is a mixed-number fraction; 1 is a whole number, and $\frac{2}{4}$ is a fraction. A mixed-number fraction can be changed into an improper fraction by multiplying the denominator (4) times ($\times$) the whole number (1) and adding the numerator (2). $4 \times 1 = 4 + 2 = 6$. Now make 6 the new numerator (top number) with the same denominator (4) and you get $\frac{6}{4}$, an improper fraction. Being able to convert mixed-number fractions into improper fractions is useful when you have to multiply proper and improper fractions together.

Reduced Fractions. Reducing fractions is a way to make fractions "simpler" and easier to use. **Reduced fractions** have been changed to their lowest common denominator. This means that both the top number (numerator) and the bottom number (denominator) of a fraction have been divided evenly by the same number. For example, the part of a dollar ($\frac{25}{100}$, or 25 cents out of 100 cents in a dollar) is also equal to $\frac{1}{4}$ of a dollar. To change $\frac{25}{100}$ into $\frac{1}{4}$, *divide both* the numerator and the denominator by the largest number possible that will go evenly into both numbers. In this example both 25 and 100 can be divided evenly by 25. You have just *reduced* this fraction to its lowest common denominator! When you are working with a drug dosage problem, wouldn't it be easier to work with $\frac{1}{4}$ rather than with $\frac{25}{100}$? The final dosage answer is the same either way.

If you find it hard to think of a large number that can be divided evenly into both the numerator and the denominator, start with several small numbers. For example, in $\frac{25}{100}$ each number can be divided evenly by 5. This answer, $\frac{5}{20}$, can then be divided by 5 again to get to $\frac{1}{4}$. Does this make sense? Do whatever is easier for you. The final answer is the same.

Reducing Special Fractions. How do you manage fractions with larger numbers, such as $\frac{240}{120}$? You could reduce it the way it is (dividing 240 by 120), and the answer is 2. There is a way to make it a little easier. Because *both* the top number (numerator) and the bottom number (denominator) end in *zero*, you can "chop off" both zeros and be left with $\frac{24}{12}$. By chopping off the zeros, you are actually dividing both the numerator (240) and the denominator (120) by 10, resulting in a new numerator of 24 and a new denominator of 12. The answer is still 2 because you divided both the numerator and the denominator by 10. *However, be careful because this shortcut only applies to zeros.* You can use it with any number of zeros as long as there are an *equal* number of them on both the top and bottom of a fraction. For example, $\frac{3500}{4600}$ can be chopped off to $\frac{35}{46}$. The answer to reducing both fractions is the same! When reducing a fraction by 10, chop off one zero from both the numerator and the denominator. For example, this reduces $\frac{30}{50}$ to $\frac{3}{5}$. When reducing a fraction by 100, chop off two zeros from both the numerator and the denominator. For example, this reduces $\frac{300}{500}$ to $\frac{3}{5}$. When reducing a fraction by 1000, chop off three zeros from both the numerator and the denominator (for example, $\frac{3000}{5000}$ is reduced to $\frac{3}{5}$).

 Memory Jogger

The value of a proper fraction is always less than 1; for example, $\frac{1}{5}$.

 Memory Jogger

The value of an improper fraction is always greater than 1; for example, $100\overline{)125}$, or 1.25.

 Try This!

TT-1 Change these mixed-number fractions into improper fractions.

a. $1\frac{3}{4}$ c. $4\frac{1}{5}$

b. $2\frac{5}{8}$ d. $6\frac{7}{8}$

Answers are at the end of this chapter.

 Try This!

TT-2 Reduce each of these fractions to their lowest common denominators.

a. $\frac{10}{24}$ c. $\frac{36}{84}$

b. $\frac{50}{100}$ d. $\frac{9}{15}$

Answers are at the end of this chapter.

 Memory Jogger

When dividing a fraction with both the top and bottom numbers ending in zero, you can chop off the same number of zeros from both numbers.

 Try This

TT-3 How many zeros can you chop and drop?

a. $\frac{230}{3500}$ c. $\frac{20}{500}$

b. $\frac{1400}{10}$ d. $\frac{500}{100}$

Answers are at the end of this chapter.

Memory Jogger

When the numerator of a fraction is 1, the bigger the denominator, the smaller the fraction.

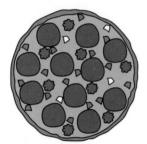

Whole pizza
(1/1)

1/2 pizza
slice

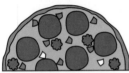

1/4 pizza   1/8 pizza
slice   slice

FIGURE 3-2 Fraction sizes.

Try This!

TT-4 Which fraction represents the largest part of the whole for a and b? What is the lowest common denominator for each set of three fractions?

a. $\dfrac{1}{2}$, $\dfrac{3}{4}$, or $\dfrac{7}{8}$

b. $\dfrac{1}{5}$, $\dfrac{5}{15}$, or $\dfrac{6}{45}$

Which fraction represents the smallest part of the whole for c and d? What is the lowest common denominator for each set of three fractions?

c. $\dfrac{1}{3}$, $\dfrac{1}{5}$, or $\dfrac{1}{6}$

d. $\dfrac{1}{2}$, $\dfrac{3}{8}$, or $\dfrac{3}{4}$

Answers are at the end of this chapter.

Comparing Fractions

There may be times when you must compare several drugs and determine which dose is the strongest (or weakest). What if the dose comes in $\frac{1}{4}$, $\frac{1}{2}$, and $\frac{1}{8}$ strengths? How are you going to decide which is the strongest dose?

If the numerators (top numbers) are all 1, you can just think of slices of a pizza. Would you get a bigger slice if you had $\frac{1}{8}$ or $\frac{1}{4}$ of the pizza? Figure 3-2 shows the comparison of sizes by fractions. Don't be fooled into thinking that the biggest denominator gives the biggest slice. It is actually the other way around! As you can see in Figure 3-2, if the numerators are all the same (in this case they are all equal to 1), the *smallest* denominator gives the biggest slice (or the strongest dose).

But what if the denominators AND the numerators are different? Consider the fractions $\frac{2}{3}$ and $\frac{3}{4}$. How can these fractions be compared? Because they are different, you cannot compare them until you first rewrite the fractions to find the lowest common denominator. As you recall from the section on reducing fractions, this means that, to be able to compare the two strengths, you first have to convert both of them to the same denominator. Once you convert them to the same denominator, you can figure out exactly how they are related by comparing their numerators.

The best way to make them have a common denominator is to determine the *lowest* bottom number that both can be divided into evenly. For 3 and 4, that number is 12. To determine the lowest common denominator, start writing all the multiples of both denominators. Multiples of 3 are 3, 6, 9, 12, 15, 18, and so on because $1 \times 3 = 3$, $2 \times 3 = 6$, $3 \times 3 = 9$, $4 \times 3 = \mathbf{12}$, $5 \times 3 = 15$, and $6 \times 3 = 18$. Multiples of 4 are 4, 8, 12, 16, 20, 24, and so on because $1 \times 4 = 4$, $2 \times 4 = 8$, $3 \times 4 = \mathbf{12}$, $4 \times 4 = 16$, $5 \times 4 = 20$, and $6 \times 4 = 24$. When you compare the multiples of 3 with the multiples of 4, the first number that appears on both lists is **12.** For denominators of 3 and 4, then, the lowest common denominator is 12. This means that you will now use 12 as the *new* denominator for both fractions. Now, take each original denominator (3 and 4) and divide it into 12. Take each answer and multiply it by its numerator. That number becomes the *new* numerator for each fraction. For example, for the first fraction $\frac{2}{3}$, when you divide the new denominator 12 by the old denominator (3), you get 4. Now multiply the old numerator (2) by 4, and you get 8. So when the common denominator is 12, $\frac{2}{3}$ is equal to $\frac{8}{12}$. Those of you who love math may have noticed that the cross products are equal (2×12 is equal to 3×8)! This will tell you that your answer is correct.

Next try the fraction $\frac{3}{4}$. Did you get $\frac{9}{12}$? Now that both the original fractions have the same denominator ($\frac{8}{12}$ and $\frac{9}{12}$), you can easily see which one is the strongest or biggest ($\frac{9}{12}$)! Do you see that $\frac{9}{12}$ (or $\frac{3}{4}$) has more parts of the whole ($\frac{12}{12}$) than $\frac{8}{12}$ (or $\frac{2}{3}$), and so it is the strongest dose?

Adding Fractions

Adding fractions that have the same denominator is as simple as adding whole numbers. The math symbol for addition is a plus sign (+). When adding fractions that have the same denominator, you only add the numerators (top numbers). For example, when adding $\dfrac{2}{4} + \dfrac{1}{4}$, just add the numerators ($2 + 1 = 3$) and place that answer (the sum) on top of the original denominator. (The denominator does not change.) The result is $\dfrac{2}{4} + \dfrac{1}{4} = \dfrac{3}{4}$. You can add any amount of fractions with the same denominators in this way. For example, the answer to the addition problem $\dfrac{2}{6} + \dfrac{2}{6} + \dfrac{4}{6} + \dfrac{5}{6}$ is $\dfrac{13}{6}$. When the sum of fractions is an improper fraction, convert it to a mixed fraction. In this case the answer ($\frac{13}{6}$) can be converted to the mixed-number fraction of $2\frac{1}{6}$.

Adding fractions that have different denominators requires that they all first be converted to the same lowest common denominator, just as is necessary when comparing fractions. Then the numerators can be added in the same way as for fractions that started out with the same denominators. How would you add $\dfrac{1}{2} + \dfrac{4}{5} + \dfrac{3}{4}$? First, calculate the multiples of each denominator. For the denominator of 2 the multiples are 2, 4, 6, 8, 10, 12, 14, 16, 18, **20**, 22, 24, and so on. For the denominator of 5 the multiples are 5, 10, 15, **20**, 25, 30, 35, and so on. The numbers 10 and 20 are common to both 2 and 5. However, the multiples of 4 are 4, 8, 12, 16, **20**, 24, 28, and so on. The number 10 is not a multiple of 4, but **20** is a multiple of all three denominators. So **20** is now our common denominator. To make the fraction $\frac{1}{2}$ have a common denominator of 20, multiply both its numerator (1) and its denominator (2) by 10 to get $\frac{10}{20}$. To make the fraction $\frac{4}{5}$ have a common denominator of 20, multiply both its numerator (4) and its denominator (5) by 4 to get $\frac{16}{20}$. To make the fraction $\frac{3}{4}$ have a common denominator of 20, multiply both its numerator (3) and its denominator (4) by 5 to get $\frac{15}{20}$. Next add $\frac{10}{20}+\frac{16}{20}+\frac{15}{20}$, which equals $\frac{41}{20}$. Then change this improper fraction to the mixed-number fraction of $2\frac{1}{20}$.

Subtracting Fractions

The need to subtract fractions is rare for drug calculations or drug preparation, so this review of subtracting fractions is brief. Not only is subtracting fractions rare in drug calculation, negative numbers are not used. This means that you would not need to subtract the larger numerator from the smaller numerator.

The math symbol for subtraction is a minus sign (–). When subtracting two fractions that have the same denominator (bottom number), subtract the smaller numerator (top number) from the larger one. For example, when subtracting $\frac{2}{4}-\frac{1}{4}$, simply subtract 1 from 2 (2 – 1) and place that answer on the original denominator. The result is $\frac{2}{4}-\frac{1}{4}=\frac{1}{4}$.

Subtracting fractions that have different denominators first requires their conversion to the same lowest common denominator, just as you did when adding fractions with different denominators. After they have been converted to the lowest common denominator, the numerators can be subtracted in the same way as for fractions that began with the same denominators. For example, to subtract $\frac{4}{7}-\frac{2}{5}$, first find the lowest common denominator (as described under "Comparing Fractions" on p. 48), which is 35. Then multiply the numerators by the amount needed to make their denominators become 35. (That would be 5 for the first fraction and 7 for the second fraction.) Multiply the numerator (4) in $\frac{4}{7}$ by 5 and place that number on the new denominator to get $\frac{20}{35}$. Then multiply the numerator (2) in $\frac{2}{5}$ by 7 and place that number on the new denominator to get $\frac{14}{35}$. Subtract $\frac{14}{35}$ from $\frac{20}{35}$ ($\frac{20}{35}-\frac{14}{35}=\frac{6}{35}$).

Multiplying Fractions

Multiplying fractions is fairly straightforward. The math symbol for multiplication is "×." Look at all the fractions in an equation that you need to multiply. For example, multiply $\frac{3}{9}\times1\frac{5}{6}$. First make sure that all the fractions are reduced to their lowest possible terms (but you do not have to find the lowest *common* denominator). So reduce $\frac{3}{9}$ to $\frac{1}{3}$. Then see if there are any mixed-number fractions and change them to improper fractions. For this example, change the mixed-number fraction $1\frac{5}{6}$ into an improper fraction ($6\times1+5=\frac{11}{6}$). Now you have $\frac{1}{3}\times\frac{11}{6}$. To get the answer, simply multiply all the numerators (top numbers) straight across the top (1 × 11 = 11). Doing this makes a *new* numerator. Now do the same thing with the denominators (3 × 6 = 18). Doing this makes a *new* denominator. The new total is now $\frac{11}{18}$. That's it!

Dividing Fractions

Fractions that need to be divided are usually written out with the math symbol for division (÷), (for example, $\frac{5}{8}$ divided by $\frac{2}{3}$, or $\frac{5}{8}\div\frac{2}{3}$). To divide these fractions, flip

 Try This!

TT-5 Add these fractions. If a sum is an improper fraction, convert it to a mixed-number fraction.

a. $\frac{1}{7}+\frac{5}{7}$ c. $\frac{6}{8}+\frac{1}{8}+\frac{3}{8}+\frac{5}{8}$

b. $\frac{1}{5}+\frac{2}{5}+\frac{1}{5}$ d. $\frac{1}{4}+\frac{2}{4}+\frac{3}{4}$

Answers are at the end of this chapter.

 Try This!

TT-6 Add these fractions. If the sum is an improper fraction, convert it to either a whole number or a mixed-number fraction. Reduce the answers to their lowest common denominators.

a. $\frac{4}{7}+\frac{2}{5}$ c. $\frac{1}{2}+\frac{1}{6}+\frac{1}{5}$

b. $\frac{3}{4}+\frac{1}{3}+\frac{5}{6}$ d. $\frac{2}{9}+\frac{1}{3}+\frac{3}{5}$

Answers are at the end of this chapter.

 Try This!

TT-7 Subtract these fractions. If a fraction is a mixed-number fraction, first convert it to an improper fraction. Reduce answers to their lowest common denominators.

a. $\frac{4}{5}-\frac{1}{5}$ c. $\frac{3}{4}-\frac{1}{4}$

b. $1\frac{1}{3}-\frac{2}{3}$ d. $2\frac{1}{2}-1\frac{1}{2}$

Answers are at the end of this chapter.

 Try This!

TT-8 Subtract these fractions. If a fraction is a mixed-number fraction, first convert it to an improper fraction. Reduce answers to their lowest common denominators.

a. $\frac{3}{4}-\frac{2}{3}$ c. $\frac{4}{5}-\frac{1}{3}$

b. $2\frac{2}{3}-1\frac{1}{2}$ d. $2\frac{1}{2}-\frac{3}{4}$

Answers are at the end of this chapter.

 Try This!

TT-9 Multiply these fractions.

a. $1\frac{3}{4}\times5\frac{6}{7}$ c. $\frac{3}{4}\times9\frac{11}{16}$

b. $2\frac{2}{4}\times6\frac{7}{8}$ d. $\frac{1}{2}\times10\frac{1}{3}$

Answers are at the end of this chapter.

(invert) the second fraction so the problem now reads $\frac{5}{8} \times \frac{3}{2}$. Multiply across the numerators and denominators as you did when multiplying two fractions. The answer is $\frac{15}{16}$. If possible, reduce the fraction answer to its lowest terms. In this case, $\frac{15}{16}$ cannot be reduced further.

If your division involves a whole number to be divided by a fraction (for example, $2 \div \frac{3}{4}$), change the whole number 2 into a fraction by putting it over 1. The whole number 2 is the fraction $\frac{2}{1}$. (Remember that all whole numbers can be expressed as fractions by putting the whole number over 1.) Therefore the problem is now $\frac{2}{1} \div \frac{3}{4}$.

After you invert (flip) the second fraction, the problem is $\frac{2}{1} \times \frac{4}{3} = \frac{8}{3}$. Reduce this fraction to $2\frac{2}{3}$. That's it!

Dividing a fraction by a whole number works the same way. For the problem $\frac{1}{3} \div 4$, first convert it to $\frac{1}{3} \div \frac{4}{1}$ and flip (invert) the second fraction, converting the problem to $\frac{1}{3} \times \frac{1}{4}$. The answer is $\frac{1}{12}$!

DECIMALS

A **decimal**, like a fraction, describes parts of a whole. Decimals and fractions are related because decimals can be written as fractions and fractions can be written as decimals. To understand how to change from one to the other, you must first understand that the place value of decimals is based on multiples of 10. We will talk about the relationship between fractions and decimals a little later.

The key to understanding decimals is to understand the way they are written. A **decimal point** is the dividing point between whole numbers and parts of numbers in a system based on units of 10 (Table 3-1). It is located between the whole number and the part of the whole number.

Any number to the *left* of a decimal point is a *whole* number. So the whole number 125 is written from left to right as 1 one hundred, 2 tens, and 5 ones (or right to left as 5 ones, 2 tens, and 1 one hundred). By now you do this instinctively because you started doing it in first grade!

Any number to the *right* of the decimal point is a *part* of the whole number. So the decimal 0.25 is 25 parts of 100 because the place value of the 5 is hundredths, and 0.025 is 25 parts of a thousand because the third place after the decimal point (in this case the 5) has a place value of thousandths. The place to the right or left of the decimal determines the value of a number.

When working with drug dosages, *always* put a zero *before* the decimal point of any number less than 1 to indicate that there are no whole parts (for example, write .5 mg as 0.5 mg). When you are tired, reading a fax order, or reading an order written on no-carbon-required (NCR) paper, the numbers may not be clear; a decimal point could easily be missed, leading to a serious drug dosage error.

Never put any extra zeros, known as *trailing zeros*, at the end of a decimal when writing a drug dose. Trailing zeros are useless and can be confusing. For example, although 0.25 is equal to 0.250, 0.250 could be easily misread as 250 instead of 25 parts when measuring drugs. Always chop off those trailing zeros to the right of the decimal point (but only the *end* zeros).

Adding and Subtracting Decimals
Adding and subtracting decimals is exactly the same as adding and subtracting whole numbers. The key to ensuring that you obtain the correct answer when adding or subtracting decimals is to keep the decimal points in all the numbers that you are adding in the same position. For example, when adding 7.25, 9.3, and 11.71, position the decimal points as shown in the following problem.

 Try This!

TT-10 Divide these fractions.

a. $3 \div \frac{1}{2}$　　c. $5\frac{1}{4} \div \frac{6}{8}$

b. $\frac{3}{4} \div \frac{1}{2}$　　d. $10 \div \frac{2}{3}$

Answers are at the end of this chapter.

 Memory Jogger

Decimal places are always written in (and represent) multiples of 10.

 Did You Know?

The beginning of the word decimal is Latin for ten *(dec-)*.

 Clinical Pitfall

The places to the right or left of the decimal point determine the value of a number. So always put a zero before the decimal point of any proper fraction written as a decimal. If you don't, 0.25 g of a drug written as .25 could be misread as 25 g of a drug: a BIG overdose. For example, an adult morphine dose of 5 mg is normal, but a pediatric morphine dose might be .5 mg and should be written as 0.5 mg. If this dose is read as 5 mg, it is 10 times the normal dose, which could be lethal.

QSEN: Safety

Table 3-1   **Decimal Table and Conversions**

WORD DESCRIPTION	NUMBER	FRACTION
Hundred thousands	100,000	$\frac{100,000}{1}$
Ten thousands	10,000	$\frac{10,000}{1}$
Thousands	1,000	$\frac{1,000}{1}$
Hundreds	100	$\frac{100}{1}$
Tens	10	$\frac{10}{1}$
Ones/units	1	$\frac{1}{1}$
Decimal point	.	
Tenths	0.1	$\frac{1}{10}$
Hundredths	0.01	$\frac{1}{100}$
Thousandths	0.001	$\frac{1}{1,000}$
Ten thousandths	0.0001	$\frac{1}{10,000}$
Hundred thousandths	0.00001	$\frac{1}{100,000}$
Millionths	0.000001	$\frac{1}{1,000,000}$

$$7.25$$
$$+9.3$$
$$+11.71$$
$$\overline{28.26}$$

Follow the same procedure when subtracting decimals (for example, 42.22 from 98.61).

$$98.61$$
$$-42.22$$
$$\overline{56.39}$$

Multiplying Decimals
Multiplying decimals is almost as easy as multiplying whole numbers. The only difference is that your answer has to contain the right number of decimal places for it to make sense. The key is to count the total number of decimal places (the number of digits after the decimal point) in the whole problem and then make sure that the same amount of decimal places are in the answer. So you do not need to keep track of the decimals until you have an answer!

To multiply 2.4 × 4, treat the numbers as 24 × 4 and multiply, which equals 96. Now add the number of decimal places in both numbers. There is only one decimal place for this problem (it is in 2.4). Starting from the far right of 96, count one space to the left and place the decimal point; 9.6 is the correct answer. Try multiplying a

 Try This!

TT-11 Decimals as parts of a whole:
a. 0.3 = How many parts of a whole?
b. 0.75 = How many parts of a whole?
c. 5.1 = How many whole numbers, and how many parts of a whole?
d. 2.2 = How many whole numbers, and how many parts of a whole?
Answers are at the end of this chapter.

Try This!

TT-12 Multiply these decimals.
a. 100 × 0.25
b. 51.2 × 2.1
c. 15.5 × 10
d. 40.5 × 2.4
   Answers are at the end of this chapter.

decimal by another decimal. For example, when multiplying 2.4 × 3.6, treat it as 24 × 36; 964 is the correct answer. Add the number of decimal places in both numbers that were multiplied. There is one decimal place in 2.4 and one decimal place in 3.6, for a total of two decimal places. Starting from the far right of 964, count two spaces to the left and place the decimal point; 9.64 is the correct answer. Now multiply 4.3 × .21 by treating it as 43 × 21, with 903 being the answer. There are three decimal places in the number being multiplied (one in 4.3 and two in .21). So starting from the far right of 903, count spaces to the left, and place the decimal point for 0.903 as the correct answer. Remember, just as when you multiply whole numbers, it is important to line up your numbers properly when you are doing the problem without a calculator.

Dividing Decimals

Let's start by dividing a decimal by a whole number: $\frac{36.48}{2}$, or, to put it another way, $2\overline{)36.48}$ or 36.48 ÷ 2. The number being divided (or divided into) is 36.48 and is known as the **dividend**. The number doing the dividing (in this case 2) is the **divisor**. The answer to a division problem is the **quotient**.

The problem works like any other division problem except that *you must be sure that the decimal point in the answer is placed exactly above the one in the dividend.* So first put the decimal point for the answer *exactly above* the one in the dividend (36.48):

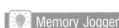

Memory Jogger

Divisor × Quotient (answer)
= Dividend
(if you divided correctly).

$2\overline{)36.48}$ Then complete the division: $2\overline{)36.48}^{18.24}$ Does this make sense?

To check division, multiply the divisor (2) and the quotient (18.24). Your answer should equal the dividend (36.48). If you don't get the dividend, your division was wrong, and you must redo it.

Dividing a decimal by a decimal is a little harder, but the principle is the same. Keep in mind that you always have to *divide by a whole number.* If your divisor is a decimal, you have to move the decimal point all the way to the right to make it a whole number. Whatever you do to the divisor, you also must do to the dividend. So move the decimal point in the dividend the *same number* of decimal spaces. For example, in the problem $\frac{32.4}{1.6}$ or $1.6\overline{)32.4}$, moving the decimal point in the divisor all the way to the right involves moving it one place: changing 1.6 to the whole number 16. Now move the decimal point in the dividend (32.4) one place to the right (an equal number of places) so 32.4 becomes 324, giving you $16\overline{)324}$. Divide as usual, and you should get $16\overline{)324.00}^{20.25}$. Check your answer in the same way as mentioned previously: multiply the divisor (16) and the answer (quotient, 20.25). The result should equal the dividend (324).

Dividing a whole number by a decimal also requires moving the decimal points to make things even. In a whole number, the decimal point is located at the *end* of the number. For example, the whole number 4 actually equals 4. Using $\frac{4}{2.5}$, which is the same as $2.5\overline{)4}$ or 4 ÷ 2.5, move the decimal point one place to the right in the divisor. *Add* a decimal place *after* 4 and move it one place to the right, making it 40. The resulting problem is $25\overline{)40.0}$. Now work the problem the way you would any division problem. Did you get $25\overline{)40.0}^{1.6}$? To divide a whole number by a decimal, add as many extra zeros to the whole number after the decimal as you need until the division ends or repeats. For drug calculations, you will not need to work a decimal problem through more than the thousandth (third) place.

Memory Jogger

Add as many extra zeros (decimal places) to the right of the dividend (whole number) as you need to make the answer accurate.

Try This!

TT-13 Divide these decimals.
a. 630 ÷ 0.3
b. 0.125 ÷ 0.5
c. 2.5 ÷ 0.75
d. 10 ÷ 0.25
   Answers are at the end of this chapter.

Changing Fractions into Decimals

Decimals and fractions are related because they are both parts of a whole. For example, decimals change the fraction $\frac{25}{100}$ into 0.25 (see Table 3-1). Because both decimals and fractions are a part of the whole, you can change fractions into decimals and decimals into fractions. You do this every time you turn $\frac{25}{100}$ into 0.25. To do this, just divide the numerator (in this case 25) by the denominator (in this case 100). This step is written as $100\overline{)25}$ or $25 \div 100$. To divide, place a decimal point after the 25 and add zeros until the division ends. The answer is .25, but when writing drug dosages, remember to write it as 0.25 to avoid any confusion.

Changing Decimals into Fractions

To change a decimal to a fraction, drop the decimal point and make this number the numerator (top number) of the fraction. The denominator (bottom number) of the fraction is the place value of the last digit (number) of the decimal. Determine the place value of the last number (digit) after the decimal point. For example, the decimal 0.25 is 25 parts of 100 because the place value of the 5 is hundredths. Then reduce the fraction to its lowest terms. For example, to change 0.25 to a fraction, drop the decimal point and make 25 the numerator. The denominator becomes 100 because the place value of the 5 in 0.25 is hundredths and 0.25 is 25 out of 100 (see Table 3-1). Therefore the fraction is written as $\frac{25}{100}$ and is reduced to $\frac{1}{4}$. Another example is the conversion of the decimal 5.017 into a fraction. It becomes $5\frac{17}{1000}$ because the place value of the 7 in .017 is thousandths.

ROUNDING PARTS OF NUMBERS

When giving drugs, it may be necessary to decide how many milliliters to give if your calculated dose is uneven. For example, if you get an answer such as 2.17 mL, you must decide whether to give 2 mL or more than 2 mL because the .17 is part of the next whole number. How do you decide which number to give? Usually liquid dosages are rounded to the tenth place rather than to a whole number.

The key concept in rounding decimals is to remember the number **5**! Any answer that ends in a number *below* .05 is *rounded down* to the next lower tenth. Any answer that ends in the number .05 or higher is *rounded up* to the next higher tenth. So if your answer is 2.82 mL, you give 2.8 mL *(rounded down)*. If your answer is 2.17 mL, you give 2.2 mL *(rounded up)*. In clinical practice with drugs that come in tablet form, there is an exception. Some tablets can be cut in half.

PERCENTS

You are probably familiar with percents from using them to decide how much money to tip a waiter in your favorite restaurant (10%, 15%, or 20%). **Percent** expresses a number as part of a hundred. The word *percent* literally means "for each hundred." In health care, percents are used to calculate drug doses and the strength of solutions (for example, the percent [%] of salt in a salt-and-water solution).

Percents express the same idea as a fraction or decimal. They can be written as a whole number (20%), a mixed-number fraction ($12\frac{1}{2}$%), a decimal (0.9%), or a proper fraction ($\frac{1}{2}$%).

Converting a Percent to a Decimal

Let's say we have a 9% salt solution. To change 9% to a decimal, drop the percent sign and multiply the number in the percent by 0.01. The 9% can then be written as 0.09, or 9 parts salt per 100 parts of water. A 0.9% salt solution (commonly called "normal saline" in the health care setting) when multiplied by 0.01 results in 0.009 or 0.9 parts of salt per 100 parts of water (also 9 parts of salt per 1000 parts of water). You can also change the 9% to a decimal just by moving the decimal point that is behind the 9 two places to the *left*. Thus 9% = 0.09 (see Table 3-1).

To change a decimal to a percent, reverse the process by moving the decimal point two places to the *right* (for example, 0.09 = 9%).

Be careful to move the decimal point in the correct direction. Moving it in the wrong direction can result in a serious error. Work it out or *call the pharmacist if you are not sure*.

 Memory Jogger

To turn a fraction into a decimal, always divide the numerator (top number) by the bottom number (denominator).

 Try This!

TT-14 Change the following fractions to decimals and the decimals to fractions.

a. $\frac{3}{4}$
b. 0.55
c. 0.075
d. 1.25
e. $\frac{7}{8}$

Answers are at the end of this chapter.

 Clinical Pitfall

The exception to the rounding principle is when you get an answer of exactly half (0.5 or $\frac{1}{2}$) of a tablet. If the tablet can be cut, give $\frac{1}{2}$ tablet (see guidelines under Dosage and Calculation problems).

QSEN: Safety

 Try This!

TT-15 Work to three places and then round to two places.

a. $\frac{58.4}{33}$
b. $\frac{6}{3.4}$
c. $\frac{27.5}{3.4}$
d. $\frac{25.4}{5}$

Answers are at the end of this chapter.

 Did You Know?

Percent comes from Latin and means "for each hundred."

 Clinical Pitfall

Moving the decimal point in the wrong direction is hazardous to your patient. If it is moved in error to the right, the dose will be too large and may cause serious or even lethal side effects. If it is moved in error to the left, the dose will be too small to be effective.

QSEN: Safety

Converting a Percent to a Fraction

The process of converting a percent to a fraction is the same whether you have a whole number, a mixed number, or a fraction of a percent.

To convert a whole number percent to a fraction, drop the percent sign and divide the percent whole number by 100. For example, to convert 20% to a fraction, drop the percent sign and divide 20 by 100 ($\frac{20}{100}$). Reduce this number to its lowest common denominator, $\frac{1}{5}$. So 20% of a pizza is the same as $\frac{1}{5}$ of a pizza (remember that 5% of a pizza is the same as $\frac{1}{20}$ of a pizza).

To convert a mixed number to a fraction, first drop the percent sign and change the mixed number to an improper fraction. Then divide that fraction by 100. So to convert $12\frac{1}{2}$% to a fraction, convert it to an improper fraction ($\frac{25}{2}$) and divide that

fraction by 100: $\frac{25}{2} \div \frac{100}{1} = \frac{25}{2} \times \frac{1}{100} = \frac{25}{200}$, which can then be reduced to $\frac{1}{8}$. So

12.5% or $12\frac{1}{2}$% of a pizza is $\frac{1}{8}$ of a pizza!

You can use the same process to make a fraction of a percent. For example, to express $\frac{1}{4}$% as a fraction, divide it by 100 (which means multiplying it by $\frac{1}{100}$).

$\frac{1}{4} \times \frac{1}{100} = \frac{1}{400}$, a mere crumb of a pizza!

Finding the Percentage of a Number

Let's begin with what you already know: 50% of a number is $\frac{1}{2}$ of that number, right? In other words, 50% of 84 is 42. How did you get that answer? You either multiplied 84 by 0.50 or you divided 84 by 2.

What is 30% of 150? This "word" problem is the same as the one you just did in your head. You already know that 30% is equal to 0.3. So to find 30% of 150, just multiply 150 × 0.3. The answer is 45! Remember to count the total number of decimal places and put the decimal in the correct place in your answer.

SOLVING DOSAGE AND CALCULATION PROBLEMS

INTRODUCTION

In some health care settings, most drugs come from the pharmacy in the correct dose, ready to give to the patients. However, remember that you are the *last check* in the system and are responsible for making sure that the patient not only gets the right drug but also gets the right dose. Always read each drug order carefully, watching for decimal points and zeros.

Sometimes a drug dose that you have on hand does not equal what you *want* to administer to the patient. You will need to calculate the correct drug dose from what you *have* on hand. The first thing you must do is write down all the information that you have and then *label* each number (that is, categorize each number as either *have* or *want*). For example, if you *have* Catapres (clonidine) 0.1 mg and you *want* to give 0.2 mg, first label all the information. Then you may proceed to plug the numbers into the following formulas and do the math. *Finally, do the DIMS (does it make sense?) test to see if the answer makes sense!* You can use these formulas only when the drug dose that you have on hand is in the same measurement unit (for example, milligrams and milligrams) as the drug dose that you want to give.

Oral Drugs

Formula 1. This formula works for drug calculations involving dry pills (tablets, capsules, caplets). If the drug order is for 440 mg of naproxen and you have tablets that each contain 220 mg of naproxen, how many tablets should you give? Here is the easy way to know: divide the number you *want* by the number you *have*.

$$\frac{Want}{Have} = \text{Number of tablets to give!}$$

So, $\frac{440 \text{ mg}}{220 \text{ mg}} = (\text{chop off the end zeros}) \frac{44}{22} = 2 \text{ tablets!}$

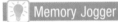 **Try This!**

TT-16 Convert the following percents into fractions.

a. $\frac{1}{2}$%   c. $5\frac{3}{4}$%

b. 3%   d. 2.5%

Answers are at the end of this chapter.

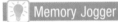 **Try This!**

TT-17 Find the percentages of the whole numbers.
a. 25% of 300
b. 10% of $5.00
c. 0.2% of 10
d. 300% of 5

Answers are at the end of this chapter.

! Drug Alert!

Administration Alert

Whenever you read a drug order, check and double check carefully for decimal points and zeros.

QSEN: Safety

Memory Jogger

You can use the calculation formulas only when the drug dose that you have on hand is in the same measurement unit as the drug dose you want to give.

What happens if the dose of diazepam (Valium) you *want* is 15 mg and you *have* Valium 10-mg tablets? Use the formula:

$$\frac{15 \text{ mg}}{10 \text{ mg}} = 1\frac{1}{2} \text{ tablets}$$

You can cut a tablet in half and give a half tablet only if the tablet is scored. A **scored tablet** is one that has a line etched into it marking the exact center (Figure 3-3). Cutting (or breaking) a tablet along this line gives you two halves of equal known dosages. If you cut or break a tablet that is not scored, the dose will not be correct, and you will have uneven halves. If tablets are not scored, call the pharmacy to see if the drug comes either in a smaller strength or as a liquid.

Other types of drugs that should not be cut or broken include capsules, long-acting or sustained-release capsules or tablets, and enteric-coated tablets. Cutting a capsule allows the powder or tiny beads inside to spill. Long-acting or sustained-release drugs are made so that small amounts of drug are released continuously throughout the day. Cutting this type of drug allows all of the drug to enter the patient's system rapidly and may cause an overdose. Enteric-coated drugs are meant to dissolve and be absorbed in the intestine rather than in the stomach. Cutting or crushing these drugs not only may cause stomach irritation, but the acid in the stomach may inactivate the drugs so they won't work. Always look up any new drug or one you are not familiar with to see if there is any reason that it should not be cut.

Formula 2. This formula works for drug calculations involving oral liquids. These drugs may be called a *suspension* or an *elixir* (an old word for an alcohol-based liquid).

$$\frac{Want}{Have} \times \text{Liquid} = \text{Amount of liquid to give}$$

If an order reads, "Give Benadryl (diphenhydramine) 50 mg," and the diphenhydramine liquid comes in 25 mg/5 mL, 5 mL is the amount of liquid in one dose that you have on hand. In this example:

$$\frac{50 \text{ mg}}{25 \text{ mg}} \times 5 \text{ mL} = 2 \times 5 \text{ mL} = \text{Give 10 mL}$$

Be sure to label both the numerator and the denominator of the formula to double check that the two dosage measurements you are working with are the same.

Drugs Given by Injection

There are three major types of injectable drugs: *intramuscular (IM),* which is injected into a muscle; *subcutaneous,* which is injected into the fat below the skin; and *intradermal (ID),* which is injected just under the top part of the skin. All three types are *parenteral* forms of drug delivery that do not go through the gastrointestinal tract (see Chapters 1 and 2 for more information about parenteral drug delivery). These drugs may come in either single-dose containers (syringes, vials, or ampules) or multiple-dose bottles (vials).

All injectable drugs are liquids, so they follow the same formula as formula 2 for liquid drugs. For example, the unit-dose syringe that you *have* contains meperidine (Demerol) 100 mg/mL, and you are ordered *(want)* to give 50 mg IM. How should you set up the problem? You would set it up the same way as for other liquid drugs.

$$\frac{Want}{Have} \times \text{Liquid} = \text{Amount to pull up into a syringe}$$

$$\frac{50 \text{ mg}}{100 \text{ mg}} \times 1 \text{ mL} = \frac{1}{2} = 0.5 \text{ mL IM}$$

A

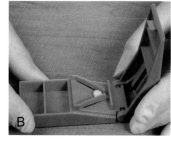
B

FIGURE 3-3 A, A scored tablet. **B,** A cutter for scored tablets.

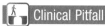 **Clinical Pitfall**

Do not attempt to cut drugs that come in these forms:
- Tablet that is not scored
- Capsule
- Gelcap
- Enteric-coated (EC) tablet
- Long-acting (LA) or sustained-release (SR) tablet

QSEN: Safety

 Try This!

TT-18 How many tablets should you give?
a. *Want* digoxin (Lanoxin) 0.25 mg; *Have* digoxin 0.125 mg
b. *Want* alendronate sodium (Fosamax) 5 mg; *Have* alendronate 10 mg
c. *Want* alprazolam (Xanax) 1.5 mg; *Have* alprazolam 0.5 mg
d. *Want* diphenhydramine (Benadryl) 75 mg; *Have* diphenhydramine 25 mg
   Answers are at the end of this chapter.

 Try This!

TT-19 How many milliliters should you give?
a. *Want* dextromethorphan (Robitussin) 7 mg; *Have* dextromethorphan 3.5 mg/5 mL
b. *Want* acetaminophen (Tylenol) 240 mg; *Have* acetaminophen 80 mg/2.5 mL
c. *Want* ibuprofen (Advil) 100 mg; *Have* ibuprofen 50 mg/1.25 mL
d. *Want* doxylamine (Aldex) 25 mg; *Have* doxylamine 6.25 mg/mL
   Answers are at the end of this chapter.

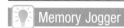 **Memory Jogger**

When dividing a fraction with both the top number (numerator) and the bottom number (denominator) ending in zero, the same number of zeros can be chopped off of both numbers.

Try This!

TT-20 How many milliliters should you give by injection?
a. *Want* hydromorphone (Dilaudid) 1 mg; *Have* a unit-dose syringe with 4 mg/mL
b. *Want* heparin 5000 units; *Have* a unit-dose syringe with 10,000 units/mL
c. *Want* trimethobenzamide 200 mg; *Have* a 20-mL vial with 100 mg/mL
d. *Want* morphine 15 mg; *Have* 50-mL vial with 10 mg/mL
Answers are at the end of this chapter.

 Try This!

TT-21 Express the following problems as a fractional proportion.
a. If 3 boats have 6 sails, then 9 boats have 18 sails.
b. If 1 case of IV fluids holds 12 bags, then 3 cases hold 36 bags.
c. If 5 mL have 325 mg of acetaminophen, then 2 mL have 130 mg.
d. If 1 mL has 2 mg of hydromorphone (Dilaudid), then 5 mL have 10 mg of hydromorphone.
Answers are at the end of this chapter.

 Memory Jogger

Remember to label your problem correctly or you might not know what the answer you get actually means!

 Try This!

TT-22 How many milliliters should you give?
a. *Want* dextromethorphan (Robitussin) 7 mg; *Have* dextromethorphan 3.5 mg/5 mL
b. *Want* ibuprofen (Advil) 100 mg; *Have* ibuprofen 50 mg/1.25 mL
c. *Want* digoxin (Lanoxin) 0.03 mg; *Have* digoxin 0.05 mg/1 mL
d. *Want* hydromorphone (Dilaudid) 1 mg; *Have* hydromorphone 2 mg/1 mL
Answers are at the end of this chapter.

USING PROPORTIONS TO SOLVE FOR *X*

A fraction uses a division line (called a *bar*) or slash to describe a mathematic relationship between two numbers (for example, $\frac{1}{2}$ or ½). A **proportion** describes an *equal* mathematical relationship between two *sets* of numbers (for example, $\frac{1}{2} = \frac{2}{4}$). If you look closely, you will see that, when you multiply *diagonally* across the equal sign, 1 × 4 *equals* 2 × 2! Another way of thinking of the proportion is that 1 is related to 2 in the same way as 2 is related to 4.

You can use proportions to solve for *X*, the unknown, as an alternate approach to drug calculations, especially if you don't want to memorize a formula. When you write a proportion as a set of fractions, be careful to label each piece of the equation. For example:

$$\frac{1 \text{ case}}{12 \text{ bottles}} = \frac{3 \text{ cases}}{36 \text{ bottles}}$$

Notice that in the fractions, *both* numerators identify the number of "cases," and *both* denominators identify the number of bottles. All fractional proportions must be set up this way for you to obtain the correct answer.

What if a piece of the proportion is missing? This is what happens when the prescriber orders a drug strength that is different from the one you have on hand. To figure out how many of the drug tablets you have on hand will be equal to the strength that is ordered, set up a proportion to solve for the missing piece.

For example, an order reads, "Give 500 mg of Primidone by mouth (orally)," and you have on hand primidone 250 mg per one caplet. How many caplets will you have to give the patient to equal 500 mg? Set the problem up as:

$$\frac{250 \text{ mg}}{1 \text{ caplet}} = \frac{500 \text{ mg}}{X \text{ caplets}}$$

The *X* is what you need to give. By figuring out the "*X*" correctly, both sides of the proportion will be equal. You can cross out ("cancel") the word "mg" in the proportion equation because they are both known numbers. That leaves you with the word "caplets" as the missing part of the proportion. Therefore your answer must be the number of *caplets* needed.

Maybe you can do this in your head, but you need to understand how you get the 2 caplets. First, cross multiply to set up the equation 250 *X* = 500. An easy way to work the problem is to remember that any time you bring the number in front of the *X* (250 in this case) across the equals sign (or bring the 250 to the other side of the equals sign), it means *divide*.

$$\text{So, } X = \frac{500}{250} = 2 \text{ caplets}$$

Solving liquid drug problems by proportion involves two steps, but they are relatively easy. First label what you *have* and what you *want*, as usual. Then, set up the proportion. For example, you *want* to give diphenhydramine (Benadryl) 100 mg, and you *have* diphenhydramine 50 mg per mL. How would the proportion be set up?

Step 1:

$$\frac{50 \text{ mg}}{1 \text{ mL}} = \frac{100 \text{ mg}}{X \text{ mL}} \text{ (cancel the mg)}$$

$$50 X = 100 \text{ or } \frac{100}{50} \text{ (chop the zeros); } 5 X = 10 \text{ or } \frac{10}{5}; 10 \div 5 = 2$$

Step 2: Take the answer from step 1 and multiply that times the liquid dose that you have:

$$(\text{Liquid} = 1 \text{ mL}): 2 \times 1 \text{ mL} = 2 \text{ mL}$$

Get Ready for Practice!

Key Points

- The top number of a fraction is the numerator.
- The bottom number of a fraction is the denominator.
- If the numerator of a fraction is 1, then the larger the denominator, the smaller a part of the whole it is.
- A whole number is turned into a fraction by making the whole number the numerator and making "1" the denominator.
- Reducing fractions to their lowest terms (1 is the only number that can be evenly divided into the numerator and the denominator) helps simplify working with fractions.
- Adding fractions that have the same denominator involves only adding the numerators; the denominator remains the same.
- Adding fractions that have different denominators requires calculating the lowest common denominator, changing the numerators to proportionately match their new denominators, and adding the numerators.
- Subtracting fractions that have the same denominator involves only subtracting the smaller numerator from the larger numerator; the denominator remains the same.
- Subtracting fractions that have different denominators requires calculating the lowest common denominator, changing the numerators to proportionately match their new denominators, and subtracting the smaller numerator from the larger numerator.
- Multiplying fractions involves multiplying the numerators with one another and then multiplying the denominators with one another.
- When dividing fractions, the second fraction is inverted and multiplied by the first fraction.
- When dividing a fraction with both the top number and the bottom number ending in one or more zeros, the same number of zeros can be "chopped off" *both* numbers.
- Decimal places are always written in multiples of 10.
- The places to the right or left of the decimal determine the value of a number.
- Place a zero before the decimal point of any proper fraction written as a decimal.
- Never put a meaningless zero at the end of a decimal.
- To change a fraction into a decimal, always divide the bottom number into the top number.
- To check division of a decimal, multiply the divisor by your answer. If the division was performed correctly, you will get the dividend.
- Moving the decimal point in error to the right will make a drug dose too high and may cause serious or even lethal side effects.
- Moving a decimal point in error to the left will make a drug dose too small to be effective.
- If your drug calculation for tablets results in a decimal number less than 0.5, round down to the next lowest whole number. If the calculation results in a decimal number greater than 0.5, round up to the next highest whole number.
- Do not attempt to cut a tablet that is not scored, a capsule, a gelcap, a drug that is enteric coated, or one that is long acting.
- Urge a patient to drink a full glass of water whenever he or she takes a tablet or capsule unless fluids must be restricted because of another medical problem.
- When reading a drug order, check and double check carefully for decimal points and zeros.
- Remember to label proportion problems so that you know the correct units for your final answer.

Additional Learning Resources

evolve Be sure to visit your Evolve website (http://evolve.elsevier.com/Workman/pharmacology/) for additional online resources.

[SG] Go to your Study Guide for additional learning activities to help you master this chapter content.

Review Questions

See the Answer Keys—In-text Review Questions for answers to these questions.

1. In the formula $X = \dfrac{100}{25}$, which element of the formula represents the denominator?
   - **A.** X
   - **B.** =
   - **C.** The top number
   - **D.** The bottom number

2. Why is $\frac{165}{33}$ an "improper" fraction?
   - **A.** The answer is an odd number.
   - **B.** Neither number can be divided evenly by 2.
   - **C.** The numerator is greater than the denominator.
   - **D.** The denominator is greater than the numerator.

3. Which fraction represents the whole number 16?
   - **A.** $\dfrac{16}{1}$
   - **B.** $\dfrac{16}{16}$
   - **C.** $\dfrac{1}{16}$
   - **D.** $\dfrac{16}{2}$

4. What fraction accurately represents $4\frac{1}{2}$?
   - **A.** $\dfrac{9}{2}$
   - **B.** $\dfrac{5}{16}$
   - **C.** $\dfrac{16}{5}$
   - **D.** $\dfrac{8}{1}$

5. Which fraction is reduced to its lowest terms?

   A. $\dfrac{5}{25}$

   B. $\dfrac{17}{29}$

   C. $\dfrac{2}{8}$

   D. $\dfrac{12}{16}$

6. What is the lowest common denominator for this series of fractions: $\frac{3}{4}, \frac{1}{4}, \frac{3}{5}$?

   A. 12
   B. 15
   C. 20
   D. 30

7. What is the sum of the fractions $\frac{3}{4}, \frac{1}{4}$, and $\frac{3}{5}$?

   A. $\dfrac{32}{20}$ or $1\dfrac{3}{5}$

   B. $\dfrac{35}{20}$ or $1\dfrac{3}{4}$

   C. $\dfrac{64}{40}$ or $1\dfrac{3}{5}$

   D. $\dfrac{70}{40}$ or $1\dfrac{3}{4}$

8. What is the quotient of $\dfrac{1}{3} \div \dfrac{1}{2}$?

   A. $\dfrac{1}{6}$

   B. $\dfrac{1}{3}$

   C. $\dfrac{2}{3}$

   D. $\dfrac{6}{1}$

9. In the equation $75.5 \div 125.5 = 0.6016$, which element is the divisor?

   A. 0.6016
   B. 75.5
   C. 125.5
   D. $\div$

10. What is the quotient of $26.4 \div 16.22$ rounded to the tenth place?

    A. 0.163
    B. 1.628
    C. 16.280
    D. 162.800

11. Which number expresses the fraction $\frac{5}{8}$ as a decimal?

    A. 0.625
    B. 40.05
    C. 1.6
    D. 0.2

12. How much is 18% of 52?

    A. 2.889
    B. 9.36
    C. 288.89
    D. 936

13. The drug and dose prescribed are prednisone 20 mg. The dose of the drug on hand is prednisone 3-mg tablets. What is the relationship between the dose prescribed and the dose on hand?

    A. There is no relationship.
    B. Dose on hand is greater than dose prescribed.
    C. Dose prescribed is greater than dose on hand.
    D. Dose on hand is proportional to dose prescribed.

14. A patient is ordered 1000 mg of penicillin orally. Available are 250-mg tablets. How many tablets should you give to the patient?

    A. $\dfrac{1}{4}$ of a tablet

    B. $\dfrac{1}{2}$ of a tablet

    C. 2 tablets
    D. 4 tablets

15. Which response expresses the relationship "50 mL of morphine contains 500 mg of morphine" as a proportion?

    A. 1 mL of morphine contains 5 mg of morphine.
    B. 5 mL of morphine contains 100 mg of morphine.
    C. 10 mL of morphine contains 50 mg of morphine.
    D. 15 mL of morphine contains 150 mg of morphine.

16. You are ordered to give a patient with an allergic reaction 60 mg of diphenhydramine (Benadryl) by IM injection. The vial contains 10 mL of diphenhydramine solution with a concentration of 25 mg/mL. Exactly how many milliliters of diphenhydramine should you give to this patient? _____ mL

Answers to *Math Check* Problems

MC-1 Change these mixed-number fractions into improper fractions.

a. $3\dfrac{5}{8} = \dfrac{29}{8}$

b. $7\dfrac{1}{3} = \dfrac{22}{3}$

MC-2 Reduce each of these fractions to their lowest common denominators.

a. $\dfrac{25}{75} = \dfrac{1}{3}$

b. $\dfrac{115}{130} = \dfrac{23}{26}$

MC-3 How many zeros can you chop and drop?

a. $\dfrac{180}{2200}$ Chop off one zero from the top and bottom to

make $\{\dfrac{18}{220}\}$ (reduced to $\{\dfrac{9}{110}\}$).

b. $\dfrac{50,000}{100,000}$ Chop off four zeros from the top and bottom to

make $\dfrac{5}{10}$ (reduced to $\dfrac{1}{2}$).

MC-4 Which fraction represents the largest part of the whole for a and b? What is the lowest common denominator for each set of three fractions?

a. $\dfrac{1}{3}, \dfrac{10}{15},$ or $\dfrac{12}{24}$?

$\dfrac{10}{15}$ is the largest part of the whole ($\dfrac{2}{3}$).

The lowest common denominator is 3.

b. $\dfrac{2}{4}, \dfrac{6}{8},$ or $\dfrac{3}{24}$?

$\dfrac{6}{8}$ is the largest part of the whole. The lowest common

denominator for these fractions is 8.
Which fraction represents the smallest part of the whole for c and d? What is the lowest common denominator for each set of three fractions?

c. $\dfrac{6}{8}, \dfrac{6}{12},$ or $\dfrac{2}{3}$?

$\dfrac{6}{12}$ is the smallest part of the whole. The lowest common

denominator is 24.

d. $\dfrac{8}{9}, \dfrac{1}{3},$ or $\dfrac{3}{27}$?

$\dfrac{3}{27}$ is the smallest part of the whole. The lowest common

denominator for these fractions is 3.

MC-5 Add these fractions. If a sum is an improper fraction, convert it to either a whole number or to a mixed-number fraction.

a. $\dfrac{1}{3} + \dfrac{2}{3} + \dfrac{3}{3} = \dfrac{6}{3} = 2$

b. $\dfrac{9}{9} + \dfrac{5}{9} + \dfrac{7}{9} + \dfrac{4}{9} = \dfrac{25}{9} = 2\dfrac{7}{9}$

MC-6 Add these fractions. If the sum is an improper fraction, convert it to either a whole number or a mixed-number fraction. Reduce the answers to their lowest common denominators.

a. $\dfrac{2}{3} + \dfrac{6}{12} + \dfrac{6}{8} = \dfrac{46}{24}$; reduced to $1\dfrac{22}{24}$; further reduced to $1\dfrac{11}{12}$

b. $\dfrac{1}{9} + \dfrac{3}{4} + \dfrac{2}{3} = \dfrac{4}{36} + \dfrac{27}{36} + \dfrac{24}{36} = \dfrac{55}{36}$; reduce to $1\dfrac{19}{36}$

MC-7 Subtract these fractions. If a fraction is a mixed-number fraction, first convert it to an improper fraction. Reduce answers to their lowest common denominators.

a. $\dfrac{5}{6} - \dfrac{2}{6} = \dfrac{3}{6}$; reduce to $\dfrac{1}{2}$

b. $2\dfrac{5}{6} - 1\dfrac{3}{6} = \dfrac{17}{6} - \dfrac{9}{6} = \dfrac{8}{6} = 1\dfrac{2}{6} = 1\dfrac{1}{3}$

MC-8 Subtract these fractions. If a fraction is a mixed-number fraction, first convert it to an improper fraction. Reduce answers to their lowest common denominators.

a. $\dfrac{7}{8} - \dfrac{2}{3} = \dfrac{21}{24} - \dfrac{16}{24} = \dfrac{5}{24}$

b. $6\dfrac{1}{3} - 2\dfrac{1}{2} = \dfrac{19}{3} - \dfrac{5}{2} = \dfrac{38}{6} - \dfrac{15}{6} = \dfrac{23}{6} = 3\dfrac{5}{6}$

MC-9 Multiply these fractions.

a. $1\dfrac{22}{24} \times \dfrac{1}{2} = \dfrac{47}{24} \times \dfrac{1}{2} = \dfrac{47}{48}$

b. $4\dfrac{5}{8} \times \dfrac{2}{3} = \dfrac{37}{8} \times \dfrac{2}{3} = \dfrac{74}{24} = 3\dfrac{2}{24}$; reduce to $3\dfrac{1}{12}$

MC-10 Divide these fractions.

a. $\dfrac{7}{8} \div \dfrac{2}{3} = \dfrac{7}{8} \times \dfrac{3}{2} = \dfrac{21}{16}$ or $1\dfrac{5}{16}$

b. $6\dfrac{3}{4} \div 2\dfrac{1}{3} = \dfrac{27}{4} \div \dfrac{7}{3} = \dfrac{27}{4} \times \dfrac{3}{7} = \dfrac{81}{28}$ or $2\dfrac{25}{28}$

MC-11 Decimals as parts of a whole:
a. 0.50 = 50 parts of 100
b. 2.48 = 2 whole numbers and 48 parts of 100

MC-12 Multiply these decimals.
a. $16.5 \times 0.5 = 165 \times 5 = 825$, two decimal places, final answer is 8.25
b. $1.2 \times 1.2 = 12 \times 12 = 144$, two decimal places, final answer is 1.44

MC-13 Divide these decimals.
a. $52.8 \div 12 = 120\overline{)528}$, then divide $120\overline{)528}^{\,4.4}$

b. $1.4 \div 1.4 = 14\overline{)14}$, then divide $14\overline{)14}^{\,1}$

MC-14 Change the following fractions to decimals and the decimals to fractions.

a. $0.065 = \dfrac{65}{1000}$; reduced to $\dfrac{13}{200}$

b. $\dfrac{300}{650} = 650\overline{)300}$ (or $65\overline{)30}$) $= 0.4615$

MC-15 Work to three places and then round to two places.

a. $\dfrac{128.5}{80} = 80\overline{)128.5} = 80\overline{)128.500} = 1.505 = 1.51$

b. $\dfrac{26.8}{13.4} = 13.4\overline{)26.8} = 134\overline{)268} = 2$

MC-16 Convert the following percents into fractions.

a. $\dfrac{2}{3}\% = \dfrac{2}{3} \div \dfrac{100}{1} = \dfrac{2}{3} \times \dfrac{1}{100} = \dfrac{2}{300}$ reduced to $\dfrac{1}{150}$

b. $7\% = 7 \div 100 = \dfrac{7}{100}$ (cannot be reduced further)

MC-17 Find the percentages of the whole number.
a. 0.6% of 50 = $0.006 \times 50 = 0.3$
b. 20% of 120 = $0.2 \times 120 = 24$

MC-18 How many tablets should you give?

a. *Want* carvedilol 25 mg; *Have* carvedilol 6.25 mg:

$$\frac{25\,mg}{6.25\,mg} = 4\ tablets$$

b. *Want* estrogen 0.0625 mg; *Have* estrogen 0.125 mg

tablet: $\dfrac{0.0625\,mg}{0.125\,mg} = \dfrac{1}{2}$ tablet

MC-19 How many milliliters should you give?

a. *Want* diphenhydramine (Benadryl) 50 mg; *Have* diphenhydramine 25 mg/5 mL:

$$\frac{50\,mg}{25\,mg} \times 5\ mL = 2 \times 5\ mL = give\ 10\ mL$$

b. *Want* chloral hydrate syrup 100 mg; *Have* chloral hydrate syrup 500 mg/5 mL: $\dfrac{100\,mg}{500\,mg} \times 5\,mL = \dfrac{1}{5} \times 5\,mL = give\ 1\ mL$

MC-20 How many milliliters should you give by injection?

a. *Want* penicillin 50,000 units; *Have* penicillin 1,000,000 units/50 mL:

$$\frac{50{,}000\ units}{1{,}000{,}000\ units} \times 50\ mL = \frac{1\ unit}{20\ units} \times 50\ mL =$$

inject 2.5 mL

b. *Want* prochlorperazine (Compazine) 10 mg; *Have* prochlorperazine 5 mg/mL:

$$\frac{10\,mg}{5\,mg} \times 1\ mL = 2 \times 1\ mL = inject\ 2\ mL$$

MC-21 Express the following problems as a fractional proportion.

a. If one box of eggs has 18 eggs, then two boxes have 36 eggs. $\dfrac{1}{18} = \dfrac{2}{36}$

b. If one chewable tablet of diphenhydramine contains 12.5 mg, then four chewable tablets have 50 mg.

$$\frac{1\ tablet}{12.5\,mg} = \frac{4\ tablets}{50\,mg}$$

MC-22 How many milliliters should you give?

a. *Want* carbamazepine (Tegretol) 75 mg oral suspension; *Have* carbamazepine 100 mg/5 mL

$$\frac{100\,mg}{5\,mL} = \frac{75}{X\,mL};\ (cancel\ mg),\ 100\,X = 375\ mL;$$

$$X = \frac{375}{100};\ X = 3.75\ mL,\ give\ 3.75\ mL$$

b. *Want* acetaminophen (Tylenol) 100 mg; *Have* acetaminophen 160 mg/5 mL:

$$\frac{160\,mg}{5\,mL} = \frac{100\,mg}{X\,mL};\ (cancel\ mg),\ 160\,X = 500\ mL;$$

$$X = \frac{500}{160};\ X = 3.125;\ (round\ down),\ give\ 3\ mL$$

Answers to *Try This!* Problems

TT-1 Change these mixed-number fractions into improper fractions.

a. $1\dfrac{3}{4} = \dfrac{7}{4}$

b. $2\dfrac{5}{8} = \dfrac{21}{8}$

c. $4\dfrac{1}{5} = \dfrac{21}{5}$

d. $6\dfrac{7}{8} = \dfrac{55}{8}$

TT-2 Reduce each of these fractions to their lowest common denominators.

a. $\dfrac{10}{24} = \dfrac{5}{12}$

b. $\dfrac{50}{100} = \dfrac{1}{2}$

c. $\dfrac{36}{84} = \dfrac{3}{7}$

d. $\dfrac{9}{15} = \dfrac{3}{5}$

TT-3 How many zeros can you chop and drop?

a. $\dfrac{230}{3500}$ Chop off one zero from the top and bottom to make $\dfrac{23}{350}$.

b. $\dfrac{1400}{10}$ Chop off one zero from the top and bottom to make $\dfrac{140}{1}$.

c. $\dfrac{20}{500}$ Chop off one zero from the top and bottom to make $\dfrac{2}{50}$.

d. $\dfrac{500}{100}$ Chop off two zeros from the top and bottom to make $\dfrac{5}{1}$ (or 5).

TT-4 Which fraction represents the largest part of the whole?

a. $\dfrac{1}{2}, \dfrac{3}{4},$ or $\dfrac{7}{8}$? $\dfrac{7}{8}$ is the largest part of the whole. The lowest common denominator for these fractions is 8.

b. $\dfrac{1}{5}, \dfrac{5}{15},$ or $\dfrac{6}{45}$? $\dfrac{5}{15}$ is the largest part of the whole. The lowest common denominator for these fractions is 15. (Hint: $\dfrac{6}{45}$ is not in lowest terms.)

Which fraction represents the smallest part of the whole?

c. $\dfrac{1}{3}, \dfrac{1}{5},$ or $\dfrac{1}{6}$? $\dfrac{1}{6}$ is the smallest part of the whole. The lowest common denominator for these fractions is 30.

d. $\dfrac{1}{2}, \dfrac{3}{8},$ or $\dfrac{3}{4}$? $\dfrac{3}{8}$ is the smallest part of the whole. The lowest common denominator for these fractions is 8.

TT-5 Add these fractions. If a sum is an improper fraction, convert it to a mixed-number fraction.

a. $\dfrac{1}{7}+\dfrac{5}{7}=\dfrac{6}{7}$

b. $\dfrac{1}{5}+\dfrac{2}{5}+\dfrac{1}{5}=\dfrac{4}{5}$

c. $\dfrac{6}{8}+\dfrac{1}{8}+\dfrac{3}{8}+\dfrac{5}{8}=\dfrac{15}{8}=1\dfrac{7}{8}$

d. $\dfrac{1}{4}+\dfrac{2}{4}+\dfrac{3}{4}=\dfrac{6}{4}=1\dfrac{2}{4}\left(1\dfrac{1}{2}\right)$

TT-6 Add these fractions. If the sum is an improper fraction, convert it to either a whole number or a mixed-number fraction.

a. $\dfrac{4}{7}+\dfrac{2}{5}=\dfrac{20}{35}+\dfrac{14}{35}=\dfrac{34}{35}$ (cannot be reduced further)

b. $\dfrac{3}{4}+\dfrac{1}{3}+\dfrac{5}{6}=\dfrac{9}{12}+\dfrac{4}{12}+\dfrac{10}{12}=\dfrac{23}{12}$; convert to $1\dfrac{11}{12}$

c. $\dfrac{1}{2}+\dfrac{1}{6}+\dfrac{1}{5}=\dfrac{15}{30}+\dfrac{5}{30}+\dfrac{6}{30}=\dfrac{26}{30}$; reduce to $\dfrac{13}{15}$

d. $\dfrac{2}{9}+\dfrac{1}{3}+\dfrac{3}{5}=\dfrac{10}{45}+\dfrac{15}{45}+\dfrac{27}{45}=\dfrac{52}{45}$; reduce to $1\dfrac{7}{45}$

TT-7 Subtract these fractions. If a fraction is a mixed-number fraction, first convert it to an improper fraction. Reduce answers to their lowest common denominators.

a. $\dfrac{4}{5}-\dfrac{1}{5}=\dfrac{3}{5}$

b. $1\dfrac{1}{3}-\dfrac{2}{3}=\dfrac{4}{3}-\dfrac{2}{3}=\dfrac{2}{3}$

c. $\dfrac{3}{4}-\dfrac{1}{4}=\dfrac{2}{4}$; reduce to $\dfrac{1}{2}$

d. $2\dfrac{1}{2}-1\dfrac{1}{2}=\dfrac{5}{2}-\dfrac{3}{2}=\dfrac{2}{2}=1$

TT-8 Subtract these fractions. If a fraction is a mixed-number fraction, first convert it to an improper fraction. Reduce answers to their lowest common denominators.

a. $\dfrac{3}{4}-\dfrac{2}{3}=\dfrac{9}{12}-\dfrac{8}{12}=\dfrac{1}{12}$ (cannot be reduced further)

b. $2\dfrac{2}{3}-1\dfrac{1}{2}=\dfrac{8}{3}-\dfrac{3}{2}=\dfrac{16}{6}-\dfrac{9}{6}=1\dfrac{1}{6}$

c. $\dfrac{4}{5}-\dfrac{1}{3}=\dfrac{12}{15}-\dfrac{5}{15}=\dfrac{7}{15}$ (cannot be reduced further)

d. $2\dfrac{1}{2}-\dfrac{3}{4}=\dfrac{5}{2}-\dfrac{3}{4}=\dfrac{10}{4}-\dfrac{3}{4}=\dfrac{7}{4}=1\dfrac{3}{4}$

TT-9 Multiply these fractions.

a. $1\dfrac{3}{4}\times5\dfrac{6}{7}=\dfrac{7}{4}\times\dfrac{41}{7}=\dfrac{287}{28}$; reduce to $10\dfrac{1}{4}$

b. $2\dfrac{2}{4}\times6\dfrac{7}{8}=\dfrac{10}{4}\times\dfrac{55}{8}=\dfrac{550}{32}$, or $\dfrac{275}{16}$; reduce to $17\dfrac{3}{16}$

c. $\dfrac{3}{4}\times9\dfrac{11}{16}=\dfrac{3}{4}\times\dfrac{155}{16}=\dfrac{465}{64}$; reduce to $7\dfrac{17}{64}$

d. $\dfrac{1}{2}\times10\dfrac{1}{3}=\dfrac{1}{2}\times\dfrac{31}{3}=\dfrac{31}{6}$; reduce to $5\dfrac{1}{6}$

TT-10 Divide these fractions.

a. $3\div\dfrac{1}{2}=\dfrac{3}{1}\div\dfrac{1}{2}=\dfrac{3}{1}\times\dfrac{2}{1}=\dfrac{6}{1}$ or 6

b. $\dfrac{3}{4}\div\dfrac{1}{2}=\dfrac{3}{4}\times\dfrac{2}{1}=\dfrac{6}{4}=1\dfrac{2}{4}$ or $1\dfrac{1}{2}$

c. $5\dfrac{1}{4}\div\dfrac{6}{8}=\dfrac{21}{4}\div\dfrac{6}{8}=\dfrac{21}{4}\times\dfrac{8}{6}=\dfrac{168}{24}$ or 7

d. $10\div\dfrac{2}{3}=\dfrac{10}{1}\div\dfrac{2}{3}=\dfrac{10}{1}\times\dfrac{3}{2}=\dfrac{30}{2}$ or 15

TT-11 Decimals as parts of a whole.
a. 0.3 = 3 parts of 10
b. 0.75 = 75 parts of 100
c. 5.1 = 5 whole numbers and 1 part of 10
d. 2.2 = 2 whole numbers and 2 parts of 10

TT-12 Multiply these decimals.
a. $100\times0.25=100\times25=2500$, two decimal places, final answer is 25
b. $51.2\times2.1=512\times21=10752$, two decimal places, final answer is 107.52
c. $15.5\times10=155\times10=1550$, one decimal place, final answer is 155
d. $40.5\times2.4=405\times24=9720$, two decimal places, final answer is 97.20

TT-13 Divide these decimals.

a. $630\div0.3=3\overline{)6300}$, then divide $3\overline{)6300}^{\,2100}$

b. $0.125\div0.5=5\overline{)1.25}$, then divide $5\overline{)1.25}^{\,0.25}$

c. $2.5\div0.75=75\overline{)250}$, then divide $75\overline{)250}^{\,3.33}$

d. $10\div0.25=25\overline{)1000}$, then divide $25\overline{)1000}^{\,40}$

TT-14 Change the following fractions to decimals and the decimals to fractions.

a. $\dfrac{3}{4}=4\overline{)3}=0.75$

b. $0.55=\dfrac{55}{100}$; reduced to $\dfrac{11}{20}$

c. $0.075=\dfrac{75}{1000}$; reduced to $\dfrac{3}{40}$

d. $1.25=1\dfrac{25}{100}$ or $1\dfrac{1}{4}$

e. $\dfrac{7}{8}=8\overline{)7}=0.875$

TT-15 Work to three places and then round to two places.

a. $\dfrac{58.4}{33}=33\overline{)58.4}=330\overline{)584.000}=1.769=1.77$

b. $\dfrac{6}{3.4}=3.4\overline{)6}=34\overline{)60.000}=1.764=1.76$

c. $\dfrac{27.5}{3.4} = 3.4\overline{)27.5} = 34\overline{)275.000} = 8.088 = 8.09$

d. $\dfrac{25.4}{5} = 5\overline{)25.4} = 5\overline{)25.4} = 5.08$

TT-16 Convert the following percents into fractions.

a. $\dfrac{1}{2}\% = \dfrac{1}{2} \div \dfrac{100}{1} = \dfrac{1}{2} \times \dfrac{1}{100} = \dfrac{1}{200}$

b. $3\% = 3 \div 100 = \dfrac{3}{100}$ (cannot be reduced further)

c. $5\dfrac{3}{4}\% = \dfrac{23}{4} \div \dfrac{100}{1} = \dfrac{23}{4} \times \dfrac{1}{100} = \dfrac{23}{400}$ (cannot be reduced further)

d. $2.5\% = 2.5 \div 100 = \dfrac{2.5}{100} \left(\text{can be reduced further to } \dfrac{1}{40}\right)$

TT-17 Find the percentages of the whole numbers.
a. 25% of 300 = 0.25 × 300 = 75
b. 10% of $5.00 = 0.1 × $5.00 = $.50
c. 0.2% of 10 = 0.002 × 10 = 0.02
d. 300% of 5 = 3 × 5 = 15

TT-18 How many tablets should you give?
a. *Want* digoxin (Lanoxin) 0.25 mg; *Have* digoxin 0.125-mg tablet: $\dfrac{0.25\,\text{mg}}{0.125\,\text{mg}}$ = two tablets

b. *Want* alendronate sodium (Fosamax) 5 mg; *Have* alendronate 10-mg tablet: $\dfrac{5\,\text{mg}}{10\,\text{mg}} = \dfrac{1}{2}$ tablet

c. *Want* alprazolam (Xanax) 1.5 mg; *have* alprazolam 0.5-mg tablet: $\dfrac{1.5\,\text{mg}}{0.5\,\text{mg}}$ = three tablets

d. *Want* diphenhydramine (Benadryl) 75 mg; *Have* diphenhydramine 25-mg capsule: $\dfrac{75\,\text{mg}}{25\,\text{mg}}$ = three capsules

TT-19 How many milliliters should you give?
a. *Want* dextromethorphan (Robitussin) 7 mg; *Have* dextromethorphan 3.5 mg/5 mL: $\dfrac{7\,\text{mg}}{3.5\,\text{mg}} \times 5\,\text{mL} =$ 2 × 5 mL = give 10 mL

b. *Want* acetaminophen (Tylenol) 240 mg; *Have* acetaminophen 80 mg/2.5 mL: $\dfrac{240\,\text{mg}}{80\,\text{mg}} \times 2.5\,\text{mL} =$ 3 × 2.5 mL = give 7.5 mL

c. *Want* ibuprofen (Advil) 100 mg; *Have* ibuprofen 50 mg/1.25 mL: $\dfrac{100\,\text{mg}}{50\,\text{mg}} \times 1.25\,\text{mL} = 2 \times 1.25\,\text{mL} =$ give 2.5 mL

d. *Want* doxylamine (Aldex) 25 mg; *Have* doxylamine 6.25 mg/mL: $\dfrac{25\,\text{mg}}{6.25\,\text{mg}} \times 1\,\text{mL} = 4 \times 1\,\text{mL} =$ give 4 mL

TT-20 How many milliliters should you give by injection?
a. *Want* hydromorphone (Dilaudid) 1 mg; *Have* a unit-dose syringe with 4 mg per mL: $\dfrac{1\,\text{mg}}{4\,\text{mg}} \times 1\,\text{mL} = 0.25 \times 1\,\text{mL} =$ inject 0.25 mL

b. *Want* heparin 5000 units; *Have* a unit-dose syringe with 10,000 units/mL: $\dfrac{5000\,\text{units}}{10,000\,\text{units}} \times 1\,\text{mL} = 0.5 \times 1\,\text{mL} =$ inject 0.5 mL

c. *Want* trimethobenzamide 200 mg; *Have* 20 mL vial with 100 mg/mL: $\dfrac{200\,\text{mg}}{100\,\text{mg}} \times 1\,\text{mL} = 2 \times 1\,\text{mL} =$ inject 2 mL

d. *Want* morphine 15 mg; *Have* 50-mL vial with 10 mg/mL: $\dfrac{15\,\text{mg}}{10\,\text{mg}} \times 1\,\text{mL} = 1.5 \times 1\,\text{mL} =$ inject 1.5 mL

TT-21 Express the following problems as a fractional proportion.
a. If three boats have 6 sails, then nine boats have 18 sails. $\dfrac{3}{6} = \dfrac{9}{18}$

b. If one case of IV fluids holds 12 bags, then three cases hold 36 bags. $\dfrac{1}{12} = \dfrac{3}{36}$

c. If 5 mL have 325 mg of acetaminophen, then 2 mL have 130 mg. $\dfrac{5\,\text{mL}}{325\,\text{mg}} = \dfrac{1\,\text{mL}}{65\,\text{mg}} = \dfrac{2\,\text{mL}}{130\,\text{mg}}$

d. If 1 mL has 2 mg of hydromorphone (Dilaudid), then 5 mL have 10 mg of hydromorphone. $\dfrac{1\,\text{mL}}{2\,\text{mg}} = \dfrac{5\,\text{mL}}{10\,\text{mg}}$

TT-22 How many milliliters should you give?
a. *Want* dextromethorphan (Robitussin) 7 mg; *Have* dextromethorphan 3.5 mg/5 mL: $\dfrac{3.5\,\text{mg}}{5\,\text{mL}} = \dfrac{7\,\text{mg}}{X\,\text{mL}}$; (cancel mg), 3.5 X = 35; $X = \dfrac{7}{3.5} = 2$; 2 × 5 mL = give 10 mL

b. *Want* ibuprofen (Advil) 100 mg; *Have* ibuprofen 50 mg/1.25 mL: $\dfrac{50\,\text{mg}}{1.25\,\text{mL}} = \dfrac{100\,\text{mg}}{X\,\text{mL}}$; (cancel mg), 50 X = 125; $X = \dfrac{100}{50} = 2$; 2 × 1.25 mL = give 2.5 mL

c. *Want* digoxin (Lanoxin) 0.03 mg; *Have* digoxin 0.05 mg/1 mL: $\dfrac{0.05\,\text{mg}}{1\,\text{mL}} = \dfrac{0.03\,\text{mg}}{X\,\text{mL}}$; (cancel mg), 0.05 X = 0.03; X = 0.6; 0.6 × 1 mL = give 0.6 mL

d. *Want* hydromorphone (Dilaudid) 1 mg; *Have* hydromorphone 2 mg/1 mL: $\dfrac{2\,\text{mg}}{1\,\text{mL}} = \dfrac{1\,\text{mg}}{X\,\text{mL}}$; (cancel mg), 2 X = 1 mL; X = 0.5; 0.5 × 1 mL = give 0.5 mL

Medical Systems of Weights and Measures

Objectives

After studying this chapter you should be able to:

1. Define common units of measure for liquids and solids.
2. Convert from the household and the apothecary systems of measurement to the metric system of measurement.
3. Identify the three basic units of measure in the metric system.
4. Identify the unit of measure using a prefix and a root word.
5. Convert milliliters to liters; convert liters to milliliters.
6. Convert ounces and pounds to grams and kilograms.
7. Solve dosage problems using the metric system.
8. Solve drug calculation problems using units.

Key Terms

apothecary system (ă-PŎTH-ě-kăr-ē SĬS-těm) (p. 66) A system of volume and weight measurements formerly used by physicians and pharmacists to compound and dispense drugs.

centigrade or Celsius (SĔN-tĭ-grād, SĔL-sē-ŭs) (p. 65) Metric or hospital scale of temperature measurement based on 100. Zero (0) degrees is the freezing point of water, and 100° is the boiling point of water. Normal human body temperature ranges between 36.1° and 37.8°.

dimensional analysis (dĭ-MĒN-shŭn-ăl ă-NĂL-ă-sĭs) (p. 71) A method of comparing and equating different physical quantities by using simple algebraic rules along with known conversion factors (called equivalency ratios).

equivalent (ē-KWĬV-ě-lěnt) (p. 63) To be equal in amount or to have equal value.

Fahrenheit (FĂR-ěn-hīt) (p. 65) System of temperature measurement used in the United States in which the freezing point of water is 32° above zero and the boiling point of water is 212°. Normal human body temperature ranges between 97° and 100°.

gram (g) (GRĂM) (p. 68) The basic metric unit for measurement of weight.

liter (L) (LĒ-tŭr) (p. 68) The basic metric unit for measurement of liquids.

meter (m) (MĒ-tŭr) (p. 68) The basic metric unit for measurement of length or distance.

OVERVIEW

Systems of weights and measures were invented so there could be standard ways of comparing two or more objects for size and strength. The first measuring system discussed in this chapter is the one used to check a patient's temperature. All systems that follow are used in prescribing drugs. For solving the conversion problems in this chapter, you will need to apply the math principles presented in Chapter 3, including using proportions.

For the most part, drugs are measured by weight (for example, an extra-strength Tylenol tablet contains 500 mg of drug) or liquid volume (5 mL or 1 tsp of Benadryl). For each measuring system, this chapter identifies which units are used for *dry weights* and which are used for *liquids*. After each system is presented, there will be practice problems to work so you can see exactly how each system is used.

To convert from one system to another, values that are equal to each other, known as **equivalents,** are used. You need to understand and either memorize the equivalents in each system or carry a conversion card with you so you can convert from one system to another quickly and easily. As the United States moves closer to accepting the metric system for all weights and measures, there will be less need to learn the other systems or memorize the conversions.

MATH CHECK

Some of you are more familiar than others with weights and measures, as well as converting from one system to another. Use the following math check problems to determine your understanding of specific concepts for weights and measures and your skill level in converting from one system to another. The answers to these problems are listed at the end of the chapter. If you are accurate in your math for these problems, you may not need to review some of the content in this chapter. If you have a weakness in any specific area, review the content and principles for that area.

MATH CHECK PROBLEMS

MC-1 Convert the Fahrenheit temperature to Centigrade and the Centigrade temperature to Fahrenheit.
    a. 101.4°F = _____ °C
    b. 40°C = _____ °F

MC-2
    a. Using the formula of 1 grain is equal to 65 mg, calculate the dosage in milligrams for 5 grains of aspirin. _____ mg
    b. How many minims are in 2 fluid drams? _____ minims

MC-3 Calculate the response in teaspoons or drops. (Note: "How to" math steps for conversion of *Want* versus *Have* problems are in Chapter 3.)
    a. *Want* Benadryl 2.5 mg; *Have* Benadryl 12.5 mg/5 mL _____ drops (gtts)
    b. *Want* acetaminophen 200 mg; *Have* acetaminophen 40 mg/mL _____ teaspoons

MC-4 Convert the following weights in pounds to kilograms and the weights in kilograms to pounds.
    a. 25 lb
    b. 275 lb
    c. 45 kg
    d. 80 kg

MC-5 Convert these household measures into metric equivalents, rounding to the nearest tenth when necessary.
    a. 2 tablespoons
    b. 8.8 lb
    c. 14 inches
    d. 4 ounces
    e. 5 teaspoons

MC-6 Convert these metric measures into household equivalents.
    a. 70 kg
    b. 150 mL
    c. 75 g
    d. 500 mL

MC-7 Calculate how much drug you should administer.
    a. *Want* potassium 15 mEq in extended-release tablet; *Have* potassium 5 mEq in extended-release tablet
    b. *Want* potassium gluconate 30 mEq oral solution; *Have* potassium gluconate 20 mEq/15 mL oral solution.

MC-8 Calculate how many milliliters you should give.
    a. *Want* heparin 750 units subcutaneously; *Have* heparin 1000 units/mL
    b. *Want* heparin 750 units intravenously; *Have* heparin 500 units/mL

MC-9 Calculate how many milligrams in how many teaspoons you will give to a child who weighs 28.6 lb.

Want acyclovir 20 mg/kg; *Have* acyclovir 200 mg/5 mL oral suspension.

MC-10 Using dimensional analysis and showing your work, calculate the dosages for these problems.

   a. Dilantin (phenytoin) 100 mg is prescribed to give a child orally. The drug available is Dilantin 125 mg/5 mL. How many milliliters of this solution should be administered to equal the ordered dose?
   b. A patient who weighs 154 lb is prescribed to receive 50,000 units of penicillin intravenously per kg of weight. The penicillin solution you have on hand is 1,000,000 units/25 mL. How many milliliters should you give by intravenous (IV) injection?

MEASURING SYSTEMS TEMPERATURE: FAHRENHEIT AND CELSIUS

When measuring temperature, the symbol ° is used in place of the word "degree." Many hospitals use the metric system for measuring temperature (Celsius [C]), and other health care settings use the Fahrenheit (F) system. Health care workers must be familiar with both systems of measurement. In the **Fahrenheit** system, the freezing point of water is 32° above zero, and the boiling point of water is 212°. The normal human body temperature ranges between 97° and 100°. The **centigrade** or **Celsius** system is based on the number 100. Zero (0) degrees is set as the freezing point of water, and 100° is used for the boiling point of water. Normal human body temperature ranges between 36.1° and 37.8°.

Digital thermometers are often used to check body temperature and can be set for either system. For learning purposes, picture the old mercury thermometers such as the one shown in Figure 4-1. As you can see in the figure, there is a big difference in ranges between centigrade (Celsius) and Fahrenheit temperatures. To change from one system to another, use the following two equations or a conversion chart. Conversion is often necessary because patients usually report their temperatures from home using a thermometer with a Fahrenheit scale.

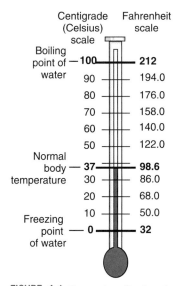

FIGURE 4-1 Comparing Centigrade to Fahrenheit values with a mercury thermometer.

Equation 1: Fahrenheit to Centigrade

$$(\text{Fahrenheit temperature} - 32) \times \frac{5}{9} = \text{Degrees Centigrade}$$

First, subtract 32° from 102° (102° − 32°) for an answer of 70 and plug that number into the formula:

$$70 \times \frac{5}{9}$$

Multiply 70 by 5, which equals 350. Divide 350 by 9, which equals 38.88°.

   If the answer has more than one decimal place, round to the nearest tenth of a degree (for example, 38.9°, not 38.88°).

Equation 2: Centigrade to Fahrenheit

$$(\text{Centigrade temperature}) \times \frac{9}{5} + 32 = \text{Degrees Fahrenheit}$$

Place the centigrade temperature of 41°C into the formula:

$$41 \times \frac{9}{5} + 32$$

Table 4-1	Apothecary Measurement System and Equivalents for the Metric and Household Systems of Measure		
APOTHECARY	**METRIC EQUIVALENT**		**HOUSEHOLD EQUIVALENT**
Dry Measure (Smallest to Largest)			
1 grain (gr)	60-65 milligrams (mg)		—
15-16 grain (gr)	1 gram (g)		0.035 ounce (oz) dry weight
Liquid Measure (Smallest to Largest)			
1 minim (m) = 1 drop			
15-**16** minims	1 milliliter (mL)		
60-**65** minims = 1 fluid dram (dr)	4-5 milliliters (mL)		1 teaspoon (tsp)
4 fluid drams	15 milliliters (mL)		1 tablespoon (Tbs)
8 fluid drams	30 milliliters (mL)		2 tablespoons (T) 1 fluid ounce

Try This!

TT-1 Convert the Fahrenheit temperature to Centigrade and the Centigrade temperature to Fahrenheit.
a. 97°F = _____ °C
b. 103.8°F = _____ °C
c. 35°C = _____ °F
d. 39.2°C = _____ °F
Answers are at the end of this chapter.

Try This!

TT-2 Convert the apothecary measures into metric equivalents and the metric equivalents into apothecary measures.
a. 1/4th of a grain is how many mg? ____mg
b. 8 minims is how many mL? _____mL
c. 60 mL is how many fluid drams? ____fluid drams
d. 2 grams is how many grains? _____grains
Answers are at the end of this chapter.

? Did You Know?

Tableware teaspoons and tablespoons used for eating are names indicating only that the two spoon types are different in size. They do not reflect the actual liquid amount that either one can hold, and they do not hold the same volume from one brand of tableware to another.

Multiply 41 by 9, which equals 369. Divide 369 by 5, which equals 73.8. Add 32, which makes the answer 105.8.

If the answer has more than one decimal place, round to the nearest tenth of a degree (for example, 100.6°, not 100.59°).

APOTHECARY SYSTEM FOR DRUG MEASUREMENTS

In earlier times, the **apothecary system**, which is a system of volume and weight measurements, was used by physicians and pharmacists to compound and dispense drugs. Table 4-1 lists apothecary abbreviations and equivalents. This system is less precise than the metric system and is no longer used to compound or dispense drugs in North America. For example, in the apothecary liquid measure system, 1 minim is equal to one drop, and 15 to 16 minims are equal to 1 milliliter (mL). However, drops are of different sizes, so not all droppers deliver 1 mL as 15 or 16 drops. Another example is the measurement of solids in grains (gr). The variance making this measurement less precise is that 1 gr is equal to 60 to 65 milligrams (mg). Some drugs, such as morphine, were converted from grains to mg using the formula that 1 grain is equal to 60 mg. Other drugs, such as aspirin, were converted from grains to milligrams using the formula that 1 grain is equal to 65 mg. Although Table 4-1 shows the variance, the number shown in bold (unless a math problem specifies otherwise) is the accepted standard set by the U.S. Pharmacopeia.

HOUSEHOLD SYSTEM FOR LIQUID AND DRY MEASUREMENTS

You have probably cooked at one time or another and have had to measure ingredients for a recipe. This same household system is the often used by patients when they are taking *liquid* drugs at home.

The household system uses drops (gtts), teaspoons (tsp), tablespoons (Tbs), ounces (oz), and cups (c) to measure liquids. Note that a liquid ounce is *not* equal to a dry ounce such as flour. In cooking, liquid ounces are measured in a one-piece measuring cup (often made of glass), and dry ounces are measured in nested cups (Figure 4-2). In health care, liquid drugs have their own special measuring tools. Table 4-2 lists household abbreviations and equivalents.

The only *dry* measures used in the household system for health care purposes are ounces and pounds. Patients usually report their weight in pounds (lb). The reported weight often must be converted to kilograms (kg) in the hospital or other health care setting.

ABBREVIATION	MEANING	EQUIVALENT
Table 4-2 Abbreviations and Equivalents for the Household System of Measure		
Dry Measure (Smallest to Largest)		
oz	Ounce	16 oz = 1 lb
lb	Pound	1 lb = 16 oz
Liquid Measure (Smallest to Largest)		
gtts	Drops	60 gtts = 1 tsp
tsp	Teaspoon	3 tsp = 1 Tbs
Tbs	Tablespoon	2 Tbs = 1 oz
fl oz	Fluid ounce	8 oz = 1 c 16 oz = 1 pt 32 oz = 1 qt 64 oz = ½ gal 128 oz = 1 gal
c	Cup	2 c = 1 p 4 c = 1 qt 8 c = ½ gal 16 c = 1 gal
pt	Pint	2 pt = 1 qt 4 pt = ½ gal 8 pt = 1 gal
qt	Quart	4 qt = 1 gal
gal	Gallon	1 gal = 4 qt
Length (Smallest to Largest)		
in	Inch	12 in = 1 ft
ft	Foot	3 ft = 1 yd 5280 ft = 1 mile
yd	Yard	1 yd = 3 ft 1760 yd = 1 mile

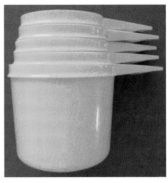

FIGURE 4-2 Nested cups used to measure dry ingredients in the household system.

⚠ Drug Alert!

Teaching Alert

Teach patients who are taking liquid drugs to buy and use only measuring tools that are designed and calibrated for liquid drugs rather than using tableware spoons to measure liquid drugs.

QSEN: Safety

⚠ Drug Alert!

Administration Alert

When using a dropper to administer liquid drugs, place it into the side of the patient's mouth rather than in the middle, where it can move down the throat too quickly and cause choking.

QSEN: Safety

⚠ Drug Alert!

Administration Alert

Always double check the amount of drug in any measuring device against the amount ordered to prevent giving an overdose.

QSEN: Safety

◎ Try This!

TT-3 Calculate the response in teaspoons or drops. (Note: "How to" math steps for conversion of *Want* versus *Have* problems are in Chapter 3.)
a. *Want* ampicillin 500 mg; *Have* ampicillin 250 mg/tsp
b. *Want* guaifenesin 50 mg; *Have* guaifenesin 100 mg/60 gtts
c. *Want* milk of magnesia 1 Tbs; *Have* milk of magnesia 1 tsp
   Answers are at the end of this chapter.

Larger liquid household measures include the pint, quart, and gallon. These larger measures are discussed later in the chapter under the metric system.

Patients often use the teaspoons and tablespoons from tableware to measure liquid drugs. However, these spoons are *not* accurate, and patients should be instructed *not* to use them to measure drugs. It is best to use measuring tools that are designed and *calibrated* (marked in accurate units) for liquid drugs. These include the dropper, oral syringe, medication spoon, and small medicine cup (see Figure 2-3 in Chapter 2). All of these can be purchased in any pharmacy or drugstore and even in many grocery stores.

Droppers are marked in both teaspoons and milliliters (mL; metric). Check the drug order carefully to determine which measurement is correct.

The most common device for measuring oral drugs in the hospital is the *oral syringe* (similar to a dropper). Oral syringes are marked in both teaspoons and milliliters. The rubber stopper is small enough to be aspirated (inhaled) into the lungs, so be sure to remove the stopper before you attempt to use the syringe.

Medication spoons have calibrated hollow handles and are useful for giving small doses between 1 and 2 tsp (5 to 10 mL). Mark the desired dose with your finger and hold the spoon at eye level to ensure that the dose you pour is accurate.

Medicine cups are useful to measure and give liquid doses from 1 tsp to 1 oz. The cup is marked around its sides in teaspoons, tablespoons, and ounces. Note that the ounce is marked "FL OZ" to indicate that this cup is for liquids only. The other marks indicate the liquid unit of the metric system: the milliliter (mL).

To use the cup accurately, fill while holding it at eye level. Either place the cup on a table and bend to look straight at the mark or hold it up to your eyes as you fill it

| Box **4-1** | **Metric Equivalents** |

DRY		**LIQUID**		**LENGTH**	
1 kg	= 1000 g	1 L	= 1000 mL	1 m (meter)	= 100 cm
1 g	= 1000 mg				= 1000 mm
	$= \dfrac{1}{1000}$ kg	1 mL	$= \dfrac{1}{1000}$ L	1 cm	= 10 mm
					$= \dfrac{1}{100}$ meter
1 mg	$= \dfrac{1}{1000}$ g			1 mm	$= \dfrac{1}{10}$ cm
					$= \dfrac{1}{1000}$ meter

(see Figure 2-4 in Chapter 2). Looking down at the mark or from an angle will result in an inaccurate dose.

METRIC SYSTEM

Most of the world uses the metric system for all types of measuring. It is the most used system worldwide for drug prescriptions because it is accurate even in small doses. The metric system is based on the number 10 and uses the decimal system (multiples of 10). (See Chapter 3 for a review of decimals.) In giving drugs, only a few of the possible metric measurements are used. For a more complete discussion of the metric system, consult a mathematics text. This system is not difficult, and you *can* learn it!

Metric Basics

The three basic units of the metric system are the **meter** (length), the **liter** (liquid), and the **gram** (weight). Each of these three words forms the *root* (that part or parts of a multiple-part word that indicates the basic meaning) of every metric measuring unit. Always look for these root words in each metric measurement. They indicate whether you are measuring a length, liquid volume, or weight. For example:

- Your height can be measured in either inches or centi*meters*.
- Your weight can be measured in pounds or kilo*grams*.
- Penicillin is prescribed in 250-milli*gram* tablets.
- A household quart is slightly less than a *liter*.

Box 4-1 lists basic metric equivalents.

Just as in decimals, there are measurements for *less than* and *more than* the basic unit. These descriptive words are called *prefixes* because they come before the root of a word. Which prefix is attached to the root explains how much larger or smaller each unit is in relation to the basic unit. For example, weight can be written in *kilo*grams, in which a kilogram is 1000 times heavier or *larger* than a gram. Drugs are often prescribed using the *milli*gram, which is 1000 times *smaller* than a gram. See Table 4-3 for a list of the prefixes most commonly used in health care, listed from large to small.

Metric Abbreviations

The basic metric unit abbreviations are meter (m), liter (L), and gram (g). Note that the "L" for liter is capitalized to avoid confusion with other abbreviations. Table 4-3 lists the abbreviations most often used.

The metric units for liquids are used for liquid oral drugs and intravenous (IV) fluids. The metric units for weight are used for drug doses and to weigh objects, including the human body. Two prefixes for weights are very small, the microgram (mcg) and the nanogram (ng). Both micrograms and nanograms are the exceptions to the "three decimal place" rule discussed in Chapter 3.

Memory Jogger

Remember from the drug dosage calculations that **L** stood for liquid dose. This will help you to remember that liters (L) are a way of measuring liquids.

Drug Alert!

Administration Alert

The milligram is 1000 times stronger than the microgram. Confusion could lead to a BIG overdose. If any drug dose order is written using an abbreviation, always clarify with the prescriber which unit is meant before giving the drug.

QSEN: Safety

Table 4-3   Metric Prefixes and Abbreviations

PREFIX	ABBREVIATION	MEANING
Weight (Gram) (g)		
kilo	kg	1000 g
milli	mg	0.001 or $\frac{1}{1000}$ of a gram
micro	mcg	0.000001 or $\frac{1}{1,000,000}$ of a gram $\frac{1}{1000}$ of a milligram
nano	ng	0.000000001 or $\frac{1}{1,000,000,000}$ of a gram
Liquids (Liter)		
deci	dL	100 mL 0.1 or $\frac{1}{10}$ of a liter
milli	mL	0.001 or $\frac{1}{1000}$ of a liter
Length (Meter)		
kilo	km	1000 meters
centi	cm	0.01 or $\frac{1}{100}$ of a meter
milli	mm	0.001 or $\frac{1}{1000}$ of a meter

Box 4-2   Household-to-Metric Equivalents

DRY WEIGHT		LIQUID	
1 oz	= 30 g (30,000 mg)	15 gtts	= 1 mL
16 oz	= 1 lb = 454 g	1 tsp	= 5 mL
		1 Tbs	= 15 mL
2.2 lb	= 1 kg	2 Tbs	= 30 mL
LENGTH		1 fl oz	= 30 mL
1 in	= 2.54 cm	8 fl oz	= 1 c = 240 mL
1 ft	= 30.48 cm	1 pt	= 500 mL (slightly less) = 0.5 L (slightly less)
		1 qt	= 1000 mL (slightly less) = 1 L

SWITCHING BETWEEN HOUSEHOLD AND METRIC SYSTEMS

You are often the medical interpreter for your patients and must be able to quickly switch or convert between metric and household measurements. Only practice will make you comfortable with the conversion (switching) process. Begin with the smaller equivalents and move to the larger ones. Box 4-2 shows household-to-metric equivalents. Remember that metric measurements are precise, and household measurements are only approximate, at best. When using household measuring instruments for drugs, the dose is not exact. One of the most common switching situations is changing a patient's weight between pounds and kilograms. One kilogram is equal to 2.2 lb. So a person's weight in kilograms is *always* less than half of his or

 Memory Jogger

Because 1 kg is equal to 2.2 lb, a person's weight in kilograms is less than half his or her weight in pounds.

Try This!

TT-4 Convert the following weights in pounds to kilograms and the weights in kilograms to pounds.

a. 98 lb   f. 68 kg
b. 52 lb   g. 12 kg
c. 315 lb   h. 122 kg
d. 2.9 lb   i. 52 kg
e. 147 lb   j. 80 kg

Answers are at the end of this chapter.

Drug Alert!

Administration Alert

Switching from one measuring system to another is only approximately right. Always apply the DIMS test ("does it make sense?") when converting between systems. If an answer does not make sense to you (for example, give 50 tsp), redo the math and ask for help.

QSEN: Safety

Try This!

TT-5 Convert these household measures into metric equivalents, rounding to the nearest tenth when necessary.

a. 250 lb   d. 4 Tbs
b. 12 oz (liquid) e. 2 tsp
c. 17 in

Answers are at the end of this chapter.

Try This!

TT-6 Convert these metric measures into household equivalents.

a. 45 g   d. 100 kg
b. 90 mL   e. 780 g
c. 1500 mL

Answers are at the end of this chapter.

Try This!

TT-7 Calculate how much drug you should administer.

a. *Want* potassium 16 mEq in extended-release tablet; *Have* potassium 8 mEq in extended-release tablet
b. *Want* potassium 10 mEq effervescent tablet; *Have* potassium 20 mEq scored effervescent tablet
c. *Want* potassium 10 mEq in an oral solution; *Have* potassium 20 mEq dissolved in 8 oz of water

Answers are at the end of this chapter.

---

her weight in pounds. To obtain the kilogram weight, first weigh the patient on a standard pound scale and then *divide* this number by 2.2. For example, a patient who weighs 232 lb weighs 105.45 kg (round to 105.5 kg). A patient who weighs 120 lb weighs 54.5 kg. To change weight in kilograms to pounds, *multiply* the kilogram number by 2.2. For example, the patient who weighs 90 kg weighs 198 lb. The infant who weighs 1.6 kg weighs 3.5 lb.

MILLIEQUIVALENT MEASURES

Milliequivalents (mEq) are used to measure electrolytes. *Electrolytes* are minerals and chemicals in the body that have a positive or negative charge. The electrolytes most often calculated in milliequivalents are potassium chloride (KCl), potassium phosphate (KPO_4), potassium gluconate, sodium, and different types of IV calcium (Ca^{++}). The electrolyte most often prescribed is KCl, which can be given orally or mixed with IV fluid. Whichever way it is given, it is irritating to the body.

Potassium can be given as a tablet, an extended-release tablet, an effervescent (fizzy) tablet, in a liquid, as a powder, or dissolved in IV fluids. The different types are *NOT interchangeable*. Do not substitute a different potassium type for the one prescribed.

Although drugs measured and prescribed in milliequivalents sound different from those measured and prescribed in milligrams, the dosage calculations are performed exactly the same way. Once again, you are determining the amount of tablets or milliliters to administer based on what you *want* versus what you *have* on hand. (If necessary, review drug dosage calculations in Chapter 3.) For example, the order reads "potassium chloride (Slow-K) 40 mEq orally," and you have Slow-K tablets that contain 20 mEq/tablet. Divide the number you *want* by the number you *have*.

$$\frac{Want}{Have} = \text{Number of tablets to give! } Want \text{ 40 mEq; } Have \text{ 20 mEq.}$$

$$\text{So, } \frac{40\,\text{mEq}}{20\,\text{mEq}/1\,\text{tablet}} = (\text{chop off the end zeroes})\frac{4}{2} = 2 \text{ tablets!}$$

UNIT MEASURES

Drugs measured in units come in either plain or international units. The most common drugs measured in units are insulin and heparin (a drug to reduce blood clotting). Others include injectable penicillin and some vitamins.

Insulin

Insulin is a drug used by some patients with diabetes to replace the insulin their bodies no longer make. (Chapter 13 has more information about diabetes and insulin.) The drug insulin is very concentrated and requires special syringes. The most common insulin syringe holds 50 units in one small 0.5-mL syringe. Each unit on the syringe is marked up to 50. However, there are many different types of insulin syringes. Some are measured up to 100 units, and others are measured up to 500 units. These syringes *cannot* be interchanged with one another or with noninsulin syringes. Carefully check the concentration of insulin in the bottle with the type of syringe chosen to make sure that you have the correct syringe. Do not go by the color of the syringe to determine whether the syringe is a 50-unit insulin syringe. *There is no common color for insulin syringe types.* Check the specific markings on the syringe rather than going by the color of the cap, needle hub, or box label. If the incorrect dose of insulin is given, severe hypoglycemia and death can result. Chapter 13 discusses safe insulin administration in detail.

Heparin

Heparin is a fast-acting anticoagulant (drug to slow or prevent blood clotting) that leaves the body quickly. A discussion of heparin and heparin-like drugs can be found in Chapter 20.

Heparin is only given by subcutaneous injection or into an IV site. It comes in single- and multiple-dose vials. In addition, weaker solutions of heparin are available already loaded in single-use syringes. Strengths of heparin vary from 10 units/mL to 40,000 units/mL.

Although drugs measured and prescribed in units sound different from those measured and prescribed in milligrams, the dosage calculations are performed exactly the same way. Once again, you are determining the milliliters to administer based on what you *want* versus what you *have* on hand. (If necessary, review drug dosage calculations in Chapter 3.) For example, the order reads "heparin 2000 units subcutaneously," and you have heparin 5000 units/mL. Divide the number you *want* by the number you *have*.

$$\frac{Want}{Have} = \text{Number of milliliters!}$$

Want 2000 units, *Have* 5000 units

$$\frac{2000}{5000/\text{mL}}(\text{chop the zeroes}) = \frac{2}{5} = 0.4\ \text{mL}$$

TWO-STEP DRUG DOSAGE CALCULATIONS

When you have two measurements that are in different systems, dosage calculation becomes a two-step problem similar to the proportion calculations presented in Chapter 3. First find how the two measurements are related to one another.

The equivalent tables shown earlier will help convert one measurement into another. For example, dextromethorphan comes in solutions of 3.5 mg per 5 mL (or written as a ratio of $\frac{3.5\ \text{mg}}{5\ \text{mL}}$). You want to give 7 mg, but you need the final dose expressed in teaspoons. How do you determine how many teaspoons to give?

The Household-to-Metric Equivalents table (see Box 4-2) tells us that 1 tsp = 5 mL.

Step 1: Convert the system you *have* into the system you *want* using proportion calculations.

$$1\ \text{tsp} = 5\ \text{mL, then } 3.5\ \text{mg} = 5\ \text{mL} = 1\ \text{tsp}$$

Step 2: Plug the numbers into the formula for liquids.

$$\frac{Want}{Have} \times Liquid = \frac{7\ \text{mg}}{3.5\ \text{mg}} \times 1\ \text{tsp} = 2\ \text{tsp}$$

DIMENSIONAL ANALYSIS

Instead of using ratio and proportion to solve dosage problems, some people use dimensional analysis. **Dimensional analysis** is a method of comparing and equating different physical aspects and quantities by using simple algebraic rules along with known conversion factors (called *equivalency ratios*). Although this type of mathematical calculation is more commonly used in engineering computations when several different dimensions are being compared, it can be applied to dosage calculations; however, it does require additional steps. Only physical quantities measuring the same phenomenon can be solved this way; physical quantities such as length, speed, weight, and, importantly, dosage size conversions can be determined using this math problem-solving technique. Dimensional analysis is often used to convert from one set of measurement units to another set of units via conversion factors in such a way that unwanted units are canceled out and a person comfortable with the calculation can always account for these units.

A simple example of this method is how many pounds are in 20 kilograms of a given substance? One kilogram is equivalent to 2.2 lb (in medical measurement), so

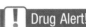

Drug Alert!

Administration Alert

To prevent insulin dose errors, check the specific markings on the syringe rather than relying on the color of the cap, needle hub, or box label.

QSEN: Safety

Drug Alert!

Administration Alert

Always write out the word *unit* or the words *international units*.

QSEN: Safety

Try This!

TT-8 Calculate how many milliliters you should give.
a. *Want* heparin 7500 units subcutaneously; *Have* heparin 10,000 units/mL
b. *Want* heparin 1000 units; *Have* heparin 5000 units/mL
c. *Want* heparin 300 units/kg body weight; *Have* heparin 20,000 units/mL. The patient weighs 250 lb.
   Answers are at the end of this chapter.

Try This!

TT-9 Calculate how many milligrams in how many teaspoons you should give to an infant who weighs 7 lb.
   Want amoxicillin 50 mg/kg; *Have* amoxicillin 50 mg/mL (Remember to round up or down.)
   Answers are at the end of this chapter.

the conversion factor from kilograms to pounds is 2.2 pounds per kilogram (2.2 lb/kg). So multiplying the 20 kilograms by the conversion factor, 20 kg × 2.2 lb/kg, or expressed as the following equation:

$$\frac{20\ kg}{1} \times \frac{2.2\ lb}{1\ kg}\ (\text{now cancel out the kg because this unit is in both the}$$

$$\text{numerator and the denominator}),\ \frac{20}{1} \times \frac{2.2\ lb}{1} = \frac{44\ lb}{1} = 44\ lb$$

As you can see, the kilogram unit is canceled out through simple algebra.

What about going the other way? How many kilograms are in 315 pounds? Flip the conversion factor over, so 1 kg/2.2 lb, multiply the weight in pounds by the new conversion factor, 315 lb × 1 kg/2.2 lb, which results in 143.2 kg. The equation would look like this:

$$\frac{315\ lb}{1} \times \frac{1\ kg}{2.2\ lb}\ (\text{cancel the pound units}) = \frac{315}{1} \times \frac{1\ kg}{2.2} = \frac{315\ kg}{2.2} = 143.2\ kg$$

Once again, the weight unit (this time pounds unit) was factored out.

These two simple examples highlight how this method could be used for longer problems and how it allows the practitioner to keep an eye on the units involved.

Here is a dosage example:

A patient who weighs 220 lb is prescribed a dose of medication at 12.5 mg/kg of body weight. The concentration of the medication on hand is 125 mg/mL, and the patient wants to take the medication orally, by teaspoon. How many teaspoons of medication will the patient need to take per dose?

Use the following dimensional analysis steps for the conversions and accounting:

Step 1: 1 kg = 2.2 lb, so the weight conversion ratio is 1 kg/2.2 lb; the patient weighs 100 kg, 220 lb × 1 kg/2.2 lb or

$$\frac{220\ lb}{1} \times \frac{1\ kg}{2.2\ lb} = \text{the patient weighs 100 kg}$$

Step 2: The weight (amount) of medication needed based on body mass is 12.5 mg/kg × 100 kg = 1250 mg or

$$\frac{12.5\ mg/kg}{1} \times \frac{100\ kg}{1} = \frac{1250\ mg}{1} = 1250\ mg$$

Step 3: 1 tsp = 5 mL, so the volumetric conversion ratio is 5 mL/tsp
The concentration in teaspoons is now 125 mg/mL × 5 mL/tsp = 625 mg/tsp or

$$\frac{125\ mg}{1\ mL} \times \frac{5\ mL}{1\ tsp}\ (\text{cancel out the mL}) = \frac{625\ mg}{1\ tsp} = 625\ mg/tsp$$

Step 4: The final dose in teaspoons is 1250 mg divided by 625 mg/tsp = 2 tsp or

$$\frac{1250\ mg}{625\ mg/tsp}\ (\text{cancel out the mg}) = \frac{1250}{625/tsp} = 2\ teaspoons$$

Steps 1 and 3 were conversions in which dimensional analysis was explicitly used. Steps 2 and 4 were simple calculations, but using dimensional analysis to solve for them allows for a higher degree of accountability and understanding of the units involved.

 Try This!

TT-10 Using dimensional analysis and showing your work, calculate the dosages for these problems.
a. Heparin 25 units is ordered to be administered subcutaneously. The solution available is heparin 40 units/mL. How many mL of this solution should be administered to equal the correct ordered dose?
b. A patient (an infant) who weighs 22 lb is prescribed to receive 50,000 units of penicillin intravenously per kg of weight. The penicillin solution you have on hand is 1,000,000 units/50 mL. How many mL should you give by IV injection?
Answers are at the end of this chapter.

Get Ready for Practice!

Key Points

- A liquid ounce is not equal to a dry ounce.
- Always double check the amount of drug in a measuring device with the amount ordered to prevent giving an overdose.
- The apothecary measurement system is less precise and not used for drug measurement in North America.
- The household measurement system is not as precise as the metric system.
- Do not substitute one type of potassium for another.
- When calculating doses for drugs that are manufactured in milliequivalents or units, determine the amount of tablets or milliliters to administer based on what you *want* versus what you *have* on hand, in the same way as for drugs manufactured in milligrams.
- To prevent insulin dose errors, check the specific markings on the syringe rather than going by the color of the cap, needle hub, or box label.
- Always write out the word *unit* or the words *international units* rather than using abbreviations.

Additional Learning Resources

evolve Be sure to visit your Evolve website (http://evolve.elsevier.com/Workman/pharmacology/) for additional online resources.

SG Go to your Study Guide for additional learning activities to help you master this chapter content.

Review Questions

See the Answer Keys—In-text Review Questions for answers to these questions.

1. Which measure or amount is closest to 1 fluid dram?
   - A. 1 fluid ounce
   - B. 1 tablespoon
   - C. 1 teaspoon
   - D. 16 minims
2. A patient is to receive 650 mg of aspirin. How many grains would this be?
   - A. 5
   - B. 10
   - C. 30
   - D. 65
3. If there are 60 gtts in a teaspoon, how many gtts are there in a tablespoon?
   - A. 600
   - B. 300
   - C. 180
   - D. 120
4. You prepare to mix dry amoxicillin into a solution by adding 150 mL of water to the bottle containing the dry amoxicillin. How many ounces of water will you add to the bottle?
   - A. 5
   - B. 10
   - C. 30
   - D. 50

5. A patient is to take 30 mg of a drug that comes as 5 mg/tsp. How many tablespoons is this? _____ Tbs
6. Which unit is the basic measure of liquid in the metric system?
   - A. Dram
   - B. Gram
   - C. Liter
   - D. Meter
7. Which weight is the *smallest*?
   - A. 1 kg
   - B. 10 mg
   - C. 100 mcg
   - D. 1000 g
8. Convert 0.7 L into milliliters. _____ mL
9. The patient weighs 115 lb. Convert this weight to kilograms. _____ kg
10. The drug and dose prescribed is cortisol 40 mg by injection. The dose available is 50 mg/mL. How many milliliters will you draw up into the syringe? _____ mL
11. The patient is to receive 15,000 units of heparin intravenously. The vial contains heparin 20,000 units/mL. How many milliliters will you draw up into the syringe? _____ mL

Answers to *Math Check!* Problems

MC-1 Convert the Fahrenheit temperature to Centigrade and the Centigrade to Fahrenheit.
a. 101.4°F = 38.6°C
b. 40°C = 104°F

MC-2
a. Using the formula of 1 grain is equal to 65 mg, calculate the dosage in mg for 5 grains of aspirin. <u>325</u> mg
b. How many minims are in 2 fluid drams? <u>130</u> minims

MC-3
Calculate the response in teaspoons or drops. (Note: "How to" math steps for conversion of *want* versus *have* problems are in Chapter 3.)
a. *Want* Benadryl 2.5 mg; *Have* Benadryl 12.5 mg/5 mL <u>15</u> drops (gtts) or 1 mL
b. *Want* acetaminophen 200 mg; *Have* acetaminophen 40 mg/mL <u>1</u> teaspoon

MC-4 Convert the following weights in pounds to kilograms and the weights in kilograms to pounds.
a. 25 lb = 11.36 kg
b. 275 lb = 125 kg
c. 45 kg = 99 lb
d. 80 kg = 176 lb

MC-5 Convert these household measures into metric equivalents, rounding to the nearest tenth when necessary.
a. 2 tablespoons = 30 mL
b. 8.8 lb = 4 kg
c. 14 inches = 35.56 cm
d. 4 ounces (liquid) = 120 mL
e. 5 teaspoons = 25 mL

MC-6 Convert these metric measures into household equivalents.
a. 70 kg = 154 lb
b. 150 mL = 5 ounces
c. 75 g = 2.5 ounces (dry weight)
d. 500 mL = 1 pint liquid

MC-7 Calculate how much drug you should administer.
a. *Want* potassium 15 mEq in extended-release tablet; *Have* potassium 5 mEq in extended-release tablet. Administer three tablets.
b. *Want* potassium gluconate 30 mEq oral solution; *Have* potassium gluconate 20 mEq/15 mL oral solution. Administer 22.5 mL.

MC-8 Calculate how many milliliters you should give.
a. *Want* heparin 750 units subcutaneously; *Have* heparin 1000 units/mL. Give 0.75 mL.
b. *Want* heparin 750 units intravenously; *Have* heparin 500 units/mL. Give 1.5 mL.

MC-9 Calculate how many milligrams in how many teaspoons you will give to a child who weighs 28.6 lb. *Want* acyclovir 20 mg/kg. Have acyclovir 200 mg/5 mL oral suspension.
A 28.6-lb child weighs 13 kg. Total dose wanted = 13 (kg) × 20 (mg) = 260 mg.
If 5 mL contain 200 mg, then 1 mL contains 40 mg. 260 mg divided by 40 mg/mL = 6.5 mL of drug to be administered.

MC-10 Using dimensional analysis and showing your work, calculate the dosages for these problems.
a. Dilantin (phenytoin) 100 mg is prescribed to give a child orally. The drug available is Dilantin 125 mg/5 mL. How many milliliters of this solution should be administered to equal the ordered dose?

$$\frac{100\ mg}{1} \div \frac{125\ mg}{5\ mL} = \frac{100\ mg}{1} \times \frac{5\ ml}{125\ mg}\ (\text{cancel the mg})$$

$$= \frac{500\ ml}{125} = 4\ mL$$

b. A patient who weighs 154 lb is prescribed to receive 50,000 units of penicillin intravenously per kilogram of weight. The penicillin solution you have on hand is 1,000,000 units/25 mL. How many milliliters should you give by IV injection?
Step 1 Convert the patient's weight in pounds to kilograms.

$$\frac{154\ lb}{1} \times \frac{1\ kg}{2.2\ lb}\ (\text{cancel the pounds}) = \frac{154\ kg}{2.2} = 70\ kg$$

Step 2 Calculate the amount of penicillin needed based on the patient's weight in kilograms.

$$\frac{50,000\ units}{1\ kg} \times \frac{70\ kg}{1}\ (\text{cancel out the kilograms})$$

$$= \frac{3,500,000\ units}{1} = 3,500,000\ units$$

Step 3 Convert penicillin to units per milliliter.

25 mL = 1,000,000 units. So 1,000,000 divided by 25 = 40,000 units per mL.

$$\frac{1,000,000\ units}{25\ mL} = 40,000\ units\ per\ mL$$

Step 4 Using the conversion factor of 40,000 units per milliliter, the desired dose of 50,000 units/kg, and the patient's weight in kilograms, calculate the volume of drug to administer in milliliters. Multiply the patient's weight by 50,000 units and divide the total by 40,000 = 87.5 mL.

$$\frac{50,000\ units}{1} \times \frac{70\ kg}{1} = 3,500,000\ units\ \frac{3,500,000\ units}{40,000\ units/mL}$$

(cancel out the units) = 87.5 mL

Answers to *Try This!* Problems

TT-1 Convert the Fahrenheit temperature to Centigrade and the Centigrade to Fahrenheit.
a. 97°F = 36.1°C
b. 103.8°F = 39.9°C
c. 35°C = 95°F
d. 39.2°C = 102.6°F

TT-2 Convert the apothecary measures into metric equivalents and the metric equivalents into apothecary measures.
a. 1/4th of a grain is how many mg?
   15 mg
b. 8 minims is how many milliliters?
   0.5 mL
c. 60 mL is how many fluid drams?
   16 fluid drams
d. 2 grams is how many grains?
   30 grains

TT-3 Calculate the response in teaspoons or drops.
a. *Want* ampicillin 500 mg; *Have* ampicillin 250 mg/tsp
   2 tsp = 500 mg
b. *Want* guaifenesin 50 mg; *Have* guaifenesin 100 mg per 60 gtts
   50 mg in 30 gtts or in 0.5 tsp
c. *Want* milk of magnesia 1 Tbs; *Have* milk of magnesia 1 tsp
   3 tsp of milk of magnesia = 1 Tbs

TT-4 Convert the following weights in pounds to kilograms and the weights in kilograms to pounds.
a. 98 lb = 44.5 kg
b. 52 lb = 23.6 kg
c. 315 lb = 143.2 kg
d. 2.9 lb = 1.3 kg
e. 147 lb = 66.8 kg
f. 68 kg = 149.6 lb
g. 12 kg = 26.4 lb
h. 122 kg = 268.4 lb
i. 52 kg = 114.4 lb
j. 80 kg = 176 lb

TT-5 Convert these household measures in metric equivalents, rounding to the nearest tenth when necessary.
a. 250 lb = 113.6 kg
b. 12 oz (liquid) = 360 mL
c. 17 in = 43.2 cm
d. 4 Tbs = 60 mL
e. 2 tsp = 10 mL

TT-6 Convert these metric measures into household equivalents.
a. 45 g = 1.5 oz (dry weight)
b. 90 mL = 3 oz
c. 1500 mL = 1 qt and 1 pt, or 6 c
d. 100 kg = 220 lb
e. 780 g = 1.7 lb

TT-7 Calculate how much drug you should administer.
a. *Want* potassium 16 mEq in extended-release tablet; *Have* potassium 8 mEq in an extended-release tablet

$$\text{Give two extended-release tablets.}$$

b. *Want* potassium 10 mEq effervescent tablet; *Have* potassium 20 mEq scored effervescent tablet

$$\text{Give one half } (\tfrac{1}{2}) \text{ of the effervescent tablet.}$$

c. *Want* potassium 10 mEq in an oral solution; *Have* potassium 20 mEq dissolved in 8 oz of water as an oral solution

$$\text{Give 4 oz of the oral solution.}$$

TT-8 Calculate how many milliliters you should give.
a. *Want* heparin 7500 units subcutaneous; *Have* heparin 10,000 units/mL

$$\frac{7500}{10,000/\text{mL}} = \frac{75}{100} = 0.75\,\text{mL}$$

b. *Want* heparin 1000 units; *Have* heparin 5000 units/mL

$$\frac{1500}{5000/\text{mL}} = \frac{1}{5} = 0.2\,\text{mL}$$

c. *Want* heparin 300 units/kg body weight; *Have* heparin 20,000 units/mL. The patient weighs 250 lb.

$$250\,\text{lb} = 250 \text{ divided by } 2.2 = 113.6\,\text{kg, round to } 114\,\text{kg}$$

$$114\,\text{kg} \times 300\,\text{units} = \text{need } 34,200\,\text{units}$$

$$34,200 \text{ divided by } 20,000 = 1.71\,\text{mL, round to } 1.7\,\text{mL}$$

TT-9 Calculate how many milligrams in how many teaspoons you should give to an infant who weighs 7 lb.
Want amoxicillin 50 mg/kg; *Have* amoxicillin 50 mg/mL
 (Remember to round up or down.)

$$7\,\text{lb} = 3.18\,\text{kg, round to } 3.2\,\text{kg}$$

$$50\,\text{mg} \times 3.2\,\text{kg} = 160\,\text{mg; want } 160\,\text{mg}$$

$$5\,\text{mL} = 1\,\text{tsp}; 50\,\text{mg/mL} = 250\,\text{mg/5 mL (1 tsp)}$$

$$\frac{160}{250} \times 1\,\text{tsp} = 0.64\,\text{tsp; not easy to measure, better to use}$$
$$\text{a medicine dropper (in mL)}$$

$$\frac{Want}{Have} \times 1\,\text{mL} = \frac{160\,\text{mg}}{50\,\text{mg}} \times 1\,\text{mL} = 3.2\,\text{mL}$$

TT-10 Using dimensional analysis and showing your work, calculate the dosages for these problems.
a. Heparin 25 units is ordered to be administered subcutaneously. The solution available is heparin 40 units/mL. How many milliliters of this solution should be administered to equal the correct ordered dose?

$$\frac{25\,\text{units}}{1} \div \frac{40\,\text{units}}{1\,\text{mL}} = \frac{25\,\text{units}}{1} \times \frac{1\,\text{mL}}{40\,\text{units}}$$

$$(\text{cancel out the units}) = \frac{25\,\text{mL}}{40} = 0.625\,\text{mL}$$

$$\text{Round down to 0.6 mL.}$$

b. A patient (infant) who weighs 22 lb is prescribed to receive 50,000 units of penicillin intravenously per kg of weight. The penicillin solution you have on hand is 1,000,000 units/50 mL. How many milliliters should you give by intravenous injection?
Step 1: Convert the patient's weight in pounds to kilograms.

$$\frac{22\,\text{lb}}{1} \times \frac{1\,\text{kg}}{2.2\,\text{lb}} \ (\text{cancel out the lb}) = \frac{22}{1} \times \frac{1\,\text{kg}}{2.2} = \frac{22\,\text{kg}}{2.2} = 10\,\text{kg}$$

Step 2: Calculate the amount of penicillin needed based on the infant's body mass.

$$\frac{50,000\,\text{units}}{1\,\text{kg}} \times \frac{10\,\text{kg}}{1} \ (\text{cancel out the kg}) = \frac{50,000\,\text{units}}{1} \times \frac{10}{1}$$
$$= 500,000\,\text{units}$$

Step 3: Convert penicillin to units per milliliter.

$$50\,\text{mL} = 1,000,000 \text{ units. So } 1,000,000 \text{ divided by}$$
$$50 = 20,000 \text{ units per mL.}$$

$$\frac{1,000,000\,\text{units}}{50\,\text{mL}} = 20,000 \text{ units per mL}$$

Step 4: Using the conversion factor of 20,000 units per milliliter, the desired dose of 50,000 units/kg, and the infant's weight in kilograms, calculate the volume of drug to administer in milliliters. Multiply the patient's weight by 50,000 units and divide the total by 20,000
= 25 mL.

$$\frac{50,000\,\text{units}}{1} \times \frac{10}{1} = 500,000\,\text{units} \quad \frac{500,000\,\text{units}}{20,000\,\text{units/mL}}$$
$$(\text{cancel out the units}) = 25\,\text{mL}$$

Dosage Calculation of Intravenous Solutions and Drugs

Objectives

After studying this chapter you should be able to:

1. Identify three common problems of intravenous (IV) therapy.
2. Explain how the size of an IV fluid drop determines the flow rate for IV fluid infusion.
3. List the parts of an order for IV fluids that are necessary to determine the correct infusion rate.
4. Correctly calculate IV drug infusion problems when provided with the volume, hours to be infused, and drip factor.
5. Use the "15-second" rule to determine an IV flow rate.
6. List the required parts of a valid IV therapy order.

Key Terms

administration set (ăd-mĭn-ĭ-STRĀ-shŭn SĔT) (p. 77) The tubing and drip chamber used to administer an IV drip.

drip chamber (DRĬP CHĂM-bŭr) (p. 77) The clear cylinder of plastic attached to the IV tubing. It is filled no more than halfway so you can see the fluid dripping.

drip rate (DRĬP RĀT) (p. 78) The number of drops per minute needed to make an IV solution infuse in the prescribed amount of time.

drop factor (DRŎP FĂK-tŭr) (p. 77) The number of drops (gtts) needed to make 1 mL of IV fluid. The larger the drop, the fewer drops needed to make 1 mL.

duration (dŭr-Ā-shŭn) (p. 76) How long in minutes or hours an IV infusion is ordered to run.

extravasation (ĕks-tră-vă-SĀ-shŭn) (p. 79) Condition in which an IV needle or catheter pulls from the vein and causes

tissue damage by leaking irritating IV fluids into the surrounding tissue.

flow rate (FLŌ RĀT) (p. 77) How fast an IV infusion is prescribed to run—the number of mL delivered in 1 hour.

infiltration (ĭn-fĭl-TRĀ-shŭn) (p. 79) Condition in which an IV needle or catheter pulls from the vein and begins to leak IV fluids into the surrounding tissue, resulting in tissue swelling.

infuse (infusion) (ĭn-FYŪZ) (p. 76) To run IV fluids into the body.

volume (VŎL-yŭm) (p. 76) Amount of fluids ordered (for example, 1000 mL).

VI (p. 78) IV pump abbreviation for "volume infused."

VTBI (p. 78) IV pump abbreviation for "volume to be infused."

OVERVIEW

Administering intravenous (IV) fluids (IV therapy) is another parenteral drug delivery method. When delivered intravenously, the fluids, along with any drugs, go directly into a vein and thus *immediately* into the bloodstream. This process is called an **infusion**, which means to run (**infuse**) IV fluids into the body. IV fluids may be given alone to hydrate the patient, or they may be used to place drugs directly into the patient's system. The **volume** is the amount of fluids ordered, and the **duration** is how long in minutes or hours an IV infusion is ordered to run.

Fluids given intravenously (by IV) are also used for drugs that would not be absorbed if taken by mouth. However, because IV drugs act immediately, there is the potential for an immediate and severe problem if there is an adverse drug reaction. As discussed in Chapter 1, an *adverse drug reaction* is a severe, unusual, or life-threatening patient response to a drug that requires intervention.

How fast an IV infusion is prescribed to run depends on the reason for having it. For example, if a patient is dehydrated, the prescriber might want to run the fluids faster than if the IV is present just in case a problem occurs. So not only must you

Memory Jogger

IV infusions are ideal for drugs or fluids that:
- Must get into the patient's system quickly.
- Need to be given at a steady rate.
- Are patient controlled (such as IV drugs for pain).

know how fast an IV is prescribed to run, you must know *why* IV therapy was prescribed.

IV MECHANICS

The IV **flow rate** is how fast the IV infusion is prescribed to run (that is, the number of milliliters delivered in 1 hour). The rate of an IV depends on the diameter of the tubing. Compare the tubing to a straw. A fat straw will suck up a larger amount of soda in 10 seconds compared with a thinner straw in the same 10 seconds. When you use your finger to make the soda drip out of the straw, the fatter the straw, the larger the drop. Ten fat drops have more fluid in them than 10 thin drops. The same principle applies to IV fluids. Tubing with a larger diameter will let bigger drops into the vein and a larger amount of fluid into the body. The number of drops needed to make a milliliter of fluid is called the **drop factor.**

The diameter of the tubing varies according to the tubing manufacturer. Tubing sizes are divided into macrodrip and microdrip and have different types of drip chambers. A **drip chamber** is the clear cylinder of plastic attached to the IV tubing. It is filled not quite halfway so you can see the fluid dripping (Figure 5-1). The complete set of tubing and drip chamber used to administer an IV is the **administration set.** A *microdrip* tubing set delivers very small drops. It is most often used for children, older patients, and patients who cannot tolerate a fast infusion rate or a high volume of fluids. On the other hand, *macrodrip* sets deliver larger drops and are used when fast infusion rates or larger quantities of fluids or drugs are needed. Figure 5-1 shows the difference in drop size between a macrodrip chamber and a microdrip chamber.

Each company puts its drop factor (sometimes called *drip factor*) on every IV fluid administration set. Depending on the brand, macrodrip tubing delivers 10 drops/mL, 15 drops/mL, or 20 drops/mL. Every microdrip tubing is 60 drops/mL, regardless of who makes it. *You must use the drop factor in every IV calculation.* Figure 5-2 shows different IV tubing administration sets. Administration sets for blood transfusions are larger to prevent damage to blood cells and also have some differences in the drip chamber. This chapter does not discuss administering blood or blood products; however, flow rate calculations for any blood product are the same as for any other type of IV fluid.

IV drug therapy is an invasive procedure that requires a prescriber's order (prescription). Always double check the order before starting the procedure. Remember that the order must contain the specific drug or IV solution to be infused, the dosage or volume, the duration, and the rate of infusion.

Memory Jogger

The larger the diameter of the IV tubing, the larger the drops.

Memory Jogger

For an order to start IV therapy to be valid, it must contain the specific drug or IV solution to be infused, the dosage or volume, the duration, and the rate of infusion.

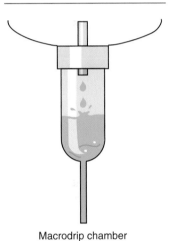

Macrodrip chamber

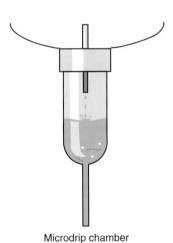

Microdrip chamber

FIGURE 5-1 Drop size differences between a macrodrip chamber and a microdrip chamber on IV tubing.

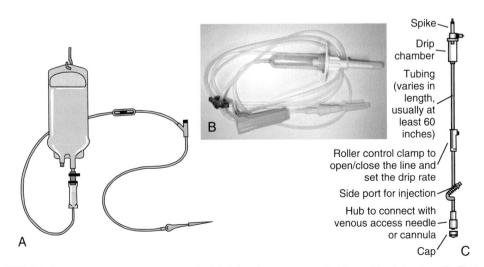

Spike

Drip chamber

Tubing (varies in length, usually at least 60 inches)

Roller control clamp to open/close the line and set the drip rate

Side port for injection

Hub to connect with venous access needle or cannula

Cap

A   B   C

FIGURE 5-2 IV tubing administration sets. **A,** Administration set connected to an IV solution bag. **B,** Photo of an actual IV tubing administration set. **C,** Detail of IV tubing administration set.

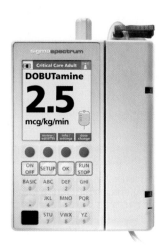

FIGURE 5-3 Example of an IV infusion pump. (Copyright © Baxter Healthcare Corp., Deerfield, IL)

 Memory Jogger

The four basic parts of IV fluid regulation are what type of fluid, how much (volume), for how long (duration), and how fast the fluids should be infused (rate).

 Memory Jogger

Adding the VI and the VTBI should equal the total amount of fluid that was in the bag when it was first hung.

REGULATING IV FLUIDS

IV therapy involves calculating the **drip rate,** the number of drops per minute needed to make the IV infuse in the prescribed amount of time. Calculations for drip rates are precise and must be made carefully. Although IV infusion rates can be controlled by adjusting the roller clamp, the vast majority of IV fluids today are regulated by either a pump or a controller. A *controller* is a simple device that uses gravity to control the flow of an IV. An *IV infusion pump* is a computer-based machine that pushes fluid into the vein by low pressure. The buttons used to program an IV pump are much like the ones you use to work the remote control to your television. Figure 5-3 shows an example of an IV infusion pump. All pumps have at least the following buttons:

- **ON/OFF** switch
- **Start/Enter**
- **STOP**
- **Delete or Clear**
- **Direction arrows:** ↑↓→←
- **Silence (MUTE)**
- **IV lock** (prevents patients and visitors from tampering with the IV pump)
- **Primary** (controller for the main IV bag—the bag hanging at the lowest point)
- **IVPB** (piggyback or secondary bag controller—the bag hanging at the highest point)

Because each brand of control device differs, always read and follow the manufacturer's directions. Even if you are not directly responsible for starting or maintaining the IV infusion, you may be responsible for checking that it is running smoothly and on time.

To understand the basics of IV fluid regulation, you need to understand these four important concepts:

- *What:* What type of fluid should be infused
- *Volume:* How much of the fluid should be infused
- *Duration:* For how long the fluid should be infused
- *Rate:* How fast the fluid should be infused

For example, a prescription reads "1000 mL of normal saline (NS) to be infused over 8 hours." The order already gives you the "What," "Volume," and "Duration." Using this information, you can determine the flow rate. As you prepare the IV infusion, check the clock to determine the start and stop time.

Once you know what type of fluids to give, how much, and for how long, you can use this information to program the pump. Just remember that the accuracy of the pump depends on the information that you punch into it. Remember "GIGO!": "Garbage in, garbage out!" *If you make an error programming the pump, at least one factor will be incorrect, and a drug administration error will result.*

Be sure to understand all the abbreviations that are used and that may show up on the IV monitor screen. For example, a pump may use the abbreviations "VI" and "VTBI." The **VI** stands for "volume infused" and tells you how much has been infused up to that minute. **VTBI** means the "volume to be infused" or the amount that is left in the bag at any point. As the VI increases, the VTBI decreases. At any given time, if you add what has been infused (VI) to what is left in the bag (VTBI), you should have the total amount of fluid that was prescribed.

How will you know how much is really in the IV bag at any time during the infusion? Figure 5-4 shows a standard IV bag for NS (0.9% saline in water). In this illustration, the black markings on the clear plastic bag are repeated in the box next to the bag so that you can read them more easily. Note that there are numbers with horizontal lines going down the right side of the bag (and the label). These numbers indicate how much fluid has been infused from the bag. For example, if the fluid line of solution in the bag is even with the line next to the number 4, 400 mL have been infused, and 600 mL (1000 mL − 400 mL) remain in the bag to be infused.

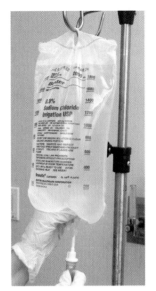

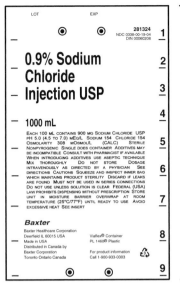

LOT   EXP

281324
NDC 0338-00-19-04
DIN 00060208

0.9% Sodium Chloride Injection USP

1000 mL

EACH 100 mL CONTAINS 900 mg SODIUM CHLORIDE USP PH 5.0 (4.5 TO 7.0) mEQ/L SODIUM 154 CHLORIDE 154 OSMOLARITY 308 mOSMOL/L (CALC) STERILE NONPYROGENIC SINGLE DOSE CONTAINER ADDITIVES MAY BE INCOMPATIBLE CONSULT WITH PHARMACIST IF AVAILABLE WHEN INTRODUCING ADDITIVES USE ASEPTIC TECHNIQUE MIX THOROUGHLY DO NOT STORE DOSAGE INTRAVENOUSLY AS DIRECTED BY A PHYSICIAN SEE DIRECTIONS CAUTIONS SQUEEZE AND INSPECT INNER BAG WHICH MAINTAINS PRODUCT STERILITY DISCARD IF LEAKS ARE FOUND MUST NOT BE USED IN SERIES CONNECTIONS DO NOT USE UNLESS SOLUTION IS CLEAR FEDERAL (USA) LAW PROHIBITS DISPENSING WITHOUT PRESCRIPTION STORE UNIT IN MOISTURE BARRIER OVERWRAP AT ROOM TEMPERATURE (25°C/77°F) UNTIL READY TO USE AVOID EXCESSIVE HEAT SEE INSERT

Baxter

Baxter Healthcare Corporation
Deerfield IL 60015 USA
Made in USA
Distributed in Canada by
Baxter Corporation
Toronto Ontario Canada

Viaflex® Container
PL 1460® Plastic

For product information
Call 1-900-933-0303

1 2 3 4 5 6 7 8 9

These numbers correspond to the volume (× 100) already infused. So, when the fluid level in the bag is even with the number 4, 400 mL of the solution has infused and 600 mL remains in the bag.

FIGURE 5-4 An IV solution bag (1000 mL) with the label from the bag enlarged and illustrated on the right. (Photo from Perry, A., & Potter, P. (2009). *Clinical nursing skills & techniques* (7th ed.) St. Louis: Mosby.)

Mark the top line of the bag with the *start time* (the actual time when the IV infusion is started) and put a thick line with a pen or marker on the bag in 1-hour segments down the volume line, just like a ruler. Each hour marked should be right next to the volume to be infused for that hour. End with the *stop time*, the time when the IV bag is supposed to be empty (fluid is totally infused).

Always calculate both the start and stop times, and mark the IV bag, even when it is on a controller or pump. Many things can happen to disturb the flow rate. For example, the tubing may kink, or the IV needle may get out of place and lead to infiltration. **Infiltration** is a condition that occurs when an IV needle or catheter pulls from the vein and begins to leak (infiltrate) IV fluids into the surrounding tissue. This condition prevents the patient from receiving the right dose of fluid or drug and causes swelling in the surrounding tissues. When the fluid or drug that infiltrates is irritating and leads to tissue damage or loss, the condition is called **extravasation**. Figure 5-5 shows the appearance of the tissue around an IV infusion that has infiltrated and the appearance of tissue where extravasation has occurred.

Never speed up an IV infusion to make up for lost time when the infusion is behind schedule. Playing "catch up" can cause fluids to enter the patient too quickly. This can lead to fluid overload and other complications.

An IV infusion on a pump or controller can develop flow problems just as an IV without a pump can. A controller stops dripping if it encounters an obstruction. On the other hand, a pump actually uses pressure to push the drops in to get past the blockage. *This means that pumps can continue to push in drops even if the needle is no longer in the vein.* Thus if an infiltration has occurred, a controller stops, but a pump continues to push IV fluid into the surrounding tissue. All pumps have a set limit to the pressure that can be used. This limit is displayed on the IV screen (for example, "Limit 600 mm Hg" [millimeters of mercury]). If the IV pump has to exert more pressure than the 600 mm Hg of pressure that was set to force the fluid into the vein, it will BEEP—loudly!

IV CALCULATIONS

For you to correctly calculate the flow rate, every IV prescription must include (1) the total volume to be infused, and (2) the length of time the IV should run (in hours). You can then use the particular drop factor of the tubing that you are using to calculate how many *drops per minute* are needed to make the IV infuse in the ordered

---

! Drug Alert!

Administration Alert

Always calculate both the start and stop times and then mark the IV bag, even when the IV is on a controller or pump.

QSEN: Safety

Clinical Pitfall

Never speed up an IV to make up for lost time when the infusion is behind schedule.

QSEN: Safety

Memory Jogger

If an infiltration has occurred, a controller stops, but a pump can continue to push IV fluid into the surrounding tissue.

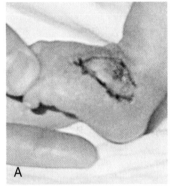

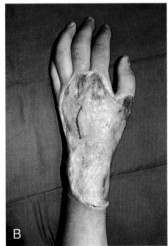

FIGURE 5-5 Appearances of tissues after IV infiltration **(A)** and after extravasation **(B)**. (**A** from Hockenberry, M.J., & Wilson, D. (2006). *Wong's nursing care of infants and children* (8th ed.). St. Louis: Mosby; **B** from Weinzweig, J., & Weinzweig, N. (2005). *The mutilated hand*, St. Louis: Mosby.)

time. All IV rates that are controlled using the control roller or the control slide on the tubing are calculated by drops per minute. Some pump rates are calculated by drops per minute, and others are programmed by the pump computer in terms of milliliters per hour to be infused.

Now that you know the theory, let's work with the formula.

Macrodrip Formula

The basic formula for determining how fast to run an IV infusion is $\dfrac{\text{Drop factor}}{\text{Minutes}}$.

Now let's break it down to make it easier.

Step 1: An IV infusion of 1000 mL is prescribed to run for 8 hours.

First find out how many milliliters should run in 1 hour *(flow rate)*. It is much easier to work with 1 hour than with 8 hours!

$$\text{Divide 1000 by 8:} \frac{1000}{8} = 125 \text{ mL/1 hr. Does it make sense (DIMS)?}$$

Step 2: Now calculate how many drops per minute are needed to make the IV infuse at 125 mL/hr (or 125 mL/60 minutes). This depends on the drop factor (drops/mL) of the IV tubing and drip chamber.

$$\frac{\text{Volume (milliliters)}}{\text{Time (minutes)}} \times \text{Drop factor (drops/milliliters)} = \text{Drops per minute}$$

You check the label information on the administration set and find that the drop factor is 15.

$$\frac{125}{60} \times 15 = 2.08 \times 15 = 31.2 \text{ drops/minute, round down to 31 drops/minute.}$$

The Macrodrip Tubing Shortcut

Now that you know the macrodrip formula, here is a shorter way to calculate the drops per minute with macrodrip tubing. Because all of the diameters of tubing and drip chamber (10, 15, or 20) can be evenly divided into 60, you can use this relationship to calculate drip rates. Let's use these to calculate the original prescription of 1000 mL to infuse over 8 hours, which equals 125 mL/hr.

- Sets with 10 gtts/mL, divide milliliters per hour by 6 (because 6 × 10 = 60 minutes); 125 ÷ 6 = 12.5 drops/minute, round to 13 drops/minute
- Sets with 15 gtts/mL, divide milliliters per hour by 4 (because 4 × 15 = 60 minutes); 125 ÷ 4 = 31.2 drops/minute, round to 31 drops/minute
- Sets with 20 gtts/mL divide milliliters per hour by 3 (because 3 × 20 = 60 minutes); 125 ÷ 3 = 41.6 drops/minute, round to 42 drops/minute

Get the idea?

Microdrip Formula

The microdrip formula is much easier. When using microdrip tubing, the drop factor of 60 drops/mL is the same as the number of minutes in 1 hour (60). Using the same formula as for macrodrip, you can see that the two 60s cancel each other out.

$$\frac{125}{60} \times \frac{60}{1} \text{ (drop factor)} = \frac{125}{1} = 125 \text{ microdrops/minute}$$

This is why the flow rate for microdrip tubing always equals the drop rate. Just calculate the milliliters needed per hour, and you have the drops per minute!

The 15-Second Rule

To see if the drip rate (for example, 42 gtts/min) is accurate, technically you should stand at the bedside and count the drops in the drip chamber for a full minute. When you are busy, a minute can seem like a long time! Because a minute has 60 seconds,

Try This!

TT-1 Calculate the milliliters to be infused in 1 hour given each of the following prescriptions.
a. 500 mL in 4 hours
b. 250 mL in 1 hour
c. 1000 mL in 6 hours
d. 1000 mL in 24 hours
   Answers are at the end of this chapter.

Try This!

TT-2 Use the macrodrip tubing shortcut to calculate the drip rate for each of these prescriptions.
a. 1000 mL D₅W in 6 hours, drop factor 10
b. 500 mL lactated Ringer's in 5 hours, drop factor 15
c. 1000 mL NS in 24 hours, drop factor 20
   Answers are at the end of this chapter.

Try This!

TT-3 Calculate the drops per minute needed to get the right volume per hour for each of these prescriptions.
a. 500 mL D₅W in 24 hours with microdrip tubing
b. 1000 mL lactated Ringer's in 12 hours, drop factor = 15
c. 250 mL D₅W in 2 hours, drop factor = 20
   Answers are at the end of this chapter.

you can divide the drop rate by 4, round off the answer, and then count that number of drops for 15 seconds. Your answer will be close to what it would have been if you had counted for the whole 60 seconds. For example, if the drop rate is the 31 gtts/min using the macrodrip tubing shortcut, divide 31 by 4: $\dfrac{31}{4} = 7.75$, and round that up to 8.

If you count 8 gtts when you count for 15 seconds, the IV infusion rate is correct! Be sure to check the IV rate every time that you are in the room. It only takes 15 seconds! Remember that this method only works for *manually* controlled IV bags, not those on a pump.

Memory Jogger

Remember that the 15-second drip rate check works only for *manually* controlled IV bags, not those on a pump.

Try This!

TT-4 Calculate the 15-second drip rate for each of these problems.
a. 20 gtts/min
b. 56 gtts/min
c. 28 gtts/min
Answers are at the end of this chapter.

Get Ready for Practice!

Key Points

- Always double check the order before starting an IV infusion.
- For an order to start IV therapy to be valid, it must contain the specific drug or IV solution to be infused, the dosage or volume, the duration, and the rate of infusion.
- IV infusions are ideal for drugs or fluids that must get into the patient's system quickly, need to be given at a steady rate, or are patient controlled (such as IV drugs for pain).
- The four basic parts of IV regulation are what type of fluid, how much (volume), for how long (duration), and how fast the fluids should be infused (rate).
- The rate of an IV infusion depends on the diameter of the tubing. The larger the diameter of IV tubing, the larger the drops.
- Because each brand of IV pump or control device differs, always read and follow the manufacturer's directions.
- Always calculate both the start and stop times and then time-tape the IV bag, even when it is on a controller or pump.
- Never speed up an IV to make up for lost time when the infusion is behind schedule.
- Adding the VI and the VTBI should equal the total amount of fluid that was in the bag when it was first hung.
- Remember that the 15-second drip rate check works only for *manually* controlled IV bags, not those on a pump.

Additional Learning Resources

 Be sure to visit your Evolve website (http://evolve.elsevier.com/Workman/pharmacology/) for additional online resources.

SG Go to your Study Guide for additional learning activities to help you master this chapter content.

Review Questions

See the Answer Keys—In-text Review Questions for answers to these questions.

1. Which is a common health problem resulting from IV therapy?
   A. The patient is more likely to gain weight when receiving IV therapy.
   B. Adverse drug reactions happen more quickly with IV drugs.
   C. Patients are required to stay in bed during IV therapy.
   D. IV drugs cost more than oral drugs.
2. Why does a drop factor of 10 result in a faster infusion at the same number of drops per minute than a drop factor of 15?
   A. A drop factor of 10 is a bigger individual drop than a drop factor of 15.
   B. An infusion set with a drop factor of 10 has more drops per milliliter than an infusion set with a drop factor of 15.
   C. An infusion set with a drop factor of 10 has macrotubing, and an infusion set with a drop factor of 15 has microtubing.
   D. An infusion set with a drop factor of 15 has macrotubing, and an infusion set with a drop factor of 10 has microtubing.
3. Which parts of an order are needed to correctly calculate the flow rate?
   A. Drop factor, drop rate
   B. Specific fluid, number of hours
   C. Specific fluid, total volume to be infused
   D. Total volume to be infused, number of hours
4. Calculate the flow rate for 1000 mL of dextrose 5% in NS to be infused over 6 hours. The tubing that is available has a drop factor of 20 gtts/mL.
   _____ gtts/min

5. A patient's IV infusion is supposed to have a drip rate of 31 gtts/min. You count 6 gtts/15 seconds. What is your best action?
   A. Nothing; the IV flow rate is correct.
   B. Increase the drip rate to 8 gtts/15 seconds.
   C. Increase the drip rate to 10 gtts/15 seconds.
   D. Decrease the drip rate to 4 gtts/15 seconds.
6. Which parts of a written order for IV therapy are needed for it to be a valid order?
   A. Drop factor, flow rate, IV site
   B. Specific fluid, number of hours, drop rate
   C. Specific fluid, total volume to be infused, number of hours
   D. Total volume to be infused, number of hours, specific drop factor
7. Calculate the starting volume of an infusing solution that has a VI of 150 mL and a VTBI of 350 mL. _____mL

Critical Thinking Activities

See the Answer Keys—Critical Thinking Activities for answers to these activities.

The patient is a 10-lb infant who is dehydrated from vomiting. The order reads 240 mL NS IV over 4 hours.
1. What parts of this order make it valid?
2. What is the safest IV infusion drip chamber to use for this infusion with this patient? Explain the rationale for the safest choice.
3. Calculate the following using the safest drip chamber for this patient.
   a. mL/hour
   b. mL/min
   c. drops/min
   d. 15-second drip rate
4. Is this patient at risk for extravasation should the infusion infiltrate into the tissues? Explain why or why not.

Answers To *Try This!* Problems

TT-1 Calculate the milliliters to be infused in 1 hour given the following orders.

a. 500 mL in 4 hours: $\dfrac{500}{4}$ = 125 mL in 1 hour

b. 250 mL in 1 hour: $\dfrac{250}{1}$ = 250 mL in 1 hour

c. 1000 mL in 6 hours: $\dfrac{1000}{6}$ = 166.66 mL, round to 167 mL in 1 hour

d. 1000 mL in 24 hours: $\dfrac{1000}{24}$ = 41.66 mL, round to 42 mL in 1 hour

TT-2 Calculate the drip rate using the macrodrip tubing shortcut.
a. 1000 mL D$_5$W in 6 hours, drop factor 10:

$\dfrac{1000}{6}$ = 167 mL/hr ÷ 6 = 28 gtts/min

b. 500 mL lactated Ringer's in 5 hours, drop factor 15:

$\dfrac{500}{5}$ = 100 mL/hr ÷ 4 = 25 gtts/min

c. 1000 mL NS in 24 hours, drop factor 20:

$\dfrac{1000}{24}$ = 42 mL/hr ÷ 3 = 14 gtts/min

TT-3 Calculate the drops per minute needed to get the right volume per hour.
a. 500 mL D$_5$W in 24 hours with microdrip tubing

$\dfrac{500}{24}$ = 20.8 mL/hr, round up to 21 mL/hr and 21 gtts/min

b. 1000 mL lactated Ringer's in 12 hours, drop factor = 15

$\dfrac{1000}{12}$ = 83.33 mL/hr, round down to 83 mL per hour

$\dfrac{\text{Volume (milliliters)}}{\text{Time (minutes)}}$ × drop factor (drops per milliliter)

= drops per minute

$\dfrac{83}{60}$ × 15 = 1.38 × 15 = 20.7 gtts/min, round up to

21 gtts/min
c. 250 mL D$_5$W in 2 hours, drop factor = 20

$\dfrac{250}{2}$ = 125 mL/hr

$\dfrac{\text{Volume (milliliters)}}{\text{Time (minutes)}}$ × drop factor (drops per milliliter)

= drops per minute

$\dfrac{125}{60}$ = 2.08 × 20 = 41.6 gtts/min, round up to 42 gtts/min

TT-4 Calculate the 15-second drip rate for each of these problems.
a. 20 gtts/min = 5 gtts/15 seconds
b. 56 gtts/min = 14 gtts/15 seconds
c. 28 gtts/min = 7 gtts/15 seconds

chapter

Anti-Inflammatory Drugs

6

http://evolve.elsevier.com/Workman/pharmacology/

Objectives

After studying this chapter you should be able to:

1. List the names, actions, usual adult dosages, possible side effects, and adverse effects of commonly prescribed corticosteroids and nonsteroidal anti-inflammatory drugs (NSAIDs).
2. Describe what to do before and after giving corticosteroids and NSAIDs.
3. Explain what to teach patients taking corticosteroids and NSAIDS, including what to do, what not to do, and when to call the prescriber.
4. Describe life span considerations for corticosteroids and NSAIDs.
5. List the names, actions, usual adult dosages, possible side effects, and adverse reactions of commonly prescribed antihistamines and leukotriene inhibitors.

6. Describe what to do before and after giving antihistamines and leukotriene inhibitors.
7. Explain what to teach patients taking antihistamines or leukotriene inhibitors, including what to do, what not to do, and when to call the prescriber.
8. List the names, actions, usual adult dosages, possible side effects, and adverse effects of commonly prescribed disease-modifying antirheumatic drugs (DMARDs).
9. Describe what to do before and after giving DMARDs.
10. Explain what to teach patients taking DMARDs, including what to do, what not to do, and when to call the prescriber.
11. Describe life span considerations for DMARDs.

Key Terms

antihistamines (ăn-tē-HĬS-tĕ-mēnz) (p. 93) Drugs that reduce inflammation by preventing the inflammatory mediator histamine from binding to its receptor site; same as histamine blockers or histamine antagonists.

anti-inflammatory drugs (ăn-tī-ĭn-FLĂM-ĕ-tōr-ē DRŬGZ) (p. 85) Drugs that prevent or limit inflammatory responses to injury or invasion.

corticosteroids (kŏr-tĭ-kō-STĔR-ōydz) (p. 86) Drugs similar to natural cortisol that prevent or limit inflammation by slowing or stopping inflammatory mediator production.

disease-modifying antirheumatic drugs (dĭ-zēz MŎD-ĭ-fī-ĭng ăn-tĭ-ROO-mă-tĭk DRŬGZ) (p. 96) Drugs that reduce the

progression and tissue destruction of the inflammatory disease process by inhibiting tumor necrosis factor.

histamine (HĬS-tĕ-mēn) (p. 93) A chemical made by the body that binds to its receptor sites and causes inflammatory responses.

inflammation (ĭn-flă-MĀ-shŭn) (p. 83) A syndrome of tissue and blood vessel responses to injury or invasion.

nonsteroidal anti-inflammatory drugs (NSAIDs) (non-stĕr-ŌY-dŭl ăn-tī-ĭn-FLĂM-ĕ-tōr-ē DRŬGZ) (p. 89) Anti-inflammatory drugs that are not similar to cortisol but prevent or limit the tissue and blood vessel responses to injury or invasion by slowing the production of one or more inflammatory mediators.

Inflammation, also called the *inflammatory response*, is the normal reactions of tissues and blood vessels in response to injury or invasion. It is nonspecific, which means that the same tissue responses occur with any type of injury or invasion, regardless of the location on the body or what caused the response to start. Thus inflammation triggered by a scald burn to the hand is the same as inflammation triggered by bacteria in the middle ear. The size and severity of the inflammation depends on the intensity, severity, duration, and extent of the injury or invasion. For example, a splinter in the finger triggers inflammation only at the splinter site.

A burn injuring 60% of the skin surface triggers inflammation involving the entire body.

Inflammatory responses start tissue actions that cause visible and uncomfortable symptoms. Despite the discomfort, these actions are important in ridding the body of harmful organisms and helping repair damaged tissue. However, if the inflammatory response is excessive, tissue damage may result.

A confusing issue about inflammation is that this process occurs in response to tissue injury and invasion by organisms. An *infection* is an invasion of the body by microorganisms that cause harm. Infection usually occurs with inflammation, but inflammation can occur without infection. Examples of inflammation without infection include sprained joints and blisters. Examples of inflammation caused by noninfectious invasion include hay fever and other allergic reactions. Inflammation with infection includes appendicitis, viral hepatitis, and bacterial pneumonia, among many others. So inflammation does not always mean that an infection is present.

REVIEW OF RELATED PHYSIOLOGY AND PATHOPHYSIOLOGY

An inflammatory response is called a *syndrome* because it occurs in a predictable series of steps and stages. The response is the same, regardless of the triggering event. Responses at the tissue level cause the five signs and symptoms of inflammation: warmth, redness, swelling, pain, and decreased function.

STAGE I: VASCULAR

Stage I involves white blood cells (WBCs) and changes in blood vessels. Injured tissues and WBCs in the area release *mediators,* which are body chemicals such as histamine, leukotriene, prostaglandins, kinins, and cytokines that cause and prolong inflammatory responses. Some mediators act on blood vessels in the area of injury or invasion, causing changes. These changes include dilation of the blood vessels and capillary leak (also called *capillary leak syndrome*). These responses cause swelling, redness, and warmth of the tissues. The increased blood flow brings oxygen, nutrients, and more WBCs to injured tissues. Some mediators, such as bradykinin and substance P, cause pain. Other mediators work on WBCs to enhance and prolong the inflammatory response. These mediators include leukotriene and *tumor necrosis factor (TNF)*.

STAGE II: EXUDATE

In stage II large numbers of WBCs are created, and an *exudate* (tissue drainage) commonly called *pus* is formed. At this stage the total number of WBCs in the blood can increase up to five times above normal and indicates that an inflammatory response is taking place (see Table 1-5 in Chapter 1 for normal blood cell counts).

During this phase a cascade reaction starts to increase the inflammatory response (Figure 6-1). This action begins by converting fat from broken cell membranes into arachidonic acid, which then enters the cyclo-oxygenase (COX) pathway. *Cyclo-oxygenase (COX)* is an enzyme important in converting body chemicals into mediators of inflammation that continue the inflammatory response in the tissues. Many anti-inflammatory drugs stop this cascade by preventing COX from converting arachidonic acid into mediators.

STAGE III: TISSUE REPAIR

Although stage III is completed last, it begins at the time of injury. This process is very important in helping the injured tissue regain function. WBCs secrete chemicals that trigger the remaining healthy cells to divide. In tissues such as the heart that are unable to divide and replace damaged heart cells with new heart cells, WBCs trigger new blood vessel growth and scar tissue formation. Because scar tissue is only a patch and does not behave like normal tissue, loss of function occurs wherever damaged tissues are replaced with scar tissue.

Memory Jogger

Infection usually is accompanied by inflammation, but inflammation can occur without infection.

Memory Jogger

The five signs and symptoms of inflammation are warmth, redness, swelling, pain, and decreased function.

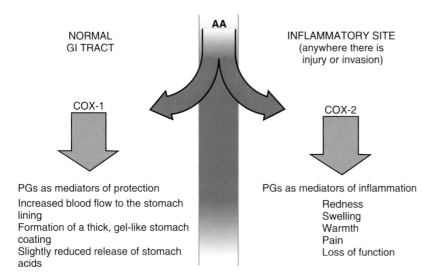

NORMAL
GI TRACT

AA

INFLAMMATORY SITE
(anywhere there is
injury or invasion)

COX-1

COX-2

PGs as mediators of protection
Increased blood flow to the stomach
lining
Formation of a thick, gel-like stomach
coating
Slightly reduced release of stomach
acids

PGs as mediators of inflammation
Redness
Swelling
Warmth
Pain
Loss of function

AA = Arachidonic acid PGs = Prostaglandins
COX-1 = Cyclo-oxygenase 1 COX-2 = Cyclo-oxygenase 2

FIGURE 6-1 Arachidonic acid cascade and mediator production.

This stage can be harmful if it lasts too long. For example, some diseases cause inflammation in the lungs and trigger scar tissue growth there. If too much scar tissue forms in the lungs, oxygen cannot enter the body, and the person dies of respiratory failure. When large amounts of TNF are released, such as in many chronic inflammatory diseases, tissues, especially bone and cartilage cells, are destroyed.

Although inflammation is an important protective response, it can cause problems. Inflammation is uncomfortable, reduces function while it is occurring, and can cause tissue damage if it is prolonged. **Anti-inflammatory drugs** that prevent or limit inflammatory responses to injury or invasion are prescribed to increase comfort and prevent tissue-damaging complications. These drugs are used as therapy for many common acute problems such as asthma, allergic reactions, and local or systemic irritation.

In addition to managing acute inflammatory problems, anti-inflammatory drugs can help manage autoimmune health problems. Autoimmunity is caused by inappropriate inflammatory and immune responses when WBC actions and products are directed against healthy normal cells and tissues. These responses are similar to normal inflammatory responses against invading organisms, but these reactions are now directed against normal body cells.

Examples of autoimmune diseases include systemic lupus erythematosus, polyarteritis nodosa, scleroderma, rheumatoid arthritis, autoimmune hemolytic anemia, psoriasis, and ankylosing spondylitis. For some of these diseases, tumor necrosis factor (TNF) causes progressive and permanent damage. Anti-inflammatory drugs are commonly used along with symptomatic treatment for autoimmune disorders.

Anti-inflammatory drugs also can help prevent rejection of transplanted organs. Because the transplanted organ is often donated by a person who is not an identical sibling to the *recipient* (person receiving the donated organ), the body considers the donated organ to be foreign material and generates inflammatory responses to destroy and remove it. Some anti-inflammatory drugs are used to suppress these responses so that the transplanted organ can continue to function in the recipient's body.

TYPES OF ANTI-INFLAMMATORY DRUGS

There are many anti-inflammatory drugs. Some must be prescribed, and others are available over the counter. The five main categories of anti-inflammatory

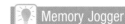
Memory Jogger

Excess scar tissue formation from prolonged inflammation is more harmful than helpful.

Memory Jogger

Types of drugs for treatment of inflammation are:

- Corticosteroids
- NSAIDs
- Antihistamines
- Leukotriene inhibitors
- DMARDs

Did You Know?

Your body makes corticosteroids as different types of cortisol.

Do Not Confuse

prednisoLONE *with* **predniSONE** *or* **methylprednisolone**

An order for prednisolone can be confused with prednisone or methylprednisolone. All three drugs are types of cortisol, but methylprednisolone is more potent and can be given parenterally. Prednisone is available in oral form only. Prednisolone is given orally and is more potent than prednisone.

QSEN: Safety

drugs include corticosteroids, nonsteroidal anti-inflammatory drugs (NSAIDs), antihistamines, leukotriene inhibitors, and disease-modifying antirheumatic drugs (DMARDs).

CORTICOSTEROIDS

Corticosteroids are drugs similar to natural cortisol that prevent or limit inflammation by slowing or stopping all known pathways of inflammatory mediator production. These drugs are the most powerful of all the drugs used for inflammation.

The cortisol that adrenal glands make has many functions necessary for life. Natural cortisol also helps control inflammatory responses. Corticosteroids may be taken in many ways:

- Orally or parenterally
- By inhalation for asthma and other inflammatory problems of the airways
- Topically for skin problems
- Injected into joints
- Rectally for hemorrhoids
- In drops for eye problems

Chapter 21 discusses the use of inhaled corticosteroids for respiratory problems. Chapter 29 discusses how to place drugs in the eye.

When taken orally or given parenterally, corticosteroids have many side effects and adverse effects. For this reason, corticosteroids are usually prescribed for only a short period of time. However, if the inflammation cannot be controlled with less powerful drugs, they may need to be taken for weeks or months. When needed for long periods of time, the goal is for the patient to take the lowest dose of corticosteroids that will control the inflammation so side effects and complications can be minimized. There are dozens of brands and strengths of corticosteroids. They all work the same way and have the same effects. Only those used most commonly are listed in the following table. Be sure to consult a drug handbook for more information about a specific drug.

Dosages for Common Corticosteroids

Drug	Dosage
Oral Corticosteroids	
betamethasone (Betnelan ♣, Betnesol ♣, Celestone)	0.5-7 mg orally daily
dexamethasone (Decadron, Dexasone ♣)	2-20 mg orally daily (dose and schedule depend on the disorder)
prednisoLONE	5-40 mg orally daily
predniSONE (Apo-Prednisone ♣)	5-60 mg orally daily in two doses (⅔ morning, ⅓ evening)
Parenteral Corticosteroids	
cortisone acetate (Cortone ♣)	*Adults:* 20-300 mg IM daily *Children:* 1-5 mg/kg IM daily
dexamethasone (Decadron, Deronil ♣, Dexasone ♣, Hexadrol)	*Adults:* 1-80 mg IM or IV daily *Children:* 0.03-0.2 mg/kg IM or IV daily
hydrocortisone (Solu-Cortef)	*Adults:* 25-125 mg IM 2-4 times daily *Children:* Dose for children not established
methylprednisoLONE (Duralone, Medalone, Solu-Medrol)	*Adults:* 10-60 mg IM or IV 2-4 times daily, depending on disorder *Children:* 0.03-0.5 mg/kg IM or IV daily
Topical Corticosteroids	
hydrocortisone (Ala-Cort, Dermacort, Lanacort) triamcinolone (Aristocort, Kenalog, Oracort, Triderm)	Most topical corticosteroids are available in strengths of 0.05% or 0.1% creams, ointments, and lotions. There is no specific amount of drug prescribed. A thin layer is applied on the affected skin area 2-3 times daily.

| Box 6-1 | Common Side Effects of Systemic Corticosteroids |

AFTER 1 WEEK OF THERAPY
- Acne
- Sodium and fluid retention
- Elevated blood pressure
- Sensation of "nervousness"
- Difficulty sleeping
- Emotional changes, crying easily

WITHIN A MONTH AFTER THERAPY
- Weight gain
- Fat redistribution (moon face and "buffalo hump" between the shoulders)
- Increased risk for gastrointestinal ulcers and bleeding
- Fragile skin that bruises easily
- Loss of muscle mass and strength
- Thinning scalp hair
- Increased facial and body hair
- Increased susceptibility to colds and other infections
- Stretch marks

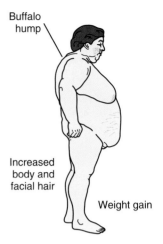

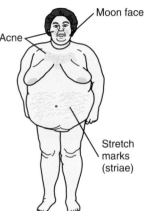

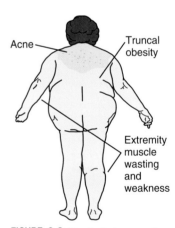

FIGURE 6-2 Physical changes from long-term corticosteroid therapy, known as a "Cushingoid" appearance.

How Systemic Corticosteroids Work

Corticosteroids decrease the production of all known body chemical mediators that trigger inflammation. They also slow the production of WBCs in the bone marrow. Because WBCs are the source of the mediators that trigger inflammation, this action also helps reduce inflammation. Corticosteroids have main effects and side effects in all cells and tissues.

Intended Responses
- Swelling at the site of inflammation is reduced.
- Redness and pain at the site of inflammation are reduced.
- The body area affected by inflammation demonstrates increased function.

Side Effects. Because systemic corticosteroids enter and affect every type of body cell, they have many side effects. The most common are listed in Box 6-1 and shown in Figure 6-2. Most side effects do not occur with just one dose of corticosteroids but may be present as soon as 5 to 7 days after starting drug therapy. Other side effects may not be present for up to a month or more of therapy. The higher the dose of corticosteroids, the sooner the side effects appear, and the more severe they are. Many side effects change the patient's appearance ("Cushingoid appearance" as shown in Figure 6-2), which may cause distress. The good news is that most of these side effects and body changes return to normal after therapy stops, although it may take a year or longer. Stretch marks shrink but are permanent.

Adverse Effects. Three important adverse effects are adrenal gland suppression, reduced immune function, and delayed wound healing. These can occur in anyone taking systemic corticosteroids for a long period of time. For this reason corticosteroids are taken for systemic inflammation only if the inflammation is severe and cannot be controlled in other ways.

The adrenal glands normally make cortisol. How much cortisol is made each day is determined by how much cortisol is already circulating in the blood. If there are less than normal amounts of cortisol in the blood, the adrenal glands produce and release more cortisol. If there are higher than normal levels of cortisol in the blood, the adrenal glands reduce production of cortisol. When blood levels of cortisol are very high, the adrenal glands stop producing it, and the cells of the adrenal glands *atrophy* (shrink).

Memory Jogger

Most long-term side effects of systemic corticosteroid therapy, including those affecting appearance, eventually return to normal after therapy is stopped.

Common Side Effects

Systemic Corticosteroids

Hypertension

Acne

Insomnia

Nervousness

| Box **6-2** | Signs and Symptoms of Acute Adrenal Insufficiency |

- Acute confusion
- Profound muscle weakness
- Slow, irregular pulse
- Hypotension
- Abdominal pain
- Nausea and vomiting
- Salt craving
- Weight loss
- Low blood glucose levels (hypoglycemia, less than 70 mg/dL)
- Low serum sodium levels (hyponatremia, less than 130 mEq/L)
- High serum potassium levels (hyperkalemia, more than 5.5 mEq/L)
- Low serum cortisol levels (less than 3.0 mcg/dL)

 Clinical Pitfall

If a patient has been taking a systemic corticosteroid drug for a week or longer, he or she must not suddenly stop taking the drug.

QSEN: Safety

Memory Jogger

It is possible for an infection to be present without symptoms when a person is taking systemic corticosteroids.

Clinical Pitfall

Never substitute one corticosteroid for another because strengths vary.

QSEN: Safety

To the body, corticosteroid drugs look very much like cortisol. When a person is taking corticosteroids, the blood levels of the drug are high. This high level fools the adrenal glands into stopping their production of cortisol and shrinking (Figure 6-3). These atrophied adrenal glands become a problem if the person suddenly stops taking corticosteroids. The adrenal glands will begin making cortisol again, but this process takes weeks to months. As a result, the person who suddenly stops taking systemic corticosteroids has no circulating cortisol, which is necessary for life, and could die from the effects of *acute adrenal insufficiency*. (Box 6-2 lists the signs and symptoms of acute adrenal insufficiency.) Instead of stopping corticosteroid drugs suddenly when therapy is no longer needed, the patient must slowly decrease the doses over time. This process is called *tapering*, and it allows the adrenal gland cells to gradually resume the process of making cortisol.

Because systemic corticosteroids reduce WBC numbers and the inflammatory response, the person taking these drugs is at greater risk for infection. When inflammation is reduced, the symptoms of infection may not be obvious. Infection symptoms (fever, redness, pain, pus, or drainage) are caused by the same mediators that cause inflammation. When corticosteroids block their production, an infection may be present but not produce obvious symptoms.

Inflammation begins the process of wound healing. Reducing inflammation with corticosteroids reduces this response and slows cell growth. These actions delay wound healing, which also increases the risk for infection.

What To Do *Before* Giving Corticosteroids

Check the dose and the specific drug name carefully. *Different types of corticosteroids are not interchangeable because the strength of the drugs varies.* For this reason, drug doses must be recalculated by the prescriber if it is necessary to switch from one corticosteroid to another.

Check for symptoms of infection (for example, fever, drainage, foul-smelling urine, productive cough, or redness around an open skin area) and report any symptoms to the prescriber. Systemic corticosteroids may make an existing infection worse.

Check the patient's blood pressure and weight. Corticosteroids cause sodium and water retention that can lead to high blood pressure (hypertension) and weight gain.

What To Do *After* Giving Corticosteroids

Check vital signs at least once per shift for changes in blood pressure or temperature elevation. Examine the skin for bruises or tears that indicate the skin is becoming more fragile. Minimize the use of tape and be gentle when handling the patient to avoid skin trauma and bleeding. Weigh the patient weekly to monitor for fluid retention.

What To *Teach* Patients About Corticosteroids

The most important information to teach a patient who is taking systemic corticosteroids is not to stop taking the drug suddenly. If the patient is ill and unable to keep the drug down, he or she should call the prescriber so the drug can be given parenterally. Also tell the patient to wear a medical alert bracelet or to carry a card stating that corticosteroids are taken daily. This allows health care personnel to take steps to prevent adrenal insufficiency if the patient should suddenly become ill or hurt and is unable to communicate.

Tell the patient to take the corticosteroid in the morning or, if the dose is higher, to take two thirds of the dose in the morning and one third before bedtime. This schedule is close to the way the adrenal glands normally release cortisol.

Tell the patient to take corticosteroids with food to help prevent stomach ulcers. Teach him or her to avoid crowds and people who are ill because resistance to infection is decreased.

Issues with Topical Corticosteroids

Topical corticosteroids are used to relieve itching and skin rashes that occur with skin inflammation. These drugs work like systemic corticosteroids, but their effects are largely confined to the skin area where the drug is applied. They come in creams, ointments, pastes, lotions, foams, and gels of various strengths. The stronger drugs require a prescription; weaker drugs are available over the counter.

Topical corticosteroids can be absorbed through the skin and have some systemic effects. Teach the patient to apply a thin layer to only the areas that need treatment. Topical corticosteroids lower immunity in the area where they are applied. This means that if there is a skin infection and topical corticosteroids are applied in that area, the infection can spread to surrounding areas more easily. For this reason, do not apply a topical corticosteroid if there is any question that the skin is infected rather than just being irritated or having a rash.

Life Span Considerations for Corticosteroids

Pediatric Considerations. Corticosteroids are prescribed for children who have severe or chronic inflammatory problems. Children are at risk for the same corticosteroid side effects as adults, even stomach ulcers.

Considerations for Pregnancy and Lactation. Severe inflammatory responses during pregnancy can be treated with corticosteroids, although the drug does cross the placenta. Babies born to mothers taking the drug through the last 3 months of pregnancy tend to be smaller than normal. Because this drug group can cross into breast milk, mothers who must take corticosteroids long term are encouraged to stop breastfeeding because the baby will have the same side effects as the mother.

Considerations for Older Adults. The increased risk for infection can be very serious in older adults, who may have age-related reduced immune function. The older patient taking systemic corticosteroids must take extra precautions to avoid infection. In addition, because the skin of an older adult is thinner than that of a younger adult, lower strengths of topical corticosteroids should be used. Teach the older adult the importance of using only a thin layer of a topical corticosteroid. Another side effect of systemic corticosteroid therapy is an increase in blood glucose level. Because the older adult is more likely to have diabetes than a younger adult, this side effect may make controlling diabetes in an older adult much more difficult. For an older adult who is prescribed a systemic corticosteroid and who has diabetes, both diet and diabetic drug therapy may need to be changed while the patient is on corticosteroid therapy.

NONSTEROIDAL ANTI-INFLAMMATORY DRUGS

Nonsteroidal anti-inflammatory drugs (NSAIDs) are anti-inflammatory drugs that are not similar in chemical structure to cortisol but prevent or limit the tissue and blood

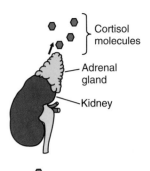

Cortisol molecules
Adrenal gland
Kidney

Low blood levels of cortisol cause a series of reactions that increase adrenal output of cortisol

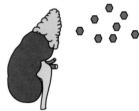

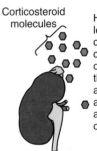

Corticosteroid molecules

High blood levels of corticosteroids cause a series of reactions that shrink the adrenal gland and reduce adrenal output of cortisol

FIGURE 6-3 Corticosteroid influence on adrenal production of cortisol.

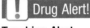 **Drug Alert!**

Teaching Alert

Teach the patient to take corticosteroids with food to help prevent stomach problems.

QSEN: Safety

 Clinical Pitfall

Never apply a topical corticosteroid to a skin area that may be infected.

QSEN: Safety

vessel responses to injury or invasion by slowing the production of one or more inflammatory mediators. Some of these drugs are available only by prescription; others are available over the counter. NSAIDs usually are taken for pain and inflammation. They are used to treat many health problems, including fever, arthritis and other rheumatologic disorders, gout, systemic lupus erythematosus, pain after surgery, menstrual cramps, and blood clots.

There are many different NSAIDs. They can first be placed into a class on the basis of whether they inhibit the enzyme COX-1 or COX-2. Then they are further separated into groups on the basis of specific chemical makeup. All NSAIDs work in similar ways but vary in some side effects. The listings in the following table describe only the most common drugs in each class. Be sure to consult a drug handbook for more information about a specific NSAID.

 Do Not Confuse

ketorolac *with* Ketalar

An order for ketorolac can be confused with Ketalar. The drug ketorolac is an anti-inflammatory drug that can be given orally or parenterally. Ketalar is a type of anesthetic agent.

QSEN: Safety

Dosages for Common COX-1 Inhibitors

Drug Class	Drug Examples	Dosage
Salicylic acid	aspirin (for example, Bayer Aspirin, Bufferin, Ecotrin, Entrophen ♣)	*Adults:* 325-650 mg orally 3-4 times daily *Children:* 80-320 mg orally 3-4 times daily, depending on size
Propionic acid	ibuprofen (Advil, Motrin, Actiprofen ♣)	*Adults:* 200-800 mg orally 3-4 times daily *Children:* 50-100 mg orally 3-4 times daily
	naproxen (Aleve, Anaprox, Naprosyn, Naprosyn E ♣, Naprox ♣, Naxen ♣)	*Adults:* 220-440 mg orally twice daily *Children over age 2 years:* 20 mg/kg/day orally, not to exceed 1000 mg in a day
	oxaprozin (Daypro)	*Adults:* 600-1800 mg orally once daily *Children:* 600-1200 mg orally once daily
Acetic acid	indomethacin (Indameth ♣, Indocid ♣, Indocin, Indochron ER, Nu-Indo ♣)	*Adults/Children:* 50-200 mg orally or by suppository daily
	nabumetone (Relafen)	*Adults:* 500-1000 mg orally once or twice daily Dosage not established for children
	ketorolac (Toradol)	*Adults:* 10-60 mg orally every 6 hr daily; 15-30 mg IM or IV every 6 hr Dosage not established for multiple doses for children
Fenamic acid	mefenamic acid (Ponstel)	*Adults:* 250 mg orally every 6 hr Dosage not established for children
	meclofenamic acid (Meclomen)	*Adults:* 50-100 mg orally every 6 hr Dosage not established for children
Enolic acid	piroxicam (Apo-Piroxicam ♣, Feldene, Novopirocam ♣)	*Adults:* 20 mg orally once daily Dosage not established for children

Dosages for Common Cox-2 Inhibitors

 Do Not Confuse

Celebrex *with* Celexa

An order for Celebrex can be confused with Celexa. Celebrex is an anti-inflammatory drug. Celexa is an antidepressant.

QSEN: Safety

Drug	Dosage
celecoxib (Celebrex)	*Adults:* 100-400 mg orally daily *Children weighing less than 25 kg:* 50 mg orally twice daily *Children weighing more than 25 kg:* 100 mg orally twice daily
meloxicam (Mobic)	*Adults:* 7.5-15 mg orally once daily Dosage and safety not established for children

How NSAIDs Work

The main action of NSAIDs is to inhibit the action of the COX enzyme that helps to make many of the different types of prostaglandins inside each cell (see Figure 6-1). *Prostaglandins* are a family of chemicals made by the body. Some prostaglandins have what are called "housekeeping" cell jobs, helping cells and tissues remain healthy and functional. COX-2 is an enzyme found only in inflammatory cells. Its purpose is to help make all the mediators of the inflammatory response, including prostaglandins, leukotriene, and kinins. *Leukotriene* is a chemical made by the body that binds to its receptors and maintains an inflammatory response. *Kinins* are a group of chemicals made by the body that cause some of the signs and symptoms of inflammation, especially pain. The most common one is bradykinin. These mediators are responsible for creating all of the uncomfortable signs and symptoms of inflammation. Most NSAIDs suppress both the COX-1 and COX-2 forms of the enzyme, so production of the helpful housekeeping mediators along with the inflammatory mediators is slowed. This means that these drugs cause side effects that are related to a reduction in the housekeeping mediators.

Intended Responses

- Redness and pain at the site of inflammation are reduced.
- Swelling and warmth at the site of inflammation are reduced.
- Body function in the area affected by inflammation is increased.
- Fever is reduced.

Side Effects. Because COX-1 NSAIDs reduce the activity of the COX-1 and COX-2 enzymes, some normal healthy cell functions are affected. For example, all COX-1 NSAIDs reduce platelet clumping and blood clotting. In fact, aspirin is often prescribed just for this action. However, just one dose of aspirin can reduce blood clotting for up to a week. Other NSAIDs reduce blood clotting only for the duration of the drug therapy. Blood clotting returns to normal within 24 to 48 hours after stopping the drug. Because anyone taking a COX-1 NSAID is at increased risk for bleeding in response to slight injuries, surgery, or dental work, these drugs are discontinued before planned invasive procedures.

COX-1 NSAIDs can irritate the stomach lining and the rest of the gastrointestinal (GI) tract. The stomach is irritated when the drug touches it directly and again when the drugs are absorbed into the blood. This can lead to development of serious bleeding ulcers and pain in the GI tract.

All the NSAIDs except aspirin can reduce blood flow to the kidney and slow urine output. This action can lead to high blood pressure and kidney damage. In addition, the action of the COX-1 NSAIDs on the kidney is exactly the opposite of the angiotensin-converting enzyme (ACE) inhibitor drugs for high blood pressure and can make them less effective (see Chapter 16).

Because COX-2 NSAIDs mostly suppress the COX-2 pathway (see Figure 6-1), which allows the normal housekeeping functions of the COX-1 pathway to continue, they have fewer side effects than COX-1 NSAIDs. *However, if a patient takes more than the prescribed dose, the side effects are the same as for COX-1 NSAIDs.* These drugs do not affect platelet action and blood clotting, so bruising and gum bleeding are not expected side effects.

Adverse Effects. In addition to possible kidney damage, common adverse effects of NSAIDs are the induction of asthma and allergic reactions. People who are sensitive to one NSAID are likely to be sensitive to all of them. In addition, taking two or more different NSAIDs at the same time increases the side effects and the risk for adverse effects.

Celecoxib (Celebrex) is made from a chemical similar to the sulfa drug type of antibiotic. A patient who is allergic to sulfa drugs is likely to also be allergic to celecoxib.

Drug Alert!

Teaching Alert

Teach patients not to increase the dose of a COX-2 inhibitor drug because the risk for side effects similar to those of COX-1 inhibitors is greatly increased.

QSEN: Safety

Common Side Effects

NSAIDs

Bleeding problems   GI ulcers, GI pain   Fluid retention

Hypertension

Another adverse reaction that was responsible for removing other COX-2 NSAIDs from the market was an increase in heart attacks and strokes among patients taking these drugs. COX-2 NSAIDs increase clot formation in the small arteries of the heart and brain, especially when these arteries are narrowed by atherosclerosis or cigarette smoking. These drugs should be avoided by any patient who has angina, smokes, or has undergone coronary artery bypass graft surgery (CABG).

The higher the dose of NSAIDs and the longer they are taken, the more likely they are to trigger an adverse effect. Except for low-dose aspirin, most NSAIDs should not be taken daily for longer than 1 week for common aches and pains. For chronic diseases such as arthritis, the drugs may need to be taken much longer. When NSAIDs are needed long term, the patient is urged to find the lowest dose that still reduces his or her inflammation and pain.

What To Do *Before* Giving NSAIDs

Carefully check the order for NSAIDs to be given parenterally. The main NSAID approved for IV use is ketorolac (Toradol).

Before giving celecoxib, ask whether the patient has an allergy to sulfa antibiotics. A patient who is allergic to sulfa drugs is likely also to be allergic to celecoxib.

Always ask the patient whether he or she has had any problems with aspirin or any other over-the-counter NSAID. If the patient reports a previous problem with NSAIDs, do not give this drug without checking with the prescriber.

Give the drug at the time the patient is eating or shortly after a meal. When possible, have the patient drink a full glass of water or milk with the drug.

Tell the patient not to chew an NSAID capsule or an enteric-coated tablet because it will ruin its stomach-protective properties.

Check the patient's blood pressure because NSAIDs can cause the patient to retain sodium and water, leading to higher blood pressure. If the patient is taking an ACE inhibitor for high blood pressure, NSAIDs can reduce its effectiveness and make heart failure and hypertension worse.

What To Do *After* Giving NSAIDs

Bleeding risk increases within several hours after a dose of a COX-1 NSAID. Examine the patient's gums, mucous membranes, and open skin areas (around IV sites) during each shift for bleeding. Look for bruises and for pinpoint purple-red spots (petechiae). Check urine, stool, or emesis for bright red blood, coffee-ground material, or other indications of bleeding.

In addition to the general actions listed in Chapter 2, when giving an NSAID to a patient who has never taken a drug from this family before, check his or her blood pressure, breathing pattern, and pulse oximetry hourly after the first dose of an NSAID in case he or she is sensitive to it. Immediately report any breathing difficulty, drop in blood pressure, or decrease of 5% or more in oxygen saturation. Any of these signs and symptoms may indicate hypersensitivity to the drug.

What To *Teach* Patients About NSAIDs

To avoid GI side effects, teach the patient to always take an NSAID with food or on a full stomach. Tell the patient not to chew an NSAID capsule or an enteric-coated tablet because doing so will ruin its stomach-protective properties. Teach him or her to check bowel movements for the presence of bright red blood or dark, tarry-looking material that would indicate bleeding somewhere in the GI tract. Tell the patient to immediately report such symptoms to the prescriber.

Because COX-1 NSAIDs reduce blood clotting, teach the patient to check the gums daily while taking the drug for bleeding, especially after toothbrushing or flossing. Tell the patient to let the dentist know that he or she takes NSAIDs before any dental procedure is performed.

Teach the patient not to take aspirin and other NSAIDs when also taking warfarin (Coumadin). These two drug types reduce blood clotting in different ways, so the patient would be at extreme risk for excessive bleeding and stroke.

Clinical Pitfall

Do not give celecoxib (Celebrex) to a patient who is allergic to the sulfa drug type of antibiotics.

QSEN: Safety

Drug Alert!

Teaching Alert

Teach the patient to avoid chewing or crushing an NSAID capsule or enteric-coated tablet.

QSEN: Safety

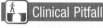

Clinical Pitfall

COX-1 NSAIDs, especially aspirin, should not be taken with warfarin (Coumadin).

QSEN: Safety

The most important precaution to teach patients taking celecoxib (Celebrex) is to take the drug exactly as prescribed. At higher doses, these drugs also inhibit the COX-1 enzymes, which can make the adverse reactions and side effects the same as for the COX-1 NSAIDs.

Teach patients to weigh themselves at least twice each week in the morning before eating or drinking anything. Instruct them to wear similar clothes each time so the weight is not changed by different types of clothing. Show them how to keep a record of their weight. Instruct them to tell the prescriber about a weight gain of more than 3 lb in a week. Also teach them how to check the ankles for swelling (which could mean heart failure, especially if it is present in the morning).

Life Span Considerations for NSAIDs

Pediatric Considerations. With the exception of ibuprofen, NSAIDs are not recommended for children. In particular, aspirin and COX-2 NSAIDs are to be avoided in children. One problem with aspirin is an association with the development of Reye's syndrome, which may occur when aspirin is given to a child who has a viral infection. *Reye's syndrome* is a liver disease that can lead to coma, brain damage, and death. Aspirin and NSAIDs may be given to children with some chronic inflammatory diseases.

 Clinical Pitfall

Avoid giving aspirin to children to prevent Reye's syndrome.

QSEN: Safety

Considerations for Pregnancy. The stronger NSAIDs, particularly indomethacin and celecoxib, should be avoided during the last 3 months of pregnancy because they may cause early closure of a blood vessel (the ductus arteriosus) important to fetal circulation and oxygenation.

Considerations for Older Adults. The older adult is at higher risk for cardiac problems when taking NSAIDs. Except for aspirin, these drugs cause salt and water retention that can lead to fluid overload and high blood pressure. Both of these problems increase the risk for heart attack and heart failure. Teach older adults taking NSAIDs to carefully monitor their weight, pulse, and urine output. Teach them the signs and symptoms of heart failure (weight gain; ankle swelling; and shortness of breath, especially when lying down).

ANTIHISTAMINES

Antihistamines, or histamine antagonists, are drugs that reduce inflammation by preventing the inflammatory mediator histamine from binding to its receptor. **Histamine** is a chemical mediator made by the body that binds to its receptor sites and causes changes that lead to inflammatory responses. There are two known types of histamine receptors. H_1 receptors are located in blood vessels and respiratory mucous membranes. H_2 receptors are located in the stomach lining. When histamine binds to H_1 receptors, tissue changes occur, causing blood vessel dilation, swelling, decreased blood pressure, poor heart contractions, narrowed airways, increased mucus production, and the formation of hives on the skin. When histamine binds to H_2 receptors, stomach acid production increases, and the risk for stomach ulcers is greatly increased. Drugs that specifically block H_2 receptors in the stomach are discussed in Chapter 23.

Histamine is the main mediator of inflammation and capillary leak. Leukotriene, another mediator that binds to a receptor, works with histamine to keep the inflammatory response going once it has started. The drugs used to slow or stop an inflammatory reaction once it has started or to prevent one from starting are the antihistamines and leukotriene blockers. Both are most commonly used for inflammation triggered by allergic reactions such as hives, watery eyes, and runny nose. In addition, one of the antihistamines, diphenhydramine (Benadryl), is given during anaphylaxis and other severe systemic allergic reactions.

 Memory Jogger

Histamine and leukotriene are major mediators of inflammation.

Many antihistamines are H_1 histamine blockers. Those most commonly prescribed are listed in the following table. Be sure to consult a drug handbook for information about a specific antihistamine.

🔁 **Do Not Confuse**

Zyrtec *with* Zyban or Zantac

An order for Zyrtec can be confused with Zyban or Zantac. Zyrtec
is an H₁ histamine blocker. Zyban
(bupropion) is an antidepressant
used to help people stop smoking.
Zantac (ranitidine) is an H₂ histamine blocker used to help heal
stomach ulcers and prevent
esophageal reflux.

QSEN: Safety

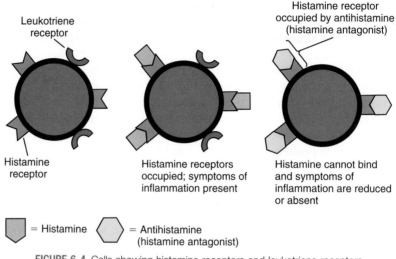

FIGURE 6-4 Cells showing histamine receptors and leukotriene receptors.

Dosages for Common Antihistamines

Drug	Dose
cetirizine (Zyrtec)	*Adults:* 5-10 mg orally daily *Children:* 2.5-5 mg orally daily
diphenhydramine (Allerdryl 🍁, Benadryl)	*Adults/Children:* 12.5-50 mg orally or IV every 6 hr
fexofenadine (Allegra)	*Adults:* Prescription 180 mg orally once daily; OTC 60 mg orally twice daily *Children 6-11 years:* 30 mg orally twice daily
loratadine (Claritin)	*Adults:* 10 mg orally daily *Children:* 5 mg orally daily

Common Side Effects

H₁ Histamine Blockers

Sleepiness

Dry mouth

Blurred vision

Tachycardia

Urinary
retention

How Antihistamines Work

Antihistamines, or histamine antagonists, bind to H₁ histamine receptor sites in mucous membranes of the respiratory tract and in blood vessels, heart muscle, and the skin. This binding prevents the histamine produced by the body from binding to its receptors, thus slowing or stopping the tissue effects of inflammation (Figure 6-4).

Intended Responses
- Blood vessels do not dilate.
- Swelling is reduced.
- Mucus and other nasal, eye, and respiratory secretions are reduced.
- Narrowed airways widen.
- Hives decrease in size and itchiness.

Side Effects. Many antihistamines cause some degree of drowsiness. Each one varies in this side effect, and every person reacts differently. For some people, even a low dose causes severe drowsiness; for others, little or none occurs. Drinking alcohol when taking an antihistamine worsens the side effect of drowsiness.

Most antihistamines cause some degree of anticholinergic side effects of dry mouth, increased heart rate, increased blood pressure, dilated pupils, and urinary retention. The severity depends on which drug is used or prescribed and how the person responds.

🚶 **Clinical Pitfall**

Do not give antihistamines to a
patient who has glaucoma, prostate enlargement, hypertension, or
urinary retention.

QSEN: Safety

Adverse Effects. For some people the pressure inside the eye *(intraocular pressure)* can become too high while taking antihistamines. This is a dangerous situation and can make glaucoma worse or even lead to blindness.

Allergic reactions to antihistamines are rare but can occur. A patient who has had a bad reaction to one antihistamine may be at risk for allergic reactions to others.

Antihistamines that induce sedation should not be given during an acute asthma attack. This is not because the drug causes asthma but because it can make the patient so drowsy that he or she may not be alert enough to work at breathing.

What To Do *Before* Giving Antihistamines

Ask if the patient is being treated for glaucoma, high blood pressure, or prostate enlargement. Antihistamines are contraindicated for a patient with any of these problems because these drugs could make these conditions worse.

Check to see what other drugs are prescribed for the patient. Opioids, sedatives, muscle relaxants, and barbiturates all increase the drowsy effect of antihistamines. If it is necessary to give an antihistamine to a patient who is taking any of these drug types, it should not be given within 4 hours of these drugs.

What To Do *After* Giving Antihistamines

In addition to the actions listed in Chapter 2, check the patient's pulse, blood pressure, and respiratory rate at least every 4 hours for the first 8 hours after giving the first dose an antihistamine. Notify the prescriber if heart rate becomes irregular, blood pressure changes significantly from the patient's baseline, or respiratory rate falls below 10 breaths/minute and stays low.

What To *Teach* Patients About Antihistamines

Teach patients to avoid alcoholic drinks when taking antihistamines. Instruct them to avoid driving or operating dangerous or heavy machinery within 6 hours of taking these drugs.

Urge the patient to contact the prescriber immediately about vision changes or pain over the eyebrows, which could mean an increase in intraocular pressure.

Teach the male patient who has prostate problems to make sure that he is urinating about as much fluid in a day as he is drinking. Urinary retention can be made worse by antihistamines. If he notices a sudden decrease in urine output or feels an urgent need to urinate and is unable to, he should contact his prescriber.

Remind the patient with asthma not to take antihistamines during an acute asthma attack at home because the drug could cause enough sleepiness to impair the ability to breathe.

LEUKOTRIENE INHIBITORS

Leukotriene is another body chemical that triggers and sustains inflammatory responses. It is found inside many types of WBCs. When it is released, it binds to leukotriene receptors and triggers the symptoms of inflammation (see Figure 6-4).

How Leukotriene Inhibitors Work

Leukotriene inhibitors work in several ways to prevent an allergy episode. Zileuton (Zyflo) prevents leukotriene production within WBCs. Montelukast (Singulair) and zafirlukast (Accolate) block the leukotriene receptors on cells. As a result of these drugs, a person with allergies has less of an inflammatory response.

Clinical Pitfall

Do not give an antihistamine that causes drowsiness to a patient who is having an acute asthma attack.

QSEN: Safety

Drug Alert!

Interaction Alert

When giving an antihistamine to a patient who is also taking opioids, sedatives, muscle relaxants, or barbiturates, avoid giving the antihistamine within 4 hours of these drugs.

QSEN: Safety

Do Not Confuse

Zyflo *with* Zyban or Zyrtec

Zyflo is a leukotriene blocker used to reduce allergic reactions. Zyban is an antidepressant used to help people stop smoking. Zyrtec is an antihistamine also used to reduce inflammation and allergic reactions.

QSEN: Safety

Dosages for Common Leukotriene Inhibitors

Drug	Dosage
montelukast sodium (Singulair)	*Adults:* 10 mg orally daily *Children:* 4 mg orally daily
zafirlukast (Accolate)	*Adults:* 20 mg orally twice daily *Children:* 10 mg orally twice daily
zileuton (Zyflo CR)	*Adults and children over 12 years:* 1200 mg orally twice daily after morning and evening meals

Common Side Effects
Leukotriene Inhibitors

Headache

Abdominal pain

Intended Responses
- Swelling of oral, nasal, eye, and respiratory mucous membranes is reduced.
- Secretions are reduced.
- Narrowed airways are opened.

Side Effects. Side effects of therapy with leukotriene inhibitors include headache and abdominal pain.

Adverse Effects. The major adverse effects of leukotriene inhibitors are liver impairment and allergic reactions, including hives and anaphylaxis. Both of these responses are rare.

What To Do *Before* Giving Leukotriene Inhibitors
Leukotriene inhibitors, especially zileuton, can cause liver impairment. Therefore, before giving the first dose, ask the patient about any previous liver problems or *jaundice* (yellowing of the skin, sclera, or mucous membranes), tenderness in the liver area of the abdomen (right upper quadrant), nausea, or fatigue. Check baseline liver function tests for comparison after the patient has been taking the drug for several months. Table 1-3 lists normal liver function tests.

What To Do *After* Giving Leukotriene Inhibitors
Regularly assess the patient for signs and symptoms of decreased liver function, including constant fatigue, itchy skin, and yellowing of the skin or sclera.

Assess the patient taking montelukast (Singulair) for mood changes, especially depression and suicidal thoughts.

What To *Teach* Patients About Leukotriene Inhibitors
Teach the patient to report any skin yellowing, pain over the liver area, or darkening of the urine to the prescriber.

Stress to patients taking montelukast (Singulair) to report any depression or thoughts of suicide immediately to the prescriber.

Life Span Considerations for Leukotriene Inhibitors
Pediatric Considerations. These drugs are prescribed for children who have allergies and inflammation. Care must be taken to calculate drug doses carefully to prevent an accidental overdose.

DISEASE-MODIFYING ANTIRHEUMATIC DRUGS
Disease-modifying antirheumatic drugs (DMARDs) are drugs that reduce the progression and tissue destruction of the inflammatory disease process by inhibiting tumor necrosis factor (TNF). They are used to treat many types of chronic inflammatory disorders, especially autoimmune disorders, such as rheumatoid arthritis, ankylosing spondylitis, psoriasis, psoriatic arthritis, Crohn disease, and ulcerative colitis. Most of these diseases involve excessive amounts of tumor necrosis factor (TNF), which causes severe tissue damage and destruction.

There are several drugs in this class. Most are antibodies directed against TNF. Most are administered by injection, although a few are oral drugs. The listings in the following table describe only the most commonly used DMARDs. Be sure to consult a drug handbook for more information about a specific DMARD.

Dosages for Common Disease-Modifying Antirheumatic Drugs

Drug	Dosage
adalimumab (Humira)	*Adults:* 40 mg subcutaneously every other week* *Children weighing 15-30 kg:* 20 mg subcutaneously every other week *Children weighing 30 kg or more:* 40 mg subcutaneously every other week
etanercept (Enbrel)	*Adults:* 50 mg subcutaneously weekly either as a single injection of 50 mg, or as two injections of 25 mg given 4 days apart *Children:* 0.8 mg/kg/week subcutaneously up to 50 mg

*Most common dosage and route. Dosages and routes may differ for some disorders.

How DMARDs Work

DMARDs are antibodies to TNF that work by binding to the TNF molecule and preventing it from binding to its receptor site on specific WBCs and other cells. This action prevents the cells with TNF receptors from producing substances that continue inflammatory responses that cause direct tissue destruction.

Apremilast (Otezla) is a newly approved DMARD to treat psoriatic arthritis. Its mechanism of action is different from others. It works by inhibiting the enzyme phosphodiesterase-4 (PDE4). As a result of less PDE4 and more intracellular cAMP, some inflammatory cells reduce their production of inflammatory chemicals and increase their production of some anti-inflammatory mediators. This results in reduced joint pain and swelling in adults with psoriatic arthritis. This oral drug is started at a dose of 10 mg twice daily and gradually increased to a final dose of 30 mg orally twice daily.

The major reported side effects of apremilast are gastrointestinal problems and headache. Adverse effects include depression and suicidal ideation. The drug should be used cautiously for anyone who has a history of depression. Teach the patient and family to immediately report to the prescriber any increase in depression or any suicidal ideation.

Intended Responses
- Pain and other disease symptoms are reduced.
- Physical function is improved.
- Progression of physical damage is reduced or delayed

Side Effects. The major common side effect of DMARD therapy is injection site reaction with pain, swelling, itching, and redness at the site for 3 to 5 days after the injection. For many people, the intensity of the reaction decreases after a few months of therapy. Additional common side effects are headache and nausea.

Adverse Effects. There are many potential adverse effects associated with DMARD therapy, and the patient should be educated about them before therapy is started. These drugs reduce overall immune function, thus infections of all kinds occur more easily. In addition, if the patient has had a previous viral infection or tuberculosis, DMARD therapy can allow these organisms to reactivate and the dormant infections to become active again. Such infections include tuberculosis, hepatitis, and a variety of opportunistic infections.

Most patients using DMARDs have suppression of the bone marrow with reduction of WBCs, red blood cells, and platelets. In addition to increased risk for infection, patients may become anemic and have bleeding problems.

Common Side Effects

DMARDs

Headache   Nausea   Injection site reaction

New onset or worsening of heart failure has occurred. These drugs are not recommended for anyone who has poorly controlled or severe heart failure.

Allergic reactions, although not common, have included anaphylaxis. Although these drugs are developed with human components rather than animal components, allergic reactions are still possible and can be severe.

What To Do *Before* Giving DMARDs

Assess the patient for any active infection. If an infection is present, therapy is delayed until the infection is gone. Because reactivation of tuberculosis (TB) is possible, the patient must be tested for dormant or active TB. If TB is present, it is a contraindication for DMARD therapy.

Visually inspect the drug vial or syringe. The solution should be clear and colorless. Etanercept may have a few particles in solution; adalimumab must be free of particles. Check the expiration date and do not use expired solutions. Do not mix either drug with any other drugs.

The first dose of the drug must be given by a health care professional in a setting that is equipped to handle any type of adverse reaction. If no adverse reactions occur, the patient can be taught how to self-inject the drug. Take the patient's vital signs, especially pulse, blood pressure, and oxygen saturation, before giving the first dose. Use this information as a baseline to assess for an adverse drug reaction.

What To Do *After* Giving DMARDs

After administering the first dose of a DMARD, observe the patient for at least 2 hours for any signs of an allergic reaction or any other type of adverse reaction. Keep the emergency cart close to the patient. Assess the patient's breathing pattern and blood pressure within 5 minutes and again at 15 minutes after the injection. Document any injection site responses or other symptoms that appear.

What To *Teach* Patients About DMARDs

Teach all patients receiving DMARDs the signs and symptoms of infection (e.g., fever, cough, malaise, foul-smelling drainage, pain or burning on urination). Instruct them to report any sign or symptom of infection to their prescriber immediately.

Patients who will be self-injecting the drug need to know the proper technique for subcutaneous injection. Tips on teaching patients how to self-administer a subcutaneous injection are presented in Chapter 13.

Life Span Considerations for DMARDs

Considerations for Pregnancy and Lactation. Both adalimumab and etanercept can be safely administered during any trimester of pregnancy. Because both are injected drugs and are poorly absorbed by the GI tract, there is no contraindication for breastfeeding while taking these drugs. However, other DMARDs (not discussed in this chapter), especially the oral agents lenalidomide (Revlimid), thalidomide (Thalomid), and pomalidomide (Pomalyst), are known to greatly increase the risk for birth defects (they are teratogenic). These drugs are not to be taken during pregnancy or while breastfeeding. Teach women of childbearing age who are sexually active to use two or more reliable methods of contraception when taking a drug known to cause birth defects or fetal harm.

Drug Alert!

Administration Alert

Keep the patient in the facility for at least 2 hours after the first injection of a DMARD. Assess the patient frequently for an adverse reaction, especially anaphylaxis. See Chapter 1 for the signs and symptoms of anaphylaxis.

QSEN: Safety

Drug Alert!

Teaching Alert

Warn women who are in the childbearing age-group that the drugs lenalidomide (Revlimid), thalidomide (Thalomid), and pomalidomide (Pomalyst) are known to cause severe birth defects and must not be taken during pregnancy.

QSEN: Safety

Get Ready for Practice!

Key Points

- Teach the patient taking systemic corticosteroids to *never* suddenly stop taking the drug.
- Do not substitute one type of corticosteroid for another.

- Remind patients taking systemic corticosteroids to avoid crowds and people who are ill because the effects of corticosteroids reduce a patient's immunity and resistance to infection.
- Teach patients to always take an NSAID with food or on a full stomach.

- Teach patients to never take a COX-1 NSAID, especially aspirin, if they are also taking warfarin (Coumadin).
- Do not give celecoxib (Celebrex) to a patient who is allergic to the sulfa drug type of antibiotics.
- Do not give an antihistamine known to cause drowsiness to a patient having an acute asthma attack.
- Do not give antihistamines to a patient who has glaucoma or an enlarged prostate.
- Drinking alcohol when taking antihistamines increases drowsiness.
- Warn patients who are taking antihistamines at home not to drive or operate heavy machinery within 6 hours of taking these drugs.
- Avoid giving an antihistamine within 4 hours of the time when an opioid, sedative, muscle relaxant, or barbiturate was given to the patient.
- The first dose of an injectable DMARD should always be given by a health care professional in a facility capable of handling any type of adverse reaction.
- Keep the patient receiving the first dose of an injectable DMARD in the facility for at least 2 hours after the injection, and assess him or her frequently for an adverse reaction, especially anaphylaxis.
- Use the teaching tips in Chapter 13 to instruct patients how to self-administer an injectable DMARD.
- Lenalidomide (Revlimid), thalidomide (Thalomid), and pomalidomide (Pomalyst) are known to cause severe birth defects and must not be taken during pregnancy.

Additional Learning Resources

evolve Be sure to visit your Evolve website (http://evolve .elsevier.com/Workman/pharmacology/) for additional online resources.

[SG] Go to your Study Guide for additional learning activities to help you master this chapter content.

Review Questions

See the Answer Keys—In-text Review Questions for answers to these questions.

Test Yourself on the Basics

1. A patient taking 40 mg of prednisone daily for the past 3 months is experiencing the following signs and symptoms. Which ones are most likely related to the prednisone? (Select all that apply.)
   A. Continuous drowsiness
   B. Excessive bruising
   C. Thinning scalp hair
   D. Increased dental cavities
   E. Hypoglycemia
   F Loss of appetite
   G. Blurred vision
   H. High blood pressure

2. Why are aspirin and aspirin-containing drugs avoided for use with children?
   A. Aspirin is associated with the development of Reye's syndrome.
   B. Aspirin would drop a child's body temperature below normal.
   C. Children are at higher risk for bleeding with aspirin use.
   D. A child's liver is too immature to metabolize aspirin.

3. Which anti-inflammatory drug class is similar to the natural cortisol your adrenal glands produce?
   A. Antihistamines
   B. Leukotriene inhibitors
   C. Corticosteroids
   D. Disease-modifying antirheumatic drugs

4. Which nonsteroidal anti-inflammatory drug (NSAID) is less likely to affect platelets and blood clotting?
   A. indomethacin (Indocin)
   B. salicylic acid (Aspirin)
   C. ibuprofen (Advil)
   D. meloxicam (Mobic)

5. Which drug is an H1 histamine blocker?
   A. bupropion (Zyban)
   B. cetirizine (Zyrtec)
   C. piroxicam (Feldene)
   D. ranitidine (Zantac)

6. Which side effects are commonly associated with most antihistamines? Select all that apply.
   A. Asthma
   B. Constricted pupils
   C. Diarrhea
   D. Dry mouth
   E. Drowsiness
   F. Hypertension
   G. Nausea and vomiting
   H. Urinary retention

7. What is the most common side effect of any leukotriene inhibitor?
   A. Headache
   B. Jaundice
   C. Runny nose
   D. Cigarette craving

8. How are most disease-modifying antirheumatic drugs administered?
   A. Inhalation
   B. Oral liquid
   C. Topical cream
   D. Subcutaneous injection

Test Yourself on Advanced Concepts

9. The patient who was taking an oral corticosteroid for the past month to treat a breathing problem has been tapered down and off the drug. One week later, she has all of the following changes. Which one do you report to the prescriber immediately?
   A. A 1-pound weight gain
   B. Serum potassium level of 6.2 mEq/L
   C. Continuing scalp hair loss
   D. Thick white coating on the tongue

10. The patient who had a total knee replacement is discharged to home and prescribed to take 400 mg of celecoxib (Celebrex) orally daily for the next 10 days. Which precaution is most important to teach this patient?
    A. Avoid crowds and people who are ill.
    B. Do not floss your teeth while taking this drug.
    C. Avoid alcohol and caffeine while taking this drug.
    D. Do not increase the dose or frequency of this drug.

11. Why is indomethacin (Indocin) **never** prescribed for women late in pregnancy?
    A. The drug is known to cause hand deformities and other skeletal birth defects.
    B. The drug can cause early closure of a fetal blood vessel.
    C. There is an increased risk for clot formation after delivery.
    D. There is an increased risk for premature birth.

12. Which question is most important to ask a patient before giving the first dose of an NSAID?
    A. Do you have a cold or any other symptoms of infection?
    B. Do you or any members of your family have diabetes?
    C. Have you had any recent problems with hair loss?
    D. Have you ever had an allergic reaction to aspirin?

13. The patient prescribed fexofenadine (Allegra) for a nasal allergy reports that his mouth is dry and sticky. What is your best response or action?
    A. Suggest that the patient increase his water intake.
    B. Report this reaction to the prescriber immediately.
    C. Instruct the patient to reduce the dosage of this drug.
    D. Request that the prescriber switch the patient to a nasal spray form of the drug.

14. For which patient should the antihistamine diphenhydramine (Benadryl) be avoided?
    A. 12-year-old boy who has type 1 diabetes
    B. 45-year-old woman who has osteoarthritis
    C. 65-year-old man who has an enlarged prostate
    D. 75-year-old man who is allergic to sulfa drugs

15. A man taking zileuton (Zyflo) for the past 6 months for seasonal allergies has all of the following side effects. Which one indicates a possible severe health problem related to the use of this drug?
    A. Reduced appetite
    B. Headaches
    C. Cola-colored urine
    D. Dry skin and scalp

16. When drawing up a dose of etanercept (Enbrel), you notice a few particles floating in the clear and colorless drug. What should you do?
    A. Vigorously shake the vial before drawing up the drug.
    B. Draw up and administer the drug as prescribed.
    C. Discard the drug vial and obtain a new one.
    D. Report the observation to the pharmacy.

17. A child is prescribed 20 mg of liquid diphenhydramine (Benadryl) orally. The bottle of liquid diphenhydramine has a concentration of 12.5 mg per 5 mL. Exactly how many milliliters of diphenhydramine will you give this patient? _____ mL

18. A patient is to receive 50 mg of methylprednisolone (Solu-Medrol) IV in 250 mL of normal saline. The vial contains 125 mg of the drug in 10 mL.
    How many milliliters will you inject into the 250-mg IV bag? _____ mL

Critical Thinking Activities

See the Answer Keys—Critical Thinking Activities for answers to these activities.

Julie S. is a 40-year-old woman who was recently diagnosed with ankylosing spondylitis. You are to give her the first dose of adalimumab (Humira) 40 mg by subcutaneous injection.
1. What type of drug is adalimumab?
2. How does this drug help ankylosing spondylitis?
3. What should you do before and after giving Julie her first dose of this drug? Provide a rationale for your actions.
4. What are your teaching priorities for Julie?
5. Julie asks whether she will have to stop breastfeeding her 6-month-old daughter. What is your response and why?

Drugs for Pain Control

Objectives

After studying this chapter you should be able to:

1. Describe the different types of pain-control drugs.
2. Compare the features of drugs classified as controlled substances.
3. Explain what to do before and after giving opioid drugs and nonopioid drugs for pain control.
4. List the names, actions, usual dosages, possible side effects, and adverse effects of commonly

prescribed opioid drugs and nonopioid drugs for pain control.
5. Explain what to teach patients about opioid drugs and nonopioid drugs for pain control, including what to do, what not to do, and when to call the prescriber.
6. Describe life span considerations for pain-control drugs.

Key Terms

addiction (ă-DĬK-shŭn) (p. 108) The psychologic need or craving for the "high" feeling that results from using opioids when pain is not present.

analgesics (ăn-ăl-JĒ-zē-ŭ) (p. 104) Drugs of any class that provide pain relief either by changing the perception of pain or by reducing its source.

controlled substance (kŏn-TRŌLD SŬB-stĕns) (p. 104) A drug containing ingredients known to be addictive that is regulated by the Federal Controlled Substances Act of 1970.

dependence (dē-PĔN-dĕns) (p. 108) Physical changes in autonomic nervous system function that can occur when opioids are used long term and are not needed for pain control.

nonopioid analgesic (NŎN-Ō-pē-ōyd ăn-ăl-JĒZ-ĭk) (p. 110) A drug that reduces a person's perception of pain; it is not similar to opium and has little potential for psychologic or physical dependence.

opioid analgesic (Ō-pē-ōyd ăn-ăl-JĒZ-ĭk) (p. 106) A drug containing any ingredient derived from the poppy plant (or a similar synthetic chemical) that changes a person's perception of pain and has a potential for psychologic or physical dependence.

pain (PĀN) (p. 101) An unpleasant sensory and emotional experience associated with acute or potential tissue damage; pain is whatever a patient says it is and exists whenever a patient says it does.

tolerance (TŎL-ŭr-ĕns) (p. 106) The adjustment of the body to long-term opioid use that increases the rate at which a drug is eliminated and reduces the main effects (pain relief) and side effects of the drug.

withdrawal (wĭth-DRŎ-ĕl) (p. 108) Autonomic nervous system symptoms occurring when long-term opioid therapy is stopped suddenly after physical dependence is present.

PAIN

Pain is an unpleasant sensory and emotional experience associated with tissue damage. It is common, and everyone experiences it in a different way. The best way to describe and monitor pain is through the patient's own report. Thus pain is whatever the patient says it is and exists whenever he or she says it does.

We perceive pain with all our senses. How we feel and react to pain depends on our emotional makeup along with our previous experiences with pain.

Pain is often both underreported and undertreated, leading to poor pain control. Box 7-1 lists factors that contribute to the poor reporting and treatment of pain. One factor in good pain control is recognizing the severity of the patient's pain, even when he or she cannot describe it.

How much pain the patient feels is called *pain intensity*. There are several ways to work with the patient to determine pain intensity. Figure 7-1 shows an example

 Memory Jogger

Pain is whatever the patient says it is and exists whenever he or she says it does.

Box 7-1 | **Barriers to Good Pain Management**

- Patient's and health care worker's fear of addiction
- Patient's fear of meaning of pain, for example:
  - Worsening of condition
  - Threats to independence
  - Impending death
- Patient's and health care worker's belief that pain is an expected part of aging
- Patient's fear of testing
- Health care worker's fear of "drugging the older adult"
- Health care provider's fear of overdosing a patient

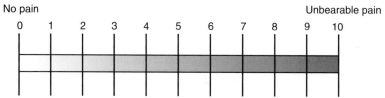

No pain   Unbearable pain

0   1   2   3   4   5   6   7   8   9   10

Patient indicates the number that matches his or her pain on the scale from 0 to 10

FIGURE 7-1 A common numeric pain distress scale.

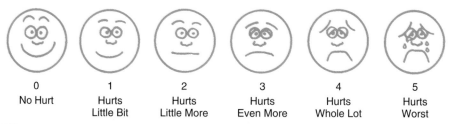

0	1	2	3	4	5
No Hurt	Hurts Little Bit	Hurts Little More	Hurts Even More	Hurts Whole Lot	Hurts Worst

FIGURE 7-2 The Wong-Baker FACES Pain Rating Scale for children and nonverbal adults. (From Hocken-berry, M. J., & Wilson, D. (2015). *Wong's nursing care of infants and children* (10th ed.). St. Louis: Mosby. Used with permission. Copyright © 2015 Mosby.)

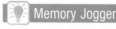
Memory Jogger

Check behaviors for pain in patients who cannot point or express pain in words.

of a common pain scale that is useful for an alert patient to rate his or her pain. When the patient cannot speak or when you are working with young children, a nonverbal scale called FACES may be used (Figure 7-2). The patient picks the face on the scale that best represents how he or she is feeling. Another scale, the FLACC (Face, Legs, Activity, Cry, Consolability) scale, is often used for infants, very young children, and any patient who cannot express pain in words or point to a face (Figure 7-3). This scale uses observations and scoring of behaviors to establish a pain intensity level.

REVIEW OF RELATED PHYSIOLOGY AND PATHOPHYSIOLOGY

PAIN ORIGIN AND TRANSMISSION

Acute pain, although uncomfortable, can be a helpful response because it tells us that something is wrong and often where it is wrong. The brain is the place where pain is actually "felt" (Figure 7-4). If you stub your toe, the damage stimulates nerve endings that send messages along a sensory nerve to the place in your brain where that particular nerve stops. The message triggers your brain to know that your toe hurts. So even though the damage causing the pain occurs in the toe, it is your brain that *perceives* the pain. If the sensory nerve between your toe and your brain were severed, you would not feel pain in your toe no matter how badly you injured it. Also, if the area of your brain that is connected to the sensory nerve of the toe were damaged or destroyed, you would not feel pain as a result of hurting your toe.

Memory Jogger

Pain perception occurs in the brain, not at the site of injury.

Category	Score		
	0	**1**	**2**
Face	No particular expression or smile	Occasional grimace or frown, withdrawn, disinterested	Frequent-to-constant quivering chin, clenched jaw
Legs	Normal position or relaxed	Uneasy, restless, tense	Kicking, or legs drawn up
Activity	Lying quietly, normal position, moves easily	Squirming, shifting back and forth, tense	Arched, rigid, or jerking
Cry	No cry (awake or asleep)	Moans or whimpers, occasional complaint	Crying steadily, screams or sobs, or frequent complaints
Consolability	Content, relaxed	Reassured by occasional touching, hugging, or being talked to, distractible	Difficult to console or comfort

Each of the five categories–(F) Face, (L) Legs, (A) Activity, (C) Cry, (C) Consolability–
is scored from 0-2, which results in a total score between 0 and 10.

FIGURE 7-3 The FLACC (Face, Legs, Activity, Cry, Consolability) pain rating scale for infants and patients who are not alert.

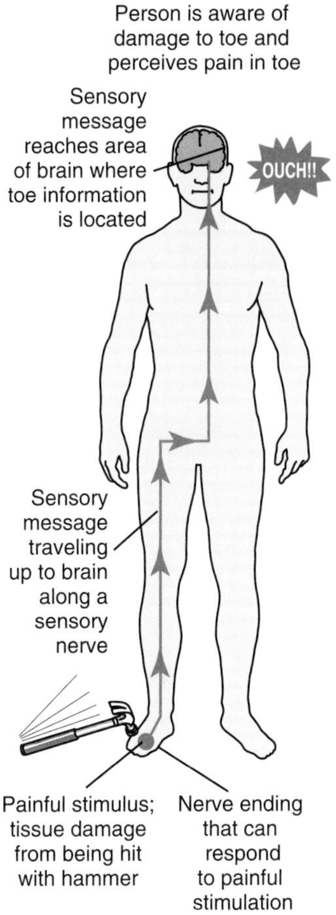

Nociceptors are sensory nerve endings that, when activated, trigger the message sent to the brain that allows the perception of pain (Figure 7-5). Nociceptors can be activated when body chemicals called *mediators* bind to them. The mediators for pain include substance P ("P" is for "pain") and many of the same mediators that cause the symptoms of inflammation, especially bradykinin (see Chapter 6). When mediators are released from damaged tissue (such as when you stub your toe), they bind to the nociceptors and activate them (see Figure 7-5). Once activated, the receptor starts electrical changes that send the message along the nerve to the brain. Other ways that the receptors can be triggered include changing their shapes (by stretching or applying pressure), exposing them to extreme heat or cold, and reducing the oxygen level in the tissue surrounding them. Different types of nerve fibers transmit pain messages to the brain. These fibers differ in how fast they transmit the message, where they are located, and what type of pain sensation is transmitted. This is one reason why not all pain drugs work in the same way and why some drugs are effective in relieving one type of pain and not effective at all for another.

PAIN PERCEPTION

Different nerve fibers end in different areas of the brain. This means that the brain perceives pain on different levels. Some fibers pass through areas of the brain where emotions and memories are stored, allowing emotions, memories, and behavior to affect pain perception. Because nerve fibers pass through many body areas on the way to the brain and interact with other nerves, the perception of pain location is not always direct. For a more complete discussion of information on pain transmission and pain types, refer to a physiology or pathophysiology textbook.

Each person's pain perception is different. The smallest amount of tissue damage that makes a person aware of having pain is known as the *pain threshold*. It is the point that a person first feels any pain. The pain threshold is different for every person and varies from one body site to another. Most drugs used for pain control change (raise) the patient's pain threshold.

Related to pain threshold is *pain tolerance,* which is a person's ability to endure or "stand" the pain intensity. Behavioral and emotional factors as well as physical factors affect a person's pain tolerance. This makes pain tolerance unique to each person. Pain tolerance is so personal that you cannot determine a person's level of pain on the basis of behavior. You must always ask patients about their pain. Just because a person tolerates pain does not mean that he or she isn't suffering!

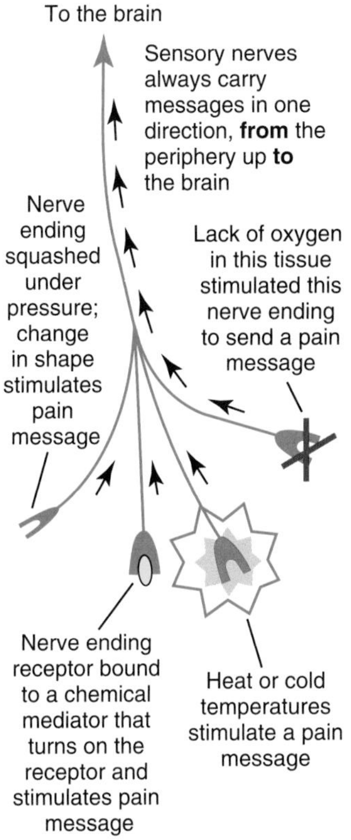

Person is aware of damage to toe and perceives pain in toe

Sensory message reaches area of brain where toe information is located

OUCH!!

Sensory message traveling up to brain along a sensory nerve

Painful stimulus; tissue damage from being hit with hammer

Nerve ending that can respond to painful stimulation

FIGURE 7-4 A sensory pathway for pain perception.

To the brain

Sensory nerves always carry messages in one direction, **from** the periphery up **to** the brain

Nerve ending squashed under pressure; change in shape stimulates pain message

Lack of oxygen in this tissue stimulated this nerve ending to send a pain message

Nerve ending receptor bound to a chemical mediator that turns on the receptor and stimulates pain message

Heat or cold temperatures stimulate a pain message

FIGURE 7-5 Sensory nerve endings (nociceptors) triggered by different types of stimuli to send pain messages to the brain.

Memory Jogger

Different types of nerve fibers are responsible for the type of pain felt and which type of pain drug is most effective at relieving the pain.

Clinical Pitfall

Do not assume that a patient who is tolerating pain well is comfortable.

Memory Jogger

Common physiologic changes with acute pain include elevated heart rate, blood pressure, and respiratory rate; cool, clammy skin; dry mouth; restlessness; and inability to concentrate.

Memory Jogger

The four most common sources of chronic pain are:
• Neck and back pain
• Arthritis pain
• Migraine headaches
• Nerve pain

Clinical Pitfall

Do not rely on changes in vital signs to indicate the intensity of chronic pain.

QSEN: Safety

Clinical Pitfall

Do not rely on nondrug therapies alone for pain control.

QSEN: Safety

TYPES OF PAIN

Pain is divided into types on the basis of its cause, how long it lasts, and whether it is present continuously or comes and goes *(intermittent)*. The three main types of pain are acute, chronic, and cancer.

Acute pain has a sudden onset, an identifiable cause, a limited duration, and improves with time even when it is not treated. It is the most common pain type; typical causes include trauma, surgery, heart attack, inflammation, and burns. Acute pain usually triggers the physical responses of elevated heart rate, respiratory rate, and blood pressure. Skin becomes cool and clammy with increased sweating of the hands and feet. The mouth becomes dry, and usually the pupils of the eyes dilate. A person's behavioral responses to acute pain often include restlessness, inability to concentrate, general distress, and a sense that something bad is happening (a sense of *impending doom*).

Chronic pain is present daily for 6 months. It persists or increases with time, may not have an identifiable cause, and does not trigger the physiologic responses associated with acute pain. This means that a person with chronic pain can have severe pain intensity without changes from the normal ranges for heart rate, breathing rate, or blood pressure. Chronic pain may hurt less on some days than others but is always present. Causes may be difficult to find.

Cancer pain has many causes and is complex. This means that more than one pain strategy and often more than one type of drug for pain control are needed. The patient with cancer often receives traditional pain-control drugs but at much higher doses than those prescribed for other types of pain. The drug therapy plan may include every type of pain-control drug given in combination to ensure adequate pain relief. Drug therapy for cancer pain must be tailored to each patient for the most effective pain control.

GENERAL ISSUES RELATED TO ANALGESIC DRUG THERAPY

Pain is the number one health problem that drives people to seek medical help. It interferes with every aspect of a person's life and may decrease the quality of life. Pain control involves many different approaches. Drug therapy is one approach. *Usually the nondrug therapies for pain control are used along with drug therapy, not in place of it.*

Analgesics are drugs of any class that control pain either by changing the perception or by reducing the source of pain. Different types of drugs are used for pain control based on how they work. These include opioids and nonopioid miscellaneous drugs. Different types of pain respond differently to each drug type.

All analgesic drugs provide some degree of pain relief, but some drugs are stronger than others. It may take a greater amount of a weaker drug to provide the same amount of pain relief that a stronger drug provides.

Drugs prescribed for pain control have traditionally been ordered on a PRN, or "as needed," basis, usually with a range of doses permitted (for example, "Give morphine sulfate 2 to 6 mg IV every 4 to 6 hours PRN"). Such drug orders, known as *range orders,* are not always effective for controlling acute pain because there is too much variation in the timing and dose of the drug. Patients often try to go as long as possible before accepting another dose, or health care workers may stick to the lowest doses and the longest durations.

Better pain-control plans involve two techniques: doses are given on a schedule around the clock to prevent complete elimination of the drug before the next dose, or the patient is given a machine to "punch in" a small intravenous (IV) dose whenever the need arises. This is called *patient-controlled analgesia (PCA).* Sometimes these two techniques are used at the same time for personalized and effective pain control.

Many drugs used for pain control have ingredients that may be addictive. In the United States any drug that contains ingredients known to be addictive is classified by the federal government as a **controlled substance** and is regulated by the Federal Controlled Substances Act of 1970. This act classifies controlled substances into five

Table 7-1	Classification of Controlled Substances (United States)	
SCHEDULE	**DESCRIPTION**	**EXAMPLES**
I	High potential for abuse No accepted medical use in treatment in United States Lack of accepted safety for use of the drug or other substance under medical supervision	More than 80 drugs or substances of which the following are the most well known: Alpha-acetylmethadol; gamma-hydroxybutyric acid (GBH); heroin; lysergic acid diethylamide (LSD); marijuana; mescaline; peyote; "quaaludes"
II	High potential for abuse Currently accepted use for treatment in United States Abuse may lead to severe psychologic dependence or physical dependence	More than 30 drugs or substances of which the following are the most well known: Amphetamines; cocaine; codeine; fentanyl; hydromorphone (Dilaudid); meperidine (Demerol); methadone; methylphenidate (Ritalin); morphine; oxycodone (Percodan); pentobarbital; secobarbital
III	Potential for abuse is less than the drugs or substances in schedules I and II Currently accepted medical use for treatment in the United States Abuse may lead to moderate or low physical dependence or high psychologic dependence	Most drugs are compounds containing some small amounts of the drugs from schedule II along with acetaminophen or aspirin such as Tylenol No. 3 or No. 4, Fiorinal Other drugs include anabolic steroids such as testosterone preparations and sodium oxybate [Xyrem], a drug containing GHB for use with the sleep disorder narcolepsy
IV	Low potential for abuse relative to the drugs or substances in schedule III Currently accepted medical use for treatment in the United States Abuse may lead to limited physical dependence or psychologic dependence relative to the drugs or substances in schedule III	Include diet drugs with propionic acid Other well-known drugs include benzodiazepines (lorazepam [Ativan], flurazepam [Dalmane], diazepam [Valium], midazolam [Versed], alprazolam [Xanax]); chloral hydrate; paraldehyde; pentazocine (Talwin); phenobarbital
V	Low potential for abuse relative to the drugs or substances in schedule IV Currently accepted medical use in the United States Abuse may lead to limited physical dependence or psychologic dependence relative to the drugs or substances in schedule IV	Include cough preparations with small amounts of codeine and drugs for diarrhea that also contain small amounts of opioids such as diphenoxylate with atropine (Lomotil)

Data from United States Drug Enforcement Administration, Title 21, Section 812.

schedules based on how likely they are to result in addiction. The drugs most likely to lead to addiction are in schedule I. Those with the least potential for addiction are in schedule V. Table 7-1 describes and lists examples of drugs in each category.

The federal government requires that all schedule II and some schedule III drugs be carefully controlled. These drugs require a prescription written by a state-approved prescriber with a registered number from the Drug Enforcement Administration (DEA). These drugs are stored in a locked area of the facility and unit, and each drug dose is carefully tracked. On hospital units, these drugs are counted at the change of every shift, and each prescribed dose must be "signed out" for a particular patient. States vary in whether licensed practical nurses (LPNs) and licensed vocational nurses (LVNs) are permitted to administer any or all schedule drugs.

 Memory Jogger

Analgesics include:
- Opioids
- Nonopioid miscellaneous drugs

 Clinical Pitfall

Pain drugs have varying strengths and dosages to achieve the same level of pain relief.

QSEN: Safety

Memory Jogger

In the United States drugs and drug products with the highest potential for addiction or abuse are classified as schedule I; those with the lowest potential for addiction or abuse are classified as schedule V.

 Drug Alert!

Action/Intervention Alert

Check the patient's pain level 30 minutes after giving a pain-control drug and then hourly.

QSEN: Safety

Many drug types can be used as analgesia for pain control. Each type has both different and common actions and effects. The *intended response* of all pain-control drugs is to reduce pain. In addition to the practices listed for drug administration in Chapter 2, general responsibilities for safe administration of drugs for pain control are listed in the following paragraphs. Specific responsibilities are listed with each individual drug class.

Responsibilities before administering pain-control drugs include checking the patient's pain intensity using the pain scale preferred by your workplace (see Figures 7-1 through 7-3). Checking the pain level before you give a drug helps to determine how effective the drug is in relieving the patient's pain.

Check to see when the patient last received the drug for pain control. Giving doses too close together can lead to more side effects or toxic levels. Giving doses too far apart can lead to more suffering for the patient. If the patient is to receive a drug on a regular schedule rather than PRN, try to keep on schedule even if the patient is sleeping or is not reporting pain. *A sleeping patient is not necessarily comfortable or pain free.*

Responsibilities after administering a pain-control drug include asking how much pain relief the patient has received as a result of the drug. This helps to determine whether the drug is right for the patient's pain, if the dose needs to be changed, or if the pain-control strategy must be adjusted. Check pain relief after 30 minutes and then hourly until the next dose is scheduled.

Teach the patient taking a pain-control drug that the best pain relief occurs when drugs are taken on a regular schedule rather than PRN. If the patient thinks that the pain is improving and less drug is needed, tell him or her first to reduce the dose but to maintain the schedule. If the pain continues to improve, the time between doses may be increased. Remind the patient that addiction will not occur if the drugs are taken to relieve pain.

OPIOIDS (NARCOTICS)

Opioid analgesics, also called *narcotics,* are drugs that contain any ingredient derived from the poppy plant (or a similar synthetic chemical) that change a person's perception of pain and have the potential for psychologic or physical dependence. All opioids work in the same way and have similar side effects. The main difference among various types of opioids is the strength of the drug.

Prescribed opioids can be addictive and generally are classified by the U.S. federal government as schedule II drugs. They also have a high potential for abuse that can lead to psychologic or physical dependence. (When an opioid is combined in smaller dosages with other drugs, the combination may be classified as a schedule III drug.) The fear of addiction to opioids is one cause of poorly treated pain. In addition, opioids are *high-alert drugs* that have an increased risk of causing patient harm if used in error. The error may be giving too high a dose, giving too low a dose, giving a dose to a patient for whom it was not prescribed, and not giving it to a patient for whom it was prescribed.

Although most opioids are prescribed for pain control, there are other conditions for which opioids may be used. Some other uses for opioids include controlling coughing, reducing diarrhea, and reducing respiratory difficulties at the end-of-life and with end-stage chronic respiratory diseases.

An issue that can occur with longer-term opioid use is drug tolerance. **Tolerance** is the adjustment of the body to long-term opioid use that increases the rate of drug elimination and reduces the main effect (pain relief) and side effects of the drug. It occurs with anyone who is taking opioids for a long period of time. More drug is needed to achieve the same degree of pain relief. Thus although there are recommended dosages for acute pain and short-term opioid use, dosages for long-term use can be many times more than the "standard" short-term dose as the person becomes drug tolerant. For this reason, there is no true cap or ceiling on opioid drug doses with long-term use, such as with prolonged cancer pain.

 Memory Jogger

Opioid dosages for long-term use can be many times more than the "standard" short-term dose as the person becomes drug tolerant.

The following table describes opioids most commonly used for pain control. Be sure to consult a drug reference for more information about any specific opioid. The dosages listed are those recommended for acute pain and short-term use. The dosages used for other pain types may be much higher. Opioids given parenterally are usually single-agent drugs. When given orally, opioid tablets, capsules, or liquids may contain other drugs such as acetaminophen, aspirin, or other nonsteroidal anti-inflammatory drugs (NSAIDs).

Do Not Confuse

OxyContin *with* **MS Contin**

An order for OxyContin can be confused with MS Contin. Although both drugs are opioids, the large differences in dosages make under-dosing or overdosing possible.

QSEN: Safety

Dosages for Common Opioids

Drug	Dosage
morphine ❶ (Morphine Sulfate, Duramorph, Epimorph ♣, Morphitec ♣, Roxanol, MS Contin)	*Adults:* 10-30 mg orally every 4 hr (Children's oral dose calculated individually based on the child's age, size, and pain severity) *Adults:* 5-20 mg IM or 7-10 mg IV every 4 hr *Children:* 100-200 mcg/kg IM or 50-100 mcg/kg IV every 4 hr
hydromorphone ❶ (Dilaudid, Hydrostat)	*Adults:* 2-7.5 mg orally every 3-6 hr; 1-2 mg IM every 2-3 hr; 500 mcg-1 mg IV every 3 hr as needed Safety and efficacy in children not established
meperidine ❶ (Demerol)	*Adults:* 50-150 mg orally, IM, or IV every 3-4 hr *Children:* 1.1-1.7 mg/kg orally or IM every 3-4 hr
codeine ❶ (Paveral ♣)	*Adults:* 15-60 mg orally or IM every 3-6 hr *Children:* 0.5 mg/kg orally or IM every 3-6 hr
fentanyl ❶ (Fentanyl, Actiq, Oralet) fentanyl transdermal ❶ (Duragesic)	Oral lozenges and lollipops vary in strength; check carefully *Adults:* 0.05-0.1 mg IM every 1-2 hr, or 2.5-10 mg patch every 72 hr
oxycodone ❶ (OxyContin, OxyFast, Supeudol ♣)	*Adults:* 10-160 mg orally every 12 hr
oxycodone with acetaminophen ❶ (Endocet ♣, Percocet, Tylox)	*Adults:* 1.5-10 mg orally every 4-6 hr
oxycodone with aspirin ❶ (Endodan ♣, Oxycodan, Percodan)	*Adults:* 1.5-10 mg orally every 4-6 hr
oxymorphone ❶ (Opana, Numorphan)	*Adults:* 10-20 mg orally every 4-6 hr
hydrocodone ❶ (Lortab, Vicodin)	*Adults:* 5-10 mg orally every 4-6 hr *Children:* 2-5 mg orally every 4-6 hr
hydrocodone ER (Zohydro)	*Adults:* 10 mg orally every 12 hours Safety and efficacy in children not established
hydrocodone with acetaminophen ❶ (Dolacet, Polygesic, Vicodin)	*Adults:* 5-7 mg orally every 4-6 hr *Children:* 2.5 mg orally in solution every 4-6 hr
tramadol ❶ (Ultram)	*Adults:* 50-70 mg orally every 6 hr
tapentadol (Nucynta)	*Adults:* 50-100 mg orally every 4-6 hr
(Nucynta ER)	*Adults:* 50 mg orally every 12 hr Safety and efficacy in children not established

❶ High-alert drug.

Do Not Confuse

hydromorphone *with* **morphine**

An order for hydromorphone can be confused with morphine. Although both drugs are opioids, hydromorphone is five times stronger than morphine. Giving hydromorphone in place of morphine could result in a serious overdose.

QSEN: Safety

How Opioids Work

The classic opioid is morphine. Morphine and all other opioids work by binding to opioid receptor sites in the brain and other areas. The main opioid receptors are mu (OP3), kappa (OP2), and delta (OP1). When a drug binds to and acts as an agonist at mu, the responses include pain relief, some degree of respiratory depression, some sedation, decreased intestinal motility, and pupil constriction. When a drug binds to and acts as an agonist at kappa, the responses include sedation, pupil constriction, and *dysphoria* (a state of feeling emotional or mental discomfort, restlessness, and

Do Not Confuse

tramadol *with* Toradol

An order for tramadol can be confused with Toradol. Tramadol is an oral opioid analgesic. Toradol is a nonsteroidal anti-inflammatory drug (NSAID) that can be given orally or parenterally.

QSEN: Safety

Common Side Effects

Opioids

Constipation,   Drowsiness   Flushing
Nausea/
Vomiting

Itching

Memory Jogger

Drug dependence is a physical problem; drug addiction is a psychologic problem.

Clinical Pitfall

Never substitute one opioid for another without an order from the prescriber that includes a recalculation of the dose. Strengths vary.

QSEN: Safety

anxiety). When a drug binds to and acts as an agonist at delta, the responses include some pain relief, dysphoria, and hallucinations.

Morphine binds most tightly and best to the mu receptor, acting as an agonist. This activates the mu receptors, and the person's perception of pain is altered. *Opioids only alter the perception of pain; they do nothing at the site of damaged tissue to reduce the cause of pain.* Some drugs act as an agonist at one type of opioid receptor site and, at the same time, act as an antagonist at other opioid receptor sites, providing mixed responses. The opioids that provide the best pain relief bind most strongly to the mu receptors. Agents that are strong morphine agonists include morphine, hydromorphone, oxymorphone, meperidine, fentanyl, and methadone. Those that bind moderately well to the mu receptors and provide some degree of pain relief include codeine, hydrocodone, oxycodone, and tramadol.

Drugs that are considered morphine agonist-antagonists have mixed responses. They tend to act as agonists at kappa and delta and as antagonist at mu. As a result, they provide less pain relief than pure morphine agonists and more hallucinations and dysphoria. They also produce less respiratory depression than mu agonists. These drugs include pantazocine (Talwin), butorphanol (Stadol), and nalbuphine (Nubain). They are less commonly used for pain control than are the opioids that are mu agonists.

Side Effects. The most common side effect of opioids is constipation. Some patients may have nausea and vomiting if intestinal motility is affected. Flushing and skin itching also may occur as blood vessels dilate. At higher dosages, drowsiness is common.

Adverse Effects. *Respiratory depression* is possible when opioids are used, especially at higher doses and when the drugs are given intravenously. Most patients have only mild respiratory depression, with respirations dropping to 7 to 12 breaths/minute. If severe (less than 8 breaths/minute), action must be taken to prevent hypoxia (low tissue oxygen levels).

Addiction, dependence, and *withdrawal* can occur with opioid use. **Dependence** is the physical changes in autonomic nervous system function that can occur when opioids are used long term (more than a few weeks, especially after pain is reduced or no longer present). **Addiction** is the psychologic need or craving for the "high" feeling resulting from the use of opioids when pain is not present. When opioids are needed for pain, their use seldom causes either dependence or addiction.

Withdrawal is the occurrence of autonomic nervous system symptoms when long-term opioid therapy is stopped suddenly after physical dependence is present. Symptoms include nausea, vomiting, abdominal cramping, sweating, delirium, and seizures. This reaction seldom occurs in a patient who is taking opioids for pain. It is common among people who are not in pain but who take opioids for the psychologic "high" that they can produce.

What To Do *Before* Giving Opioids

In addition to the general responsibilities related to analgesic therapy for pain (p. 104), check the dose and the specific drug name carefully. *Opioids are not interchangeable because the strength of the drugs varies. Only the prescriber can change the drug order.* Drug doses must be recalculated by the prescriber when one opioid is switched to another.

When giving the first dose of an opioid to a patient who has never taken an opioid (is opioid naïve), check the patient's respiratory rate and oxygen saturation. Opioids can cause some degree of respiratory depression.

What To Do *After* Giving Opioids

In addition to the general responsibilities related to analgesic therapy for pain (p. 104), be sure to monitor the patient's respiratory rate and oxygen saturation for indications of respiratory depression. This is especially important when the patient is receiving an opioid for the first time or when the drug dosage has been increased. If the respiratory rate is 8 or less and the patient is sleeping, try to wake him or her. First call the patient's name. If there is no response, gently shake his or her arm. Shake more firmly if needed. If the patient does not respond to these actions, use a slightly stronger trigger (without using enough force to cause harm) such as:

- Squeezing the trapezius muscle (located at the angle of the shoulder and neck muscle)
- Applying pressure to the nail bed

If the patient cannot be aroused, immediately call for help. If the patient's oxygen saturation is below 95% or is five percentage points lower than his or her normal saturation, arouse the patient and check the saturation when fully awake. If the saturation does not improve when fully awake, apply supplemental oxygen and notify the charge nurse or prescriber.

When respiratory depression is severe, the opioid effects may need to be reversed by giving an opioid blocker (antagonist) such as naloxone (Narcan, Evzio) or naltrexone (Depade, ReVia, Vivitrol). When an IV opioid blocker is given, it displaces opioids on the opioid receptors. When the opioid is off the receptors, all the effects of the opioids are reversed within 1 minute, including respiratory depression. Unfortunately the pain control effects are also reversed. Watch the patient who has received an opioid receptor blocker (antagonist) for respiratory depression closely for several hours in case respiratory depression recurs.

A patient receiving an opioid may become drowsy and is at risk for falling. Be sure to raise the side rails and place the call light button within easy reach for the patient.

When a patient is receiving opioids for several days, ask about constipation daily. Most patients taking opioids for 2 days or longer have constipation. Be sure to give any prescribed stool softeners or laxatives.

Opioids can cause a sudden lowering of blood pressure, especially when the patient changes position (*orthostatic hypotension*). Instruct the patient change position slowly.

What To *Teach* Patients About Opioids

In addition to the general precautions related to analgesic therapy for pain (p. 104), teach patients to take opioids with food rather than on an empty stomach to reduce the risk for nausea. Teach patients taking an extended release (ER) form of an oral opioid drug to swallow the capsule or tablet whole because chewing it or opening the capsule allows too much of the drug to be absorbed all at once and an overdose can occur.

Opioids cause drowsiness. Warn the patient not to drive or operate heavy machinery when taking these drugs. In addition, the patient may feel dizzy or light-headed from a sudden drop in blood pressure. Tell him or her to move slowly when rising or changing positions.

Constipation is a common side effect because opioids slow intestinal movement. If the prescriber has ordered a stool softener or laxative, urge the patient to start using these drugs before constipation occurs.

Life Span Considerations for Opioids

Pediatric Considerations. Opioid drugs are *high-alert medications* that are used for pain control in children of all ages. Dosages are calculated for each child on the basis of the child's age, size (weight in kilograms), health, and pain severity. Identifying pain intensity with a young child can be difficult but is still needed. For a child who is old enough to talk, use the FACES pain scale (see Figure 7-2) to help determine pain severity. For an infant or child too young to talk, rely on behavior to help determine pain severity such as the behaviors described in the FLACC scale (see Figure 7-3). Infants in pain cry frequently with great intensity. They do not smile, laugh, or show interest in toys and are not comforted by holding, cuddling, rocking, or a pacifier.

Memory Jogger

When an opioid blocker (e.g. naloxone) is given, all of the opioid effects are reversed, including the pain control effects.

Drug Alert!

Teaching Alert

Teach patients taking an extended release (ER) form of an oral opioid drug to swallow the capsule or tablet whole because chewing it or opening the capsule allows too much of the drug to be absorbed all at once and an overdose can occur.

QSEN: Safety

Memory Jogger

What is painful for an adult is painful for a child.

A child can have the same side effects as an adult when taking opioids. Constipation is a problem for a child, and the same steps must be taken to avoid it.

Respiratory depression can be a dangerous problem for infants or young children. When opioids are used with an infant or a small child, it is best to use an apnea monitor and/or pulse oximeter. When these devices are not available, check the patient's rate and depth of respiration at least every 15 minutes. Remember that infants and small children may have a normal respiratory rate between 30 and 40 breaths/minute. A respiratory rate of less than 20 in an infant or small child is cause for concern.

Considerations for Pregnancy and Lactation. Opioids may be prescribed to women during pregnancy. These drugs do cross the placenta and enter the fetus. The fetus can become addicted to opioids and go through withdrawal after birth. If the mother receives long-term opioid therapy or abuses heroin during pregnancy and the drug is discontinued several weeks before birth, the newborn should not have any symptoms of withdrawal. However, if the mother is still receiving long-term opioid therapy or abusing opioid drugs when the baby is born, the newborn will need special care for withdrawal.

When opioids are given to a woman in labor, the baby may have respiratory depression after delivery. If an opioid is given intravenously within an hour of delivery, the baby may need a dose of an opioid antagonist such as naloxone (Narcan) after delivery.

Breastfeeding is best avoided when a woman is taking opioid drugs for more than a couple of days. If the mother is unable to stop breastfeeding while taking the drug, teach her the strategies listed in Box 1-1 in Chapter 1, to reduce infant exposure to these drugs.

Considerations for Older Adults. In addition to the usual effects of opioids, an older adult is at risk for low vision. The pupil of the older adult does not dilate fully, and less light enters the eye, reducing vision. When the older patient takes an opioid, the pupil is even smaller than usual, reducing vision even more. This problem increases his or her risk for falling. Teach the older adult to increase room lighting to make reading easier and reduce the risk for tripping and falling over objects.

Opioids, especially meperidine (Demerol), can make the chest muscles of older adults tighter, which makes breathing and coughing more difficult. Thus the risk for pneumonia and hypoxia is greater for them. Check the respiratory rate and depth and the oxygen saturation at least every 2 hours. In addition, meperidine causes the buildup of a toxic metabolite in older adults that can result in seizures.

NONOPIOID PAIN-CONTROL DRUGS

A variety of nonopioid drugs can be used alone or with other pain-control drugs to manage special types of pain. **Nonopioid analgesics** are drugs that reduce a person's perception of pain but are not similar to opium and have little potential for psychologic or physical dependence. These additional drugs are sometimes termed *adjuvant drugs* because they enhance the pain-control features of other pain drugs. Most have other main uses and are discussed in more detail elsewhere in this text.

ACETAMINOPHEN

Acetaminophen alone (such as Abenol ♣, Atasol ♣, Panadol, Tylenol, and many others) can be effective for pain relief. It works in the brain to change the perception of pain and reduces the sensitivity of pain receptors.

Acetaminophen is given orally in tablets, capsules, or liquids and can also be given rectally in a suppository. It is available over-the-counter as a single drug or combined with other substances such as caffeine and aspirin (Excedrin). It also is combined with other pain-control drugs, especially opioids. The usual adult dose is 325 to

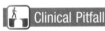

[!] Drug Alert!

Action/Intervention Alert

If a mother receives an opioid during labor, watch her newborn closely for the first 2 to 4 hours after birth for any sign of respiratory depression.

QSEN: Safety

Clinical Pitfall

Avoid the use of meperidine in the older adult.

QSEN: Safety

650 mg every 4 to 6 hours and should not exceed 3 g/day. For children the usual dose is 7 to 15 mg/kg every 4 hours.

A new formulation of acetaminophen can be given intravenously. This drug, OFIRMEV, is indicated in an acute care setting for mild to moderate pain in patients over 2 years old. The drug should be administered only as a 15-minute infusion, not as a bolus.

Important Issues

Because oral acetaminophen is available without a prescription, many people believe that it has no side effects or adverse effects. However, one of its metabolites can be toxic when taken at high doses or too often, especially to the liver, which can be damaged or destroyed. With higher dosages or overdose, kidney damage also can occur. Taking this drug with alcohol greatly increases the risk for permanent liver damage.

Warn patients that many over-the-counter drugs for colds, headache, allergies, and sleep aids also contain acetaminophen, as do a variety of drugs prescribed for pain. The acetaminophen in these drugs must be figured into the maximum daily dose of 3 g along with any separate acetaminophen. Remind patients not to drink alcoholic beverages on days when they take acetaminophen or any drug containing acetaminophen.

When acetaminophen overdose occurs, the drug acetylcysteine must be given intravenously as soon as possible as an antidote to prevent liver failure. If acetylcysteine administration is delayed more than 24 hours after an acetaminophen overdose, it will not be effective in saving the liver.

Life Span Considerations for Acetaminophen

Pediatric Considerations. Acetaminophen is toxic to the liver at higher doses. *A young child should never receive an adult dose of acetaminophen.* Because acetaminophen comes in liquid forms with different strengths, it is important to teach parents to read labels carefully and not assume that the doses are the same for all liquids. Some liquid forms contain as few as 16 mg/mL, and others may contain as much as 70 mg/mL.

NONSTEROIDAL ANTI-INFLAMMATORY DRUGS

Nonsteroidal anti-inflammatory drugs (NSAIDs) are one type of nonopioid analgesic. NSAIDs can help manage pain associated with inflammation, bone pain, cancer pain, and soft tissue trauma. These drugs act at the tissue where pain starts and do not change a person's perception of pain. Chapter 6 provides a complete discussion of the actions and uses of NSAIDs as well as the patient care responsibilities.

ANTIDEPRESSANTS

Older and newer antidepressants have been found to reduce some types of chronic pain and cancer pain. The most common antidepressant drugs used for pain control are amitriptyline (Apo-Amitriptyline ✦, Elavil), nortriptyline (Pamelor), paroxetine (Paxil), and sertraline (Zoloft). They are usually given orally, and the doses for pain control can be different from those used to treat depression. Antidepressants help increase the amount of natural opioids (endorphins and enkephalins) in the brain and also reduce the depression that can occur with chronic pain. Usually the patient must take one of these drugs for 1 or 2 weeks before he or she feels any relief from pain. Chapter 27 provides a complete discussion of the actions and uses of antidepressant drugs as well as the patient care responsibilities.

ANTICONVULSANTS

Certain anticonvulsants (drugs that reduce seizure activity) have been found to reduce some types of chronic pain and cancer pain, especially neuropathic pain (nerve pain with tingling and burning) and migraine headaches. The two most common anticonvulsant drugs used for pain control are gabapentin (Neurontin) and

 Clinical Pitfall

Acetaminophen can be toxic to the liver and should not be taken by anyone with liver health problems.

QSEN: Safety

 Drug Alert!

Teaching Alert

Teach parents to read the label on liquid acetaminophen bottles for infants and small children carefully and ensure that the correct dose is given for the child's size. Teach parents to telephone the nearest pharmacy and talk with the pharmacist to ensure that the dose is correct if they are not confident in their own calculations.

QSEN: Safety

pregabalin (Lyrica). They appear to work by reducing the rate of electrical transmission along sensory nerves and may also affect pain perception. The doses for pain control are often higher than those used to control seizures. Chapter 25 provides a complete discussion of the actions and uses of anticonvulsant drugs as well as the patient care responsibilities.

MUSCLE RELAXANTS

Skeletal muscle relaxants are another group of drugs that are used in combination with other drugs for pain control when part of the pain experience includes muscle spasms. A variety of drugs have the effect of relaxing skeletal muscles and reducing pain. The most common ones used for this purpose are the carbamates and the cyclobenzaprines. Both of these drug groups work by depressing the central nervous system (CNS) and produce significant sedation. A more complete discussion of the actions, dosages, and side effects of these drugs is presented in Chapter 30.

Get Ready for Practice!

Key Points

- Pain is whatever the patient says it is and exists whenever he or she says it does.
- Acute pain usually triggers the stress response of the body and results in changes in a patient's vital signs; chronic pain often does not.
- Giving pain-control drugs on a regular schedule rather than on a PRN basis is likely to provide better pain relief.
- A sleeping patient may still have pain. Do not skip a regularly scheduled dose of a drug for pain control just because the patient is sleeping.
- Opioids only alter the perception of pain; they do nothing at the site of the damaged tissue to affect the cause of the pain.
- Physical dependence, addiction, and withdrawal are rare when opioids are taken by a patient who is in pain.
- Use an apnea monitor and pulse oximeter to monitor the breathing effectiveness of an infant or small child receiving opioids.

Additional Learning Resources

evolve Be sure to visit your Evolve website (http://evolve.elsevier.com/Workman/pharmacology/) for additional online resources.

SG Go to your Study Guide for additional learning activities to help you master this chapter content.

Review Questions

See the Answer Keys—In-text Review Questions for answers to these questions.

Test Yourself on the Basics

1. Which type of pain drug has the highest risk for development of physical or psychological dependence?
   A. Opioids
   B. NSAIDs
   C. Antidepressants
   D. Nonopioids

2. Which opioid drug should be avoided for older adults?
   A. Morphine
   B. Methadone
   C. Demerol
   D. Oxycodone

3. Which vital sign is most important to monitor after giving a patient a dose of morphine for severe pain?
   A. Blood pressure
   B. Heart rate
   C. Respiratory rate
   D. Oral temperature

4. For which common side effect must you monitor on a daily basis for any patient taking any opioid drug for pain?
   A. Confusion
   B. Constipation
   C. Tachycardia
   D. Diarrhea

5. How can you assess pain in an infant?
   A. Use a number-based pain scale.
   B. Ask the parents if they think the infant is in pain.
   C. Monitor the infant using the FLACC scale.
   D. Use a pain scale with faces to determine severity of the pain.

Test Yourself on Advanced Concepts

6. Which side effects or adverse effects are associated with opioid analgesics? (Select all that apply.)
   A. Aggression
   B. Slow, shallow respirations
   C. Constipation
   D. Widely dilated pupils
   E. High blood glucose levels
   F. Nausea and vomiting
   G. Irregular heartbeat
   H. Liver failure

7. Which teaching point is essential for older adults prescribed an opioid drug for pain control?
   A. Report the presence of constipation to the prescriber.
   B. Take any prescribed stool softeners at bedtime.
   C. Increase room lighting to decrease the risk of falling.
   D. Always take this drug on an empty stomach.

8. Why is morphine categorized in the United States as a schedule II drug rather than a schedule I drug?
   A. It has a high potential for abuse.
   B. It has a currently accepted use for treatment.
   C. It is a synthetic product rather than a naturally occurring substance.
   D. It is usually combined with nonopioid drugs when used for pain control.

9. What is the most important action to take after administering any drug for pain?
   A. Ask the patient whether the pain interferes with sleep.
   B. Assess the patient's susceptibility for drug abuse.
   C. Ask the patient to rate his or her level of pain relief.
   D. Remind the patient that dependence is possible.

10. Which opioid analgesic has the lowest normal recommended dosages?
    A. Codeine (Paveral)
    B. Morphine (Duramorph)
    C. Meperidine (Demerol)
    D. Hydromorphone (Dilaudid)

11. For which class of drug used for pain control in a small child should an apnea monitor and pulse oximetry be used to assess for respiratory depression?
    A. Aspirin
    B. Opioids
    C. Acetaminophen
    D. Nonsteroidal anti-inflammatory drugs

12. Which drug is available as an oral lozenge or lollipop?
    A. Codeine
    B. Tramadol
    C. Fentanyl
    D. Hydrocodone

13. What is the most important precaution to teach the parents of a 1-year-old child taking acetaminophen (Tylenol) for pain?
    A. "Watch your child closely for slowing of the rate and depth of breathing."
    B. "Be sure to call the prescriber if your child develops tremors of the hand."
    C. "Read the label carefully for the correct amount of liquid drug to give your child."
    D. "Check your child's pain level using the FACES pain scale before and after you give the drug."

14. What is the most important precaution to teach a patient taking acetaminophen orally for pain?
    A. Drink 8 ounces of water with each tablet.
    B. Avoid drinking alcohol while on this drug.
    C. Avoid driving or operative heavy equipment while on this drug.
    D. Be sure to wear sunscreen, a hat, and protective clothing when outdoors.

15. A 3-year-old child is to receive 250 mg of acetaminophen (Tylenol). The liquid you have on hand has a drug concentration of 160 mg/5 mL.
    A. How many milliliters is the correct dose for this child? _____ mL
    B. How many milliliters is the correct dose if the liquid has a concentration of 100 mg/5 mL? _____ mL

16. An adult patient is prescribed to receive 750 mcg of hydromorphone intravenously. The IV solution you have on hand has a concentration of 1 mg/mL. How many milliliters is the correct dose for this patient? _____mL

Critical Thinking Activities

See the Answer Keys—Critical Thinking Activities for answers to these activities.

Mrs. Black is a 55-year-old woman who has had chronic low back pain for about 5 years, for which she takes 440 mg of naproxen sodium orally twice daily. She now has an acute exacerbation of her back pain after tripping on the stairs and has been prescribed fentanyl (Duragesic) 100 mcg/hr for the next 72 hours.

1. What type of drug is naproxen sodium?
2. What type of drug is fentanyl (Duragesic)?
3. Is it okay for this patient to continue to take the naproxen sodium at the same time she takes the fentanyl? Why or why not?
4. How is fentanyl (Duragesic) 100 mcg/hr administered?
5. What are the adverse effects of this drug?

Anti-Infectives: Antibacterial Drugs

http://evolve.elsevier.com/Workman/pharmacology/

Objectives

After studying this chapter you should be able to:

1. List the names, actions, usual adult dosages, possible side effects, and adverse effects of the different types of antibacterial drugs.
2. Describe what to do before and after giving any of the different types of antibacterial drugs.
3. Explain what to teach patients taking any of the different types of antibacterial drugs, including what to do, what not to do, and when to call the prescriber.
4. Describe life span considerations for the different types of antibacterial drugs.

Key Terms

antibiotic resistance (ăn-tĭ-bī-Ŏ-tĭk rē-ZĬS-těns) (p. 134) The ability of a bacterium to resist the effects of antibacterials.

bactericidal (băk-tēr-ĭ-SĪD-ŭl) (p. 115) A drug that reduces the number of bacteria by killing them directly.

bacteriostatic (băk-tēr-ē-ō-STĂT-ĭk) (p. 115) A drug that reduces the number of bacteria by preventing them from dividing and growing rather than directly killing them.

cell wall synthesis inhibitors (p. 120) A class of antibacterial drugs that kills susceptible bacteria by preventing them from forming strong, protective cell walls.

drug generation (DRŬG jĕn-ŭr-Ā-shŭn) (p. 121) Stage of drug development in which later generations are changed slightly to improve their effectiveness or means of administration.

fluoroquinolones (flŏr-ō-KWĬN-ă-lōnz) (p. 132) A group of drugs from the DNA synthesis inhibitor class that enter bacterial cells and prevent bacteria reproduction by suppressing the action of two enzymes important in making bacterial DNA.

metabolism inhibitors (mă-TĂS-bo-lizm ĭn-HĬB-ĭ-tŏrs) (p. 130) A class of antibacterial drugs that interfere with bacterial reproduction by preventing the bacteria from making folic acid.

protein synthesis inhibitors (PRŌ-tēn SĬN-thē-sĭs ĭn-HĬB-ĭ-tŏrs) (p. 124) A large class of antibacterial drugs that includes aminoglycosides, macrolides, and tetracyclines, which prevent bacteria from making proteins important to their life cycles and infective processes.

spectrum of efficacy (SPĔK-trŭm of ĔF-ĭ-kĕ-sē) (p. 116) A measure of how many different types of bacteria a drug can kill or prevent from growing.

susceptible organisms (sŭ-SĔP-tĭ-bŭl ŌR-găn-ĭ-zĭmz) (p. 116) Bacteria or other organisms that either can be killed by or have their reproduction reduced by an antibacterial drug.

virulence (VĬR-ŭl-ĕns) (p. 115) The measure of how well bacteria can invade and spread despite a normal immune response.

One of the most important advances in health care was the development of "antibiotic" drugs to treat infectious bacterial diseases—diseases that had previously led to death or permanent health problems. An *infection* is an invasion by microorganisms that disturbs the normal environment of the body and causes harm or disease. Infection agents include bacteria, viruses, fungi, protozoa, and other microorganisms. Bacterial infections are the most common cause of disease, sepsis, and death worldwide.

REVIEW OF RELATED PHYSIOLOGY AND PATHOPHYSIOLOGY

Humans interact constantly with various types of bacteria. Some of these bacteria are harmless, and others are or can become *pathogenic*, which means these bacteria can cause infection, systemic disease, and tissue damage. Some bacteria are nonpathogenic. *Nonpathogenic bacteria* coexist with us, causing no systemic disease or tissue damage and are considered normal flora. *Normal flora* are the nonpathogenic

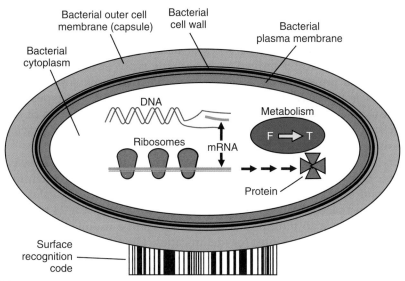

FIGURE 8-1 The surface of a bacterium, its membrane, and its internal features. $F \rightarrow T$, metabolic conversion of folic acid to thymine.

bacteria that we always have on skin, mucous membranes, and in the digestive tract. They provide protection by "crowding out" pathogenic organisms and preventing them from entering the body. These bacteria are kept in check by our immune system. *Opportunistic bacteria* cause disease and tissue damage only in someone whose immune system is not working well. So there are differences in bacteria that make some types more dangerous to humans than others.

BACTERIAL FEATURES

Bacteria are single-cell organisms that have their own genetic material (DNA and genes), cytoplasm, some organelles, and membranes. Unlike human cells, bacterial cells may also have several layers of membranes, cell walls, and capsules or coats (Figure 8-1). Bacterial types vary in their ability to invade a person and avoid that person's immune and inflammatory responses. The **virulence** of bacteria is a measure of how well they can invade and spread despite a normal immune response. Bacteria are also classified according to whether they change color when a dye called *Gram stain* is applied. Those that change color are called *gram-positive*, and those that do not are called *gram-negative*. In general, gram-negative bacteria are more virulent and harder to kill or control because they are surrounded by a protective capsule.

ANTIBACTERIAL THERAPY

Despite all of the body's barriers to infection, sometimes bacteria make it past these protections and enter your body where they multiply, damage tissues, and cause disease. Some bacterial infections are minor and can be cured by the immune system. Others are more severe and could cause serious harm and even death. (Usually more virulent bacteria cause more serious infections.) Antibacterial drugs are used to prevent bacteria from spreading infection throughout your body and causing severe damage.

BACTERICIDAL AND BACTERIOSTATIC DRUGS

Some antibacterial drugs are **bactericidal**, which means that they kill bacteria directly. Other antibacterial drugs are **bacteriostatic**, which means that they prevent bacteria from reproducing until the body's own white blood cells (WBCs) and antibodies get rid of them. So if a person's immune system is not working well, he or she would benefit from a bactericidal drug and not a bacteriostatic drug. Some drugs are bactericidal at high dosages but are only bacteriostatic at lower dosages.

 Memory Jogger

Pathogenic bacteria are those that can cause damage or tissue disease. Nonpathogenic bacteria do not cause disease or damage unless they overgrow or are present in a susceptible body area. Opportunistic bacteria cause disease or tissue damage only when the immune system is impaired.

 Memory Jogger

Not all types of bacteria are equal in their ability to cause disease after infection.

 Memory Jogger

Bactericidal drugs directly kill bacteria, whereas bacteriostatic drugs stop them from reproducing while the immune system kills the bacteria.

SPECTRUM OF EFFICACY

Antibacterial drugs are sometimes described by their **spectrum of efficacy,** which is a measure of how many different types of bacteria the drug can kill or prevent from growing. Each drug is judged by how many types of bacteria are susceptible to it. **Susceptible organisms** are bacteria or other organisms suppressed by it. A *narrow-spectrum antibacterial drug* is effective against only a few types of bacteria. An *extended-spectrum antibacterial drug* is effective against more types of bacteria. A *broad-spectrum antibacterial drug* is effective against a wide range of bacteria, both gram-positive and gram-negative.

Identifying the type of bacteria causing an infection is important for selecting the appropriate drug to treat the infection. The most common method to identify bacteria is culture and sensitivity (C&S). Culturing bacteria means to transfer it from an infected site and place it in a sterile nutritious broth to grow for 24 to 48 hours. By allowing the bacteria to multiply, more bacteria can be examined microscopically and tested with other procedures for identification. Culturing may be done alone or along with sensitivity testing (which is more expensive). When sensitivity testing is included, discs containing a specific antibacterial drug are placed in the culture with the bacteria. When a drug is effective against the bacteria, the bacteria do not grow in the area where the disc was placed.

A perfect antibacterial drug would kill bacteria and not harm the patient's body in any way. There are no perfect drugs. Because bacteria have some of the same features as human cells (such as DNA and genes, proteins, and cellular metabolism), some of the drug effects on bacteria also have the same effects on your cells. The goal of antibacterial drug therapy is to use a dose that kills the bacteria or suppresses its growth as much as possible without serious harm to the patient. However, sometimes, when an infection is life threatening, it may be necessary to use higher doses or combinations of drugs that together have more serious side effects.

GENERAL ISSUES IN ANTIBACTERIAL THERAPY

Many different drug types are used for antibacterial therapy. Each type has both distinctive and common actions and effects. A discussion of general side effects, adverse effects, and responsibilities for antibacterial drugs follows. Intended responses, specific side effects, adverse effects, and responsibilities are listed with each individual drug class.

The intended responses for all antibacterial drugs are the disappearance of signs and symptoms of infection and the eradication of the infectious bacteria. Body temperature is expected to return to normal, WBC counts are expected to remain between 5000 and 10,000 cells/mm^3, and there should be no drainage and redness in the area of infection.

Side effects common to all antibacterial drugs include intestinal disturbances that can range from an increase in the number of bowel movements to severe diarrhea. This is considered an *expected side effect*, not an allergic reaction. The reason these drugs cause diarrhea is that, in addition to killing the infecting bacteria, they also kill some of the normal intestinal flora that help with food digestion. The normal flora are helpful and nonpathogenic as long as they stay only in the intestinal tract. When their numbers decline, less food is digested and moves out more quickly as diarrhea.

Another side effect resulting from the loss of normal flora in the mouth and vagina is *yeast* infections. In the mouth this is known as *thrush*. Thrush makes food taste bad and can cause gum disease. In the vagina the infection causes a white, cheesy discharge and intense itching. Remember that antibacterial therapy is waging a "bug war" against pathogenic bacteria that often kills off some of the good bacteria of normal flora. When this happens, other bug armies that live in small numbers in human, such as fungi and yeast, take over temporarily.

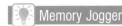

Memory Jogger

The goal of antibacterial therapy is to kill bacteria or prevent their reproduction without harming the patient.

Memory Jogger

When normal flora are killed by antibiotic therapy, common problems the patient may develop include diarrhea and the overgrowth of yeast in the mouth and vagina.

Adverse effects that are possible with any antibacterial drug include severe allergic reactions and anaphylaxis, especially when the drug is given intravenously. The major symptom of an allergic reaction to an oral drug is a skin rash that may appear days after starting the drug. A more severe allergic reaction to an intravenous (IV) drug is difficulty breathing and shock, which is called *anaphylaxis*. If not recognized and treated quickly, anaphylaxis can lead to vascular collapse, shock, and death.

Pseudomembranous colitis is a complication of antibacterial therapy that causes severe inflammation in areas of the colon (large intestine). Other names for this problem include *antibiotic-associated colitis* and *necrotizing colitis*. The cause of the problem is the overgrowth of an intestinal organism called *Clostridium difficile* (also known as "*C. diff*"). This organism is not killed by most antibacterial drugs, and it can take over the patient's intestinal tract when normal flora are killed off. This organism releases a powerful toxin that damages the intestines. The lining of the colon becomes raw and bleeds. Other symptoms include watery diarrhea, the constant feeling of the need to move the bowels, abdominal cramps, low-grade fever, and bloody stools. Patients can lose so much water and so many electrolytes in the watery diarrhea that they become dehydrated. When this problem occurs, the drug should be stopped. Although any antibacterial drug can cause pseudomembranous colitis if it is taken long enough, the more powerful drugs allow it to happen sooner.

Before giving any antibacterial drug, ask the patient if he or she has any drug allergies. Notify the prescriber if the patient has an allergy to the drug. If he or she does have an allergy to a drug and is to receive it anyway, check with the prescriber about first giving the patient diphenhydramine and epinephrine to reduce any serious reaction. Place the emergency cart close to the door of the patient's room.

Antibacterial drugs often suppress the growth of WBCs in the bone marrow. Check the patient's WBC count before drug therapy begins and use the value as a baseline in detecting side effects and gauging the drug's effectiveness. Table 1-5 in Chapter 1 lists the normal values for blood cells.

Also check the patient's vital signs (including temperature) and mental status before starting any antibacterial drug. These too can be used to detect side effects and gauge drug effectiveness.

Many IV antibacterial drugs can interact with other drugs and irritate the tissues. Make sure that the IV infusion is running well and has a good blood return. In addition, either flush the line before giving the antibacterial or use fresh tubing to give it. Double check the recommended infusion rate for the specific drug. Most should be given slowly over at least 30 to 60 minutes. Some may need to be given by slow continuous infusion for 8 hours or longer.

After giving an antibacterial drug, ask the patient about the number of daily bowel movements and their character. Although all antibacterial drugs change the normal flora of the intestines and can cause diarrhea, this symptom is also a sign of the more serious *pseudomembranous colitis*. The diarrhea of colitis is more watery and intense.

When giving the first IV dose of an antibacterial drug, check the patient every 15 minutes for any signs or symptoms of an allergic reaction (hives at the IV site, low blood pressure, rapid irregular pulse, swelling of the lips or lower face, the patient feeling a "lump in the throat"). If the patient is having an anaphylactic reaction, your first priority is to prevent any more drug from entering him or her. Stop the drug from infusing but keep the IV access open. If the drug is infusing high into the IV tubing, change the tubing after stopping the drug and do not let any drug remaining in the tubing run into the patient.

Monitor the patient for the effectiveness of the antibacterial drug in treating the infection. Signs and symptoms of a resolving infection include reduced or absent fever; no chills; wound drainage that is no longer thick, foul smelling, brown, green, or yellow; wound edges that are not red and raw-looking; and a WBC count that is in the normal range (see Table 1-5 in Chapter 1).

Check the patient's mouth daily for a white, cottage cheese–like coating on the gums, roof of the mouth, or insides of the cheeks. This substance is an overgrowth of yeast called thrush.

Memory Jogger

Signs and symptoms of an anaphylactic reaction to a drug are:
- Tightness in the chest
- Trouble breathing
- Low blood pressure
- Hives around the IV site
- Swelling of the face, mouth, and throat
- Hoarse voice
- Weak, thready pulse
- A sense that something bad is happening.

Drug Alert!

Action/Intervention Alert

If a patient appears to be having anaphylaxis from an IV drug, prevent any more drug from entering the patient but maintain the IV access.

QSEN: Safety

Memory Jogger

Teach patients to take any anti-bacterial drug exactly as prescribed and for as long as prescribed.

Because many IV antibacterial drugs are irritating to tissues and veins, check the IV site at least every 2 hours for symptoms of phlebitis, which include a change in blood return, any redness or pain, or the feeling of hard or "cordlike" veins above the site. If such problems occur, follow the policy of your agency concerning removal of the IV access.

Teach patients receiving an antibacterial drug to take the drug for as long as it was prescribed. Some patients stop taking the drug as soon as they feel better, which can lead to a recurrence of the infection and the development of resistant bacteria.

For all antibacterial therapy, it is important to keep the blood level high enough to affect the bacteria causing the infection. Therefore teach the patient to take the drug evenly throughout a 24-hour day. If the drug is to be taken twice daily, teach the patient to take it every 12 hours. For three times a day, teach the patient to take it every 8 hours. For four times a day, teach the patient to take it every 6 hours. Help the patient plan a schedule that is easy to remember and keeps the drug at the best blood levels.

If a rash or hives develop while taking an antibacterial drug, remind the patient to stop taking the drug and call the prescriber immediately. Explain that this is a sign of drug allergy. Tell the patient to call 911 immediately if he or she has trouble breathing or has the feeling of a "lump in the throat" because these are signs of a more serious allergic reaction.

TYPES OF ANTIBACTERIAL DRUGS

Antibacterial drugs are classified according to how they kill bacteria or how they stop or slow bacterial reproduction. The four major classes of antibacterial drugs are cell wall synthesis inhibitors, protein synthesis inhibitors, metabolism inhibitors, and DNA synthesis inhibitors. Within each class there are several types of drugs. Table 8-1 lists the actions of the different types of antibacterial drugs. Figure 8-2 shows the specific areas of a bacterium that are targeted by different types of antibacterial drugs. The decision to use one type of drug over another is based on whether the

Table 8-1   Actions of Antibacterial Agents

DRUG TYPE	MAJOR ACTIONS	DRUG EXAMPLES
Cell wall synthesis inhibitors (bactericidal)	Bind to cell wall proteins and prevent them from being incorporated into bacterial cell walls Inhibit the bacterial enzyme needed to cross-link the cell wall components, making the walls loose Activate enzymes called *autolysins* in the bacterial cell walls, which eat holes in the walls, making them leaky	**Penicillins** amoxicillin (Amoxil, Amoxicot, Apo-Amoxi ♣, Biomox, Moxilin) amoxicillin; clavulanate potassium (Augmentin, Clavulin ♣) penicillin G benzathine (Bicillin LA) penicillin G (Pfizerpen) penicillin V potassium (Apo-Pen-VK ♣, Nadopen-V ♣, Pen-V, BeePen-VK, Veetids) ticarcillin/clavulanate (Timentin) **Cephalosporins** cefazolin (Ancef, Kefzol) cefdinir (Omnicef) ceftriaxone (Rocephin) cephalexin (Apo-Cephalex ♣, Biocef, Keflex, Keftab, Novo-Lexin ♣, Nu-Cephalex ♣) **Monobactams** aztreonam (Azactam) **Carbapenems** ertapenem (Invanz) imipenem/cilastatin (Primaxin) meropenem (Merrem) **Others** vancomycin (Vancocin)

Table 8-1   **Actions of Antibacterial Agents—cont'd**

DRUG TYPE	MAJOR ACTIONS	DRUG EXAMPLES
Protein synthesis inhibitors (bacteriostatic or bactericidal)	Bind to the large (50S) subunit of ribosomes, preventing them from "reading" the mRNA Bind to the small (30S) subunit of ribosomes, preventing them from "reading" the mRNA Bind to the enzyme needed to bring the amino acids into contact with the mRNA and linking them together	**Aminoglycosides** amikacin (Amikin) gentamicin (Cidomycin ✿, Garamycin, Gentacidin) streptomycin **Macrolides** azithromycin (Zithromax, Zmax) clarithromycin (Biaxin) erythromycin (Apo-Erythro ✿, E-Mycin, Erycette, Erymax, Erythromid ✿, Romycin) erythromycin lactobionate (Erythrocin, Lactobionate) **Tetracyclines** demeclocycline (Declomycin) doxycycline (Adoxa, Apo-Doxy ✿, Atridox, Doryx, Dox-Caps, Doxycin ✿, Monodox, Novodoxyclin ✿, Vibramycin) minocycline (Arestin, Dynacin, Minocin, Vectrin) tetracycline (Ala-Tet, Apo-Tetra ✿, Brodspec, Novotetra ✿, Nu-Tetra ✿, Panmycin, Sumycin, Tetracon) **Lincosamide** clindamycin (Cleocin) **Oxazolidinone** linezolid (Zyvox) **Streptogramins** dalfopristin/quinupristin (Synercid)
Metabolism inhibitors (bacteriostatic)	Suppress the activity of an enzyme needed to convert other substances (PABA and pteridine) into folic acid in bacteria; as a result, the bacteria do not have enough folic acid to be able to make DNA and grow	**Sulfonamides** sulfadiazine sodium sulfisoxazole (Gantrisin, Soxazole ✿, Truxazole) **Trimethoprim** (Primsol, Trimpex) **Combination Drugs** trimethoprim/sulfamethoxazole (Apo-Sulfatrim ✿, Bactrim, Bethaprim, Novo-Trimel ✿, Nu-Cotrimex ✿, Roubac ✿, Septra, Sulfatrim, Uroplus, SMX-TMP)
DNA synthesis inhibitors (bactericidal)	Enter bacterial cells and suppress the action of two enzymes (gyrase and topoisomerase) important in allowing the bacteria to make DNA	**Fluoroquinolones** ciprofloxacin (Ciloxan, Cipro) gatifloxacin (Tequin) gemifloxacin (Factive) levofloxacin (Levaquin) lomefloxacin (Maxaquin) moxifloxacin (Avelox) ofloxacin (Floxin)

PABA, Para-aminobenzoic acid.

bacterium causing the infection is known (by culture and/or sensitivity testing), how serious the infection is, which drugs are known to kill it or slow its growth, how well the patient's immune system is working, the patient's overall health (especially kidney, liver, and bone marrow function), and whether the patient has any known drug allergies.

PENICILLINS, CEPHALOSPORINS, AND OTHER CELL WALL SYNTHESIS INHIBITORS

The first antibacterial drug developed for general use was penicillin. It was originally a natural product made from bread mold. Some penicillins are still made as a product

 Memory Jogger

The four classes of antibacterial drugs are:
- Cell wall synthesis inhibitors
- Protein synthesis inhibitors
- Metabolism inhibitors
- DNA synthesis inhibitors

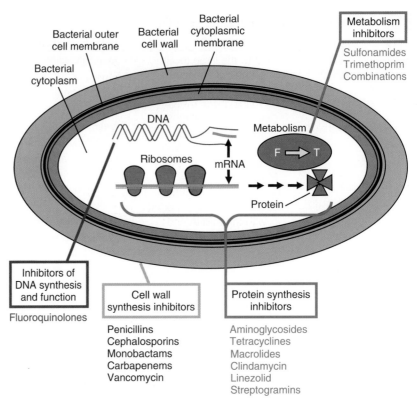

FIGURE 8-2 Bacterial targets of different types of antibacterial drugs. *F → T*, metabolic conversion of folic acid to thymine.

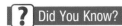

? Did You Know?

In 1929 mold was discovered to be effective in killing bacteria.

of mold, and others are made synthetically from chemicals. In addition to penicillin, this drug class includes the cephalosporins, carbapenems, monobactams, and vancomycin. The carbapenems and vancomycin are powerful drugs available only by injection and have serious side effects.

How Cell Wall Synthesis Inhibitors Work

Some bacteria have a cell wall, and others do not (see Figures 8-1 and 8-2). **Cell wall synthesis inhibitors** are a class of antibacterial drugs that kill susceptible bacteria by preventing them from forming strong, protective cell walls. Although the penicillins are just one type of drug in this class, many people refer to any cell wall synthesis inhibitor as a "penicillin-like drug."

These drugs usually act in at least one of three ways. Think of a cell wall as made up of individual bricks known as penicillin-binding proteins (PBPs), with mortar between the bricks holding the wall together tightly. One way these drugs interfere with cell walls is that they bind to the bricks, keeping them from being placed in the wall. The second way these drugs work is by preventing the mortar from being made, which results in the bricks just lying loosely on top of each other so the wall is easy to break. The third way these drugs work is by activating an enzyme that punches holes in the wall. So even though a wall may be formed, it is leaky and does not protect the bacteria.

Cell wall synthesis inhibitors are most effective against bacteria that divide rapidly and are usually found on the skin and mucous membranes, respiratory tract, ear, bone, and blood. Some infections for which penicillins, cephalosporins, and other cell wall synthesis inhibitors are prescribed include strep throat, tonsillitis, otitis media, simple urinary tract infections, wound infections, upper and lower respiratory infections, prostatitis, and gonorrhea. They also may be used for sepsis and Lyme disease. The more powerful drugs in this class such as the carbapenems and vancomycin are used for severe infections such as sepsis, endocarditis, abscesses, and infections that involve multiple types of bacteria.

Memory Jogger

Penicillin and other cell wall synthesis inhibitors are effective only against bacteria that have a cell wall because that is the target of the actions of these drugs.

Box 8-1	Cephalosporins by Drug Generation

FIRST GENERATION (EXTENDED SPECTRUM)
cefazolin (Ancef, Kefzol)
cephalexin (Biocef, Keflex)
cephradine (Velosef)

SECOND GENERATION (BROAD SPECTRUM)
cefaclor (Ceclor)
cefditoren (Spectracef)
cefoxitin (Cefoxitin, Mefoxin)
cefuroxime (Ceftin, Kefurox, Zinacef)
loracarbef (Lorabid)

THIRD GENERATION (BROAD SPECTRUM)
cefdinir (Omnicef)
cefixime (Suprax)
cefotaxime (Claforan)
cefotetan (Cefotan)
cefpodoxime (Vantin)
ceftazidime (Ceptaz, Fortaz, Tazicef, Tazidime)
ceftibuten (Cedax)
ceftizoxime (Cefizox)
ceftriaxone (Rocephin)

FOURTH GENERATION (BROAD SPECTRUM)
cefepime (Maxipime)

Cell wall synthesis inhibitors have been around longer than other types of antibacterial drugs. Some, especially the cephalosporins, have more than one drug generation. **Drug generation** refers to the stage of development of a drug in which later generations are changed slightly to improve their effectiveness or means of administration. For example, the cephalosporins have four drug generations. Box 8-1 lists the cephalosporins in each generation.

The activity of penicillin and some other cell wall synthesis inhibitors can be enhanced when other agents are added to the drug. For example, penicillin can be destroyed by a bacterial enzyme called *beta-lactamase*, which makes bacteria that have this enzyme resistant to penicillin. Combining penicillin with clavulanic acid (clavulanate) inhibits this bacterial enzyme and reduces penicillin resistance even though clavulanic acid has little if any antibiotic effect on the bacteria. An agent that improves the activity of imipenem is cilastatin. Without cilastatin, imipenem is rapidly metabolized in the kidney and excreted. Cilastatin slows this metabolism and allows the imipenem to remain in the body longer for better antibacterial action.

There are many types of cell wall synthesis inhibitors, and within each type there are dozens of different brands and strengths. They all work in similar ways and have similar effects. The penicillins and cephalosporins are most often prescribed. The monobactams, carbapenems, and vancomycin are more powerful and prescribed less often. Only the drugs most commonly prescribed and those most often used in acute care settings are listed in the following table. Be sure to consult a drug reference for more information about a specific drug in this class.

Dosages for Common Cell Wall Synthesis Inhibitors

Drug	Dosage
Penicillins	
amoxicillin (Amoxil, Amoxicot, Apo-Amoxi ♣, Biomox, Moxilin, Novamoxin ♣) (Moxatag ER)	*Adults:* 250-500 mg orally every 8 hr *Children:* 20 mg/kg orally every 8 hr *Adults and Children over 12 years:* 775 mg orally once daily
amoxicillin/clavulanic acid (Amoclan, Augmentin, Clavulin ♣, Novo-Clavamoxin ♣)	*Adults:* 250-500 mg orally every 8 hr *Children:* 20 mg/kg orally every 8 hr
penicillin G benzathine (Bicillin LA, Megacillin ♣)	*Adults:* 1.2 million units intramuscular (IM) once as a single dose *Children:* 300,000-600,000 units IM as a single dose
penicillin G (Pfizerpen)	*Adults:* 1-4 million units IM or IV every 6 hr *Children:* 40,000-50,000 units/kg IM or IV every 6 hr

Continued

Dosages for Common Cell Wall Synthesis Inhibitors—cont'd

Drug	Dosage
penicillin V potassium (Apo-Pen-VK ♦, Nadopen-V ♦, NuPen ♦, Pen-V, VeePen, Pen-VK, V-Cillin-K, Veetids)	*Adults:* 250-500 mg orally every 6 hr *Children:* 250 mg orally twice daily
ticarcillin/clavulanic acid (Timentin)	*Adults:* 3 g IV every 4-6 hr *Children:* 50 mg/kg IV every 6 hr
Cephalosporins	
cefazolin (Ancef, Kefzol)	*Adults:* 500 mg to 1 g IM or IV every 6-8 hr *Children:* 25-100 mg/kg IM or IV every 8 hr
cefdinir (Omnicef)	*Adults & Children over 43 kg:* 300 mg orally every 12 hr *Children less than 43 kg:* 7 mg/kg orally every 12 hr
ceftriaxone (Rocephin)	*Adults:* 1-2 g IM or IV daily *Children:* 50-75 mg/kg IM or IV every 12 hr
cephalexin (Apo-Cephalex ♦, Bio-Cef, Keflex, Keftab, Novo-Lexin ♦, Nu-Cephalex ♦)	*Adults:* 250-500 mg orally every 6 hr *Children:* 8-25 mg/kg orally every 6 hr
Monobactams	
aztreonam (Azactam, Cayston)	*Adults:* 500 mg to 2 g IM or IV every 8-12 hr *Children:* 30 mg/kg IM or IV every 6-8 hr
Carbapenems	
ertapenem (Invanz)	*Adults:* 1 g IV or IM daily *Children older than 3 months:* 15 mg/kg IV or IM every 12 hr
imipenem/cilastatin (Primaxin)	*Adults:* 250 mg-1 g IM or IV every 6-8 hr; 500-750 mg IM every 12 hr *Children:* 25 mg/kg IM or IV every 6 hr
meropenem (Merrem)	*Adults:* 500 mg-1 g IV every 6-8 hr *Children:* 20-30 mg/kg IV every 8 hr
Others	
vancomycin (First-Vancomycin, Vancocin)	*Adults:* 500 mg IV every 6 hr or 1 g IV every 12 hr *Children:* 10 mg/kg IV every 6 hr

Common Side Effects

Penicillins and Cephalosporins

Diarrhea   Itchiness

Common Side Effects

Carbapenems and Vancomycin

IV site   Reduced   Reduced
reaction   kidney   hearing
               function

Side Effects. Most cell wall synthesis inhibitors have fewer side effects than other types of antibacterial drugs. Part of the reason for this is that human cells have no cell walls, so they are not targeted by these drugs. But remember that all drugs have some side effects. The cell wall synthesis inhibitors, especially penicillin, are more likely to cause allergic reactions.

The more powerful drugs in this class, especially vancomycin, have more side effects. These include nausea and vomiting, fever, chills, "red man syndrome" (with rash and redness of the face, neck, upper chest, upper back, and arms), pain at the injection site, reduced hearing, and greatly reduced kidney function.

Adverse Effects. *The carbapenems may cause central nervous system changes, including confusion and seizures.*

The cephalosporins, carbapenems, and vancomycin can greatly reduce kidney function. If a patient is being treated with two or more drugs from this class or with an aminoglycoside (discussed later), the risk for kidney damage and kidney failure increases.

What To Do *Before* Giving Cell Wall Synthesis Inhibitors

In addition to the general responsibilities related to antibacterial therapy (pp. 116-118), when giving a cell wall synthesis inhibitor for the first time, ask whether the patient has any known drug allergies, especially to the drug prescribed. If a patient is allergic to penicillin, the risk for a cephalosporin allergy is increased.

Oral cephalosporins are poorly absorbed with iron supplements and antacids. If a patient is receiving either of these drugs, the cephalosporin should be given 1 hour before or 4 hours after the dose of iron or antacid.

If a patient will receive IV penicillin, check that the injectable form can be given intravenously. One type of injectable penicillin, procaine penicillin, contains a local anesthetic and is not an IV drug. This drug is milky white rather than clear.

If a patient is to receive a carbapenem, ask whether he or she has ever had seizures. If so, notify the prescriber because this drug lowers the seizure threshold.

Vancomycin is given only intravenously and has many adverse effects if given too fast. These include low blood pressure; a histamine release that causes dilation of blood vessels and a red appearance to the face, neck, chest, back, and arms (red man syndrome); and cardiac dysrhythmias. To reduce the risk for these problems, vancomycin should be given over at least 60 minutes and never as a bolus or a "push" dose. This drug is highly toxic to the ears and kidneys.

What To Do *After* Giving Cell Wall Synthesis Inhibitors

In addition to general responsibilities related to antibacterial therapy (pp. 117-118), check the patient hourly for the first 4 hours after the first oral dose and every 15 to 30 minutes for the first 2 hours after receiving the first IV dose. Remember that drugs from this class are more likely to cause an allergic reaction than are other types of antibacterials.

What To *Teach* Patients About Cell Wall Synthesis Inhibitors

In addition to the general care needs and precautions related to antibacterial therapy (p. 118), teach patients to take cephalosporins at least 1 hour before or 4 hours after iron or an antacid.

If a patient is taking a liquid oral form of penicillin or a cephalosporin, instruct him or her to keep the drug tightly closed and refrigerated to prevent loss of drug strength. Teach the patient to shake the suspension well just before measuring the drug.

Life Span Considerations for Cell Wall Synthesis Inhibitors

Pediatric Considerations. Cell wall synthesis inhibitors are used for infants and children with bacterial infections susceptible to these drugs. One of the most common drugs given to children is amoxicillin for ear infections. The more powerful drugs (carbapenems, monobactams, and vancomycin) are used only for extremely serious infections.

Considerations for Pregnancy and Lactation. Penicillins and most of the cephalosporins have a low likelihood of increasing the risk for birth defects or fetal harm and can be used to treat infections during pregnancy. The more powerful drugs (carbapenems, monobactams, and vancomycin) have a low to moderate likelihood of increasing the risk for birth defects or fetal harm and are also used, when needed, during pregnancy. All of these drugs pass into breast milk and will affect a nursing infant, possibly causing the infant to develop a drug allergy. These drugs are usually prescribed for only 5 to 14 days, and the breastfeeding mother should be urged to reduce infant exposure to the drug (see Box 1-1 in Chapter 1).

Considerations for Older Adults. The carbapenems and vancomycin can be both *ototoxic* (causing hearing problems) and *nephrotoxic* (causing kidney problems) at higher doses or when taken for many days in a row. Older adults are more sensitive to these problems than younger adults. Be alert for a decrease in hearing or having the patient tell you he or she has a "ringing" in the ears *(tinnitus)*. Intake and output should be monitored daily, especially if the patient is also taking another drug known to affect kidney function.

Action/Intervention Alert

Watch closely if a patient who is receiving a cephalosporin is allergic to penicillin. These drugs are similar, and an allergy to one often means an allergy to the other. Remember, diarrhea is NOT an allergic reaction.

QSEN: Safety

Clinical Pitfall

Never give procaine penicillin intravenously.

QSEN: Safety

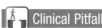

Administration Alert

Give IV vancomycin over at least a 60-minute period.

QSEN: Safety

AMINOGLYCOSIDES, MACROLIDES, TETRACYCLINES, AND OTHER PROTEIN SYNTHESIS INHIBITORS

Protein synthesis inhibitors are a large class of antibacterial drugs with several main subtypes, including aminoglycosides, macrolides, and tetracyclines. By slowing protein synthesis, these drugs prevent bacteria from making proteins important to their life cycles and infective processes. If any of the pieces and processes (such as gene expression, DNA replication, ribosome activity, and linking amino acids into a protein chain) needed for protein synthesis are not working, the bacterium cannot make the protein it needs. As a result, it will either die or not be able to reproduce. Protein synthesis inhibitors work on different parts of this entire process to stop the bacterium from being able to live and reproduce (see Table 8-1).

How Protein Synthesis Inhibitors Work

Aminoglycosides actually go through the cell membrane and enter the bacterium. This process uses a transport system that requires oxygen. After entering, the drug binds to the ribosomes and prevents amino acids from forming proteins (see Figure 8-2). Without these important proteins, bacteria, especially those that use oxygen, usually die.

Macrolides also enter the bacterium through the cell membrane and bind to ribosomes (see Figure 8-2). The results are the same; no bacterial protein is made, and the bacteria either die or are unable to reproduce. At higher dosages with susceptible organisms, the macrolides are bactericidal. However, at usual and lower dosages, the macrolides are bacteriostatic. Macrolides have no effect on bacteria that do not require oxygen.

Tetracyclines also enter the bacterium through the cell membrane. To get inside, they must be brought in by a special transporter on the surface of the bacterium or through a special porin channel. If a bacterium does not have either of these entry mechanisms, it is not affected by tetracycline. Once inside the bacterium, tetracyclines act in two ways to inhibit protein synthesis (see Figure 8-2). However, their actions on protein synthesis are usually only bacteriostatic rather than bactericidal except at high concentrations.

Clindamycin also uses two actions to inhibit protein synthesis. Both actions slow bacterial protein synthesis. This drug is usually bacteriostatic but can be bactericidal in high doses. *Linezolid* (Zyvox) prevents translation of mRNA into protein. It is bacteriostatic against *staphylococci* and *enterococci* and is bactericidal against most strains of *streptococci*. The *streptogramin* in current use is made up of two streptogramin antibiotics (dalfopristin and quinupristin [Synercid]) that work together to inhibit protein synthesis at both the beginning and the end of the process. This drug has many side effects, and its use is limited to severe systemic infections that are life threatening and resistant to vancomycin.

Each group of protein synthesis inhibitors is described separately in the following table. Within each group the listings include only the drugs on the list of 100 most commonly prescribed drugs and those most often used in acute care settings. Be sure to consult a drug reference for more information about a specific drug in this drug group.

⇄ **Do Not Confuse**

Amikin *with* anakinra

An order for Amikin can be confused with anakinra. Amikin is an antibacterial drug, whereas anakinra is a biologic agent for rheumatoid arthritis.

QSEN: Safety

Dosages for Common Aminoglycosides

Drug	Dosage
amikacin (Amikin)	*Adults and Children:* 5 mg/kg IM or IV every 8 hr
gentamicin (Cidomycin ♣)	*Adults:* 1-2 mg/kg IM or IV every 8 hr *Children:* 2-2.5 mg/kg IM or IV every 8 hr
streptomycin	*Adults:* Tuberculosis: 15 mg/kg/day IM once daily (maximum 1 g); 25-35 mg/kg IM 2-3 times weekly (maximum 1.5 g) *Children:* Tuberculosis: 20-40 mg/kg IM or IV once daily or 25-30 mg/kg IM 2-3 times weekly (maximum 1.5 g)

The aminoglycosides are powerful antibacterial drugs given intravenously or intramuscularly that have some uncomfortable side effects and serious adverse effects. They are most commonly used for burns, central nervous system infections, joint and bone infections, intra-abdominal infections, peritonitis, and sepsis. Streptomycin is also used in the treatment of tuberculosis.

Dosages for Common Macrolides

Drug	Dosage
azithromycin (Zithromax, Zmax)	*Adults:* 500 mg orally first day, 250 mg orally daily days 2-5 *Children:* 12 mg/kg orally once daily for 5 days
clarithromycin (Biaxin, Biaxin XL, Clarithromycin Extended Release)	*Adults:* 250-500 mg orally every 12 hr; extended release 500 mg orally once daily *Children:* 7.5 mg/kg orally every 12 hr
erythromycin (Apo Erythro ♣, E-mycin, Erycette, Erymax, Erythromid ♣, Romycin)	*Adults:* 250-500 mg orally every 6-12 hr *Children:* 5-12.5 mg/kg orally every 6-12 hr

The *macrolides* are antibacterial drugs that have extended- to broad-spectrum effects. Depending on the bacteria type and the blood level of drug, they are usually bacteriostatic but can be bactericidal with susceptible organisms. Usually higher doses are needed for bactericidal effects. These drugs work well against common infections of the skin, mucous membranes and other soft tissues, chlamydial infections, and respiratory infections, and are prescribed for patients who are allergic to penicillins or cephalosporins. The macrolides are used for legionnaires' disease, diphtheria, and mycobacterial infections.

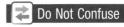

Do Not Confuse

Vibramycin *with* ribavirin

An order for Vibramycin can be confused with ribavirin. Vibramycin is an antibacterial drug, whereas ribavirin is a strong antiviral agent known to cause birth defects.

QSEN: Safety

Dosages for Common Tetracyclines

Drug	Dosage
demeclocycline (Declomycin)	*Adults:* 150 mg orally every 6 hr or 300 mg orally every hr *Children:* 7-13 mg/kg (total) orally divided over 2-4 doses daily
doxycycline (Adoxa, Apo-Doxy ♣, Atridox, Doryx, Dox-Caps, Doxycin ♣, Monodox, Novodoxyclin ♣, Vibramycin)	Oral and IV doses: *Adults:* 100 mg orally every 12 hr first day, then 100 mg once daily *Children:* 2.2 mg/kg orally every 12 hr first day, then 2.2 mg/kg once daily
minocycline (Arestin, Dynacin, Minocin, Myrac, Solodyn)	Oral and IV doses: *Adults:* 200 mg first dose, then 100 mg every 12 hr *Children:* 4 mg/kg first dose, then 2 mg/kg every 12 hr
tetracycline (Ala-Tet, Apo-Tetra ♣, Brodspec, Emtet, Novotetra ♣, Nu-Tetra ♣, Panmycin, Sumycin, Tetracon)	*Adults:* 500 mg orally every 6-12 hr *Children:* 6.25-12.5 mg/kg orally every 6 hr

The *tetracyclines* are broad-spectrum drugs that are bacteriostatic against most of the organisms that are sensitive to penicillins. Because they are bacteriostatic and not bactericidal, tetracyclines should be given only to patients with healthy immune systems. They are often prescribed for patients who are allergic to penicillins or cephalosporins. Infections most responsive to tetracyclines are acne, urinary tract infections, skin and mucous membrane infections, gonorrhea, upper and lower respiratory tract infections, sexually transmitted infections, Rocky Mountain spotted fever, syphilis, Lyme disease, and typhoid fever. In addition, they are used to prevent anthrax after exposure to the bacteria.

Dosages for Other Protein Synthesis Inhibitors

Drug	Dosage
Lincosamides	
clindamycin (Cleocin, Dalacin C ✦)	*Adults:* 150-450 mg orally every 6 hr; 300 mg IM or IV every 6, 8, or 12 hr *Children:* 2-4 mg/kg orally every 6 hr; 20-40 mg IM or IV (total) divided into 3-4 doses
Oxazolidinones	
linezolid (Zyvox)	Oral and IV doses: *Adults:* 600 mg every 12 hr *Children:* 10 mg/kg every 12 hr
Streptogramins	
dalfopristin/quinupristin (Synercid)	*Adults/Children:* 7.5 mg/kg IV (over 60 min) every 12 hr for at least 7 days

Common Side Effects
Aminoglycosides

Nausea/Vomiting   Rash   Fever

Lethargy

Common Side Effects
Macrolides

Nausea/Vomiting,   Photosensitivity
Diarrhea, Loss of
appetite

Common Side Effects
Tetracyclines

Nausea/   Photosensitivity   Sore tongue
Vomiting,
Diarrhea

Memory Jogger

Drugs that have adverse effects on the kidneys (nephrotoxic) almost always have adverse hearing and balance effects (ototoxic) on the ears.

The three remaining types of protein synthesis inhibitors are very powerful drugs with more severe side effects. These drugs are reserved for treating severe or life-threatening infections that do not respond well to other types of antibacterial drugs. The oxazolidinone and streptogramin classes are usually reserved for treating infections from *vancomycin-resistant enterococcus (VRE)* or *methicillin-resistant Staphylococcus aureus (MRSA)*. They are also used for infected diabetic foot ulcers. The third class, the lincosamides, in addition to topical therapy for acne, is used orally and parenterally for severe infections such as peritonitis, cellulitis, abscesses, malaria, and pneumonia caused by *Pneumocystis jiroveci*. The usual doses for all three drug types may be greatly increased when the infection is life threatening.

Side Effects. *Aminoglycosides* often cause nausea, vomiting, rash, lethargy, fever, and increased salivation. They also can increase the number of eosinophils (a type of WBC) in the blood. When given intravenously, these drugs are irritating to the vein.

Macrolides have side effects that occur more in the GI tract. They include nausea, vomiting, abdominal pain, diarrhea, loss of appetite, and changes in taste sensation. These drugs greatly increase sun sensitivity (*photosensitivity*), making serious sunburns possible.

Tetracycline side effects include nausea, vomiting, diarrhea, a sore tongue (*glossitis*), and rash. These drugs greatly increase sensitivity to the sun, making serious sunburns possible. Rarely do they cause esophageal irritation and ulcer formation. Although all antibacterial drugs can result in yeast overgrowth in the mouth and vagina, tetracycline is more likely to have this effect early in the course of treatment.

Clindamycin can cause rash, pain and redness at the injection site (when the drug is given intramuscularly) and thrombophlebitis in the vein where the drug infuses.

Linezolid constricts blood vessels and can raise blood pressure in patients who have high blood pressure. Other side effects include nausea, diarrhea, and headaches.

Streptogramin side effects include muscle and joint pain, pain and inflammation at the IV site, rash, nausea, and vomiting.

Adverse Effects. *Aminoglycosides* are highly toxic to the ears and kidneys, causing hearing loss and reduced kidney function when taken in high doses or for long periods. This is because the tissues that make up the inner ear and the nephrons of the kidney both come from the same tissue layer in the embryo. Because these tissues are similar in structure, both are at risk for damage by the same drugs.

Macrolides interfere with the metabolism of many drugs. For some such as digoxin, macrolides keep the drug in the blood longer so digoxin side effects occur faster. Macrolides also increase the effects of warfarin (Coumadin), increasing the risk for bleeding. Combining other drugs such as pimozide, astemizole, terfenadine, and ergotamine with a macrolide increases the risk for life-threatening cardiac dysrhythmias.

Parenteral forms of macrolides are irritating to veins and tissues. Symptoms of liver irritation or other problems have also been reported.

Tetracyclines can raise pressure inside the brain *(intracranial pressure)*. Symptoms occurring with this adverse reaction include dizziness, blurred vision, confusion, and ringing in the ears *(tinnitus)*.

In high doses tetracyclines can decrease kidney function and increase liver enzyme levels. These problems resolve when the drug is discontinued, but drugs from this class should be used with caution for any patient with reduced liver or kidney function.

Clindamycin can reduce liver function and decrease WBC counts. When clindamycin is given too rapidly by IV infusion, shock and cardiac arrest may occur.

Linezolid reduces blood cell counts, especially red blood cells and platelets, and causes damage to the optic nerve. Usually these problems occur only in patients who have been taking the drug for longer than 28 days.

Streptogramin increases the blood levels of many drugs, which can then lead to adverse effects of these drugs even when the patient is taking them at normal doses.

What To Do *Before* Giving Protein Synthesis Inhibitors

In addition to the general responsibilities related to starting antibacterial therapy (p. 117), these specific responsibilities are important before giving protein synthesis inhibitors.

Aminoglycosides. Check the patient's current laboratory work, especially blood urea nitrogen (BUN) and serum creatinine levels because aminoglycosides are toxic to the kidneys (see Table 1-4 in Chapter 1). If laboratory values are higher than normal before starting the drug, the risk for kidney damage is greater. Use these data as a baseline to determine whether the patient develops kidney problems while taking aminoglycosides.

Assess the patient's hearing by whispering a phrase with your back turned toward the patient. Document how loudly you need to repeat the phrase until the patient hears it and can repeat it back correctly to you. Use this data as a baseline to determine whether the patient's hearing changes after taking the drug.

Make sure that the aminoglycoside is well diluted before giving it IV. Give the drugs slowly over 30 to 60 minutes to reduce the risk for vein irritation and adverse cardiac effects.

Macrolides. If a patient is prescribed a macrolide, check to see whether he or she is also taking digoxin, warfarin, pimozide, astemizole, terfenadine, or ergotamine. If so, notify the prescriber immediately because macrolides change the metabolism of these drugs, which can cause adverse effects.

When giving these drugs IV, infuse them slowly. For example, it is recommended that erythromycin be infused by slow continuous drip over 8 to 12 hours.

Tetracyclines. Food, antacids, and dairy products prevent oral tetracycline from being absorbed. Give drugs from this class 1 hour before or 2 hours after a meal. Do not give with milk. Give the patient a full glass of water to drink with tetracycline capsules or tablets, and urge him or her to drink more fluids throughout the day to prevent irritation to the esophagus.

Check the dosages for doxycycline and minocycline carefully because they are lower than for other tetracyclines and other types of antibacterial drugs.

 Drug Alert!

Administration Alert

Only use solutions of erythromycin that were mixed less than 8 hours earlier.

QSEN: Safety

 Drug Alert!

Administration Alert

Check the dosages for doxycycline and minocycline carefully because they are lower than for other tetracyclines and other types of antibacterial drugs.

QSEN: Safety

Other Protein Synthesis Inhibitors. Check the patient's current laboratory work, especially BUN and serum creatinine levels, because clindamycin, linezolid, and streptogramin are toxic to the kidneys. If these values are higher than normal before starting the drug, the risk for kidney damage is greater.

All three drugs are known to cause vein irritation and phlebitis. Give them slowly over 30 to 60 minutes (or as prescribed) to reduce the risk for vein irritation and cardiac side effects.

When mixing and diluting streptogramins, use only dextrose 5% in water because a precipitate will form in anything else. The IV line used to give these drugs must either be fresh or flushed with only dextrose 5% in water and never with sodium chloride or heparin.

What To Do *After* Giving Protein Synthesis Inhibitors

In addition to the general responsibilities related to antibacterial therapy (pp. 117-118), see the specific responsibilities listed below by drug group for what to do after giving protein synthesis inhibitors.

Aminoglycosides. Assess the patient's hearing daily as described on p. 127 and compare the findings to the patient's hearing before a drug from this class is started.

To determine whether the drug is effective and because aminoglycosides can also *cause* a fever as a side effect, check the patient's temperature every 4 to 8 hours.

Because these drugs are toxic to the kidneys, examine the patient's intake and output record daily to determine whether urine output is within 500 mL of the total fluid intake. If blood work was done for kidney function, especially BUN and creatinine levels, compare the values before and after the drug was started (see Table 1-4 in Chapter 1). If the levels rise above the normal range, notify the prescriber.

Macrolides. For a patient taking a macrolide for the first time or for a patient with known cardiac rhythm problems, assess his or her heart rate and rhythm at least every shift during macrolide therapy. If a new change in rhythm develops, check the patient again in 15 minutes. If the change in rhythm persists or recurs, notify the prescriber.

Tetracyclines. Tetracyclines increase the effects of warfarin (Coumadin). Check the patient who is also taking warfarin daily for any signs or symptoms of increased bleeding such as bleeding from the gums, presence of bruising or petechiae, oozing of blood around IV insertions or other puncture sites, or the presence of blood in urine or stool.

Other Protein Synthesis Inhibitors. Check the blood pressure of a patient taking linezolid at least every shift. This drug can raise blood pressure, especially in patients who already have high blood pressure or are taking other drugs that also raise blood pressure.

What To *Teach* Patients About Protein Synthesis Inhibitors

In addition to the general care needs and precautions related to antibacterial therapy (p. 118), these specific teaching points for protein synthesis inhibitors are important.

Macrolides. Teach patients to take macrolides with food or within 1 hour of having eaten to reduce some of the intestinal side effects. Instruct patients not to chew or crush tablets or capsules. Remind patients to avoid taking other drugs without the prescriber's knowledge.

Teach patients taking either macrolides or tetracyclines to avoid direct sunlight, use sunscreen, and wear protective clothing (including a hat) whenever they are in the sun to prevent a severe sunburn. Remind them to avoid tanning beds and salons.

Drug Alert!

Administration Alert

Mix the parenteral form of streptogramins only with dextrose 5% in water.

QSEN: Safety

Drug Alert!

Teaching Alert

Teach patients taking macrolides or tetracyclines to protect themselves from sun exposure because these drugs greatly increase sun sensitivity, even among people with dark skin.

QSEN: Safety

If the patient also takes warfarin (Coumadin), remind him or her to keep all appointments to check blood clotting. Macrolides, especially erythromycin, increase the effects of warfarin, which can greatly increase the risk for bleeding.

Tetracyclines. Teach patients to drink a full glass of water with the tetracycline capsules or tablets and to drink more fluids throughout the day to prevent irritation to the esophagus.

Food and milk interfere with absorption of oral tetracyclines. Teach the patient to take these drugs 1 hour before or 2 hours after meals and to not take the drug with milk.

Other Protein Synthesis Inhibitors. Teach patients to drink a full glass of water with oral clindamycin and to drink more fluids throughout the day to prevent irritation to the esophagus.

Linezolid can raise blood pressure, sometimes to dangerous levels. When foods containing tyramine are eaten while a patient is taking linezolid, very high blood pressure can result. (Tyramine is a metabolite of the amino acid tyrosine and can cause the release of excess amounts of dopamine, epinephrine, and norepinephrine.) Teach patients to avoid tyramine-containing food such as aged cheese, smoked meats, pickled food, beer, red wine, soy, and sauerkraut while taking this drug.

Life Span Considerations for Protein Synthesis Inhibitors

Pediatric Considerations. *Aminoglycosides* can cause severe respiratory depression in infants and children. In addition, because infants and children have immature kidney function, the risk for kidney damage is greater.

The use of *tetracyclines* during tooth development in infancy and early childhood can cause a permanent yellow-gray discoloration of the teeth and make the tooth enamel thinner. Therefore these drugs should not be used in children younger than 8 years of age except for anthrax exposure or a serious infection that is not likely to respond to other antibacterial drugs.

Considerations for Pregnancy and Lactation. IV and intramuscular (IM) *aminoglycosides* have a moderate to high likelihood of increasing the risk for birth defects or fetal harm (except for gentamicin, which has a moderate likelihood) and should not be given to pregnant women unless the infection is life threatening and the organisms are susceptible only to these drugs. Because these drugs are known to cause hearing loss and reduced kidney function, a woman should not breastfeed while taking them.

Most *macrolides* have a low likelihood of increasing the risk for birth defects or fetal harm and can be taken during pregnancy if needed. These drugs pass into breast milk and affect the infant, often causing colic and diarrhea. Because they are usually prescribed for only 5 to 14 days, teach breastfeeding women to reduce infant exposure to the drug (see Box 1-1 in Chapter 1).

Tetracyclines have a moderate to high likelihood of increasing the risks for birth defects or fetal harm. Their use during tooth development in the last half of pregnancy and infancy can cause a permanent yellow-gray discoloration of the teeth and make the tooth enamel thinner. Therefore these drugs should not be used during pregnancy or when breastfeeding except for anthrax exposure or a serious infection that is not likely to respond to other antibacterial drugs.

Considerations for Older Adults. *Aminoglycosides* are both ototoxic and nephrotoxic at higher doses or when taken for many days in a row. Doses are usually lowered for the older adult. *Macrolides* may be ototoxic in older adults who are also taking a high ceiling or "loop" diuretic such as furosemide (Lasix). Be alert for patient reports of reduced hearing or tinnitus. Monitor the intake and output of older adults daily, especially if they are also taking other drugs known to affect kidney function.

 Clinical Pitfall

Tetracyclines should not be used in children younger than 8 years of age because it changes tooth enamel in the developing permanent teeth.

QSEN: Safety

 Clinical Pitfall

Avoid giving drugs from the aminoglycoside or tetracycline classes to pregnant or breastfeeding women.

QSEN: Safety

METABOLISM INHIBITORS: SULFONAMIDES AND TRIMETHOPRIM

Metabolism inhibitors are a class of antibacterial drugs that interfere with bacterial reproduction by preventing the bacteria from making folic acid. This class includes sulfonamides and trimethoprim and are bacteriostatic rather than bactericidal. Although classed as antibacterial drugs, metabolism inhibitors can be effective in some infections caused by organisms other than bacteria such as shigellosis, toxoplasmosis, and pneumocystis pneumonia. They are more commonly used to treat urinary tract infections, middle ear infections, pneumonia, and infectious diarrhea. They are also helpful in treating eye, skin, and vaginal infections and infections of the perineum. Sulfonamides and trimethoprim are also available as creams, lotions, eye drops, and ointments.

How Sulfonamides and Trimethoprim Work

Bacteria need a type of folic acid to be able to make DNA and reproduce. A specific enzyme is needed to convert other substances into folic acid in bacteria. The sulfonamides and trimethoprim prevent that enzyme from converting the other substances into folic acid. As a result, bacteria do not have enough folic acid to make DNA and grow. This does not kill the bacteria; it just limits their ability to reproduce (see Figure 8-2).

The following table focuses on the oral and parenteral forms of these drugs. Be sure to consult a drug reference for more information about a specific drug in this drug group.

⮂ **Do Not Confuse**

sulfaDIAZINE *with*
sulfiSOXAZOLE

An order for sulfaDIAZINE can be confused with sulfiSOXAZOLE. Although both drugs belong to the sulfonamide class of antibiotics, their dosages are different and they are NOT interchangeable.

QSEN: Safety

Dosages for Common Sulfonamides, Trimethoprim, and Combination Drugs

Drug	Dosage
Sulfonamides	
sulfaDIAZINE sodium	*Adults:* 2-4 g orally first, then 500 mg-1 g orally every 6-8 hr *Children:* 75 mg/kg orally first, then 30-40 mg/kg orally every 6-8 hr
sulfiSOXAZOLE (Gantrisin Pediatric, Soxazole ♣)	*Adults:* 2-4 g orally first, then 1-2 g orally every 6 hr *Children:* 75 mg orally first, then 30-40 mg/kg orally every 6 hr
trimethoprim (Primsol, Proloprim)	*Adults:* 100 mg orally every 12 hr or 200 mg orally daily *Children:* 5 mg/kg orally every 12 hr
Combination Drugs	
trimethoprim/sulfamethoxazole (Apo-Sulfatrim ♣, Bacter-Aid DS, Bactrim, Bactrim DS, Bethaprim, Novo-Trimel ♣, Nu-Cotrimex ♣, Roubac ♣, Septra, Septra DS, Septra IV [only form given parenterally], Sulfatrim, Sultrex)	*Adults:* 1-2 tablets (800 mg sulfamethoxazole and 160 mg trimethoprim) orally every 12 hr *Children:* trimethoprim content: 4 mg/kg and sulfamethoxazole 20 mg/kg orally every 12 hr *IV dosage for adults and children based on trimethoprim content:* 2-2.5 mg/kg trimethoprim IV slow infusion (60 to 50 min) every 6-12 hr

Common Side Effects

Metabolism Inhibitors

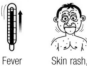

Headache   Fever   Skin rash, Photosensitivity

Side Effects. Common side effects of sulfonamides are headache, fever, rash, and increased sun sensitivity. Serious sunburns are possible while taking drugs from this class. The most common side effects of trimethoprim are headache, nausea, vomiting, and itchiness.

Adverse Effects. The sulfonamides are a type of chemical that can easily turn into crystals. Crystals that form and clump in the kidneys can cause kidney failure or kidney stones.

One of the most serious adverse effects of metabolism inhibitors is suppression of bone marrow cell division. This results in fewer red blood cells (*anemia*) and fewer

WBCs. Some patients are affected in this way only slightly; for others the suppression can be so great that they are at risk for infection.

A simple skin rash can occur with metabolism inhibitors, but more serious skin problems are also possible. These include peeling and sloughing, blister formation, and a combination of many types of skin eruptions known as *Stevens-Johnson syndrome*. This problem is serious and can lead to life-threatening losses of fluids and electrolytes (see Chapter 1).

Metabolism inhibitors should be avoided in any person who has a genetic disorder called glucose-6-phosphate dehydrogenase (G6PD) deficiency. In a patient with this health problem the drug causes red blood cells to break. G6PD deficiency is most common among African-American males and males of Mediterranean descent.

What To Do *Before* Giving Sulfonamides or Trimethoprim

In addition to the general responsibilities related to antibacterial therapy (pp. 117-118), ask patients about any known drug allergies, especially to sulfa drugs. Notify the prescriber about this issue.

If a patient is African-American or of Mediterranean descent, ask him if he or any member of his family has a genetic blood disorder. If he says yes, ask the prescriber whether a test for G6PD deficiency should be performed before starting the drug.

IV sulfamethoxazole/trimethoprim combination (Septra IV) can interact with other drugs and also can irritate tissues. Make sure that the IV infusion is running well and has a good blood return. This drug must be mixed and diluted only with dextrose 5% in water and should never be given intramuscularly. Either flush the line with dextrose 5% in water before giving the drug or use fresh tubing. Infuse Septra IV over 60 to 90 minutes.

Check the patient's current laboratory work, especially liver function tests, because these drugs are irritating to the liver (see Table 1-3 in Chapter 1). If laboratory values are higher than normal before starting the drug, the risk for liver inflammation is greater. Also check the patient's sclera and skin for yellowing *(jaundice)* because this problem occurs with liver inflammation. Use these data as a baseline to detect developing liver problems in patients taking metabolism inhibitors.

Check the patient's recent laboratory work for counts of WBCs, red blood cells, and platelets (see Table 1-5 in Chapter 1). Check the patient's skin for bruises or petechiae.

Check whether the patient is also taking a thiazide diuretic, especially if he or she is older than age 65. If a thiazide diuretic is also ordered, notify the prescriber because combining these drugs greatly increases the risk for anemia and bleeding.

Give the patient a full glass of water to drink with an oral sulfonamide or trimethoprim. Urge him or her to drink more fluids to prevent crystals from forming in the kidneys.

What To Do *After* Giving Sulfonamides or Trimethoprim

In addition to the general responsibilities related to antibacterial therapy (pp. 117-118), offer the patient a full glass of water every 4 hours (day and night) to help prevent crystals from forming in the kidney tubules.

Check the complete blood count every time it is performed to determine whether WBC, red blood cell, and platelet levels have changed (see Table 1-5 in Chapter 1).

Check the patient's skin every shift for rash, blisters, or other skin eruptions that may indicate a drug reaction. Ask whether he or she has noticed any itching or skin changes.

Check the patient daily for yellowing *(jaundice)* of the skin or sclera, which is a symptom of liver problems and red blood cell breakdown *(lysis)*. The best places to check are the whites of the eyes closest to the iris, the roof of the mouth, and the skin of the chest. Avoid checking the soles of the feet or palms of the hands, especially in patients with darker skin, because these areas often appear yellow even when the patient is not jaundiced.

Cultural Awareness

Closely watch male patients who are African-American or of Mediterranean descent for anemia and jaundice when they are receiving a metabolism inhibitor.

Memory Jogger

Ask patients about any known drug allergies, especially to sulfa drugs.

QSEN: Safety

Clinical Pitfall

Never give IV sulfamethoxazole/ trimethoprim (Septra IV) by bolus or rapid infusion.

QSEN: Safety

Drug Alert!

Administration Alert

Give patients a full glass of water to drink with an oral sulfonamide or trimethoprim.

QSEN: Safety

Cultural Awareness

In patients with darker skin, check for jaundice on the whites of the eyes closest to the iris and on the roof of the mouth. Do not look at the soles of the feet or palms of the hands.

Drug Alert!

Teaching Alert

Teach patients taking sulfon-amides or trimethoprim to protect themselves from sun exposure because these drugs greatly increase sun sensitivity, even among people with dark skin.

QSEN: Safety

Clinical Pitfall

Sulfonamides and trimethoprim should not be used during the last 2 months of pregnancy or during breastfeeding because it can cause severe jaundice in the infant.

QSEN: Safety

Do Not Confuse

Tequin *with* Tegretol or Ticlid

An order for Tequin can be con-fused with Tegretol or Ticlid. Tequin is a fluoroquinolone anti-bacterial drug. Tegretol is a drug for seizure control, and Ticlid is a platelet aggregation inhibitor.

QSEN: Safety

What To *Teach* Patients About Sulfonamides or Trimethoprim

In addition to the general care needs and precautions related to antibacterial therapy (p. 118), teach patients taking either type of drug from this class to avoid direct sun-light, use sunscreen, and wear protective clothing (including a hat) whenever they are in the sun to prevent a severe sunburn. Remind them to avoid tanning beds and salons.

Teach patients to drink a full glass of water with sulfonamide or trimethoprim tablets and to drink more fluids throughout the day to prevent crystals from forming in the urine and clogging the kidneys.

Tell patients to notify the prescriber if yellowing of the skin or eyes, a sore throat, fever, rash, blisters, or multiple bruises develop. All these problems are signs of serious adverse effects.

Life Span Considerations for Sulfonamides or Trimethoprim

Pediatric Considerations. Infants younger than 2 months of age are likely to become severely jaundiced when taking metabolism inhibitors because free bilirubin levels will rise and brain damage is possible. These drugs are not recommended for infants younger than 2 months of age except for life-threatening toxoplasmosis infections.

Considerations for Pregnancy and Lactation. Metabolism inhibitors have a low to moderate risk of increasing the risk for birth defects or fetal harm. Because these drugs can cause severe jaundice in infants, they should be avoided during the last 2 months of pregnancy to reduce the chance that the baby will be born while the mother is taking the drug. For the same reason, the breastfeeding mother should use alternate methods of infant feeding during the time that she is taking metabolism inhibitors.

Considerations for Older Adults. Metabolism inhibitors have more intense side effects, especially anemia and an increased risk for bleeding, in people older than age 65. When these drugs are taken by a person who also takes a thiazide diuretic, the risk for bleeding increases greatly.

DNA SYNTHESIS INHIBITORS: FLUOROQUINOLONES

The major DNA synthesis inhibitors are the fluoroquinolones. These drugs have many uses when taken systemically and in eye-drop and ear-drop forms. Their most common uses are for skin infections, urinary tract infections, respiratory tract infec-tions, infectious diarrhea, and gonorrhea. Fluoroquinolones also are used to prevent and treat anthrax. Be sure to consult a drug reference for more information about a specific drug in this group.

How Fluoroquinolones Work

Fluoroquinolones are DNA synthesis inhibitors that enter bacterial cells and prevent bacteria reproduction by suppressing the action of two enzymes important in making bacterial DNA. They are bactericidal to most bacteria that are sensitive to these drugs.

Dosages for Common Fluoroquinolones

Drug	Dosage (Adults Only)
ciprofloxacin (Cetraxal, Ciloxan, Cipro, Cipro XR, ProQuin XR)	250-750 mg orally every 12 hr or 1000 mg orally once daily 200-400 mg IV every 12 hr
gemifloxacin (Factive)	320 mg orally once daily
levofloxacin (Iquix, Levaquin, Quixin)	250-750 mg orally or IV daily
lomefloxacin (Maxaquin)	400 mg orally daily
moxifloxacin (Avelox, Avelox IV)	400 mg orally or IV daily
ofloxacin (Floxin)	200-400 mg orally every 12 hr

Common Side Effects. The most common fluoroquinolone side effects include rash, nausea and vomiting, abdominal pain, and muscle and joint pain. Lomefloxacin increases sun sensitivity, making serious sunburns possible.

These drugs can concentrate in urine, making the urine irritating to tissues. As a result, the patient may have pain or burning of the urethra and nearby tissues during urination. A patient who is incontinent may have skin irritation in the entire perineal area.

Adverse Effects. Fluoroquinolones can cause serious heart dysrhythmias, including prolonged Q-T interval. This serious problem is more common when the patient is also taking other drugs for dysrhythmias (such as amiodarone, quinidine, procainamide, or sotalol) or when he or she also has a low blood potassium level (*hypokalemia*).

Development of *peripheral neuropathy* is possible while taking these drugs. Signs and symptoms of this problem include tingling, burning, numbness, and pain in the hands or feet.

For a patient with diabetes, these drugs raise or lower blood glucose levels, leading to either *hyperglycemia* or *hypoglycemia*.

A rare adverse effect of fluoroquinolones is the rupture of a tendon, most often in the shoulder, hand, wrist, or heel (Achilles tendon). This complication is most likely to occur in an older patient who is also taking a corticosteroid.

What To Do *Before* Giving Fluoroquinolones

In addition to the general responsibilities related to antibacterial therapy (p. 117), remember that the oral forms of some fluoroquinolones are poorly absorbed with iron supplements, multivitamins, and antacids. Give fluoroquinolones at least 2 hours before or 4 hours after the dose of a multivitamin, iron, or antacid.

Check whether the patient also takes amiodarone, quinidine, procainamide, or sotalol. If so, notify the prescriber immediately because taking any of these drugs with fluoroquinolones can lead to serious dysrhythmias.

When mixing or diluting parenteral forms of this drug, use only sterile dextrose 5% in water, normal saline, lactated Ringer's, or 5% sodium bicarbonate. Do not use sterile water.

Give patients a full glass of water to drink with oral fluoroquinolone capsules or tablets and urge them to drink more fluids throughout the day. This action prevents forming a concentrated amount of drug in the urine that can irritate the urethra and perineum. Even the parenteral forms of the drug can concentrate in the urine. Make sure that patients receiving the drug by IV infusion also have a good fluid intake.

What To Do *After* Giving Fluoroquinolones

In addition to the general responsibilities related to antibacterial therapy (pp. 117-118), assess the heart rate and rhythm every 4 hours during therapy of a patient who either has known cardiac dysrhythmias or is taking a fluoroquinolone for the first time. If a new change in rhythm develops, check the patient again in 15 minutes. If the change persists or recurs, notify the prescriber.

For a patient who also has diabetes, check the blood glucose level even more often than usual.

What To *Teach* Patients About Fluoroquinolones

In addition to the general care needs and precautions related to antibacterial therapy (p. 118), remind patients who also take warfarin (Coumadin) to keep all appointments to check blood clotting. Fluoroquinolones increase warfarin levels and the risk for bleeding.

Because oral fluoroquinolones are poorly absorbed when taken with vitamin supplements, iron supplements, or antacids, teach patients to take the fluoroquinolone at least 2 hours before or 4 hours after taking a multivitamin, iron supplement, or antacid.

Common Side Effects
Fluoroquinolones

Rash   Nausea, Abdominal pain   Headache

Muscle and joint pain

 Clinical Pitfall

Do not give any fluoroquinolone as a bolus or by intramuscular or subcutaneous routes.

QSEN: Safety

 Clinical Pitfall

Do not use sterile water to mix or dilute IV forms of fluoroquinolones.

QSEN: Safety

⚠ **Drug Alert!**
Intervention Alert

Check patients with diabetes often for hypoglycemia or hyperglycemia because fluoroquinolones can cause quick changes in blood glucose levels.

QSEN: Safety

Drug Alert!

Teaching Alert

Teach patients taking fluoroquinolones to protect themselves from sun exposure because these drugs greatly increase sun sensitivity, even among people with dark skin.

QSEN: Safety

Teach patients to drink a full glass of water with oral fluoroquinolone capsules or tablets and to drink more fluids throughout the day to prevent the forming of a concentrated amount of drug in the urine that can irritate the urethra and perineum.

Teach patients how to check their pulse and remind them to check it twice each day. Tell them to notify the prescriber if their pulse becomes irregular, if palpitations occur, or if they become dizzy.

Tell patients to stop taking the drug and see the prescriber as soon as possible if pain or swelling in a tendon or joint occurs. The risk for a tendon rupture is increased while taking the drug and for about 1 month after the drug is stopped.

Sun sensitivity greatly increases the risk for sunburn, even for people who have dark skin. Teach patients to avoid direct sunlight, use sunscreen, and wear protective clothing (including a hat) whenever they are in the sun to prevent severe sunburn. Remind them to avoid tanning beds and salons.

Life Span Considerations for Fluoroquinolones

Pediatric Considerations. The use of fluoroquinolones in infants and children younger than 18 years of age is not recommended unless the infection is life threatening and not sensitive to other drugs. Fluoroquinolones can damage bones, joints, muscles, tendons, and other soft tissues when given to patients who are still growing.

Considerations for Pregnancy and Lactation. Fluoroquinolones have a moderate likelihood of increasing the risk for birth defects or fetal harm, especially bone, joint, and tendon defects. These drugs should not be used during pregnancy. The breast-feeding mother should use alternate methods of infant feeding during the time that she is taking fluoroquinolones.

Considerations for Older Adults. Tendon rupture is seen more often in older adults taking fluoroquinolones. The tendons most often affected are in the shoulder, hand, wrist, and Achilles tendon at the heel. Taking corticosteroids at the same time as a fluoroquinolone increases the risk, but tendon rupture can occur when taking fluoroquinolones alone. Tendon rupture also can occur up to 1 month after the drug has been stopped. If the patient has pain or inflammation of a tendon or around a joint, he or she should stop the drug, stop moving or exercising that joint, and see the prescriber as soon as possible.

ANTIBACTERIAL DRUG RESISTANCE

When antibacterials are overused, prescribed for conditions not responsive to these drugs, or taken improperly, drug-resistant strains of bacteria may develop. **Antibiotic resistance** is the ability of a bacterium to resist the effects of antibacterial drugs. Bacteria that can either be killed by antibacterials or have their reproduction suppressed are called *susceptible* organisms. Those that are neither killed nor suppressed by antibacterial drugs are called *resistant* organisms. Some bacteria are resistant to one type of antibacterial drug but susceptible to other types. The concern now is that many bacteria species and strains that were once susceptible to many types of antibacterial drugs are becoming resistant to most types. When a bacterium becomes resistant to three or more different types of antibacterial drugs, it is called a *superbug* or a *multiple drug–resistant (MDR) organism.* The fear is that common bacteria that are not particularly hard to treat will become superbugs and cause "superinfections" that are difficult or impossible to control or cure. Several families of bacteria and other organisms have already become more resistant to anti-infective therapy.

Examples of resistant organisms include methicillin-resistant *Staphylococcus aureus* (MRSA), *Streptococcus pneumoniae,* multidrug-resistant tuberculosis (MDR-TB), gonorrhea, vancomycin-resistant enterococcus (VRE), vancomycin-resistant streptococcus (VRS), carbapenem-resistant enterobacteriaceae (CRE), typhoid fever, malaria, and even head lice. The infections caused by resistant organisms cost more to treat, increase the lengths of hospital stays, and lead to higher death rates.

 Memory Jogger

When antibacterial drug resistance develops, the bacteria are resistant to the drug, but the patient is not resistant to the drug. This means that if the patient should later develop an infection with a bacterium that is susceptible to the drug, the patient can then take that drug and it will be effective.

Get Ready for Practice!

Key Points

- Gram-negative bacteria are harder to kill or control with antibacterial drugs because they have a protective capsule that limits the effects of drugs.
- Diarrhea is an expected side effect of therapy with most antibacterial drugs.
- Check the patient's vital signs (including temperature) and mental status before starting an antibacterial drug.
- Check to determine which solutions can be used to dilute a particular IV antibacterial drug and which solutions or drugs should be avoided with that drug.
- For drugs that are toxic to the ears and hearing (ototoxic) such as vancomycin and the aminoglycosides, check the patient's hearing before therapy begins.
- For drugs that cause heart rhythm disturbances such as macrolides and fluoroquinolones (whether given alone or with other drugs), check the patient's heart rate for rhythm and quality for a full minute before giving the first dose of the drug.
- For drugs that increase the effects of warfarin (when the patient is also taking warfarin) such as macrolides, tetracyclines, streptogramins, and fluoroquinolones, check the patient's most recent international normalized ratio (INR) before giving the first dose of the drug.
- Give antibacterial drugs on a schedule that evenly spaces them throughout 24 hours.
- Do not give (and teach patients not to take) cephalosporins, tetracyclines, or fluoroquinolones with antacids, multiple vitamins, or iron supplements.
- For the patient taking warfarin and a macrolide, tetracycline, streptogramin, or fluoroquinolone, check the patient daily for any signs or symptoms of increased bleeding.
- Drugs that have adverse effects on the kidneys (nephrotoxic) almost always have adverse effects on the ears for hearing and balance (ototoxic).
- Urge the patient taking any antibacterial drug to stop the drug and inform the prescriber if a rash or other skin eruption develops.
- Warn patients to immediately call 911 if they begin to have difficulty breathing, a rapid irregular pulse, swelling of the face or neck, or the feeling of a "lump in the throat."
- Teach patients taking macrolides to take the drug with food or within 1 hour of having eaten.
- Teach patients taking macrolides, tetracyclines, sulfonamides, or fluoroquinolones that these drugs can cause severe sunburn, even for patients with dark skin.
- Drug types that should be avoided during pregnancy, while breastfeeding, and with infants or children unless the infection is life threatening include aminoglycosides, tetracyclines, sulfonamides, and fluoroquinolones.
- Even a patient who has never taken an antibacterial drug can have an infection with bacteria that is resistant to antibacterial drug therapy.

Additional Learning Resources

evolve Be sure to visit your Evolve website (http://evolve.elsevier.com/Workman/pharmacology/) for additional online resources.

SG Go to your Study Guide for additional learning activities to help you master this chapter content.

Review Questions

See the Answer Keys—In-text Review Questions for answers to these questions.

Test Yourself on the Basics

1. What is the most important question to ask any patient before he or she starts antibacterial therapy?
   - A. When did you last eat or drink?
   - B. Is your temperature elevated?
   - C. Do you have any known drug allergies?
   - D. How often do you drink alcoholic beverages?
2. Which aminoglycoside antibacterial drug is often prescribed to treat tuberculosis?
   - A. streptomycin
   - B. azithromycin (Zithromax)
   - C. demeclocycline (Declomycin)
   - D. trimethoprim/sulfamethoxazole (Septra)
3. Indicate which cephalosporin drugs are third generation. (Select all that apply.)
   - A. cefazolin (Ancef)
   - B. cefaclor (Ceclor)
   - C. cefdinir (Spectracef)
   - D. cefepime (Maxipime)
   - E. cefuroxime (Ceftin)
   - F. ceftriaxone (Rocephin)
   - G. cephalexin (Keflex)
   - H. cefpodoxime (Vantin)
4. Which drug group has the adverse reactions of reducing hearing and kidney function?
   - A. Macrolides
   - B. Penicillins
   - C. Cephalosporins
   - D. Aminoglycosides
5. Which drugs should be avoided for newborns and infants unless an infection is so severe that it is life threatening? (Select all that apply.)
   - A. amikacin (Amikin)
   - B. azithromycin (Zithromax)
   - C. cefdinir (Omnicef)
   - D. clarithromycin (Biaxin)
   - E. demeclocycline (Declomycin)
   - F. moxifloxacin (Avelox)
   - G. penicillin G benzathine (Bicillin LA)
   - H. trimethoprim/sulfamethoxazole (Bactrim)

6. Antibacterial drugs that are toxic to the kidneys (nephrotoxic) are more likely to be toxic to which other organ or tissue?
   A. Ears
   B. Brain
   C. Liver
   D. Lungs

7. Which antibacterial drug is most commonly associated with "red man syndrome"?
   A. amikacin (Amikin)
   B. erythromycin (E-mycin)
   C. penicillin V potassium (Pen-VK)
   D. vancomycin (Vancocin)

Test Yourself on Advanced Content

8. A patient prescribed to take oral penicillin tells you that all of the following problems occurred the last time she took penicillin. Which problem is a true allergic reaction?
   A. Strong-smelling urine
   B. Hives and rash
   C. Oral thrush
   D. Diarrhea

9. Why should a patient who has a bacterial infection and who is immunosuppressed be treated with a drug that is bactericidal rather than bacteriostatic?
   A. Bacteriostatic drugs are more likely to trigger allergic responses than are bactericidal drugs.
   B. Bactericidal drugs also prevent overgrowth of normal flora and bacteriostatic drugs do not exert this action.
   C. The effectiveness of a bacteriostatic drug relies on the patient's immune system to eradicate the infectious bacteria.
   D. The activity of bacteriostatic drugs further suppresses the immune response and increases the risk for opportunistic infections.

10. A patient who has been taking tetracycline for a week tells you that a cheesy white substance on the gums and roof of the mouth has appeared. What is your best suggestion?
    A. "Drink at least 3 liters of water each day and avoid all dairy products while you are on this drug."
    B. "Go immediately to the emergency room because this is a sign of a serious allergic reaction."
    C. "Stop taking the drug and notify your prescriber because this is a sign of the beginning of an allergic reaction."
    D. "Brush your teeth at least three times a day and use mouthwash to help clear this yeast infection."

11. When you check on a patient receiving cefazolin (Kefzol) IV 15 minutes after the drug was started, the patient tells you, "I can't swallow, my chest hurts, and I feel like something bad is going to happen, but I don't know what." What do you do first?
    A. Discontinue the IV.
    B. Notify the prescriber.
    C. Stop the drug infusion.
    D. Check the arms, chest, and back for hives or a rash.

12. What is the most important action or precaution to teach a patient prescribed to take any antibacterial drug?
    A. Always take the drug with food or milk.
    B. Always take the drug for as long as it was prescribed.
    C. Never drink caffeine or alcohol while taking an antibacterial drug.
    D. Be sure to swallow all antibacterial tablets whole rather than chewing them.

13. Which drug can cause a tendon rupture in a patient who also takes a corticosteroid daily?
    A. amikacin (Amikan)
    B. linezolid (Zyvox)
    C. vancomycin (Vancocin)
    D. levofloxacin (Levaquin)

14. Which drugs can cause photosensitivity and increase the risk for severe sunburn? (Select all that apply.)
    A. amoxicillin (Amoxil)
    B. cephalexin (Keflex)
    C. erythromycin (E-mycin)
    D. lomefloxacin (Maxaquin)
    E. minocycline (Dynacin)
    F. penicillin V potassium (Pen-VK)
    G. sulfasoxazole (Gantrisin pediatric)
    H. vancomycin (Vancocin)

15. A 1-year-old child who weighs 22 lb is to receive an intravenous dose of ticarcillin 50 mg/kg.
    a. What is this child's weight in kg?
    b. How much ticarcillin should he or she receive at 50 mg/kg?_____mg

16. Your patient is prescribed to receive 750 mg of meropenem (Merrem) by IV "piggyback" in 250 mL of normal saline. The vial of meropenem you have is a concentration of 50 mg/mL. How many milliliters of meropenem will be added to the normal saline for a 750 mg dose?_____mL

Critical Thinking Activities

See the Answer Keys—Critical Thinking Activities for answers to these activities.

The patient is a 74-year-old woman who is prescribed to take trimethoprim/sulfamethoxazole (Bactrim) for a severe urinary tract infection. The prescription says she is to take 1 tablet every 12 hours for the next 14 days. She tells you that she thinks we all take too many drugs and plans to stop taking the drug as soon as the pain and burning on urination go away.

1. What type of drug is trimethoprim/sulfamethoxazole, and how does it work?
2. Is it okay for her to stop taking this drug as soon as the symptoms are gone? Why or why not?
3. What are the side effects of this drug?
4. What precautions and actions will you teach her about this drug therapy?

Anti-Infectives: Antiviral Drugs

Objectives

After studying this chapter you should be able to:

1. List the names, actions, and usual adult dosages for antiviral and antiretroviral drugs.
2. Identify the possible side effects and adverse effects of antiviral and antiretroviral drugs.
3. Describe what to do before and after giving antiviral and antiretroviral drugs.
4. Explain what to teach patients taking antiviral and antiretroviral drugs, including what to do, what not to do, and when to call the prescriber.
5. Describe life span considerations for antiviral and antiretroviral drugs.

Key Terms

antiretroviral drugs (ăn-tī-RĔT-rō-vī-răl DRŬGZ) (p. 147) A category of antiviral drugs that suppress the replication (reproduction) of viruses (retroviruses) that use RNA as their primary genetic material instead of DNA.

antiviral drugs (ăn-tī-vī-răl DRŬGZ) (p. 139) Drugs that are virustatic against nonretroviruses and prevent them from either reproducing or releasing their genetic material.

entry inhibitors (ĔN-trē ĭn-HĬB-ĭ-tŭrz) (p. 154) A class of antiretroviral drug that prevents HIV cellular infection by blocking the CCR5 receptor on CD4+ T cells.

fusion inhibitors (FŪ-zhŭn ĭn-HĬB-ĭ-tŭrz) (p. 153) A class of antiretroviral drug that prevents HIV infection by blocking the viral docking protein (gp41) from fusing with the host cell.

human immune deficiency virus (HIV) (HYŪ-mŭn ĭm-MYŪN dĕ-FĬSH-ĕn-sē VĪ-rŭs) (p. 146) The most common retrovirus known to cause disease among humans. It is the organism known to cause HIV disease and AIDS.

integrase inhibitors (ĬN-tĕ-grāz ĭn-HĬB-ĭ-tŭrz) (p. 152) A class of antiretroviral drugs that prevent HIV infection by inhibiting the enzyme integrase, which is needed to allow insertion of viral DNA into the DNA of the human host cell.

non-nucleoside analog reverse transcriptase inhibitors (NNRTIs) (NŎN-NŪ-klē-ō-sīd ĂN-ă-lŏg TRĂN-skrĭp-tāz ĭn-HĬB-ĭ-tŭrz) (p. 150) A class of antiretroviral drugs that inhibit the action of the enzyme reverse transcriptase by binding directly to the enzyme, preventing it from converting viral RNA to DNA.

nucleoside analog reverse transcriptase inhibitors (NRTIs) (NŪ-klē-ō-sīd ĂN-ă-lŏg TRĂN-skrĭp-tāz ĭn-HĬB-ĭ-tŭrz) (p. 149) Drugs that are similar in structure to bases that form DNA. These drugs compete with real bases in HIV-infected cells and reduce viral replication.

protease inhibitors (PIs) (PRŌ-tē-āce ĭn-HĬB-ĭ-tŭrz) (p. 151) A class of antiretroviral drugs that prevent HIV replication and prevent the release of HIV particles from infected cells.

viral load (VĪ-rŭl LŌD) (p. 148) The number of viral particles in a blood sample, which indicates the degree of viral infection.

virulence (VĬR-ŭ-lĕns) (p. 138) The measure of how well a microorganism can invade and persist in growing, even when the person's body is trying to destroy or eliminate it.

virus (VĪ-rŭs) (p. 137) An intracellular, submicroscopic parasite.

virustatic (vī-rŭ-STĂ-tĭk) (p. 139) Drug actions that reduce the number of viruses present by preventing them from reproducing and growing.

Viral infections are common. Some, like a cold, are non–life threatening and require no drug therapy. Others, such as hepatitis, are more complicated and, left untreated, may cause serious damage or death. This chapter focuses on viral infections and the drugs used to prevent or control them.

VIRAL INFECTION

Viruses are intracellular, submicroscopic parasites that must infect a living host cell to reproduce. A *host* is the person infected by a virus whose cells allow viral reproduction. When viruses infect a living cell in just the right way, the resources, energy,

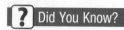 **Did You Know?**

Viruses are not capable of self-reproduction.

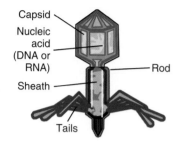

FIGURE 9-1 The basic anatomy of a common virus.

 Memory Jogger

Most common viruses must enter the body in large numbers for infection to result in disease because these viruses have a low efficiency of infection.

and machinery of that living cell are used to make new viruses. Because they are so small, viruses can more easily enter the body than bacteria and funguses can. Entrance sites include mucous membranes in the nose, conjunctiva of the eye, respiratory tract, digestive tract, and genital or urinary tract. They can also enter through broken skin, and they can be injected into the body in blood or blood products.

There are two basic types of viruses: *common viruses* (nonretroviruses) and *retroviruses*. Likewise there are two basic categories of antiviral drugs: those that work against some common viruses (*antiviral drugs*) and those that have some effect against retroviruses (*antiretrovirals*). Common viruses are discussed in this section; retroviruses are discussed later in this chapter.

REVIEW OF RELATED PHYSIOLOGY AND PATHOPHYSIOLOGY FOR COMMON VIRUSES

A *common virus* is a nonretrovirus that uses either DNA or RNA as its genetic material and has a relatively low efficiency of cellular infection. *Efficiency of infection* is the ease with which an organism causes disease through infection. This means that most common viruses must invade the body in large numbers to cause disease. These viruses are responsible for common infections such as chickenpox, shingles, measles, mumps, herpes, warts, hepatitis, and the common cold. The basic anatomy of a common virus is shown in Figure 9-1.

For viruses to cause disease after they enter the body, they must actually enter cells and use the reproductive machinery of the cell to make more viruses that then leave the cell to infect more cells. So becoming sick with a viral disease requires that many cells be infected by common viruses. Inside the body viruses can be destroyed or removed by the immune system. A healthy person will not become ill from most viruses unless the number of invading viruses overwhelms the normal protections.

Viruses that enter the body and survive must enter cells and insert their genetic material into the genetic material of the host cells. Then viral genes direct the host cell to make more viruses. These new viruses fill the cell and eventually break out of it to infect new host cells (Figure 9-2). Viral infections are not cured but are self-limiting, meaning that in a person with a healthy immune system the illness only lasts for so long. If a person's immune system is working properly, the body fights off the infection by itself. If the immune system is weak or if the body has other health problems, the person may die from the effects of the disease.

Some common viruses are stronger than others, with greater **virulence** (the measure of how well a microorganism can invade and persist in growing, even when the person's body is trying to destroy or eliminate it). One of the most virulent viruses

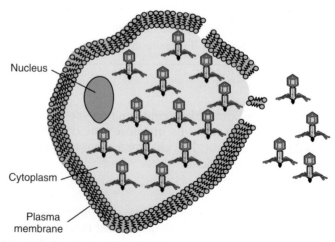

FIGURE 9-2 An infected cell generates new viruses and then opens the cell and sends newly generated viruses out to infect more host cells.

is the hepatitis B virus (HBV). Others, such as the virus group that cause the common cold, are less virulent. When more viruses are required for disease to result, the efficiency of infection for that virus is low. If fewer viruses are required to cause an infection to develop into a disease, the efficiency of infection is high.

Some common infections are minor and can be limited by the immune system. Because more severe viral infections can cause serious harm and even death, antiviral drugs are used to prevent viruses from spreading infection all through the body and causing severe damage.

GENERAL ISSUES IN ANTIVIRAL THERAPY

An important concept to remember for all antiviral drugs is that they are only viru-static. **Virustatic** drugs reduce the number of viruses by preventing them from repro-ducing and growing. They are not *virucidal* and cannot kill the virus. By keeping the number of viruses low, antiviral drugs allow the natural defenses of the body to destroy, eliminate, or inactivate them.

Antiviral drugs are virustatic drugs that prevent viruses from either reproducing or from releasing their genetic material. Drugs that are effective against common viruses do not have specific categories and may have more than one mechanism of action. Some antivirals suppress viral reproduction. Others prevent the virus from opening its coat and allowing the genetic material to be released. The exact mecha-nism of action of still other antivirals is not known.

Allergic reactions are possible with any antiviral drug. The allergy may be mild and annoying or severe and life threatening *(anaphylaxis)*. More serious reactions occur when antiviral drugs are given intravenously.

Intended responses for antiviral drugs include:
- The duration or intensity of an existing viral disease is shortened.
- Reactivation of a dormant viral infection is prevented.
- A viral infection is prevented from multiplying to the point that a disease results.

Before giving an antiviral drug, ask whether the patient has any drug allergies. If so, notify the prescriber before giving the drug.

After giving the first dose of an intravenous (IV) antiviral drug, check the patient every 15 minutes for signs or symptoms of an allergic reaction (hives at the IV site; low blood pressure; rapid, irregular pulse; swelling of the lips or lower face; the patient feeling a lump in the throat). If the patient is having an anaphylactic reaction, your first action is to prevent any more drug from entering him or her. Stop the drug from infusing but maintain the IV access. If the drug is infusing high into the IV tubing, change the tubing after stopping the drug and do not let any drug left in the tubing infuse into the patient.

Inspect the IV site at the beginning of the infusion, halfway through the infusion, and at the end of the infusion and document your findings. If redness is present or the patient reports discomfort at the site, slow the infusion and check for a blood return. Look for any redness or pain or the feeling of hard or cordlike veins above the site. If any of these problems occur, follow the policy of your facility for removing the IV line.

Teach patients receiving antiviral drugs the importance of taking the drug long enough to ensure suppression of viral reproduction. If the patient stops taking the drug as soon as he or she feels better, symptoms of infection may recur, and resistant viruses may develop. Teach the patient to take antiviral drugs exactly as prescribed and for as long as prescribed.

For all antiviral therapy it is important to keep the blood level high enough to affect the viruses causing the infection. So it is best for the patient to take the drug evenly throughout a 24-hour day. If the drug should be taken twice daily, teach the patient to take it every 12 hours. For three times a day, teach the patient to take it every 8 hours. Help the patient plan an easy-to-remember schedule that keeps the drug at the best blood levels.

 Memory Jogger

The more virulent a virus is, the fewer viruses are needed to cause infection and disease. The effi-ciency of infection is higher.

 Memory Jogger

Antiviral drugs do not kill viruses; they only suppress their reproduc-tion and growth.

 Memory Jogger

Signs and symptoms of a severe allergic reaction include hives at the IV site; low blood pressure; rapid, irregular pulse; swelling of the lips or lower face; and the patient feeling a lump in the throat.

! Drug Alert!

Action/Intervention Alert

If the patient appears to be having anaphylaxis from an IV drug, prevent more drug from entering the patient but maintain IV access.

QSEN: Safety

 ! Drug Alert!

Teaching Alert

Teach patients to take antiviral drugs exactly as prescribed and for as long as prescribed.

QSEN: Safety

Dosages for Common Antiviral Drugs

Drug	Dosage
acyclovir (Apo-Acyclovir ♣, Avirax ♣, Zovirax)	*Adults:* 5-10 mg/kg IV every 8 hr; 400 mg orally every 8 hr (genital herpes) *Children:* 10 mg/kg IV every 8 hr; 20 mg/kg orally 4 times daily (chickenpox)
adefovir dipivoxil (Hepsera)	*Adults and Children over 12 years:* 10 mg orally once daily *Children under 12 years:* Safety and efficacy have not been determined
amantadine (Symmetrel, Endantadine ♣)	*Adults/Children over 10 years:* 100 mg orally twice daily or 200 mg orally once daily *Adults over 65 years:* 100 mg orally once daily *Children under 10 years:* 2.5-4 mg/kg orally every 12 hr
ribavirin (Copegus, Moderiba, Rebetol, RibaPak, Ribasphere, RibaTab, Virazole)	*Adults/Children over 75 kg:* 600 mg orally every 12 hr *Children 60-75 kg:* 400-600 mg orally every 12 hr; other oral dosing is weight dependent *Aerosol administration:* 20 mg/mL for respiratory syncytial virus at 12-18 hr/day delivers an average of 190 mcg/L of air
oseltamivir (Tamiflu)	*Adults/Children over 40 g:* 75 mg orally every 12 hr for 5 days (dosage adjusted downward by weight for children less than 40 kg)
rimantadine (Flumadine)	*Adults/Children over 10 years:* 100 mg orally twice daily *Adults over 65 years:* 100 mg orally once daily *Children under 10 years:* 3.3 mg/kg orally twice daily (maximum 150 mg)
simeprevir (Olysio)	*Adults:* 150 mg orally once daily with other antivirals to treat hepatitis C that is "genotype 1"
valacyclovir (Valtrex)	*Adults/Children:* 1-2 g orally every 12 hr for initial treatment of herpes simplex virus 1 or 2; 500-1000 mg orally every 12 hr for management of recurrent infections
zanamivir (Relenza)	*Adults/Children over 7 years:* Two oral inhalations (one 5-mg blister per inhalation for a total dosage of 10 mg) every 12 hr for 5 days

ANTIVIRAL DRUGS

ACYCLOVIR AND VALACYCLOVIR

Acyclovir and valacyclovir are related drugs. At the cell level valacyclovir is converted to acyclovir when it is metabolized.

How Acyclovir and Valacyclovir Work

Acyclovir and valacyclovir slow viral reproduction by forming "counterfeit" DNA bases and inhibiting the enzymes needed to complete the formation of viral DNA chains. Table 9-1 lists diseases caused by these viruses. The dosages and length of therapy for these drugs depend on which virus is causing the infection, the severity of the infection, and the health of the patient's immune system. Other related drugs with actions similar to those of acyclovir include famciclovir and penciclovir.

Side Effects. Common side effects of both of these drugs are headaches, dizziness, and nausea and vomiting.

Adverse Effects. Pain and irritation at the injection site may occur with IV acyclovir, especially when the drug is given rapidly.

Both drugs can reduce kidney function and lead to kidney damage and failure. This problem is caused by the drugs precipitating in the kidney tubules, which is most likely to occur when the patient is not well hydrated.

What To Do *Before* Giving Acyclovir or Valacyclovir

In addition to the general responsibilities related to antiviral therapy (p. 139), check whether the patient takes phenytoin (Dilantin) or another drug for seizure control. Acyclovir and valacyclovir reduce the effectiveness of phenytoin, and the prescriber

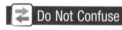

Do Not Confuse

Zovirax *with* **Zyvox**

An order for Zovirax can be confused with Zyvox. Zovirax is an antiviral drug, whereas Zyvox is an antibacterial drug used to treat methicillin-resistant *Staphylococcus aureus* (MRSA).

QSEN: Safety

Do Not Confuse

Valtrex *with* **Valcyte**

An order for Valtrex can be confused with Valcyte. Valtrex is an oral antiviral drug use to treat herpes simplex, varicella zoster, cytomegalovirus, and Epstein-Barr viruses. Valcyte is a drug for cytomegalovirus retinitis for patients with AIDS.

QSEN: Safety

Table **9-1** Diseases Caused by Specific Viruses	
VIRUS	**DISEASE**
Cytomegalovirus (CMV)	Mononucleosis Serious eye infection (retinitis) in people who are immunosuppressed
Epstein-Barr virus (EBV)	Chronic fatigue syndrome Some types of lymphoma Systemic infection in newborns and people with severe immunosuppression
Hantavirus (HV)	Hantavirus pulmonary syndrome (HPS)
Hepatitis A virus (HAV)	Hepatitis A
Hepatitis B virus (HBV)	Acute hepatitis B Chronic hepatitis B Liver failure Liver cancer
Hepatitis C virus (HCV)	Chronic hepatitis C Liver failure
Herpes simplex virus type 1 (HSV1)	Cold sores Systemic infection in newborns and people with severe immunosuppression
Herpes simplex virus type 2 (HSV2)	Genital herpes infections
Respiratory syncytial virus (RSV)	Severe respiratory infection in infants, young children, and older adults
Varicella-zoster virus (VZV)	Chickenpox Shingles
West Nile virus (WNV)	Severe infection with symptoms similar to those of encephalitis or meningitis

 Memory Jogger

Acyclovir and valacyclovir are most effective against Epstein-Barr virus, cytomegalovirus, herpes simplex virus types 1 and 2, and varicella zoster virus.

Common Side Effects

Acyclovir and Valacyclovir

Headache   Dizziness   Nausea/
                                 Vomiting

may need to adjust the phenytoin dosage to prevent seizures while the patient is on antiviral therapy.

Make sure that the IV infusion is running well and has a good blood return. Dilute parenteral acyclovir to the proper concentration with only sterile water for injection. Inspect the drug for discoloration or particles.

Acyclovir can interact with other drugs in the tubing. Either flush the line before giving acyclovir or use fresh tubing for the infusion.

Administer the drug slowly over 60 minutes to avoid kidney problems and reduce the risk for irritation at the injection site.

What To Do *After* Giving Acyclovir or Valacyclovir

In addition to the general responsibilities related to antiviral therapy (p. 139), these specific responsibilities after giving acyclovir or valacyclovir are important.

Give the patient a full glass of water to drink with oral doses and urge him or her to drink more fluids throughout the day to keep these drugs from precipitating in the kidneys. This is even more important if the patient also takes other drugs that can damage the kidney.

What To *Teach* Patients About Acyclovir or Valacyclovir

In addition to teaching patients about the general care needs and precautions related to antiviral therapy (p. 139), instruct them to drink a full glass of water with each dose of the drug and to drink at least 3 L of fluid daily.

Life Span Considerations for Acyclovir or Valacyclovir

Pediatric Considerations. Oral dosages of these drugs for children older than 2 years of age are very similar to the dosages for adults.

 Drug Alert!

Action/Interaction Alert

Acyclovir and valacyclovir reduce the effectiveness of phenytoin (Dilantin) for seizure control.

QSEN: Safety

 Drug Alert!

Administration Alert

Administer IV acyclovir as an infusion over 60 minutes.

QSEN: Safety

 Drug Alert!

Action/Intervention Alert

Ensure that patients taking acyclovir or valacyclovir drink at least 3 L of fluid daily.

QSEN: Safety

Considerations for Pregnancy and Lactation. Both acyclovir and valacyclovir have a low likelihood of increasing the risk for birth defects or fetal damage. The benefits of the use of acyclovir or valacyclovir during pregnancy should be weighed against any possible risks. These drugs appear in breast milk and can enter the infant during breastfeeding. Teach breastfeeding mothers to reduce the infant's exposure to these drugs (see Box 1-1 in Chapter 1).

Considerations for Older Adults. Dizziness, agitation, and confusion may occur as side effects. Older adults are at greater risk for these effects as a result of age-related changes in kidney function and may require more frequent monitoring of kidney function tests (see Table 1-4 in Chapter 1). These changes increase the time that acyclovir and valacyclovir remain in the body, increasing the risk for side effects. Teach older patients to avoid driving or operating heavy equipment until they know how these drugs may affect them.

ADEFOVIR DIPIVOXIL

How Adefovir Dipivoxil Works

Adefovir dipivoxil is an oral drug that acts as a counterfeit base limiting the DNA replication and reproduction of the hepatitis B virus (HBV). These actions suppress viral replication in infected cells, especially liver cells. Unlike some antiviral drugs, the duration of therapy with this drug may be many months to years long.

Side Effects. The most common side effects of adefovir dipivoxil are nausea and abdominal pain.

Adverse Effects. Adefovir dipivoxil has many adverse effects and carries a black box warning (see Chapter 1). This drug is highly liver toxic (hepatotoxic) and kidney toxic (nephrotoxic). It should be used cautiously or not at all in patients who have impaired kidney function or non–hepatitis-related liver diseases.

This drug also interacts with many other drugs, especially antiretroviral drugs. Be sure to consult a pharmacist or drug handbook for specific interactions. The majority of time, this drug is prescribed for outpatient use.

What To Do *Teach* Patients Taking Adefovir Dipivoxil

In addition to teaching patients about the general care needs and precautions related to antiviral therapy (p. 139), warn them that an acute exacerbation of hepatitis B symptoms can occur if the drug is stopped suddenly.

Tell patients to notify the prescriber if they develop yellowing of the skin or eyes, darkening of the urine, or lightening of the stools. These problems are signs of liver toxicity, a serious adverse effect of adefovir dipivoxil.

Remind patients to be aware of their urine output. Although measuring it is usually not necessary, they should be alert for an output that is significantly less than their fluid intake and report this change to the prescriber.

Warn patients not to take other drugs or supplements without checking with the prescriber because adefovir dipivoxil interacts with so many other drugs.

Because of the potential for liver damage, urge patients to avoid drinking alcohol or using acetaminophen while taking this drug.

Life Span Considerations for Adefovir Dipivoxil

Considerations for Pregnancy and Lactation. Adefovir has a moderate likelihood of increasing the risk for birth defects or fetal damage and appears in breast milk. Therefore it is not recommended that this drug be used during pregnancy unless the benefits clearly outweigh the risks. Breastfeeding is not recommended while taking this drug to avoid exposure to the infant.

Considerations for Older Adults. Adefovir dipivoxil should be used cautiously, if at all, in patients over 65 years of age. This is especially true for older adults

Memory Jogger

Adefovir dipivoxil is most effective against the hepatitis B virus.

Common Side Effects

Adefovir Dipivoxil

Nausea/Vomiting; Abdominal Pain

who are taking a variety of drugs for chronic disorders of the kidneys, liver, or heart.

AMANTADINE AND RIMANTADINE

How Amantadine and Rimantadine Work

Amantadine is an oral drug that prevents viral infection by blocking the opening of the external coating of the influenza A virus and stopping the release of viral particles into respiratory epithelial cells. These actions prevent infection and also inhibit viral replication in infected cells.

Rimantadine is similar in chemical structure and action to amantadine; however, it tends to concentrate more in respiratory tissues and less in the brain than amantadine. As a result, it has fewer nervous system side effects.

Side Effects. The most common side effects of amantadine (and to a lesser extent rimantadine) include the anticholinergic effects of blurred vision, dry mouth, and hallucinations, along with orthostatic (postural) hypotension and dizziness.

Adverse Effects. Amantadine affects the central nervous system (CNS) and may worsen glaucoma and urinary retention. It should not be taken by patients who have either of these problems. Patients who have psychiatric disorders may have an increased risk for suicidal thoughts while taking this drug. These adverse effects have been seen with rimantadine only at very high doses.

What To *Before* Giving Amantadine or Rimantadine

In addition to the general responsibilities related to antiviral therapy (p. 139), ask whether the patient has glaucoma or a problem with urinary retention, especially whether male patients have an enlarged prostate gland. Also check whether the patient has any known psychiatric problems, especially severe depression, or has attempted suicide in the past. If the patient has any of these problems, notify the prescriber before administering the drug.

What To *Teach* Patients About Amantadine or Rimantadine

In addition to teaching patients about the general care needs and precautions related to antiviral therapy (p. 139), teach them not to stand or sit up quickly because this may lower blood pressure rapidly, causing dizziness and an increased risk for falls. Also instruct them to hold onto railings when going up or down steps.

Tell the patient and family to report to the prescriber immediately any worsening of depression or thoughts of suicide.

Life Span Considerations for Amantadine or Rimantadine

Considerations for Pregnancy and Lactation. Amantadine and rimantadine have a moderate likelihood of increasing the risk for birth defects or fetal damage and appear in breast milk. Therefore it is not recommended that either of these drugs be used during the first trimester of pregnancy or by women who are breastfeeding.

Considerations for Older Adults. The dosage of either drug should be reduced for patients older than age 65 years. Both drugs can worsen heart failure and increase edema. Teach older adults taking either amantadine or rimantadine to weigh themselves daily and notify the prescriber if they have gained more than 3 lb in 2 days. Also teach older patients to measure their pulse at least once daily and notify the prescriber if it becomes more irregular or is hard to find.

RIBAVIRIN

How Ribavirin Works

Ribavirin is a "counterfeit" base that suppresses viral action and reproduction by unknown mechanisms. It is effective at suppressing many viruses; however, because

Memory Jogger

Amantadine and rimantadine are most effective against the influenza A virus.

Common Side Effects

Amantadine and Rimantadine

Dizziness   Blurred vision   Dry mouth

Hallucinations   Orthostatic hypotension

 Clinical Pitfall

Avoid giving amantadine to anyone who has glaucoma, urinary retention, or a psychiatric disorder.

QSEN: Safety

Drug Alert!

Teaching Alert

Teach the patient and family to report to the prescriber immediately any worsening of depression or thoughts of suicide.

QSEN: Safety

 Drug Alert!

Teaching Alert

Teach older adults taking amantadine or rimantadine to watch for worsening of heart failure and to report weight gain, increased swelling of the feet or legs, or a change in pulse quality or rhythm to the prescriber.

QSEN: Safety

Ribavirin is used to treat *Hantavirus*, hepatitis A, hepatitis C, respiratory syncytial virus (RSV), and West Nile viruses, among other more rare viruses. It is most often used to treat RSV infection in children and chronic hepatitis C infection (in combination with interferon).

Common Side Effects

Ribavirin

| Nausea/ Vomiting; Diarrhea | Fever | Headache |

 Clinical Pitfall

Do not permit anyone who is pregnant or breastfeeding to administer ribavirin, handle it, care for a patient taking it, or enter the room of a patient receiving the aerosolized form.

QSEN: Safety

 Drug Alert!

Interaction Alert

Ribavirin should not be given to anyone who is also receiving didanosine.

QSEN: Safety

 Drug Alert!

Administration Alert

Administer ribavirin at least 1 hour before or 2 hours after an antacid.

QSEN: Safety

---

of its severe side effects and adverse effects, it is most commonly used for viral infections that do not respond to other antiviral agents.

Side Effects. Ribavirin has many side effects. The most common include nausea, vomiting, diarrhea, fever, and headache. Additional side effects include conjunctivitis, muscle pain, fatigue, dizziness, and injection site pain or irritation (parenteral form).

Adverse Effects. *Ribavirin is a potent drug with many adverse effects, and its use is limited to patients who have severe viral infections for which no other drugs are effective.* A major adverse effect is that ribavirin is a *teratogen,* an agent that can cause birth defects. It should not be given to pregnant or breastfeeding women. It should not be handled or inhaled by anyone who is pregnant.

This drug can suppress the bone marrow production of red blood cells (RBCs) and white blood cells (WBCs), especially when it is used along with interferon therapy. As a result, the patient can be anemic and at risk for infection.

With prolonged use, ribavirin can impair the function of the liver, kidneys, heart, and ears. In addition, it may lead to some forms of cancer.

What To Do *Before* Giving Ribavirin

In addition to the general responsibilities related to antiviral therapy (p. 139), before giving ribavirin check the patient's heart rate, rhythm, and pulse quality. Also check lung function by assessing the rate and depth of respiratory effort, breath sounds, pulse oximetry, color of skin and mucous membranes, and level of consciousness. Assess kidney function by checking the most recent 24-hour intake and output and comparing the amount of urine excreted with the amount of fluids consumed. Also check the patient's current kidney tests, especially the blood urea nitrogen (BUN) and serum creatinine levels. (See Table 1-4 in Chapter 1 for a listing of normal values.) If the values are higher than normal before starting the drug, the risk for kidney damage is greater. Assess liver function by checking for yellowing *(jaundice)* of the skin, palate, or whites of the eyes and by checking liver function tests. (See Table 1-3 in Chapter 1 for a listing of normal values.) Check the patient's hearing as described in Chapter 8. Use these data as a baseline to detect changes that may result from adverse drug effects.

Because ribavirin often suppresses the growth of bone marrow cells, check the patient's most recent WBC and RBC counts before drug therapy begins. Use these data as a baseline in determining the presence of side effects and whether or not the drug is effective against the infection. (See Table 1-5 in Chapter 1 for a listing of normal values for blood cells.)

Check the patient's vital signs (including temperature and mental status) before starting ribavirin. Use this information as a baseline to determine whether any side effect or adverse effect is present and whether the drug therapy is effective against the infection.

Ribavirin can interact with didanosine (Videx), a drug used in the treatment of human immune deficiency virus (HIV). When ribavirin is used with didanosine, severe liver problems and death from liver failure can result.

When administering aerosolized ribavirin, use only the SPAG-2 aerosol generator. Read the instruction manual before using this instrument. Prepare the aerosolized form of the drug using sterile technique and following the manufacturer's directions for preparation and dilution.

Antacids interfere with absorption of oral ribavirin. Administer the ribavirin at least 1 hour before or 2 hours after an antacid has been given.

What To Do *After* Giving Ribavirin

In addition to the general responsibilities related to antiviral therapy (p. 139), monitor the patient receiving ribavirin closely for any sign of side effects or organ toxicity. Check laboratory values daily for WBC and RBC counts, bilirubin level, liver enzyme levels, and BUN and creatinine levels. Compare urine output with fluid intake. Check hearing daily. Document all changes and notify the prescriber.

What To *Teach* Patients About Ribavirin

In addition to teaching patients about the general care needs and precautions related to antiviral therapy, instruct patients to take oral ribavirin for hepatitis C at least 1 hour before or 2 hours after taking an antacid because antacids interfere with ribavirin absorption. Instruct them to contact their prescriber as soon as possible if symptoms of allergy or other adverse effects develop.

Life Span Considerations with Ribavirin

Considerations for Pregnancy and Lactation. This drug has a high likelihood of increasing the risk for birth defects and fetal damage. It should never be given to a woman who is pregnant. If a woman of childbearing age who is sexually active is prescribed ribavirin, she must use two forms of contraception. Male patients taking this drug whose partners are pregnant should use condoms to prevent exposure of the pregnant women to the drug. Pregnant women living in the household of a person taking ribavirin should not touch the drug.

Considerations for Older Adults. Ribavirin should be administered cautiously to older adults. These patients are more likely to have age-related changes in major organs and are at greater risk for organ toxicities. The older adult may be started at a lower drug dosage. Older patients taking ribavirin have a much greater risk for anemia than younger patients. Aerosolized ribavirin is not indicated for older adults.

OSELTAMIVIR AND ZANAMIVIR

How Oseltamivir and Zanamivir Work

Oseltamivir and zanamivir work by inhibiting the enzyme neuraminidase, which is needed to spread viral particles in the respiratory tract. For effective treatment oseltamivir must be taken within 12 to 48 hours, and zanamivir must be taken within 12 to 36 hours of the onset of the first influenza symptoms. These drugs shorten the duration and reduce the severity of influenza. They can also prevent influenza from developing after exposure to the virus.

Side Effects. Oseltamivir is an oral drug taken as a liquid (suspension) or capsule. The most common side effects are nausea and vomiting, diarrhea, dizziness, and headache.

Zanamivir is an inhaled drug with side effects of nausea, cough, diarrhea, headache, and nasal congestion.

Adverse Effects. Specific adverse effects of oseltamivir are rare but include worsening hyperglycemia in people who have diabetes and also can elevate liver enzyme levels. Specific adverse effects of zanamivir are rare but include breathing problems, confusion, and seizures.

What To *Teach* Patients About Oseltamivir or Zanamivir

In addition to the general care needs and precautions related to antiviral therapy (p. 139), teach patients how to take these drugs properly. Teach patients prescribed oseltamivir suspension about the proper way to mix it and take it. This drug comes with its own mixing device and measuring device.

Teach patients taking zanamivir how to use an inhaler (see Box 21-1 in Chapter 21). For this drug, remind the patient *not* to use a spacer. If the patient takes other drugs by inhalation for another breathing problem such as asthma or chronic obstructive pulmonary disease, teach him or her to use the bronchodilator *before*

Drug Alert!

Teaching Alert

Teach patients taking ribavirin to report any of the following symptoms immediately to the prescriber: rash; itching or hives; swelling of the face, lips, or tongue; trouble breathing; chest pain; fever; bluish tinge to the lips or nail beds; tremors or seizures; persistent changes in heart rate or rhythm; decrease in urine output; and feeling unusually weak or tired.

QSEN: Safety

Drug Alert!

Action/Intervention Alert

Assess the older adult taking ribavirin for indications of anemia: low RBC count, low hemoglobin level, pallor or cyanosis, fatigue, increased heart and respiratory rate, and low blood pressure.

QSEN: Safety

Memory Jogger

Oseltamivir and zanamivir are effective for prevention and treatment of influenzas A and B, and swine influenza. Oseltamivir also is used at higher dosages to treat avian influenza H5N1.

Common Side Effects

Oseltamivir

Nausea/ Vomiting; Diarrhea   Dizziness   Headache

Common Side Effects

Zanamivir

  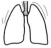

Nausea; Diarrhea   Headache   Cough

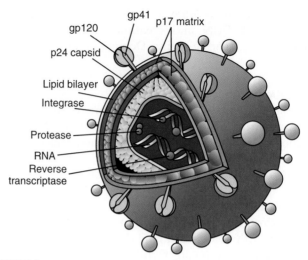

FIGURE 9-3 The components of the human immune deficiency retrovirus.

Drug Alert!

Teaching Alert

Teach patients who take other drugs by inhalation for another breathing problem to use the bronchodilator at least 5 minutes before using the zanamivir inhaler.

QSEN: Safety

Did You Know?

Everyone with AIDS has HIV infection but not everyone with HIV infection has AIDS.

Memory Jogger

The main cell type infected and destroyed by HIV infection is the CD4+ cell (helper/inducer T cell).

Memory Jogger

CD4+ T cells are the "generals" of the immune system army. When they are infected and destroyed, the person is immune deficient and cannot successfully fight off other infections.

using the zanamivir inhaler and to wait at least 5 minutes before using the zanamivir inhaler.

Teach patients and families that, if an adverse effect occurs, they should stop taking the drug and notify the prescriber as soon as possible.

RETROVIRAL INFECTION

REVIEW OF RELATED PHYSIOLOGY AND PATHOPHYSIOLOGY

A *retrovirus* is a special type of virus that always uses RNA as its genetic material and carries with it the enzymes reverse transcriptase, integrase, and protease, which allow high efficiency of cellular infection. This means that disease may result even when low levels of retroviruses enter the body. The **human immune deficiency virus (HIV)** is a retrovirus that attacks the immune system of an infected person, eventually causing him or her to have little or no immune protection. The most severe form of immune deficiency disease caused by HIV infection is known as *acquired immune deficiency syndrome (AIDS)*.

HIV has an outer layer with special "docking proteins," known as *gp41* and *gp120*, that help the virus enter cells with receptors for these proteins (Figure 9-3). Inside, the virus has its genetic material along with the enzymes reverse transcriptase and integrase. One of the cells that has receptors for the docking proteins is the *CD4+ cell, helper/inducer T cell*, or *T4 cell*. This cell directs immune system defenses and regulates the activity of all immune system cells. If HIV enters a CD4+ T cell, it can then create more virus particles.

After entering a host cell, HIV must get its genetic material into the DNA of the host cell. DNA is the genetic material of the human cell. The genetic material of HIV is RNA. To infect and take over a human cell, the genetic material must be the same. HIV carries the enzyme *reverse transcriptase* to convert HIV RNA into DNA. Then the enzyme *integrase* inserts this DNA into the human DNA of the CD4+ T cell.

HIV particles are made in the infected CD4+ T cell using the machinery of the host cell. The new virus particle is made in the form of one long protein strand. The strand is clipped with chemical scissors, an enzyme called *HIV protease*, into several small pieces. These pieces are formed into a new finished viral particle, which then leaves the infected cell to infect other CD4+ T cells (Figure 9-4).

With time the number of HIV particles overwhelms the immune system, and the patient is at risk for bacterial, fungal, and viral infections and some cancers. *Opportunistic infections* are caused by organisms that are present as part of the normal

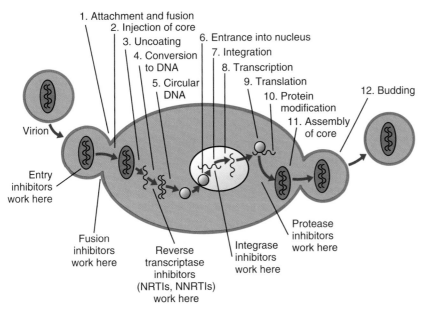

FIGURE 9-4 Sites in the life cycle of the human immune deficiency virus (HIV) in which different antiretroviral drugs work. *NRTI*, Nucleoside analog reverse transcriptase inhibitor; *NNRTI*, Non-nucleoside analog reverse transcriptase inhibitor.

environment and kept in check by normal immune function. In a person with AIDS the immune system is extremely suppressed. T-cell count falls, viral load rises, and without treatment the patient dies relatively quickly of opportunistic infections or cancer.

GENERAL ISSUES IN ANTIRETROVIRAL THERAPY

Antiretroviral drugs are a broad category of antiviral drugs that suppress the replication (reproduction) of retroviruses, which use RNA as their primary genetic material instead of DNA. The six classes of antiretroviral drugs are nucleoside analog reverse transcriptase inhibitors (NRTIs), non-nucleoside analog reverse transcriptase inhibitors (NNRTIs), protease inhibitors (PIs), integrase inhibitors, fusion inhibitors, and entry inhibitors.

A patient with HIV infection receives drugs from several classes in regimens called *cocktails* because HIV is not controlled by any one antiretroviral drug alone. This approach is termed *highly active antiretroviral therapy (HAART)*. Antiretroviral drugs are virustatic and do not kill the virus. Different types of HAART drugs are available as combination tablets containing two or three drugs to reduce the number of individual drugs that a patient may have to take.

An important issue with HAART is the development of drug-resistant mutations in the HIV organism. When resistance develops, viral replication is no longer suppressed by the drugs. Several factors contribute to the development of drug resistance to HAART, with the most important being missed drug doses. When doses are missed, the blood concentrations become lower than that needed to inhibit viral replication, allowing the virus to replicate and produce new viruses that are resistant to the drugs being used.

Any antiretroviral drug can cause an allergic reaction. It may be minor, with a rash appearing days after starting the drug, or can result in anaphylaxis. (See p. 139 for a discussion of anaphylaxis.)

Two common adverse effects of the antiretrovirals are liver toxicity and worsening hyperglycemia.

Most antiretroviral drugs interact with other drugs and food. These interactions can cause serious adverse effects and can change the activity of drugs.

 Memory Jogger

The six classes of antiretroviral drugs are:
- Nucleoside analog reverse transcriptase inhibitors (NRTIs)
- Non-nucleoside analog reverse transcriptase inhibitors (NNRTIs)
- Protease inhibitors (PIs)
- Integrase inhibitors
- Fusion inhibitors
- Entry inhibitors

 Clinical Pitfall

Do not delay, skip, or reduce HAART doses.

QSEN: Safety

Drug Alert!

Interaction Alert

Before giving antiretroviral drugs, ask the patient about all other drugs or supplements that he or she takes and then check with the pharmacist to avoid a possible drug interaction.

QSEN: Safety

 Cultural Awareness

Check for jaundice in patients with darker skin on the whites of the eyes closest to the iris and on the roof of the mouth. Do not use the soles of the feet or the palms of the hands.

 Drug Alert!

Teaching Alert

Teach patients on HAART for HIV infection the importance of taking their drugs exactly as prescribed to maintain the effectiveness of the drugs.

QSEN: Safety

Intended responses with antiretroviral therapy focus on the results of suppression of viral reproduction. These responses include:

- **Viral load** (the number of viral particles in a blood sample, which indicates the degree of viral infection) is reduced.
- Immune function is improved, as evidenced by higher CD4+ cell count; higher CD4+ to CD8+ ratio.
- The patient has fewer episodes of opportunistic infections.

Before giving an antiretroviral drug, obtain a list of all other drugs that the patient takes because antiretrovirals interact with many other drugs. Check with the pharmacist for possible interactions and the need to consult the prescriber about dosage or changing the patient's other drugs.

Ask the patient about previous allergic reactions to drugs. If a drug allergy has occurred, determine which drug or drugs caused it, the specific reactions the patient had, and how the problem was treated. Notify the prescriber of previous allergic reactions to drugs and make sure that this information is documented in the patient's chart.

Because antiretroviral therapy can lead to liver toxicity, make sure that the patient does not have a liver problem before starting these drugs. Check the patient's most recent laboratory values for liver problems (elevated liver enzyme levels). (See Table 1-3 in Chapter 1 for a listing of normal values.)

If the patient has diabetes, check his or her blood glucose level before administering an antiretroviral drug. Use this value as a baseline to monitor whether the drug is affecting the patient's blood glucose level.

Some antiretroviral drugs must be taken with food; others must be taken on an empty stomach. Check a drug reference to determine how an individual drug should be given with regard to meals.

After giving an antiretroviral drug, check the patient daily for yellowing of the skin or sclera *(jaundice),* which is a symptom of liver problems. The best places to check are the whites of the eyes closest to the iris, the roof of the mouth, and the skin of the chest. Avoid checking the soles of the feet or palms of the hands, especially in a patient with darker skin, because these areas often appear yellow even when the patient is not jaundiced.

If the patient has diabetes, check blood glucose levels more often, and assess fasting blood glucose levels whenever they are ordered. Report higher-than-normal levels to the prescriber because adjustments may be needed in the dosages of antidiabetic drugs.

Check the patient's skin every shift for rash, blisters, or other skin eruptions that may indicate a reaction to the drug. Ask the patient about any itching or skin changes.

Teach patients receiving antiretroviral therapy the importance of taking their drugs exactly as prescribed to maintain the effectiveness of HAART drugs. Even a few missed doses per month can promote drug resistance.

Remind patients that antiretroviral drugs do not kill the virus or cure the disease. These drugs only help reduce the number of viruses in the body; the person will still have HIV disease.

Teach patients to follow the manufacturer's directions for whether a specific drug should be taken with food or on an empty stomach.

Warn patients taking antiretrovirals to tell all health care providers that they are taking these drugs because of the potential for drug interactions. Teach patients not to take any over-the-counter drug or herbal supplement without consulting the antiretroviral prescriber.

Tell patients to notify the prescriber if they develop yellowing of the skin or eyes, darkening of the urine, or lightening of the stools. These problems are signs of liver toxicity, a serious adverse effect of these drugs.

Pediatric considerations include that most antiretroviral drugs and HAART therapy are used for control of the disease in HIV positive children. Two exceptions are maraviroc and raltegravir. The safety and efficacy of these drugs have not yet been established for children.

Considerations for pregnancy and lactation include that most antiretroviral drugs for HAART are recommended to be taken by HIV-positive pregnant women because the virus can cross the placenta and infect the fetus. When these drugs are taken as prescribed, they can reduce the chances of fetal infection. The woman who is HIV-positive should not breastfeed because the virus can be transferred from the mother to the infant in breast milk.

TYPES OF ANTIRETROVIRAL DRUGS

NUCLEOSIDE ANALOG REVERSE TRANSCRIPTASE INHIBITORS

How NRTIs Work
Nucleoside analog reverse transcriptase inhibitors (NRTIs) are drugs that are similar in structure to bases that form DNA. These drugs compete with real bases in HIV-infected cells and reduce viral replication. (See Figure 9-4 for where these drugs work to disrupt HIV reproduction.)

Dosages for Common NRTIs

Drug	Dosage
abacavir (Ziagen)	*Adults:* 300 mg orally twice daily or 600 mg orally once daily *Children:* 8 mg/kg orally twice daily
didanosine (ddI, Videx)	*Adults/Children over 60 kg:* 125-200 mg orally twice daily
didanosine (Videx EC)	*Adults/Children over 60 kg:* 400 mg orally once daily
emtricitabine (Emtriva)	*Adults:* 200 mg tablet or 240 mg solution orally daily *Children:* 6 mg/kg, up to 240 mg (24 mL) orally daily
lamivudine (Epivir, Epivir-HPV, 3TC)	*Adults:* 300 mg orally daily *Children:* 4 mg/kg orally every 12 hr (maximum of 150 mg)
stavudine (d4T, Zerit)	*Adults:* 40 mg orally twice daily *Children less than 60 kg:* 0.5-1 mg/kg orally every 12 hr
tenofovir (Viread)	*Adults:* 300 mg orally daily *Children:* Safe dosages have not been established
zidovudine (Apo-Zidovudine , Azidothymidine, AZT, Novo-AZT , Retrovir)	*Adults/Children over 30 kg:* 300 mg orally twice daily *Children less than 30 kg:* 9 mg/kg orally twice daily

Side Effects. Common side effects of NRTIs are nausea, headache, and increased digestive upsets when eating fatty or fried foods. Each NRTI may have more side effects. Be sure to consult a drug reference for side effects of each specific drug.

Adverse Effects. The two most common adverse effects of NRTIs are liver toxicity and peripheral neuropathy with long-term use.

Abacavir is more likely to cause hypersensitivity reactions within the first 4 weeks. This response starts with flulike symptoms and progresses to life-threatening hypersensitivity.

What To *Teach* Patients About NRTIs
In addition to teaching patients about the general care needs and precautions related to antiretroviral therapy (pp. 148-149), instruct them to avoid fatty foods and fried foods. These foods can cause digestive upsets and lead to pancreatitis when combined with NRTIs.

After long-term use patients often develop peripheral neuropathy with reduced sensation. Teach patients who have reduced sensation to prevent injury. Loss of sensation increases the patient's risk for injury because he or she may not be aware of excessive heat, cold, or pressure.

! Drug Alert!

Teaching Alert

Teach women who are HIV-positive to take prescribed antiretroviral drugs during pregnancy to prevent HIV infection in their infants.

QSEN: Safety

Do Not Confuse

lamivudine *with* lamotrigine

An order for lamivudine can be confused with lamotrigine. Lamivudine is an antiretroviral drug, whereas lamotrigine is a drug used to control seizures.

QSEN: Safety

Do Not Confuse

Retrovir *with* ritonavir

An order for Retrovir can be confused with ritonavir. Retrovir is an antiretroviral drug from the NRTI class, whereas ritonavir is an antiretroviral drug from the protease inhibitor class.

QSEN: Safety

Common Side Effects

NRTIs

Nausea, Intolerance   Headache
to fatty foods

Drug Alert!

Teaching Alert

Warn patients taking abacavir to stop the drug if flulike symptoms develop, to report the response to the prescriber, and to never restart taking the drug.

QSEN: Safety

Teach patients taking abacavir to stop the drug and notify the prescriber if flulike symptoms occur. Warn them that, if this response occurs, to never take the drug again.

Life Span Considerations for NRTIs

Considerations for Pregnancy and Lactation. NRTIs increase the risk for lactic acidosis in pregnant women. Signs and symptoms of lactic acidosis are muscle aches; tiredness and difficulty remaining awake; abdominal pain; hypotension; and a slow, irregular heartbeat.

Considerations for Older Adults. Peripheral neuropathy develops more quickly in the older adult taking NRTIs. This greatly increases the risk for falls and other injuries.

NON-NUCLEOSIDE ANALOG REVERSE TRANSCRIPTASE INHIBITORS

How NNRTIs Work

Non-nucleoside analog reverse transcriptase inhibitors (NNRTIs) are a class of antiretroviral drugs that inhibit the action of the enzyme reverse transcriptase by binding directly to the enzyme, preventing it from converting viral RNA to DNA. As a result, viral reproduction is suppressed. Figure 9-4 shows where these drugs work to disrupt HIV reproduction.

 Do Not Confuse

Viramune *with* Viracept

An order for Viramune can be confused with Viracept. Viramune is an antiretroviral drug from the NNRTI class, whereas Viracept is an antiretroviral drug from the protease inhibitor class.

QSEN: Safety

 Memory Jogger

The generic names for the common NNRTIs usually have "vir" in the middle of the name (for example, efavirenz).

Dosages for Common NNRTIs

Drug	Dosage
delavirdine (Rescriptor)	*Adults:* 400 mg orally three times daily *Children:* Safety and efficacy have not been established
efavirenz (Sustiva)	*Adults/Children over 40 kg:* 600 mg orally once daily *Children 10 to 39 kg:* 200-300 mg orally once daily at bedtime
etravirine (INTELENCE)	*Adults:* 200 mg orally twice daily *Children:* Safety and efficacy have not been established
nevirapine (Viramune)	*Adults:* 200 mg orally daily for first 14 days, then 200 mg orally twice daily *Children:* Dosages for young children based on total body surface area
rilpivirine (EDURANT)	*Adults:* 25 mg orally once daily *Children:* Safety and efficacy have not been established

Common Side Effects

NNRTIs

Rash   Nausea/
Vomiting,
Abdominal
pain   Headache

Side Effects. Common side effects of NNRTIs are rash, nausea and vomiting, headache, and abdominal pain. Additional side effects with these drugs are difficulty sleeping and vivid dreams or nightmares. Be sure to consult a drug reference for side effects associated with each specific drug.

Adverse Effects. The two most common adverse effects with NNRTIs are anemia and liver toxicity.

What To *Teach* Patients About NNRTIs

In addition to teaching patients about the general care needs and precautions related to antiretroviral therapy (pp. 148-149), tell them to notify their prescriber if they develop a sore throat, fever, different types of rashes, blisters, or multiple bruises. These problems are signs of serious adverse effects of drugs from this class.

Teach patients to take the drug at least 1 hour before or 2 hours after taking an antacid. Antacids inhibit the absorption of drugs in the NNRTI class.

Remind patients to keep all appointments for blood tests because NNRTIs can cause anemia.

 Drug Alert!

Teaching Alert

Teach patients taking NNRTIs to avoid St. John's wort because it reduces the effectiveness of these drugs.

QSEN: Safety

Life Span Considerations for NNRTIs

Considerations for Pregnancy and Lactation. Etravirine and nevirapine have a low likelihood of increasing the risk for birth defects or fetal damage and may be taken at any stage of pregnancy. Neither delavirdine nor efavirenz should be taken during pregnancy.

Considerations for Older Adults. Older adults are more likely to be taking other drugs that could interact with an NNRTI. Remind the patient to tell all health care providers about all drugs he or she takes. Also teach older adults how to take their pulse and assess it for irregularities. Remind the patient to report new irregularities to the prescriber.

PROTEASE INHIBITORS

How Protease Inhibitors Work

Protease inhibitors (PIs) are a class of antiretroviral drugs that prevent HIV replication and prevent the release of HIV particles from infected cells. HIV produces its proteins, including those needed to move viral particles out of the host cell, in one long strand. For the proteins to be active, this large protein must be broken down into separate smaller proteins through the action of the viral enzyme HIV protease. When PIs are taken into an HIV-infected cell, they make the protease enzyme work on the drug rather than on the initial large protein. Thus active proteins are not produced, and viral particles cannot leave the cell to infect other cells. (See Figure 9-4 for where these drugs work to disrupt HIV reproduction.)

Dosages for Common Protease Inhibitors

Drug	Dosage
atazanavir (Reyataz)	*Adults:* 300 mg orally daily *Children:* 7 mg/kg orally daily
darunavir (Prezista)	*Adults:* 800 mg orally twice daily *Children over 40 kg:* 600 mg orally every 12 hr *Children under 40 kg:* 450 mg orally every 12 hr
fosamprenavir (Lexiva)	*Adults:* 700 mg orally twice daily *Children:* 18 mg/kg orally twice daily
indinavir (Crixivan)	*Adults:* 800 mg orally every 8 hr *Children:* 500 mg/m^2 orally every 8 hr
lopinavir/ritonavir (Kaletra)	*Adults:* 400 mg/100 mg orally twice daily *Children:* 300 mg/75 mg per m^2 dose orally twice daily
nelfinavir (Viracept)	*Adults/Children older than 12 years:* 1250 mg orally every 12 hr or 750 mg orally every 8 hr
saquinavir (Invirase)	*Adults/Children older than 16 years:* 1000 mg orally every 12 hr *Children younger than 16 years:* 33 mg/kg orally every 8 hr
tipranavir (Aptivus)	*Adults:* 500 mg (given with ritonavir) orally twice daily *Children:* 14 mg/kg (given with ritonavir) orally twice daily

Side Effects. Common side effects of PIs are headache, diarrhea, depression, difficulty sleeping, and abdominal weight gain. Each drug may have more side effects. Be sure to consult a drug reference for side effects of each specific drug.

Adverse Effects. The most common adverse effect of PIs is liver toxicity. They also increase lipid levels, leading to hyperlipidemia, atherosclerosis, and pancreatitis.

PIs should be used cautiously in anyone who has hemophilia. They can induce uncontrolled bleeding in these patients.

Atazanavir and ritonavir can impair electrical conduction in the heart and lead to heart block, especially in a person who has an abnormally slow heart rate.

 Do Not Confuse

Viracept *with* Viramune

An order for Viracept can be confused with Viramune. Viracept is an antiretroviral drug from the PI class, whereas Viramune is an antiretroviral drug from the NNRTI class.

QSEN: Safety

 Do Not Confuse

ritonavir *with* Retrovir

An order for ritonavir can be confused with Retrovir. Ritonavir is an antiretroviral drug from the PI class, whereas Retrovir is an antiretroviral drug from the NRTI class.

QSEN: Safety

 Do Not Confuse

saquinavir *with* Sinequan

An order for saquinavir can be confused with Sinequan. Saquinavir is an antiretroviral drug from the PI class, whereas Sinequan is a drug used to treat depression and anxiety.

QSEN: Safety

 Memory Jogger

The generic names for the common PIs usually have "-navir" at the end of the name (for example, indinavir).

Common Side Effects

Protease Inhibitors

Headache | Diarrhea; Abdominal weight gain | Insomnia

Depression

 Drug Alert!

Interaction Alert

Reyataz, Prezista, Lexiva, and Invirase must be given with ritonavir, which causes a drug-drug interaction that results in higher blood levels and effectiveness.

QSEN: Safety

Darunavir and fosamprenavir both contain sulfa and should not be used for patients who have allergies to sulfa drugs.

What To *Teach* Patients About Protease Inhibitors

In addition to teaching patients about the general care needs and precautions related to antiretroviral therapy, warn them not to crush or chew capsules because these actions may cause the drug to be absorbed too rapidly and increase the risk for side effects.

Teach patients taking atazanavir or ritonavir to check their pulse for a full minute at least twice daily. They should report any changes in heart rate or regularity to the prescriber.

An herbal supplement that greatly reduces the effectiveness of PIs is St. John's wort. Warn patients to not take St. John's wort while on HIV therapy that includes any of the PIs.

Life Span Considerations for Protease Inhibitors

Considerations for Older Adults. Older adults are more likely to be taking other drugs that could interact with PIs, especially cardiac drugs and lipid-lowering drugs. Remind the patient to tell all health care providers about all drugs that he or she takes. Teach older adults how to check their pulse for irregularities. Remind them to report new irregularities to the prescriber.

INTEGRASE INHIBITORS

Integrase inhibitors are usually prescribed for people who have HIV disease, are already taking HAART, and are beginning to have increased viral load. The safety and effectiveness of these drugs in small children have not yet been established.

Dosages for Integrase Inhibitors

Drug	Dosage
dolutegravir (TIVICAY)	*Adults:* 100 mg orally daily *Children over 40 kg:* 50 mg orally daily *Children less than 40 kg:* Safety and efficacy have not been established
elvitegravir (EVG)	*Adults:* 85-150 mg orally once daily *Children:* Safety and efficacy have not been established
raltegravir (Isentress)	*Adults and children over 25 kg:* 400 mg orally twice daily *Children under 25 kg:* Safety and efficacy have not been established

How Integrase Inhibitors Work

Integrase inhibitors are a type of antiretroviral drug that prevents HIV infection by inhibiting the enzyme integrase, which is needed to allow insertion of viral DNA into the DNA of the human host cell. Without this action, viral proteins are not made, and viral replication is inhibited. (See Figure 9-4 for where these drugs work to disrupt HIV reproduction.)

Side Effects. The most common side effects of integrase inhibitors are diarrhea, rash, and insomnia. Other side effects may include dizziness, headache, nausea and vomiting, and abdominal pain.

Adverse Effects. Adverse effects of raltegravir include anemia, hyperglycemia, and muscle pain and weakness *(rhabdomyolysis)*. Although rare, muscle problems occur more often among patients who also take other drugs that can cause rhabdomyolysis (for example, the "statin" types of lipid-lowering drug).

Adverse effects of dolutegravir include elevated liver enzymes and hyperglycemia.

⚠ Drug Alert!

Teaching Alert

Teach patients taking PIs to avoid taking St. John's wort.

QSEN: Safety

Common Side Effects

Integrase Inhibitors

Diarrhea, Nausea/ Vomiting, Abdominal pain   Dizziness   Headache

⚠ Drug Alert!

Interaction Alert

When raltegravir is taken with any of the "statin" type of lipid-lowering drugs, muscle problems are more likely to occur. If patients are taking both types of drugs, assess them more frequently for muscle aches and weakness.

QSEN: Safety

What To *Teach* Patients About Integrase Inhibitors

In addition to teaching patients about the general care needs and precautions related to antiretroviral therapy (pp. 148-149), tell them not to crush or chew raltegravir tablets and to take the drug with food to reduce GI side effects. Dolutegravir can be taken with or without food.

Teach patients to report any persistent muscle pain or weakness to the prescriber as soon as possible. Tell patients to report increased fatigue, paleness, and increased heart rate or shortness of breath to the prescriber. These are symptoms of anemia.

Teach patients with diabetes to monitor blood glucose levels more closely. Adjustments in diet and diabetes drug therapy may be needed.

Life Span Considerations for Raltegravir

Pediatric Considerations. Integrase inhibitors are not approved for use in small children.

Considerations for Pregnancy and Lactation. Raltegravir has a moderate likelihood of increasing the risk for birth defects or fetal damage. It should not be used during pregnancy if the patient's viral load indicates that her traditional HAART therapy is effective. Dolutegravir has a low likelihood of increasing the risk for birth defects or fetal damage and can be part of HAART therapy during pregnancy.

Considerations for Older Adults. Older adults are more likely to be taking a "statin" type of lipid-lowering drug, which increases the risk for muscle weakness. Older adults may have loss of muscle mass and strength as a result of the aging process. These conditions increase the risk for falls.

FUSION INHIBITORS

The only drug in this category is enfuvirtide (Fuzeon). The usual dosage is 90 mg subcutaneously twice daily. It is used with other drugs as part of a HAART regimen.

How Fusion Inhibitors Work

Fusion inhibitors are a class of antiretroviral drug that prevents infection by blocking the viral docking protein (gp41) from fusing with the host cell. Without fusion, infection of new cells does not occur. (See Figure 9-4 for where these drugs work to disrupt HIV reproduction.)

Side Effects. The most common side effect of enfuvirtide is an injection site reaction (itching, warmth, swelling, bump formation, skin hardening). Other common side effects are constipation, trouble sleeping, depression, and muscle aches.

Adverse Effects. Adverse effects are peripheral neuropathy with pain and numbness of the hands and feet (most common), increased respiratory infections (including pneumonia), and liver toxicity.

What To *Teach* Patients About Enfuvirtide

In addition to teaching patients about the general care needs and precautions related to antiretroviral therapy, instruct them how to safely self-inject the drug. A 1-month supply of the drug is available in a kit that contains single-use vials, vials of sterile water for injection, preparation syringes, administration syringes, alcohol wipes, and instruction guides. Teach the patient how to prepare the drug correctly, draw it up, inject it, dispose of the needle, and store it following the instruction guide.

Teach patients the manifestations of respiratory infection (cough, shortness of breath, fever, mucus production or a change in the color of mucus from clear to yellow, green, or brown). Instruct them to report these symptoms immediately to the prescriber.

Teach patients to store unmixed vials of drug and water at room temperature, between 59° F and 86° F and to store the mixed drug and water vial in a refrigerator

Common Side Effects

Enfuvirtide

Injection site reaction Constipation Insomnia

Muscle aches Depression

Drug Alert!

Teaching Alert

Teach patients how to prepare, administer, and store enfuvirtide.

QSEN: Safety

between 36° F and 46° F for up to 24 hours. Unused mixed drug should be discarded after 24 hours.

Teach patients to assess injection sites daily for signs of infection or reactions. Remind them that if an injection site reaction occurs, they should not use that site again until it heals and the skin is normal. Instruct patients to report an injection site infection to the prescriber and to not reuse that site until the infection has completely cleared and the skin has healed.

Like the NRTIs, after long-term use of enfuvirtide, patients often develop peripheral neuropathy with reduced sensation.

Life Span Considerations for Enfuvirtide
Considerations for Older Adults. Some older adults have vision or mobility problems that make self-administration of enfuvirtide more difficult. Assess the older patient's ability to prepare the drug, draw up the correct dosage, and reach an appropriate injection site. Include a family member or other responsible person when teaching about drug preparation and administration.

ENTRY INHIBITORS
The major drug in this category is maraviroc (Selzentry). The usual dosage range for an adult is 150 to 600 mg orally twice daily.

How Entry Inhibitors Work
Entry inhibitors are a class of antiretroviral drug that prevent HIV cellular infection by blocking the CCR5 receptor on CD4+ T cells. (See Figure 9-4 for where these drugs work to disrupt HIV reproduction.) Because this drug is not effective against all HIV subtypes, the patient must first be tested to ensure that his or her HIV infection is likely to respond to this therapy.

Side Effects. Common side effects of maraviroc include muscle aches and pains, cough, diarrhea, dizziness, and trouble sleeping. Other less common side effects include rhinitis, sinusitis, depression, and numbness or tingling of the hands and feet.

Adverse Effects. The most common adverse effects of maraviroc are hypotension and liver toxicity.

What To *Teach* Patients About Maraviroc
In addition to teaching patients about the general care needs and precautions related to antiretroviral therapy, warn them not to crush or chew capsules because these actions may cause the drug to be absorbed too rapidly and increase the risk for side effects.

Teach patients about safety and low blood pressure and to change positions slowly. When they are getting out of bed, teach them to sit on the side of the bed for a few minutes and then slowly move to a standing position. If they become dizzy, they should sit back down again for a few more minutes. Tell them to use handrails when going up or down steps and to avoid driving or operating heavy equipment while dizzy.

Life Span Considerations for Maraviroc
Pediatric Considerations. Maraviroc is not approved for use in children.

Considerations for Older Adults. Older adults are more likely to develop orthostatic hypotension with maraviroc and increase the risk for falls. Stress the need to change positions slowly and use handrails when going up or down steps. Also warn older adults to not drive or operate heavy equipment until they know how maraviroc affects them.

Common Side Effects

Maraviroc

Muscle aches, Pains   Diarrhea   Dizziness

Insomnia   Cough

DRUG FOR PREEXPOSURE PROPHYLAXIS

New research for prevention of sexual transmission has resulted in the use of drug therapy for *preexposure prophylaxis* (Pr-EP). The use of the combination drug Truvada (emtricitabine and tenofovir), which contains two NRTIs, by HIV-1 negative sexual partners of known HIV-1 positive individuals appears to reduce HIV transmission. Together these two drugs have a synergistic suppressive effect on HIV activity. See the information on pp. 149-150 for a discussion of NRTIs.

Preexposure prophylaxis does not replace the standard safer sex practices recommended to prevent HIV transmission. Also, if this type of drug therapy is used in patients who become infected with HIV-1, the risk for developing drug resistance greatly increases. Therefore, remind people prescribed Truvada to use the traditional safer sex practices and to adhere to an every-3-month HIV testing schedule along with monitoring for side effects of this drug.

Get Ready for Practice!

Key Points

- Viruses are tiny intracellular parasites that are not capable of self-reproduction and must infect a living cell to reproduce.
- Most common viruses have a relatively low efficiency of cellular infection and must invade the body in large numbers to cause disease.
- A retrovirus, specifically HIV, is virulent with a high efficiency of infection.
- Antiviral and antiretroviral drugs do not kill viruses; they only suppress viral reproduction and growth. They are virustatic rather than virucidal.
- Teach patients taking antiviral or antiretroviral drugs to take them exactly as prescribed and for as long as prescribed and to not stop therapy just because they feel better.
- Women should not breastfeed while taking an antiviral or antiretroviral drug.
- Ribavirin is highly teratogenic, which means that it can cause birth defects. Do not allow a pregnant or breastfeeding woman to touch ribavirin or care for a patient taking it.
- Antiretroviral therapy is most effective when given in multiple combinations of drugs known as highly active antiretroviral therapy (HAART).
- Most antiretroviral drugs have interactions with other drugs and herbals.
- HAART drugs can cause hyperglycemia and make diabetes worse.
- Some PIs are to be taken with food, and others must be taken on an empty stomach.
- Maraviroc and raltegravir are not approved for use in children.
- Maraviroc can cause severe orthostatic hypotension and increase the risk for falls.

Additional Learning Resources

evolve Be sure to visit your Evolve website (http:// evolve.elsevier.com/Workman/pharmacology/) for additional online resources.

SG Go to your Study Guide for additional learning activities to help you master this chapter content.

Review Questions

See the Answer Keys—In-text Review Questions for answers to these questions.

Test Yourself on the Basics

1. Which result is an expected outcome of antiviral therapy?
   A. The patient develops immunity against reinfection with the same virus.
   B. The patient's natural immunity is "boosted" as a result of drug therapy.
   C. Viruses are killed upon interacting with the drug.
   D. Viral replication is suppressed.
2. For what viral infection is ribavirin most commonly used?
   A. Hepatitis B (HVB)
   B. Herpes simplex type 2 (HSV2)
   C. Respiratory syncytial virus (RSV)
   D. Late stage human immunodeficiency virus (HIV)
3. Which food, drug, or beverage should patients be taught to avoid while taking adefovir dipivoxil (Hepsera)?
   A. Acetaminophen
   B. Aspirin
   C. Caffeine
   D. Smoked meats and aged cheese
4. What is the most common side effect of drugs from the protease inhibitor class?
   A. Increased risk for leukemia
   B. Uncontrolled bleeding
   C. Injection site pain
   D. Liver toxicity
5. Which antiretroviral drug belongs to the integrase inhibitor class?
   A. darunavir (Prezista)
   B. delavirdine (Rescriptor)
   C. didanosine (Videx)
   D. dolutegravir (TIVICAY)

6. Which antiretroviral drugs are not approved for use in children? Select all that apply.
   A. atazanavir (Reyataz)
   B. efavirenz (Sustiva)
   C. emtricitabine (Emtriva)
   D. maraviroc (Selzentry)
   E. raltegravir (Isentress)
   F. rilpivirine (EDURANT)
   G. tenofovir (Viread)
   H. tipranavir (Aptivus)

Test Yourself on Advanced Concepts

7. Acyclovir (Zovirax) is prescribed for a patient who takes phenytoin (Dilantin) for seizure control. How should drug therapy for this patient be altered?
   A. The phenytoin should be stopped because it inactivates acyclovir.
   B. The phenytoin dose should be increased because acyclovir reduces its effectiveness.
   C. The acyclovir dose should be increased because phenytoin enhances the excretion of acyclovir.
   D. The oral dose of acyclovir should be separated from the oral dose of phenytoin by at least 6 hours.

8. Which health care professional should avoid caring for a patient receiving ribavirin by aerosol inhalation?
   A. A 25-year-old who is HIV positive
   B. A 29-year-old who is 2 months pregnant
   C. A 50-year-old who has herpes simplex type 2
   D. A 62-year-old receiving radiation therapy for breast cancer

9. Why does rimantadine (Flumadine) have fewer nervous system side effects than amantadine (Symmetrel)?
   A. Amantadine has a half-life that is twice as long as rimantadine.
   B. Amantadine is more effective at suppressing viral replication than rimantadine.
   C. Rimantadine is administered orally and amantadine is administered intravenously.
   D. Rimantadine concentrates more in the respiratory system and less in the brain than amantadine.

10. Which precaution is most important to teach a patient prescribed to take zanamivir (Relenza)?
    A. Avoid using a spacer.
    B. Take the drug with food or milk.
    C. Drink a full glass of water with each dose.
    D. Report any pain or redness at the injection site to the prescriber.

11. A patient who is prescribed highly active antiretroviral therapy (HAART) is flying to a wedding and will be gone 1 day. He asks if he can skip his drugs that day so that he doesn't have to show them all at the airport. What is your best response?
    A. "Yes, just 1 day off your drugs will not make any difference."
    B. "Yes, as long as you avoid direct contact with anyone who is ill."
    C. "No, even 1 day off the drugs can help the virus become drug resistant."
    D. "No, even 1 day off the drugs increases the chances that you can spread the disease."

12. Which statement made by a patient prescribed to take lamivudine (Epivir) orally daily indicates correct understanding of therapy with this drug?
    A. "I will avoid fatty foods and fried foods."
    B. "I will report flulike symptoms to the prescriber immediately."
    C. "I will avoid drinking any beverages that contain caffeine."
    D. "I will stop this drug immediately if I become pregnant."

13. A patient is prescribed to take nelfinavir (Viracept) 750 mg orally every 8 hours. How many total milligrams of the drug should this patient have in a 24-hour period? _____ mg

14. A woman is prescribed to receive 8 mg/kg of the drug acyclovir (Zovirax) intravenously. She weighs 164 lb. What is her weight in kg? _____ kg How many milligrams of the drug should she receive for an accurate dose? _____ mg

Critical Thinking Activities

See the Answer Keys—Critical Thinking Activities for answers to these activities.

The patient is a 38-year-old woman who has hepatitis B infection, probably as a result of her injection drug use when she was in her 20s. She has been drug-free for 10 years. She is now prescribed to take the antiviral drug adefovir dipivoxil (Hepsera) 10 mg orally daily. She asks how long she will have to take this drug to cure the hepatitis.

1. How does this drug work?
2. How will you answer her question about length of time she needs to take the drug?
3. What signs and symptoms for side effects and adverse effects will you teach her to report to the prescriber?
4. What specific precautions should you teach her about this drug?

Anti-Infectives: Antitubercular and Antifungal Drugs

http://evolve.elsevier.com/Workman/pharmacology/

Objectives

After studying this chapter you should be able to:

1. List the names, actions, usual adult dosages, possible side effects, and adverse effects of the four first-line drugs used to treat tuberculosis.
2. Describe what to do before and after giving antituberculosis drugs.
3. Explain what to teach patients taking antituberculosis drugs, including what to do, what not to do, and when to call the prescriber.
4. List the names, actions, usual adult dosages, possible side effects, and adverse effects of antifungal drugs.

5. Describe what to do before and after giving antifungal drugs.
6. Explain what to teach patients taking antifungal drugs, including what to do, what not to do, and when to call the prescriber.
7. Describe life span considerations for antituberculosis drugs and antifungal drugs.

Key Terms

fungicidal (fŭn-jĭ-Sī-dŭl) (p. 163) Having the ability to kill a fungus.

fungistatic (fŭn-jĭ-STĂT-ĭk) (p. 163) Having the ability to suppress fungal reproduction and growth.

fungus (FŬN-gĭs) (p. 162) A simple organism with one or more cells (such as yeasts, molds, and mushrooms) that

reproduces by spores, has walled cells, and can live peacefully with humans or infect humans and cause disease.

tuberculosis (TB) (tū-bŭr-kyū-LŌ-sĭs) (p. 157) A highly communicable disease caused by *Mycobacterium tuberculosis*.

TUBERCULOSIS

REVIEW OF RELATED PHYSIOLOGY AND PATHOPHYSIOLOGY

The most common bacterial infection worldwide is **tuberculosis (TB)**, a highly communicable disease caused by *Mycobacterium tuberculosis*. TB spreads by *aerosol transmission*, which transfers bacteria-filled droplets through the air when a person with active TB coughs, laughs, sneezes, whistles, or sings. These droplets may then be inhaled by others (Figure 10-1). Far more people are infected with the bacteria and overcome the infection than actually develop active TB.

Once inhaled, the bacteria multiply freely when they reach a susceptible site in the lungs (bronchi or alveoli) and form a primary TB lesion, which is a small, inflamed pocket of bacteria, white blood cells (WBCs), and exudate. The lesion is surrounded by more WBCs that cause a response known as *pneumonitis*. During this time many people who have an intact immune system develop immunity to the TB organism, and further growth of bacteria is controlled by confining it to the primary lesions (see Figure 10-1). These lesions usually resolve, leaving little or no residual bacteria, and may show on chest x-ray as a scar.

Only a small percentage of people initially infected with the bacteria ever develop active TB. Immune responses develop 2 to 10 weeks after the first infection with a TB organism and can be detected by a positive reaction to an

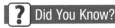

? Did You Know?

TB is the most common bacterial infection worldwide.

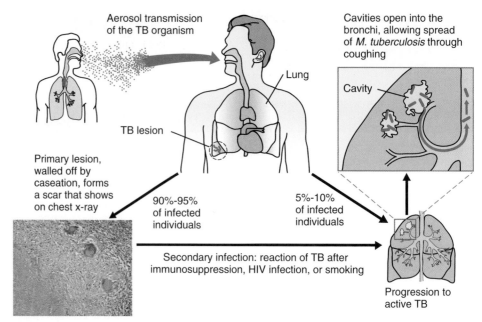

FIGURE 10-1 Primary TB infection with progression to secondary infection and active disease. *HIV,* Human immune deficiency virus; *TB,* tuberculosis. (Photo from Kumar, V., Abbas, A., Fausto, N., & Aster, J. (2009). *Robbins and Cotran pathologic basis of disease* (8th ed.). Philadelphia: Saunders. Photo courtesy Dominick Cavuoti, D.O., Dallas, Texas.)

Memory Jogger

A positive TB skin test means that the person has been infected with the bacteria at some point in his or her life but does not mean that he or she has active disease that can be spread to others.

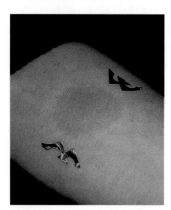

FIGURE 10-2 A positive tuberculosis skin test. The markings on either side of the test area are used to identify the skin test site and to assess the size of the reaction. (From Forbes, C. D. (2003). *Color atlas and text of clinical medicine* (3rd ed.). St. Louis: Mosby.)

Memory Jogger

Symptoms of active TB include a persistent productive cough, weight loss, poor appetite, night sweats, bloody sputum, shortness of breath, fever, aching chest pain that occurs with the cough, and chills.

intradermal TB skin test (Figure 10-2). A skin test is positive when a reddened area of 10 mm or more that is much harder than the surrounding soft tissue *(induration)* forms around the injection site. Thus most people who are exposed to TB will have a positive TB skin test but never fully develop the disease. Remember that once a TB skin test is positive, it will always be positive unless the immune system is very suppressed.

When a person is heavily exposed (often by repeated close contact with a person who has undiagnosed active TB) and has less resistance to the infection, the infection process may progress. Bacteria in the primary lesions multiply and start to kill off cells in the center of the lesion, turning it into a *necrotic* (dead tissue) mass. The mass and the area around it liquefies and is destroyed, forming a cavity (see Figure 10-1). Bacteria continue to grow in the cavity and spread into new lung areas.

TB lesions also may progress by entering the bloodstream. Once in the blood, TB can spread throughout the body and damage many organs (a disorder known as *miliary TB*). Although TB can develop in any body tissue (for example, brain, liver, kidney, bone marrow), it usually affects only the lungs.

TB is slow growing, and it may take years for symptoms to develop. A person infected with TB that is progressing beyond the initial stage cannot spread the disease to others until active symptoms occur. Active TB is diagnosed by chest x-ray, blood assay to test for the TB organism, and sputum culture.

Secondary TB is reactivation of the disease in a previously infected person whose primary lesions never completely resolved. Reactivation is more likely when immune defenses are weak, such as when a person has AIDS or is very old. Without treatment active TB can destroy so much lung tissue that death occurs.

TYPES OF DRUGS FOR TUBERCULOSIS

FIRST-LINE ANTITUBERCULAR DRUGS

The risk for TB transmission is reduced after an infectious person has received first-line anti-TB drug therapy for 2 to 3 weeks and clinical improvement occurs. However,

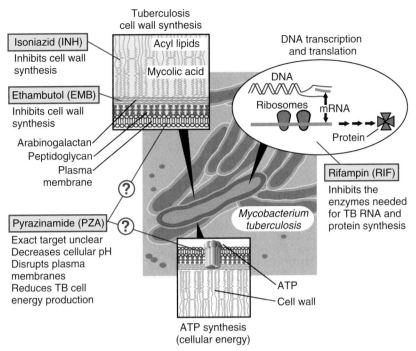

FIGURE 10-3 Probable sites of drug activity against the TB organism. *ATP*, Adenosine triphosphate; *TB*, tuberculosis.

even with initial improvement, drug therapy must continue for at least 6 months to control the disease.

Because the TB organism is slow growing, many common antibacterial drugs are not effective in controlling or killing it. Combination drug therapy is needed to treat TB and prevent its transmission. Therapy continues until the disease is under control. Current first-line therapy for TB uses isoniazid, rifampin, pyrazinamide, and ethambutol in different combinations and schedules. Some are now available in two- or even three-drug combinations. Variations of these first-line drugs along with other drug types are used when the patient either does not tolerate the standard first-line therapy or is infected with TB that is drug resistant. Control of TB depends on strict adherence to drug therapy.

How First-Line Antitubercular Drugs Work

Figure 10-3 shows where each of the first-line TB drugs works. With the exception of ethambutol, these drugs can be either *bactericidal* (kills the bacteria) or *bacteriostatic* (only suppresses bacterial growth), depending on the drug concentration within an infected site and the susceptibility of the organism.

Isoniazid works by inhibiting several enzymes important to mycobacteria metabolism and reproduction. It is able to inhibit these enzymes even when TB is dormant (in an inactive state). It is most often given as an oral drug but can be given as an intravenous (IV) or intramuscular (IM) injection.

Rifampin prevents reproduction of the TB organism by binding to the enzyme that allows RNA to be transcribed from DNA. Without this enzyme, TB cannot make the proteins needed to reproduce.

Pyrazinamide has an unknown mechanism of action but does reduce the pH of the intracellular fluid of WBCs in which the TB bacillus resides. The lower pH inhibits TB reproduction most effectively in the early stages of the disease.

Ethambutol suppresses the reproduction of TB bacteria by an unknown mechanism. It is only bacteriostatic and must be used in combination with other TB drugs.

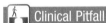 **Clinical Pitfall**

Drug therapy will not control TB unless it is continued for at least 6 months.

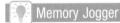 **Memory Jogger**

Strict adherence to the prescribed drug regimen is crucial for controlling TB.

Dosages for Common First-Line Antitubercular Drugs

Drug	Dosage
isoniazid (INH, Isotamine ♣, Nydrazid, PMS-Isoniazid ♣)	*Adults:* 5 mg/kg (maximum 300 mg) orally daily or 15 mg/kg (maximum 900 mg) orally twice each week *Children/Infants:* 10-15 mg/kg orally once daily
rifampin (RIF, Rifadin, Rimactane, Rofact ♣)	*Adults:* 10 mg/kg (maximum 600 mg) orally or IV daily or 2-3 times each week *Children:* 10-20 mg/kg (maximum 300 mg) orally or IV once daily or twice each week
pyrazinamide (PZA, PMS-Pyrazinamide ♣, Tebrazid ♣)	*Adults:* 15-30 mg/kg (maximum 3 g) orally daily or 50-70 mg/kg (maximum 4 g) orally twice each week *Children:* 15-30 mg/kg (maximum 2 g) orally daily
ethambutol (EMB, Etibi ♣, Myambutol)	*Adults:* 15-25 mg/kg (maximum 2.5 g) orally daily or 50 mg/kg (maximum 4 g) orally twice each week for the first 2 months of therapy *Children:* 15-25 mg/kg (maximum 2.5 g) orally daily

For adults, a new drug has been approved to use with the four standard first-line antituberculosis drugs when the disease has some degree of resistance to INH and RIF. This drug, Sirturo, is a combination of bedaquiline, pyrazinamide, and moxifloxacin. This oral drug is taken initially as 400 mg daily for 2 weeks. Then the dose is reduced to 200 mg three times weekly for the next 22 weeks. It is not approved for use in children. In addition to being liver toxic, this drug often induces cardiac changes including a prolonged QT interval on electrocardiogram.

Intended Responses
- Cough is reduced.
- Sputum production is reduced.
- Fatigue is reduced.
- Weight is gained.
- Sputum culture is negative for TB organisms.

Side Effects. Common side effects of first-line TB drug therapy are diarrhea, headache, nausea, vomiting, and difficulty sleeping.

Additional side effects of *isoniazid* include breast tenderness or enlargement (in men), loss of appetite, difficulty concentrating, and sore throat.

Specific side effects of *rifampin* include abdominal pain and urinary retention. In addition, the drug stains the skin, urine, tears, and all other secretions a reddish-orange color. Additional side effects of *pyrazinamide* include muscle aches and pains, acne, and increased sensitivity to sun or ultraviolet light.

Pyrazinamide and *ethambutol* increase the formation of uric acid, which can cause gout or make it worse.

Adverse Effects. The most common adverse effect of first-line drug therapy for TB is liver toxicity, with possible progression to permanent liver damage and failure. This risk is greatly increased if the patient drinks alcoholic beverages or uses acetaminophen while taking the drugs.

First-line drug therapy for TB has the potential to interact with many other drugs and herbal supplements. The interactions can be complex and serious.

Isoniazid can cause peripheral neuropathy with loss of sensation, especially in the hands and feet. This effect occurs most often in malnourished patients, those with diabetes, and alcoholics.

Rifampin often causes anemia. *Ethambutol* at high doses can cause optic neuritis vision changes that include reduced color vision, blurred vision, and reduced visual fields. This problem can lead to blindness. When the problem is discovered early, the eye problems are usually reversed when the drug is stopped.

Common Side Effects
First-Line Antitubercular Drugs

Diarrhea, Nausea/ Vomiting   Headache   Insomnia

Memory Jogger
Peripheral neuropathy from isoniazid therapy is caused by a deficiency of the B complex vitamins and can be prevented by increasing the intake of these vitamins during drug therapy.

What To Do *Before* Giving First-Line Antitubercular Drugs

Because drugs for TB can lead to liver toxicity, make sure that the patient has no liver problems before starting this therapy. Check the patient's most recent laboratory values for evidence of liver problems (such as elevated liver enzymes). (Refer to Table 1-3 in Chapter 1 for a listing of normal values.)

Ask male patients whether they have an enlarged prostate. Ask all patients whether they have any problem that causes urine retention. If so, report this problem to the prescriber before giving TB drugs.

Because rifampin can lead to anemia, check for anemia before starting this drug. Check the patient's most recent laboratory values for anemia (low red blood cell [RBC] count, low hemoglobin level). (Refer to Table 1-5 in Chapter 1 for a listing of normal values.)

Before giving *pyrazinamide* or *ethambutol,* ask whether the patient has ever had gout. If so, other precautions need to be taken. For example, the patient should drink a full glass of water with the drug and drink at least 3000 mL of water daily.

Before giving the first dose of *ethambutol,* assess the patient's vision and document your findings in the patient's chart. Use this information to determine whether vision changes are occurring during therapy.

Patients who have memory or compliance problems or who are homeless may benefit from directly observed therapy (DOT), in which the nurse or other health care provider watches the patient swallow the drugs. This practice contributes to more treatment successes, fewer relapses, and less drug resistance.

What To Do *After* Giving First-Line Antitubercular Drugs

For IV drug forms, check the patient's vital signs and respiratory status at least every 15 minutes for the first hour. Tell the patient to immediately report any shortness of breath or change in breathing.

Check the patient daily for yellowing *(jaundice)* of the skin or sclera, which is a symptom of liver problems. The best places to check are the whites of the eyes closest to the iris, the roof of the mouth, and the chest. Review the results of liver function tests for abnormalities.

If a patient has diabetes, check blood glucose levels more frequently and assess fasting blood glucose levels or levels of hemoglobin A1C whenever they are ordered. Report higher than normal levels to the prescriber for adjustments in the dosages of antidiabetic drugs.

At each clinic visit, ask the patient about any numbness, tingling, or pain in the hands and feet. Use monofilaments to check for peripheral neuropathy.

Check intake and output. If a patient's urine output is 1000 mL less than he or she is drinking or if other symptoms of urinary retention are present (enlarged bladder, lower abdominal discomfort), notify the prescriber.

Urge patients to drink plenty of water throughout the day and night. Ask about any pain in the joints (especially the big toe, foot, or ankle) and check for any joint swelling.

What To *Teach* Patients About First-Line Antitubercular Drugs

Teach patients to keep a supply of the prescribed drugs on hand at all times. Remind them that the disease is usually no longer contagious after drugs have been taken for 2 to 3 consecutive weeks and clinical improvement is seen. However, *stress that the patient must continue taking the drugs for 6 months or longer, exactly as prescribed.*

Explain that alcoholic beverages and drugs containing acetaminophen must be avoided for the entire drug therapy period. Many TB drugs, especially taken together, are toxic to the liver. This effect is increased by alcohol and acetaminophen. Also, a patient under the influence of alcohol is less likely to remember to take the prescribed drugs.

Tell patients to notify their prescriber if yellowing of the skin or eyes, darkening of the urine, or lightening of the stools develops. These problems are signs of liver toxicity.

Drug Alert!

Interaction Alert

First-line anti-TB drugs interact with many drugs and herbal supplements. Before giving a TB drug, ask the patient about all other drugs or supplements that he or she takes; then check with the pharmacist to avoid a possible drug interaction.

QSEN: Safety

Drug Alert!

Administration Alert

When giving pyrazinamide or ethambutol, have the patient drink a full glass of water to help excrete uric acid crystals faster and prevent them from precipitating in joints or the kidneys.

QSEN: Safety

Drug Alert!

Teaching Alert

Teach all patients on TB drug therapy to avoid alcoholic beverages and acetaminophen for the entire therapy period.

QSEN: Safety

Drug Alert!

Teaching Alert

Teach patients taking isoniazid to avoid coffee, tea (including green tea), chocolate, colas, and any other forms of caffeinated drinks or "stay-awake" pills.

QSEN: Safety

 Drug Alert!

Teaching Alert

Tell patients taking ethambutol to notify their prescriber immediately if any change in vision occurs.

QSEN: Safety

 Drug Alert!

Teaching Alert

Teach patients taking TB drugs to avoid taking any other type of drugs (prescribed or over-the-counter) or supplements without first checking with the TB drug prescriber.

QSEN: Safety

Tell patients that TB drugs may cause nausea. To help prevent it, suggest taking the daily dose at bedtime.

Teach patients with diabetes to check their blood glucose level as often as prescribed and to notify their prescriber if the level is consistently out of the target range. The prescriber may need to change the antidiabetic drug dosage, schedule, or drug type.

Isoniazid can raise blood pressure to dangerous levels when taken with caffeine. Teach patients taking it to avoid coffee, tea (including green tea), chocolate, colas, and any other forms of caffeinated drinks or "stay-awake" pills.

Teach patients taking *rifampin* to expect the drug to stain the skin, urine, and all other secretions. These will have a reddish-orange tinge but will be clear to normal within a few weeks after the drug is discontinued. Soft contact lenses used at this time will become permanently stained.

Teach patients to drink at least 8 oz of water when taking these drugs and increase fluid intake to at least 3 L of water daily. Tell them to drink water throughout the day and at least one full glass of water during the night.

A TB drug regimen increases sun sensitivity (*photosensitivity*) and can cause a severe sunburn, even among patients with darker skin. Teach patients to wear protective clothing, a hat, and sunscreen when going outdoors in the sunlight.

Remind patients taking *ethambutol* to notify their prescriber immediately if any change in vision develops. Patients who have glaucoma or cataracts should be followed by an ophthalmologist during ethambutol therapy.

Warn patients to tell all other health care providers that they are taking first-line drugs for TB because of the potential for drug interactions. Warn patients to not take any over-the-counter drug without checking with the prescriber of the TB drugs.

Life Span Considerations for First-Line Antitubercular Drugs

Pediatric Considerations. With the exception of ethambutol, infants and children of any age who have active TB should take first-line anti-TB drugs. Dosages for larger children and adolescents are nearly the same as for adults.

Considerations for Pregnancy and Lactation. First-line anti-TB drugs are approved for treatment of active TB in pregnant women. The risk for liver toxicity is higher when taking TB drug therapy during pregnancy, and close monitoring of liver function is needed. In addition, the pregnant woman needs higher doses of a B-complex vitamin supplement when taking isoniazid.

First-line anti-TB drugs appear in breast milk. When possible, breastfeeding should be avoided. If breastfeeding continues during TB therapy, teach the breastfeeding mother to reduce infant exposure to these drugs. (Refer to Box 1-1 in Chapter 1.) In addition, the breastfed infant should receive supplementation with B-complex vitamins.

Considerations for Older Adults. The risk for liver toxicity is higher among older adults taking drugs for TB. In addition, although gout can occur at any age, it is more common among older adults, and many older adults are more likely to have other health problems that require fluid restriction.

Older adults may have some degree of cataract formation in one or both eyes. This condition makes visual assessment for optic neuritis more difficult. Older adults taking ethambutol should be followed monthly by an ophthalmologist during therapy.

FUNGAL INFECTIONS

REVIEW OF RELATED PHYSIOLOGY AND PATHOPHYSIOLOGY

A **fungus** is a simple organism with one or more cells (such as yeasts, molds, and mushrooms) that reproduces by spores, has walled cells, and can either live

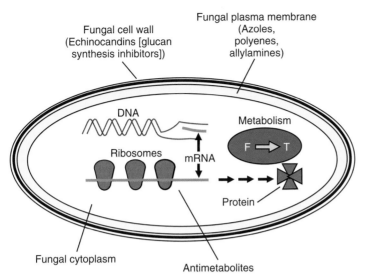

FIGURE 10-4 Sites of antifungal drug activity. *F → T*, metabolic conversion of folic acid to thymine.

peacefully with humans or infect humans and cause disease. Fungi have a thick, tough cell wall and a plasma membrane that is made of materials different from bacterial cell walls (Figure 10-4).

Fungi live in places that are moist and dark. There are more than 100,000 different types of fungi, some of which are harmless, others of which can cause infection and disease.

Because of their tough cell walls, fungi can live easily on human skin and mucous membrane surfaces and are not completely removed by usual bathing. Some types such as *Candida* are part of normal skin flora that do not cause problems unless they overgrow or enter the body. Without treatment, fungal infections remain and can become widespread, especially in people whose immune systems are not healthy. Superficial fungal infections are uncomfortable and change the appearance and function of the infected skin area. When fungal infections enter the body by inhalation or through breaks in the skin, deep fungal infections can result. With deep fungal infection, function in the affected organ is reduced, and the organ can be destroyed.

TYPES OF ANTIFUNGAL DRUGS

The thick fungal cell walls make fungi resistant to many anti-infective drugs. In addition, fungal DNA is similar to human DNA, causing antifungal drugs to often have more side effects than other types of anti-infective drugs.

DRUGS FOR SUPERFICIAL FUNGAL INFECTIONS

Treatment of superficial fungal infections of the skin or mucous membranes involves topical application of antifungal drugs. These are usually the same types of drugs used to treat deeper fungal infections but are prepared as creams, lotions, ointments, shampoos, powders, oral lozenges, and vaginal suppositories. Topical drugs are successful at clearing fungal infections that are not severe in patients with healthy immune systems. An exception is fungal infection of the fingernails or toenails. Because the fungus is under the nail, topical application is not often successful. Box 10-1 lists points to teach patients using topical antifungal therapy.

DRUGS FOR DEEP OR SYSTEMIC FUNGAL INFECTIONS

When fungal infections are deep or extensive, systemic drugs are needed to kill the fungi (**fungicidal** action) or slow their reproduction (**fungistatic** action). The classes of antifungal drugs are the azoles, polyenes, allylamines, antifungal antibiotics,

 Memory Jogger

Deep fungal infections require systemic therapy. Superficial fungal infections may be cured with topical antifungal therapy.

 Memory Jogger

Superficial fungal infections of the skin or mucous membranes are treated with topical application of antifungal drugs.

Box 10-1 Patient Teaching Tips for Topical Antifungal Agents

GENERAL
- Report any indication of an allergic reaction (new redness, swelling, blisters, or drainage) to the prescriber.
- Immediately after applying the drug, wash your hands to remove all traces of it.
- Avoid getting any antifungal drug in your eye. If the drug does get into your eye, wash the eye with large amounts of warm, running tap water and notify the prescriber.
- Use the drug exactly as prescribed and for as long as prescribed to ensure that the infection is cured.

POWDERS
- Ensure that the skin area is clean and completely dry before applying the powder.
- Hold your breath while applying to prevent inhaling the drug.
- For the foot area, be sure to apply the powder between and under your toes. Wear clean cotton socks (night and day). Change the socks at least twice daily.
- For the groin area, wear clean, close-fitting (but not tight) cotton underwear (briefs or panties).

SKIN CREAMS, LOTIONS, OINTMENTS
- Ensure that the skin area is clean and dry before applying the drug.
- Be careful to apply it only to the skin that has the infection. Keep it away from the surrounding skin.
- Apply a thin coating as often as prescribed.
- Wash and dry the area right before reapplying the next dose.
- Loosely cover the area to prevent spreading the drug to other body areas, clothing, or furniture.

ORAL LOZENGES
- Brush your teeth and tongue before using the tablet or troche.
- Let the tablet or troche completely dissolve in your mouth.
- Clean your toothbrush daily by running it through the dishwasher or soaking it in a solution of one part household bleach with nine parts water. After using bleach, rinse the toothbrush thoroughly.

VAGINAL CREAMS OR SUPPOSITORIES
- Place creams or suppositories just before going to bed to help keep them within the vagina longer.
- Wash your hands before inserting the drug.
- Insert the suppository (rounded end first) into the vagina as far as you can with your finger.
- Insert a full applicator of the cream as far into the vagina as is comfortable.
- Wash the applicator and your hands with warm, soapy water; rinse well; and dry.
- A sanitary napkin can be worn to protect your clothing and the bed from drug leakage.
- Avoid sexual intercourse during the treatment period. If you do have intercourse, the drug can create holes in a condom or damage a diaphragm and increase your risk for an unplanned pregnancy. In addition, you could spread the infection or become reinfected.
- Use the drug on consecutive days for as long as prescribed.

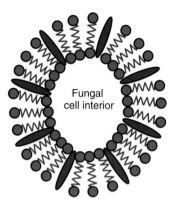

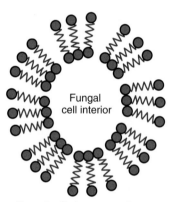

Fungal cell plasma membrane without ergosterol, which is leaky and leads to fungal cell death

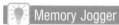

Ergosterol Phospholipid

FIGURE 10-5 Intact fungal cell plasma membrane (top) and the effects of azoles, polyenes, and allylamines on fungal cell membranes (bottom).

Memory Jogger

The major classes of antifungal drugs are:
- Azoles
- Polyenes
- Allylamines
- Antifungal antibiotics
- Antimetabolites
- Echinocandins

antimetabolites, and echinocandins. (See Figure 10-4 for where specific types of antifungal drugs work to kill or disrupt the growth of fungi.) *All systemic antifungal drugs have more side effects and adverse effects than most antibacterial drugs.* Drug dosages vary, depending on infection severity. The most common drugs in each class are discussed in this chapter. Consult a drug reference for other specific antifungal drugs.

How Antifungal Drugs Work
To reproduce and live, fungal cells must keep their plasma membranes and cell walls intact. Membranes are made up of phospholipids and ergosterol as shown in Figure 10-5. Ergosterol is a fat (lipid) similar to the cholesterol that is part of human cell

plasma membranes. The azoles, polyenes, and allylamines either prevent the fungus from making ergosterol or bind to the ergosterol and prevent it from being properly placed in the fungal membrane. As a result, the fungal membranes are leaky and allow damage to the fungus to occur. This action can prevent fungal reproduction (fungistatic) and may kill some fungi (fungicidal).

Antifungal antibiotics work by inhibiting the formation of spindle fibers, which stops the process of fungal cell division and reproduction.

Antimetabolites work by entering the fungal cell and acting as a "counterfeit" DNA base. When flucytosine is part of fungal cell DNA, it prevents fungal proteins needed for reproduction and growth from being made.

The *echinocandins* are also called *glucan synthesis inhibitors*. Fungi have a tough cell wall for protection (see Figure 10-4) that is different from the plasma membrane. This wall is made up of many substances that serve as "bricks" in the cell wall; glucan, which serves as "mortar" in the cell wall, holds the bricks tightly in place. Echinocandins stop fungal production of glucan so the mortar is thin and weak. This makes the entire fungal cell wall weak and unable to protect the fungal cell.

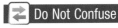 **Do Not Confuse**

Lamisil *with* **Lamictal**

An order for Lamisil can be confused with Lamictal. Lamisil is an antifungal drug, whereas Lamictal is an anticonvulsant prescribed for seizure disorders and certain psychiatric problems.

QSEN: Safety

Dosages for Common Antifungal Drugs

Drug	Dosage
Azoles	
fluconazole (Apo-Fluconazole ♣, Diflucan, Novo-Fluconazole ♣)	*Adults:* 200-400 mg orally or 200-800 mg IV daily *Children:* 6-12 mg/kg orally or IV daily
ketoconazole (Apo-Ketoconazole ♣, Extina, Nizoral, Novo-Ketoconazole ♣)	*Adults:* 200-400 mg orally once daily *Children:* 3.3-6.6 mg/kg orally once daily
itraconazole (ONMEL, Sporanox)	*Adults:* 200-400 mg orally once daily *Children:* Safety and efficacy not established
posaconazole (Noxafil, Posanol ♣)	*Adults:* 400 mg orally twice or 200 mg 3 times daily 300 mg IV twice daily first day, followed by 300 mg IV thereafter (Dosage and timing can vary depending on type and severity of fungal infection) *Children:* Safety and efficacy not established
voriconazole (Vfend)	*Adults/Children:* 6-12 mg/kg IV loading dose, then 4 mg IV every 12 hr; 200-400 mg orally every 12 hr
Polyenes	
amphotericin B "classic" ❶ (Amphocin, Fungizone)	*Adults/Children:* Dosage varies with type of infection, seriousness of infection, and patient tolerance; IV dosage not to exceed 1.5 mg/kg daily
amphotericin B lipid formulations ❶ (Abelcet, AmBisome, Amphotec)	*Adults/Children:* Dosage varies with type of infection, seriousness of infection, and patient tolerance; IV dosage not to exceed 4-6 mg/kg daily
Allylamines	
terbinafine (Apo-Terbinafine ♣, Lamisil, Novo-Terbinafine ♣)	*Adults/Children over 35 kg:* 250 mg orally daily *Children 25 to 35 kg:* 187.5 mg orally daily *Children less than 25 kg:* 125-mg oral granules
Antifungal Antibiotics	
griseofulvin (Fulvicin, Grifulvin, Gris-Peg, Grisactin)	*Adults:* 300-750 mg orally once daily (ultramicrosize) or 750-1000 mg orally once daily (microsize) *Children:* 7.3 mg/kg orally daily (ultramicrosize) or 10-11 mg/kg orally daily (microsize)
Antimetabolites	
flucytosine (Ancobon)	*Adults/Children:* 12.5-40 mg/kg orally every 6 hr

Continued

Dosages for Common Antifungal Drugs—cont'd

Drug	Dosage
Echinocandins	
anidulafungin (Eraxis)	*Adults:* 200 mg IV loading dose; then 100 mg IV daily *Children:* 3 mg/kg IV loading dose, then 1.5 mg/kg IV daily
caspofungin (Cancidas)	*Adults:* 70 mg IV loading dose, then 50 mg IV daily *Children:* 70 mg/m² IV loading dose; then 50 mg/m² IV daily
micafungin (Mycamine)	*Adults:* 100-150 mg IV daily *Children over 30 kg:* 2.5 mg/kg IV daily *Children less than 30 kg:* 3 mg/kg IV daily

❶ High-alert drug.

Common Side Effects

Antifungal Drugs

Diarrhea, Nausea/ Vomiting   Headache   Hair loss

Taste changes

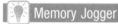 **Memory Jogger**

Antifungal drugs should be used with caution in patients who have kidney failure, liver disease, heart failure, or severe dysrhythmias.

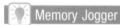 **Memory Jogger**

Amphotericin B causes renal insufficiency in all patients receiving it.

Intended Responses. The intended response to successful antifungal drug therapy is the eradication of the infection and normal function of all tissues and organs.

Side Effects. Common side effects of most antifungal drugs are changes in how food tastes, diarrhea, headache, nausea, and vomiting. Many patients taking a drug for several weeks report hair thinning. Drugs given intravenously may cause pain and redness at the injection site. Ketoconazole, voriconazole, and griseofulvin increase sun sensitivity and can lead to a severe sunburn.

Adverse Effects. Antifungal drugs have many possible adverse effects, including anemia, liver toxicity, low serum potassium levels *(hypokalemia)*, severe rashes, abnormal heart rhythms, and reduced kidney function. Most occur only at high doses or in patients with other health problems.

Skin irritation and rashes can occur with systemic antifungal therapy. Rashes may be severe with many types of lesions *(Stevens-Johnson syndrome)* (see Chapter 1). If the rashes become widespread with crusting, fever, and tissue necrosis, the condition can be life threatening.

Antifungal drugs have the potential to interact with many other drugs and herbal supplements. These interactions can be complex and serious.

Terbinafine (Lamisil) and *flucytosine* (Ancobon) can reduce WBC counts and increase the risk for infection.

The *azoles* and *amphotericin B* are all excreted by the kidney and can cause renal insufficiency. When renal insufficiency is present, the drugs are retained longer and are then more likely to cause additional severe side effects and adverse effects. If the patient is being treated with an additional drug that also impairs the kidney, the risk for kidney damage increases.

Griseofulvin, which is usually taken for 2 to 6 months to treat fungal infections of the fingernails and toenails, is associated with liver toxicity and paresthesia of the hands and feet. (Paresthesias are areas of numbness and tingling.)

Flucytosine (Ancobon) and the *echinocandins* can cause peripheral neuropathy with loss of sensation. The degree of sensation loss is related to how long the nerve-damaging drugs are used.

At very high doses the *azoles* may cause cardiac dysrhythmias, especially prolonged QT and torsades de pointes, a condition of unusual ventricular tachycardia. In addition, the drugs can interfere with cardiac drugs that are prescribed to control abnormal heart rhythms.

The *echinocandins* can increase the rate of clot formation, which increases the risk for deep vein thrombosis (DVT). DVT is most likely to occur in veins of the lower legs and pelvis. *Amphotericin B* has more adverse reactions than other antifungal drugs. For this reason systemic therapy with amphotericin B is used only for serious, life-threatening fungal infections. Common adverse effects of systemic amphotericin B include fever and chills that are so severe that this drug has been nicknamed "shake and bake." The drug dilates blood vessels, causing widespread skin flushing (known as *red man syndrome*). Hypotension and shock may occur as a result of blood vessel dilation. In addition, allergic reactions are possible, including anaphylaxis. Amphotericin B has a long half-life (15 days), and adverse effects may be present for weeks to months after the drug has been stopped.

What To Do *Before* Giving Antifungal Drugs

Because antifungal drugs may cause anemia and liver toxicity, make sure that the patient is not anemic and has no liver problems before starting these drugs. Check the patient's most recent laboratory values for anemia (low RBC count, low hemoglobin level) and liver problems (elevated liver enzyme levels). (Refer to Table 1-5 and Table 1-3 in Chapter 1 for a listing of normal values.)

Check the patient's current laboratory work, especially blood urea nitrogen (BUN) and serum creatinine levels, because these drugs can cause kidney impairment. (Refer to Table 1-4 in Chapter 1 for a listing of normal values.) Use these values as a baseline to determine whether the patient develops any kidney problems while taking an antifungal drug.

Some of the antifungal drugs should be taken with meals, whereas others should be taken on an empty stomach. Carefully plan the dosing schedule around meals. The activity of *azole* antifungal drugs can be reduced by grapefruit juice in large quantities. Do not administer an azole with grapefruit juice and limit the patient's grapefruit juice intake to no more than 24 oz per day. In addition, *ketoconazole* should not be given with drugs that reduce gastric acid such as proton pump inhibitors or histamine blockers because the drug is activated by stomach acids.

For *amphotericin B*, a test dose (1 mg IV over 20 to 30 minutes) is recommended because hypersensitivity is common. Check and recheck the exact dose to be administered each time the drug is given. Usually the first dose of amphotericin B is much smaller than the daily maintenance doses. After the first dose the drug is given either daily or every other day using gradually increasing doses.

Many health care providers prescribe premedication with specific drugs to counteract the side effects of amphotericin B. These drugs may include acetaminophen or ibuprofen to prevent or reduce fever, antihistamines (for example, diphenhydramine), IV corticosteroids (for example, hydrocortisone) to reduce blood vessel dilation, and meperidine (Demerol) to reduce or prevent excessive chills and shaking (*rigors*). Check the order to determine whether these drugs should be given in advance, and administer them at the appropriate time.

Parenteral amphotericin B must be used as soon as it is mixed. Administer the drug *slowly*, regardless of the dose.

What To Do *After* Giving Antifungal Drugs

When giving the first IV dose of an antifungal drug, check the patient every 15 minutes for any signs or symptoms of an allergic reaction (hives at the IV site, low blood pressure, rapid, irregular pulse, swelling of the lips or lower face, the patient feeling a lump in the throat). If the patient is having an anaphylactic reaction, your first action is to prevent any more drug from entering the body. Stop the drug from infusing but maintain the IV access.

Check the patient's skin every shift for rash, blisters, or other skin eruption that may indicate a reaction to the drug. Ask the patient about any itching or skin changes.

Check the patient daily for yellowing (*jaundice*) of the skin or sclera, which is a symptom of liver problems.

Check the patient's apical pulse for a full minute at least twice daily. Check whether there is a change in heart rate or regularity, document any changes, and notify the prescriber.

Check the patient's laboratory values, especially WBC counts, RBC counts, platelets, blood hematocrit, hemoglobin, BUN, creatinine, and potassium levels, every time they are taken. Compare these values with those obtained before drug therapy was started. If the potassium level is lower than 3.5 mEq/L (3.5 mmol/L) or if kidney

Memory Jogger

All patients receiving amphotericin B develop side effects, and most develop serious adverse effects. Monitor these patients very carefully because they are very sick.

Drug Alert!

Interaction Alert

Before giving an antifungal drug, ask the patient about all other drugs or supplements that he or she takes. Then check with the pharmacist to avoid a possible drug interaction.

QSEN: Safety

Drug Alert!

Administration Alert

Infuse the IV form of any azole slowly, no faster than 200 mg/hr. Flush the line only with sterile normal saline that does not contain a preservative.

QSEN: Safety

Drug Alert!

Administration Alert

Check and recheck the exact dose to be administered each time amphotericin B is given. The dose may not be the same any 2 days the drug is prescribed. It also may be different from one patient to another.

QSEN: Safety

Drug Alert!

Administration Alert

Administer parenteral amphotericin B and the echinocandins slowly, over at least 6 hours.

QSEN: Safety

Drug Alert!

Action/Intervention Alert

If the patient appears to be having anaphylaxis from an IV drug, prevent any more drug from entering the body, but maintain the IV access.

QSEN: Safety

function test values are rising, notify the prescriber. Examine the patient's intake and output record daily to determine if urine output is within 500 mL of the total fluid intake. Notify the prescriber if any blood counts are low.

With *terbinafine* or *flucytosine,* check the patient every shift for any signs of a new infection (for example, the presence of fever, drainage, foul-smelling urine, productive cough, or redness around an open skin area) and report any symptoms to the prescriber.

With *echinocandins,* check the patient's calves daily for signs of DVT (swelling, warmth, and pain or discomfort). If present, check the opposite calf and notify the prescriber.

With *amphotericin B,* check the patient's blood pressure at least every hour while the drug is infusing because the drug causes blood vessel dilation with hypotension. This can become severe enough to induce shock. Check for other symptoms of shock (pulse oximetry reading below 90%, rapid heart rate, rapid and shallow respirations, decreased urine output, change in level of consciousness). If shock symptoms are present or if blood pressure drops more than 15 mm Hg below the patient's normal level, call the Rapid Response Team and notify the prescriber immediately.

Expected side effects that usually occur during (or shortly after) the infusion with conventional IV amphotericin B include headache, chills, fever, rigors, flushing, hypotension, nausea, and vomiting. *Unlike other parenteral drugs, further slowing of the IV rate does not prevent these effects.* Assess the patient hourly for these side effects. Administer drugs as prescribed to reduce them. Even if these effects occur, it is important to attempt to administer the entire prescribed dose of amphotericin B because the infection is often life threatening.

What To *Teach* Patients About Antifungal Drugs

Warn patients taking antifungal drugs to tell all other health care providers that they are taking them because of the potential for drug interactions. Also warn patients to not take any over-the-counter drugs without consulting the prescriber of the antifungal drug.

Work with patients to make sure that they understand whether the drug is to be taken with a meal or on an empty stomach. Remind patients to avoid or minimize drinking grapefruit juice while taking an azole.

Teach patients to check their pulse for irregularities. Remind them to report new irregularities, rates faster than 100 beats per minute at rest, or rates slower than 50 beats per minute to their prescriber.

Tell patients to notify their prescriber if they develop yellowing of the skin or eyes, darkening of the urine, or lightening of the stools. These problems are signs of liver toxicity.

Tell patients to check weekly for increased fatigue, paleness, and increased heart rate or shortness of breath. These are symptoms of anemia and should be reported to their prescriber.

Teach patients to check their entire skin surface at least once daily for any rashes, blisters, or other skin changes. If skin changes occur, patients should notify their prescriber immediately.

Teach patients taking either *ketoconazole* or *voriconazole* or *griseofulvin* to avoid direct sunlight, use sunscreen, and wear protective clothing (including a hat) whenever they are in the sun to prevent a severe sunburn. In addition, tell them to avoid tanning beds and salons.

Teach patients taking *terbinafine* or *flucytosine* for more than 1 week to avoid crowds and people who are ill because resistance to infection is now decreased. Also remind them to notify their prescriber at the first sign of an infection.

Life Span Considerations for Antifungal Drugs

Pediatric Considerations. The safety and effectiveness of many systemic antifungal drugs have not been established. However, they are used cautiously in infants and children with severe fungal infections.

Administration Alert

Check the IV site during amphotericin B administration at least every 2 hours for a change in blood return, any redness or pain, or the feeling of hard or "cordlike" veins above the site. If such problems occur, follow the policy of your facility about removing the IV access.

QSEN: Safety

Teaching Alert

Teach patients taking an azole to check their pulse daily and to report new irregularities, rates faster than 100 beats per minute, or rates lower than 50 to the prescriber.

QSEN: Safety

Teaching Alert

Warn patients taking terbinafine or flucytosine for more than 1 week that they are at an increased risk for infection and should avoid crowds and people who are ill.

QSEN: Safety

Children are prescribed terbinafine for ringworm of the scalp (tinea capitis). Terbinafine is provided as granules to be sprinkled on a spoonful of pudding or other soft, nonacidic food. Tell the child to swallow the entire spoonful without chewing.

Considerations for Pregnancy and Lactation. Antifungal drugs are not recommended during pregnancy unless the fungal infection is serious or life threatening. Griseofulvin has a high likelihood of increasing the risk for birth defects or fetal damage and should never be given during pregnancy. Breastfeeding is not recommended during antifungal therapy.

Considerations for Older Adults. With *amphotericin B,* older adults may develop neurologic reactions more often. These reactions include abnormal thinking, agitation, anxiety, cerebral vascular accident, coma, confusion, depression, blurred vision, dizziness, drowsiness, hallucinations, hearing loss, and peripheral neuropathy. Assess older adults every shift for the presence of any of these changes.

With *echinocandins,* older adults are at greater risk for DVT. Use prescribed DVT prevention strategies. Assess patients daily for swelling, pain, or tenderness in the lower legs. Document positive findings and notify the prescriber.

> **!** **Drug Alert!**
>
> **Teaching Alert**
>
> Teach parents of children taking terbinafine sprinkles to avoid mixing the drug with applesauce or any acid-containing fruit or food.
>
> QSEN: Safety

Get Ready for Practice!

Key Points

- TB is spread by the airborne route, which allows droplets containing the bacteria to be exhaled when a person with active TB coughs, laughs, sneezes, whistles, or sings.
- For active TB to be controlled, the patient must adhere to combination anti-TB therapy for at least 6 months, even when symptoms are no longer present.
- A person who has a positive TB skin test will never have a negative test in the future, even after treatment has successfully controlled or eradicated the TB organism (unless he or she is profoundly immunosuppressed).
- All first-line drugs for TB can cause liver toxicity.
- All systemic antifungal drugs have more side effects and adverse effects than most antibacterial drugs.
- The most common adverse effect of antifungal therapy is anemia.
- Amphotericin B and the echinocandins are IV drugs that are usually given only in the in-patient setting. Patients receiving these drugs are usually very ill.
- Teach patients to limit intake of grapefruit juice to less than 24 oz daily while taking an azole and to not take the drug with grapefruit juice.
- Treatment with systemic amphotericin B is reserved for severe or life-threatening fungal infections.
- Amphotericin B has a long half-life (15 days), which means that side effects and adverse effects may be present for days to weeks after the drug has been stopped.
- Premedication may be prescribed before administration of amphotericin B to counteract the side effects of the drug.
- Do not administer amphotericin B at the same time as any blood product because the expected side effects of the drug may mask a transfusion reaction.

Additional Learning Resources

evolve Be sure to visit your Evolve website (http://evolve.elsevier.com/Workman/pharmacology/) for additional online resources.

SG Go to your Study Guide for additional learning activities to help you master this chapter content.

Review Questions

See the Answer Keys—In-text Review Questions for answers to these questions.

Test Yourself on the Basics

1. A patient has been admitted to the hospital with tuberculosis and is prescribed first-line drug therapy. Which drugs should you plan to teach the patient about before discharge? Select all that apply.
   - **A.** amoxicillin/clavulanate (Augmentin)
   - **B.** bedaquiline (Sirturo)
   - **C.** ethambutol (Myambutol)
   - **D.** isoniazid (Nydrazid)
   - **E.** posaconazole (Noxafil)
   - **F.** pyrazinamide (PZA)
   - **G.** raltegravir (Isentress)
   - **H.** rifampin (Rifadin)
   - **I.** vancomycin (Vancocin)
2. Which adverse effect is common to all the first-line antitubercular drugs?
   - **A.** Liver toxicity
   - **B.** Blurred vision
   - **C.** Reddish-orange urine
   - **D.** Excessive daytime drowsiness

3. Which precaution is *most important* to teach a patient who has been prescribed the four first-line anti-TB drugs?
   A. "Do not drive or operate heavy machinery while taking these drugs."
   B. "Take these drugs at night to prevent nausea and vomiting."
   C. "Do not drink alcoholic beverages while on these drugs."
   D. "Be sure to take these drugs with food."

4. Which systemic antifungal drug has the nickname "shake and bake"?
   A. anidulafungin (Eraxis)
   B. amphotericin B (Amphocin)
   C. flucytosine (Ancobon)
   D. terbinafine (Apo-terbinafine)

5. Which type of superficial fungal infection requires systemic antifungal drug therapy rather than topical antifungal drug therapy?
   A. Oral thrush
   B. Vaginal candidiasis
   C. Infection of the toenail
   D. Infection of the skin and scalp

6. Which antifungal drug is never prescribed for anyone who is pregnant because it causes birth defects?
   A. anidulafungin (Eraxis)
   B. fluconazole (Diflucan)
   C. griseofulvin (Fulvicin)
   D. micafungin (Mycamine)

7. Which precaution is important to teach a patient who is prescribed to use an antifungal cream?
   A. Wash your hands after applying the drug.
   B. Hold your breath while applying this drug.
   C. Take your pulse daily and report any irregularities immediately to the prescriber.
   D. Use a reliable method of birth control while using the drug and for 1 month after completing the drug therapy.

Test Yourself on Advanced Concepts

8. The patient taking first-line drug therapy for tuberculosis reports that his urine is now a bright reddish-orange color. What is your best response or action?
   A. Assess his skin and eyes for other indications of jaundice.
   B. Remind him to drink at least 2 to 3 L of water daily.
   C. Ask whether he has noticed any pain or burning on urination.
   D. Reassure him that this is an expected side effect of the drug therapy.

9. Why is it important to teach a patient who is taking first-line drug therapy for tuberculosis to avoid any products containing acetaminophen or Tylenol for the entire therapy period?
   A. Acetaminophen, like first-line drugs, is liver toxic and the combination worsens this adverse effect.
   B. Acetaminophen reduces the activity of first-line drugs and the dosages would need to be increased.
   C. Acetaminophen increases the activity of first-line drugs and the dosages would need to be reduced.
   D. Acetaminophen delays or inhibits the intestinal absorption of first-line drugs.

10. Which patient is most at risk for developing peripheral neuropathy as a result of taking isoniazid (Nydrazid) for tuberculosis?
    A. A 36-year-old woman who is 6 months pregnant
    B. A 45-year-old man who has gouty arthritis
    C. A 50-year-old woman who has type 1 diabetes mellitus
    D. A 65-year-old man who has a greatly enlarged prostate gland

11. The patient with tuberculosis who is prescribed the four first-line antituberculosis drugs asks how long he will have to "take all these pills." What is your best response?
    A. "When your skin test results are negative, you can stop the drugs."
    B. "You will be reevaluated to stop this therapy after 1 year."
    C. "You must take these drugs until your cough goes away."
    D. "Effective therapy requires a minimum of 6 months."

12. Why do systemic antifungal drugs used to treat deep fungal infections cause more side effects than almost any other type of anti-infective drug group?
    A. They are mostly given intravenously, which increases the speed of side effects and adverse reactions.
    B. Fungal cells have many similarities to human cells so that these drugs also exert their effects on human cells.
    C. Many antifungal drugs are actually slightly weaker forms of powerful cancer chemotherapy agents.
    D. When fungal cells are killed with these drugs, a toxic by-product is released that can damage human cells.

13. Which electrolyte value is most important to monitor for a patient who is taking a systemic antifungal drug?
    A. Calcium
    B. Chloride
    C. Sodium
    D. Potassium

14. Which precaution is most important to teach a patient who is prescribed to take an "azole" antifungal drug?
    A. Drink no more than 24 oz of grapefruit juice daily.
    B. Check your lower legs daily for the presence of swelling, pain, or tenderness.
    C. Do not drive or operate heavy equipment until you know how the drug affects you.
    D. Avoid crowds and people who are ill because you are at an increased risk for infection.

15. An adult is prescribed to receive isoniazid (INH) 5 mg/kg orally. He weighs 198 lb. What is his weight in kg? ____ kg How many mg of the drug should he receive for an accurate dose? _____ mg

16. Your patient is to receive 90 mg of amphotericin B in 500 mL of dextrose 5% in water (D_5W) to be infused over the next 4 hours. The drug solution mixed has a concentration of 5 mg/mL. How many mL of the drug solution will you add to the 500 mL of D_5W to make a dose of 90 mg? _____ mL
    How many mL per hour should the IV be infused to administer the drug over 4 hours? _____ mL/hour

Critical Thinking Activities

See the Answer Keys—Critical Thinking Activities for answers to these activities.

The patient is a 48-year-old man who is being released from prison after 15 years of incarceration. On his final physical, he is found to be 20 pounds underweight for his height and has a productive cough. He smokes three packs of cigarettes daily and is exposed to a great deal of secondhand smoke in the prison environment. On release, he is going to live with his 70-year-old aunt. A tuberculin skin test injected 3 days ago shows a 12-mm area of induration around the injection site. His records indicate that his last skin test, performed 18 months ago, did not result in any reaction. After other tests confirm that he has active TB, he is started on first-line anti-tuberculosis therapy drugs.

1. Which drugs are included in first-line therapy?
2. Would directly observed therapy be appropriate for this patient? Why or why not?
3. What are the teaching priorities for this patient?

Drugs That Affect the Immune System

Objectives

After studying this chapter you should be able to:

1. Explain the differences between active immunity and passive immunity.
2. Describe how vaccination affects immunity.
3. Explain the recommended schedules for vaccination of children and adults.
4. Describe life span considerations for vaccination.
5. List the names, actions, usual adult dosages, possible side effects, and adverse effects of drugs that suppress the immune response, including antirejection drugs.
6. Describe what to do before and after giving drugs that suppress the immune response.
7. Explain what to teach patients taking drugs that suppress the immune response, including what to do, what not to do, and when to call the prescriber.
8. Describe life span considerations for drugs that suppress the immune response.

Key Terms

acquired immunity (ă-KWĬRD ĭ-MŪ-nĭ-tē) (p. 174) An adaptive (learned) internal protection that results in long-term resistance to the effects of invading microorganisms.

active immunity (ĂK-tĭv ĭ-MŪ-nĭ-tē) (p. 177) The antibody-mediated immunity you acquire when your body actually learns to make specific antibodies in response to the presence of specific antigens.

antibody (ĂN-tĭ-bŏd-ē) (p. 175) A Y-shaped protein with areas on its "arms" that bind directly and tightly to anything that has the same specific code that triggered the B cell to respond by making specific antibodies. Also called immune globulins or immunoglobulins.

antibody titer (ĂN-tĭ-bŏd-ē TĬ-tĕr) (p. 178) A crude measurement of the presence of antibody in blood at different blood dilutions.

antigen (ĂN-tĭ-jĕn) (p. 175) Any cell, product, or protein with a code different from your own that enters your body and is recognized by your immune system as "foreign" and that will trigger your B cells to produce specific antibodies against it.

antiproliferative drugs (ĂN-tĭ-prō-LĬF-ĕr-ă-tĭv DRŬGZ) (p. 184) Drugs that slow the growth of immune system cells responsible for autoimmune diseases and for transplant rejection.

antirejection drugs (ĂN-tĭ-rē-jĕk-shŭn DRŬGZ) (p. 184) Drugs that suppress the components of the immune system responsible for rejection of transplanted tissues and organs.

artificially acquired active immunity (ăr-tĭ-FĬSH-ăl-ē ă-KWĬRD ĂK-tĭv ĭ-MŪ-nĭ-tē) (p. 177) The type of antibody-mediated immunity that is started when an antigen is deliberately placed into your body to force your B cells to make a specific antibody against it.

artificially acquired passive immunity (ăr-tĭ-FĬSH-ăl-ē ă-KWĬRD PĂ-sĭv ĭ-MŪ-nĭ-tē) (p. 180) The type of antibody-mediated immunity you would have if antibodies made by another person against an antigen were injected into your body.

attenuated vaccine (ă-TĔN-yoo-ā-tĕd văk-SĒN) (p. 177) A vaccine containing live organisms that have been modified so that they are (usually) no longer capable of reproducing or of causing disease but still retain their unique code. Also called a *live-virus* vaccine.

autoimmune disease (ŏ-tō-ĭ-MŪN dĭz-ĒZ) (p. 183) A condition in which a person's immune system sees his or her own cells and tissues as foreign and develops immunity against these body cells or tissues.

biosynthetic vaccine (BĪ-ō-sĭn-THĔT-ĭk văk-SĒN) (p. 178) A vaccine composed of science-made substances that are very similar to the parts of a virus or bacterium that causes disease.

calcineurin inhibitors (KĂL-sē-nyŭr-ĭn ĭn-HĬB-ĭ-tŭrz) (p. 185) A class of drugs that works to prevent the first phase of T-cell activation by binding to protein and forming a complex that inhibits calcineurin present in some immune system cells.

immunization (ĭ-MŪ-nĭ-ZĀ-shŭn) (p. 177) The desired outcome or response of successful vaccination in which the person actually develops immune resistance to the substance in the vaccine. Often used interchangeably with the term *vaccination*.

immunosuppressant drugs (ĬM-ū-nō-sŭ-PRĔS-ĕnt DRŬGZ) (p. 182) Drugs that inhibit or prevent the optimal or excessive functioning of immune system.

inactivated vaccine (ĭn-ĂK-tĭv-Ā-tĭd văk-SĒN) (p. 177) A vaccine composed of organisms that could cause diseases but have been killed or inactivated by heat, radiation, or chemicals that prevent the organisms from reproducing and causing disease. Sometimes called *killed vaccine*.

innate immunity (ĭn-ĀT ĭ-MŪ-nĭ-tē) (p. 173) The natural native resistance to infection provided by the general responses of inflammation. Innate immunity is nonspecific and does not require training.

monoclonal antibodies (mŏn-ō-KLŌ-năl ăn-tĭ-BŎD-ēs) (p. 185) Antibodies produced by mouse cells or a combination of mouse and human antibody–producing cells against a protein found on the surface of all human T lymphocytes (T cells).

naturally acquired active immunity (NĂ-chŭr-ăl-ē ă-KWĬRD ĂK-tĭv ĭ-MŪ-nĭ-tē) (p. 177) The type of antibody-mediated immunity that is started when your body is invaded by a foreign organism without assistance and your B cells learn to make antibodies against the invaders.

naturally acquired passive immunity (NĂ-chŭr-ăl-ē ă-KWĬRD PĂ-sĭv ĭ-MŪ-nĭ-tē) (p. 177) The type of antibody-mediated immunity you acquired as a result of antibodies transferred to you as a fetus or infant from your mother through the placenta and through breast milk.

polyclonal antibodies (pŏl-ē-KLŌ-năl ăn-tĭ-BŎD-ēs) (p. 185) Antibodies produced by other animals (usually horses and rabbits) in response to the administration of human white blood cells, especially T cells.

selective immunosuppressants (sŭ-LĔK-tĭv ĬM-ū-nō-sŭ-PRĔS-ĕnts) (p. 184) Drugs that more selectively target the immune system cells and products responsible for autoimmune diseases and transplant rejection.

toxoid (TŎK-sŏyd) (p. 178) A vaccine that contains either a modified toxin that an organism produces or an actual part of the organism.

true immunity (troo ĭ-MŪ-nĭ-tē) (p. 173) The ability of the body to recognize a specific organism when it reinvades (reexposes itself to the body's internal environment) and take steps to remove, inactivate, or destroy the invading organisms before illness can occur.

vaccination (văk-sĭn-Ā-shŭn) (p. 177) The deliberate injection or ingestion of an organism or other antigen for the intended purpose of stimulating B cells into producing antibodies specific to the antigen, resulting in immunologic resistance to any disease caused by the antigen.

vaccine (văk-SĒN) (p. 177) A biologic preparation containing the universal product code of a specific disease-causing microorganism. It can be composed of the organism itself, a part of the organism that retains its unique code, or a protein the organism produces that also contains the unique code.

Despite being exposed almost continually to disease-causing organisms, especially bacteria and viruses, we remain healthy and well more often than we are sick. The immune system working with inflammation helps our bodies learn to protect themselves from invading microorganisms that can cause diseases. As discussed in Chapter 6, inflammation and the inflammatory responses provide day-to-day, nonspecific resistance (protection) against invasion of disease-causing (pathogenic) organisms. These nonspecific responses recognize when an invading organism enters the body through the skin, mucous membranes, respiratory tract, or the gastrointestinal tract and take general steps to remove or destroy the invaders. Because these protective inflammatory responses are general and can be triggered by any invasion, they are considered **innate** (native) **immunity,** or resistance that your body can perform without training. It is called *innate* or *native* because you were born with it. It is one of the reasons that humans do not get some types of animal disorders, such as distemper or mange. These general protective responses are helpful but can be overwhelmed when organisms invade in great numbers. *Even more important is the fact that the general protective responses do not prevent us from getting sick over and over again every time our bodies are heavily invaded by the same organisms.* Thus general inflammatory responses are protective but do not provide true immunity to any specific invader. However, the general inflammatory responses are needed to work with the immune system to provide true immunity.

 Memory Jogger

Inflammation (innate immunity) helps protect the body but cannot provide true immunity to any specific disease-causing microorganism.

OVERVIEW OF THE IMMUNE SYSTEM AND IMMUNITY

True immunity is the ability of the body to recognize a specific organism when it reinvades (reexposes itself to the body's internal environment) and to take steps to remove, inactivate, or destroy the invading organisms before illness can occur. The immune system helps you develop true immunity. This system can sometimes seem confusing because it not "housed" within one organ. Instead, the immune system parts can be found in many places within the body, especially near areas where invasion and injury are more likely to occur. The main tissues of the immune system are

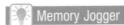

Memory Jogger

The lymphocytes provide long-lasting true immunity.

the white blood cells (WBCs), also known as leukocytes, the substances these cells produce, and tissues containing colonies of WBCs, such as lymph nodes, tonsils, intestinal tract, and the spleen. The bone marrow is the original source of WBCs, many of which then circulate throughout the body. The WBCs involved in inflammation are the neutrophils, macrophages, eosinophils, basophils, along with a tissue-based cell called a mast cell. These are the cells that provide the general innate protection against invasion. The lymphocyte family of WBCs provides true immunity but requires the assistance of inflammation to do so.

The B lymphocytes (B cells) and T lymphocytes (T cells) together are responsible for providing long-lasting true immunity so that for most types of diseases caused by infectious organisms, you actually have the disease only once. For example, if you had chickenpox (caused by the varicella zoster virus [VZV]) as a child, it is unlikely that you will develop chickenpox again even when you are tremendously reexposed to VZV. This is because the lymphocytes that were exposed to VZV when you originally got sick with the chickenpox learned to recognize VZV and developed specific immunity in the form of antibodies to that virus. Because the immune system has to *learn* to make antibodies, this type of immunity is *acquired* rather than *innate*.

Acquired immunity is an *adaptive* (learned) internal protection that results in long-term resistance to the effects of invading microorganisms. The responses are not automatic. Much of acquired immunity occurs through the processes of antibody formation by B cells and antibody actions.

ANTIBODY PRODUCTION

Antibody production is an adaptive process performed by B cells after they learn to recognize a specific invader. All WBCs can recognize an invader, and the WBCs involved in inflammation are best at it. All cells in your body have a universal product code specific to you (and any identical siblings you may have) (Figure 11-1). This code, which is officially known as your *tissue type* and the *human leukocyte antigens (HLAs)*, is genetically determined by genes you inherit from your parents. So the codes are similar among family members but only exactly the same in identical siblings (e.g., identical twins or triplets). Your immune system cells, which also have this unique "you" code, have the special ability to compare the code of any cell or protein it encounters to determine whether it is one of your cells. If the code is identical to your code, the encountered cell is considered "self," and the normal immune system takes no action against it. If the code of the encountered cell or protein is not a perfect match to your code, the immune system cells consider it an invader that is "foreign" to you (Figure 11-2). Once a foreign or invading cell is recognized, the general inflammatory cells take steps to eliminate, neutralize, or destroy it. If you are heavily invaded by infectious organisms and get sick, the general inflammation cells help the lymphocytes also recognize the organisms as

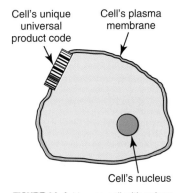

Cell's unique universal product code   Cell's plasma membrane

Cell's nucleus

FIGURE 11-1 Human cell with unique universal product code.

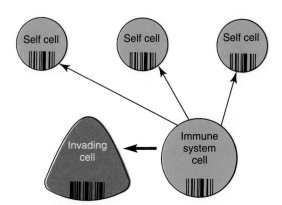

Self cell   Self cell   Self cell

Invading cell   Immune system cell

FIGURE 11-2 Immune system cell recognizing an invading or foreign cell by differences in its universal product code. (Modified from Ignatavicius, D. D., & Workman, M. L. (2016). *Medical-surgical nursing: Patient-centered collaborative care* [8th ed.]. St. Louis: Saunders.)

foreign so that they can start specific antibody production to 1) limit how long you are sick with this disease and 2) prevent you from ever becoming sick from the same infection again.

Any cell, product, or protein with a code different from your own that enters your body and is recognized by your immune system as foreign is an **antigen** to you. Usually the general WBCs first recognize the antigen as foreign. Some of these WBCs bring the invading antigen into contact with fresh, "unsensitized" lymphocytes. The T cell helps the B cell learn exactly how the invading antigen's code is different from your code. This is called *sensitizing* the B cell against a specific antigen. Then the sensitized B cell starts making and releasing antibodies that will bind only to cells or products that carry that specific invader's code. An **antibody** is a Y-shaped protein with areas on its "arms" that bind directly and tightly to anything that has the same specific code that triggered the B cell to make the antibody to begin with. (Other names for antibodies are *immune globulins* and *immunoglobulins*.) Each B cell learns to make only one specific type of antibody that can only recognize and bind to one specific antigen. Figure 11-3 outlines this process.

When you are invaded by so many chickenpox viruses that you actually get sick with the chickenpox, many fresh unsensitized B cells in your body start learning to make anti-chickenpox antibodies. Not a lot of anti-chickenpox antibodies are made at this time, but the ones that are made are important in helping you get well in 5 to 10 days so that your chickenpox disease does not last for several months. The most important part about B cells becoming sensitized against an antigen and learning to make a specific antibody is that they always remember how to make those

> **Memory Jogger**
>
> B-cell recognition of antigens is the trigger for B cells to begin making antibodies.

1. Invasion of the body by new antigens in sufficient numbers to stimulate an immune response.

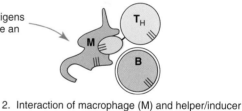

2. Interaction of macrophage (M) and helper/inducer T cell (T$_H$) in the processing and presenting of the antigen to the unsensitized "virgin" B lymphocyte (B).

3. Sensitization of the virgin B lymphocyte to the new antigen.

7. On reexposure to the same antigen, the sensitized lymphocytes and their progeny produce large quantities of the antibody specific to the antigen. In addition, new "virgin" B lymphocytes become sensitized to the antigen and also begin antibody production.

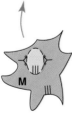

6. Antibody binding causes cellular events and attracts other leukocytes to the complex. The interaction of other leukocytes along with the cellular events results in the neutralization, destruction, or elimination of the antigen.

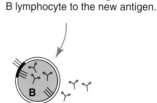

4. Antibody production by the B lymphocyte. These antibodies are directed specifically against the initiating antigen. The antibodies are released from the B lymphocyte and float freely in the blood and some other fluids.

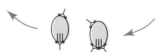

5. Antibodies bind to the antigen, forming an immune complex.

FIGURE 11-3 The steps involved in making antibodies for immunity. (From Ignatavicius, D. D., & Workman, M. L. (2016). *Medical-surgical nursing: Patient-centered collaborative care* [8th ed.]. St. Louis: Saunders.)

antibodies. Also, all future cells produced by these sensitized B cells (known as plasma cells) are not really "fresh." They are born sensitized and already know how to make the specific antibody. So with time, you have millions of B cells sensitized against the chickenpox virus. When you are reexposed to the chickenpox virus later in life, even when the exposure is huge, you will not get sick with the chickenpox because all those sensitized B cells produce enormous amounts of anti-chickenpox antibodies. These antibodies bind to the invading chickenpox viruses and act to destroy, eliminate, or neutralize them so that you do not actually get sick again with the chickenpox. You now have *antibody-mediated immunity* to chickenpox. In fact, with every reexposure to the chickenpox virus, you become more and more immune to it. This great protection continues until your immune system is damaged (by drugs, diseases, or environmental agents) or just plain wears out as you age.

A special feature about antibody-mediated immunity is the antibodies made by B cells are released into the blood and other body fluids. This means that the antibodies can go where they are needed most in the body, such as sites of invasion. Also, because the antibodies are released into the blood, they can be taken from the blood of one person and injected into another person's body. For this reason, an older term for antibody-mediated immunity is *humoral immunity*. In addition to the blood and body fluids, B cells are heavily concentrated in the spleen, parts of lymph nodes, tonsils, and the mucosa of the intestinal tract.

ANTIBODY PROTECTION

Acquired true immunity provided by antibodies has several subtypes. These include naturally acquired immunity and artificially acquired immunity. Both types of acquired immunity can be divided into active immunity and passive immunity. Although all subtypes are helpful and provide some protection, they differ in how well they protect and how long that protection lasts. Figure 11-4 shows how the various types of immunity develop.

Naturally Acquired Immunity

Naturally acquired immunity is the type of immunity started when a person's body is invaded by a foreign organism without assistance. So when you are invaded by

Memory Jogger

All future B cells produced after sensitization are also sensitized against the specific antigen and can make antibodies.

Memory Jogger

Antibody-mediated immunity can be transferred from one person to another.

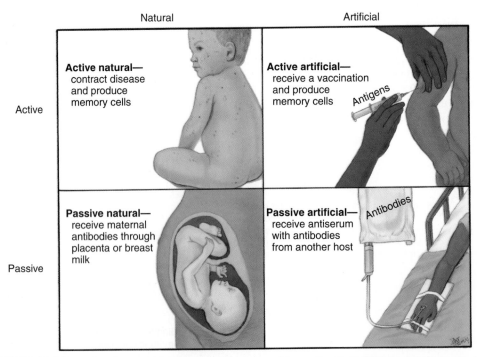

FIGURE 11-4 Examples demonstrating how different types of immunity develop. (From Applegate, E. J. (2011). *The anatomy and physiology learning system* (4th ed.). St. Louis: Saunders.)

any common cold virus, an influenza virus, or an infectious type of bacteria as a result of being exposed to someone who is sick with any of these organisms, the exposure is "natural," and your immune system has the opportunity to develop immunity against the organism even though you may get sick with this exposure. So *naturally acquired* refers to how the exposure to an invader occurs. This type of immunity can be active or passive. **Active immunity** means that your own body developed the antibodies. **Naturally acquired active immunity** is the type of antibody-mediated immunity that is started when you are invaded by a foreign organism without assistance and your B cells then learn to make antibodies against the invaders. This type of immunity is the strongest and most long lasting. It can provide good protection for many decades. **Naturally acquired passive immunity** is the type of antibody-mediated immunity you acquired as an antibody transfer from your mother through the placenta and through breast milk. Your body did not make these antibodies. This type of immunity is very important in helping to keep young infants healthy but provides protection for only a matter of months, not years.

Artificially Acquired Active Immunity

Although naturally acquired active immunity is the best type, sometimes having a person actually become ill with infectious organisms to make his or her own antibodies is not a good idea. For example, when a person catches diphtheria, he or she develops long-lasting immunity to it and will not get sick with diphtheria again. However, diphtheria has a high mortality rate, and some people who get the disease die from it. So artificially acquired active immunity is used to assist the body to learn to make antidiphtheria antibodies without having to get sick with the disease. **Artificially acquired active immunity** is the type of antibody-mediated immunity that is started when an antigen is deliberately placed into your body to force your B cells to make a specific antibody against it. This type of immunity is commonly developed in most countries with the widespread use of vaccination, starting in early childhood.

Vaccination. **Vaccination** is the deliberate injection or ingestion of an organism or other antigen for the intended purpose of stimulating B cells into producing antibodies specific to the antigen, resulting in immunologic resistance to any disease caused by the antigen. Most often vaccination involves the injection of a vaccine. A **vaccine** is a biologic preparation containing the universal product code of a specific disease-causing microorganism. The preparation can be composed of the organism itself, a part of the organism that retains its unique code, or a protein the organism produces that also contains the unique code. Although vaccination usually results in the person's B cells becoming sensitized and making the desired antibodies, this artificial method of stimulating antibody-mediated immunity is less efficient than that stimulated by naturally acquired active immunity. As a result, more than one vaccination with the same vaccine may be required and, even then, the resistance is not permanent. The person requires periodic "boosting" of the immunity with revaccination to recruit more B cells to produce the proper antibodies and to remind existing sensitized B cells to continue to make antibodies. Vaccination and immunization are often used as interchangeable terms; however, **immunization** is the desired response of successful vaccination in which the person actually develops immune resistance to the substance in the vaccine.

Types of Vaccines. Different substances are used in the vaccine preparations. Sometimes inactivated organisms (usually viruses or bacteria) are used. **Inactivated vaccines** contain organisms that could cause diseases but have been killed or inactivated by heat, radiation, or chemicals that prevent the organisms from reproducing and causing disease. Examples of inactivated vaccines include those for immunization against influenza, cholera, hepatitis A, and rabies. **Attenuated vaccines** contain live organisms that have been modified so that they are no longer capable of reproducing or of causing disease (usually) but still retain their unique code. This type of

Memory Jogger

Naturally acquired active immunity is the most effective and long-lasting type of immunologic protection.

Memory Jogger

Artificially acquired active immunity is used to help people develop immunity to a dangerous disease without the risks associated with becoming sick first.

Memory Jogger

Successful vaccination results in immunization with the development of immunologic resistance to the organism in the vaccine.

Memory Jogger

The four types of vaccines currently available are:
- Inactivated vaccines
- Attenuated vaccines
- Toxoids
- Biosynthetic vaccines

vaccine is also called a *live-virus* vaccine. Attenuating the organisms also makes them noncontagious (unless a person has very reduced immune function). Examples of attenuated vaccines include those for immunization against measles, mumps, rubella, polio, and chickenpox. **Toxoids** are vaccines that contain either a modified toxin that an organism produces or an actual part of the organism. In either case, the toxoid must have the unique code to stimulate proper antibody production. Examples of toxoid vaccines are those for immunization against tetanus, diphtheria, pertussis (whooping cough), human papilloma virus (HPV), and hepatitis B (HVB). **Biosynthetic vaccines** are those containing science-made substances that are very similar to the parts of a virus or bacterium that causes disease. Examples of biosynthetic vaccines are those for immunization against *Haemophilus influenzae* type B.

Vaccination and Boosting Schedules. For most types of vaccines used for artificially acquired active immunity, more than one injection is required on a specific schedule to ensure that adequate numbers of B cells become sensitized to the antigen and begin making antibodies. Usually, additional boosting vaccinations, which contain smaller doses of the original antigens, are needed to retain protection. For example, infants are usually vaccinated against diphtheria, tetanus, and pertussis (DTaP) with a single injection containing all three antigens at ages 2 months, 4 months, and 6 months for a total of three separate injections (doses). The vaccination is repeated as a fourth dose between the ages of 15 and 18 months, and again as a fifth dose between the ages of 4 and 6 years. An injection of a different formulation of these same three antigens (known as Tdap) is recommended again between the ages of 11 and 12 years. It is also recommended that women receive Tdap with each pregnancy and that all adults over the age of 19 years receive this vaccination every 10 years. Additional vaccinations usually given in childhood include those against fairly common infectious diseases that can have severe consequences, such as hepatitis B (HVB), *Haemophilus influenza* type B (Hib), pneumonia, polio, measles, mumps, rubella, hepatitis A (HVA), varicella, rotavirus, human papilloma virus (HPV), and meningitis. Vaccination against seasonal influenza is recommended yearly for children. (See the Evolve site for the current recommended schedules for immunizations during childhood.)

 Memory Jogger

Vaccinations must be readministered periodically as a "booster" to maintain immunologic protection.

Vaccination and immunization are not confined to childhood. Vaccines are now available to stimulate protection for adults against common infectious diseases that, although not considered as serious as the ones for which childhood vaccination is recommended, can have fatal consequences, especially for older adults and for those who have chronic illnesses. Such vaccinations are recommended to prevent seasonal influenza, various types of pneumonia, shingles (varicella), hepatitis A, and hepatitis B. Recommended vaccinations for adults against certain childhood disorders vary, depending on whether the person actually experienced any of these diseases as a child. Some adult vaccinations are recommended yearly, such as the seasonal influenza vaccine. Others are recommended on a one-dose, two-dose, or three-dose lifetime schedule. (See the Evolve site for the current adult recommended schedules for immunizations.)

 Memory Jogger

Adults need vaccination and revaccination for continued active immunity.

Other adult vaccinations may be recommended depending on the person's job or travel. Although rabies vaccination is available, it is not part of a recommended set of vaccinations because very few people are exposed to this deadly disease. For those who are, such as veterinarians and other animal handlers, the vaccine is available. People who travel or military personnel who might be expected to travel to areas of the world where some contagious diseases are more common should receive specific vaccinations against such disorders as yellow fever, cholera, typhoid, malaria, anthrax, and many others. Just like for ordinary vaccinations, usually more than one injection is required on a specific schedule to effectively result in successful immunization. Box 11-1 outlines responsibilities associated with the administration of vaccines.

So how do you know whether vaccination results in successful immunization? It is possible to know about how much of any specific antibody you have by performing a blood titer for that antibody. An **antibody titer** is a crude measurement of the

Box 11-1	Responsibilities When Administering Vaccines

STORAGE

- Upon receiving vaccines from the manufacturer:
  - Immediately unpack and store in a designated area or with a designated refrigeration device that is separate from other drugs or food.
  - Ensure refrigerator is plugged into an outlet that is serviced with emergency power and that the refrigerator is labeled "Do Not Unplug."
  - Keep all vials (opened and unopened) in their original boxes.
  - Do not store vaccine vials on the door of the refrigerator or in the freezer compartment.
  - Check the vials on a weekly basis for expired vaccines or diluents, and discard those that are expired.

BEFORE ADMINISTRATION

- Check the recommended schedule for whether the vaccination is appropriate for the patient.
- Check the expiration date on the vaccine vial and, if a diluent is to be used, also check the expiration date on the diluent vial.
- Read the package insert to determine all components of the vaccine (including preservatives), the recommended dosage, appropriate techniques and solutions for dilution, and any special instructions for administration.
- Ask whether the patient has ever had a reaction to the vaccine or any component of the vaccine.
- Ask when the patient last received this or any other vaccine.
- Ask the patient (or the parent/guardian of the patient) about any known allergies.
- Determine whether the patient is ill or has been ill within the previous 24 hours (some vaccines should NOT be given to a patient who has a fever or any type of infection).
- Using aseptic technique, draw up the appropriate dose into the syringe type recommended by the manufacturer and adjusted for patient size.
- Administer the drug using the recommended technique and site.

AFTER ADMINISTRATION

- Document the vaccination in the patient's medical record or permanent vaccination log, including:
  - Name and age of the patient
  - Name of the vaccine
  - Manufacturer, lot number, and expiration date of the vaccine
  - Dosage of the vaccine
  - Site of vaccination
  - Condition of the site
- Provide a copy of the specific vaccine's Vaccine Information Statement (VIS) developed by the Centers for Disease Control and Prevention (CDC) to the patient or parents/guardians.
- Document which version of the VIS was provided.
- Observe the patient as recommended by the manufacturer for any immediate reaction to the vaccination.
- Teach the patient what side effects to expect and which ones require immediate medical attention.

presence of antibody in your blood at different blood dilutions. For example, if you have a 0 titer for anti-chickenpox antibody (anti-VZV or varicella), you do not have any measureable antibody response even when your blood is not diluted. If you have a positive titer of 32, it means that you have enough antibody that it is still detectable even when your blood has been diluted to a ratio of 1 part blood to 31 parts diluent. Although somewhat crude, this test can indicate whether you have ever had a specific infectious disease (or have been vaccinated against it) and to what degree you are protected against the disease at the time the test was performed.

 Memory Jogger

An antibody titer can determine whether you have any immunologic resistance to an infectious disease.

Seasonal Influenza Vaccination. So why is it recommended that adults and children receive seasonal influenza vaccination every year? Doesn't the protection last longer than a year? Yes, the protection does last longer than a year. The big problem is that there are many strains of influenza. Each strain has a different unique code. If you get sick with one specific strain this year, you will develop long-lasting naturally acquired active immunity to that strain. However, if next year a different strain comes to your community (or family), you do not have any immunity against it, and, if sufficiently infected, you will get sick with the new strain of influenza. This is also true for "flu shots." When you receive an annual flu shot, the vaccination contains antigens for the three or four viruses that are predicted (by the Centers for Disease Control and Prevention [CDC]) to be the most likely ones to be prevalent this year. Receiving this vaccination allows you to develop artificially acquired active immunity to these three or four influenza strains, which will protect you against these strains for many years. However, next year the most likely strains predicted to be prevalent may not be the ones you were vaccinated against this year. So if you skip next year's vaccination you will be susceptible to the different strains of influenza and may get sick if heavily exposed.

Artificially Acquired Passive Immunity

Artificially acquired passive immunity is the type of antibody-mediated immunity you would have if antibodies made by another person (or animal) were injected into your body. Because these antibodies are foreign to you, your immune system recognizes them as foreign and eliminates them quickly. For this reason, passive immunity provides only immediate, short-term protection against a specific antigen. It is mainly used when a person is exposed to a serious disease for which he or she has little or no actively acquired immunity. The injected antibodies are expected to inactivate the invading organism or antigen.

Examples of Artificially Acquired Passive Immunity. Some adults have either never received a tetanus vaccination or have never had their childhood vaccinations boosted with tetanus toxoid. The bacterium that causes the disease tetanus (*Clostridium tetani*) is very common and can enter the body easily through contaminated large or deep wounds. Tetanus has a high mortality rate (which is why children are vaccinated against it very early in life). So if a person has a deep puncture wound (perhaps caused by a large rusty nail or a manure-covered pitchfork) and has either never been vaccinated or has not been boosted for 30 years, he or she has few or no circulating antibodies against tetanus. As a result, this person has a very high risk for developing tetanus and dying from the disease. To provide immediate protection, the person can be injected with the drug HyperTET, which is a large amount of anti-tetanus antibodies produced in other people and pooled together as a large dose. The expectation of an injection of HyperTET is that these already made antibodies will bind to the tetanus bacteria and the toxins they produce and rid the patient's body of them so that he or she does not develop the disease from this injury. However, the person should still be vaccinated later (within a week) with tetanus toxoid so that he or she can develop his or her own artificially acquired active immunity against tetanus.

Other fatal disorders for which artificially acquired passive immunity can be used to temporarily provide protection include rabies and poisonous snakebites. In the 2014 outbreak of the deadly Ebola virus disease (EVD), artificially acquired passive immunity has been used successfully in a small number of cases. The plasma from a person who had been sick with EVD and who had recovered from the disease was transfused into a patient who actively had the disease. This plasma contained a high concentration of anti-EVD antibodies. The result was that the person who received the plasma with the anti-EVD antibodies also recovered from the disease. When artificial passive immunity is attempted using plasma, the blood type of the donor and the recipient must match.

RhoGAM. Artificially acquired passive immunity can also be used to prevent problems that are not related to infections. The primary example of this use is the

Memory Jogger

For some infectious organisms, such as influenza, there are many strains, each of which requires vaccination for immunologic protection.

Memory Jogger

Artificially acquired passive immunity through the transfer of antibodies from another person or animal provides only very short-term immunologic protection.

Memory Jogger

Artificially acquired passive immunity is indicated when people are known to have been exposed to deadly diseases and their vaccination status is not known or insufficient for protection.

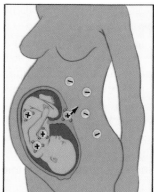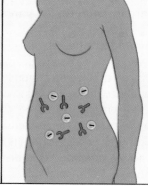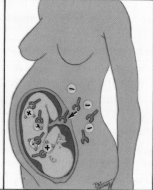

First pregnancy Rh− mother exposed to Rh+ agglutinogens.

After exposure, Rh− mother produces anti-Rh agglutinins.

Second pregnancy with Rh+ fetus. Anti-Rh agglutinins cause agglutination of fetal red blood cells.

FIGURE 11-5 How anti-Rh antibodies are generated during pregnancy with an Rh-negative mother and an Rh-positive fetus. (From Applegate, E. J. (2011). *The anatomy and physiology learning system* (4th ed.). St. Louis: Saunders.)

administration of RhoGAM (Rho D immunoglobulin) to a woman who is Rh-negative and has just given birth to an Rh-positive baby. In addition to the A, B, and O blood types, there is another protein type on some people's red blood cells (RBCs). This is the rhesus factor, most commonly known as the "Rh factor." People who have the gene for this factor have RBCs that are Rh-positive. People who do not have the gene for this factor do not have the Rh protein on their RBCs and are Rh-negative. If a person who is Rh-negative is exposed to RBCs that are Rh-positive, his or her immune system will start making anti-Rh antibodies to get rid of any Rh-positive cells.

Although maternal blood and fetal blood do not usually heavily mix during pregnancy, some of the fetus's RBCs do enter maternal circulation. This is most likely to happen during labor and delivery. If the mother is Rh-negative and the fetus is Rh-positive, the mother then starts to make anti-Rh antibodies. The first pregnancy usually does not result in many of these antibodies, and the first child is not affected. However, if the mother becomes pregnant again with another Rh-positive fetus, she makes many more anti-Rh antibodies that can cross the placenta and destroy that fetus's RBCs, which can cause major problems and death for the fetus or newborn. This problem is shown in Figure 11-5.

To prevent an Rh-negative mother's immune system from making large amounts anti-Rh antibodies, she is given a heavy dose very soon after delivery of these anti-Rh antibodies that were made in other people. These already made anti-Rh antibodies attack any remaining Rh-positive cells still circulating in the mother's blood so that her immune system cells do not have a chance to become sensitized to them and learn to make their own anti-Rh antibodies. Without the stimulation, there are few if any anti-Rh antibodies in the mother's blood during the next pregnancy so that fetus is safe from having its RBCs destroyed. To be effective, RhoGAM must be given to the Rh-negative mother (never to the Rh-positive infant) as soon as possible after delivery of every Rh-positive baby.

LIFE SPAN CONSIDERATIONS FOR VACCINATION

Pediatric Considerations

Although childhood is a time for extensive vaccination, it is also when the recommended schedules must be closely followed for best effect. Newborns have a very immature immune system and are not capable of forming a lot of antibodies at this time. This is why most vaccinations given before 6 months of age are administered as multiple doses over time. Another consideration is that a child who is sick with a viral or bacterial infection should not be vaccinated until he or she is well. This is because the child's immune system is busy making antibodies to the organism

Memory Jogger

Be sure to teach parents the importance of following the recommended schedule for all childhood vaccinations.

Memory Jogger

Urge pregnant women to receive seasonal influenza vaccination and the Tdap vaccination during every pregnancy.

Memory Jogger

Reactivation of the varicella zoster virus (VZV) is responsible for shingles.

Memory Jogger

Teach all older adults to follow the recommended schedules for vaccination and revaccination.

causing the sickness, and it may not be capable of generating sensitized B cells and antibodies to the organism(s) introduced with the vaccine.

Considerations for Pregnancy and Lactation

At one time women were not vaccinated during pregnancy. Although vaccination with immunization is best performed before pregnancy, some vaccinations can be safely administered during pregnancy.

The CDC recommends that live-virus vaccines be given at least 1 month before pregnancy and avoided during pregnancy. These include measles, mumps, rubella, polio, and chickenpox. Seasonal influenza vaccination is highly recommended during any stage of pregnancy. It is also recommended that during each pregnancy women receive the Tdap (tetanus, diphtheria, acellular pertussis) vaccination. Travel vaccination recommendations vary with the part of the world the pregnant woman expects to experience, the stage of the pregnancy, and the composition of the vaccine. A pregnant woman considering overseas travel should talk with her health care provider about vaccination safety.

Considerations for Older Adults

As a person ages, the efficiency of the immune system slowly declines. The function of already sensitized B cells is diminished and the person often does not have as many antibodies even to organisms that actually stimulated their naturally acquired active immunity. Thus older adults can become ill with diseases to which they once had immunologic protection. For example, many older adults develop "shingles," which is caused by the varicella zoster virus (VZV), the same one that causes chickenpox. However, shingles does not represent a new infection. It is a reactivation of the VZV that these people were infected with when they got chickenpox as children. The VZV stayed in their bodies and "hid out" in places where the immune system does not reach, such as the ganglia of sensory nerves. Of course, some of these VZV left those sites and went into other tissues where the person's anti-chickenpox (anti-VZV) antibodies trapped and eliminated them. As the person aged, there were fewer and fewer antibodies available to get rid of these old VZV. So when the VZV left the ganglia of sensory nerves, it traveled down the nerves and caused very painful outbreaks of shingles in the skin along the nerve tracts.

The point to this discussion is that we now know that both the naturally acquired active immunity and the artificially acquired active immunity for older adults diminishes, leaving them at least less immunologically protected and sometimes without immunologic protection. Revaccination (boosting) becomes more important with age. People over 90 years of age, sometimes called the "oldest old," are the fastest growing segment of the United States population. Many of these older adults are not aware of their loss of immunologic protection and the need for revaccination.

IMMUNOSUPPRESSIVE THERAPY

The immune system, which is protective most of the time, can overreact and cause tissue-damaging excessive responses. Some problems are acute and short term, such as a severe allergic reaction. Other problems, especially autoimmune disorders, can be chronic and very destructive. For either category of problem, therapy with **immunosuppressant drugs** that inhibit or prevent optimal functioning of the immune system may be used. Another use of immunosuppressant drugs is when the immune system is reacting normally but needs to be suppressed to reduce its normal function. This situation is most commonly associated with organ transplantation. There is nothing wrong with the immune system; however, its normal functions cause transplanted organs and tissues to be rejected. Immunosuppressive drugs are used to manage autoimmune diseases and to manage transplant rejection.

REVIEW OF RELATED PHYSIOLOGY AND PATHOPHYSIOLOGY

Autoimmune Disease

Autoimmune disease is a condition in which a person's immune system sees some of his or her own cells and tissues as "foreign" and develops immunity against these body cells or tissues. This inappropriate immunity involves lymphocyte responses and antibody formation against healthy normal cells and tissues. (Antibodies directed against self-tissues or cells are known as *autoantibodies*.) Sometimes these inappropriate immune reactions are triggered by infection or inflammation in the area, but the actual cause of autoimmune disease is not known. Immune system cells and products, such as antibodies, can form against one type of cells and cause problems only for specific tissue, organ, or system. A classic example of this type of selective autoimmune disease is myasthenia gravis in which the person makes antibodies against the acetylcholine receptor on muscle cells. As a result, transmission of nerve impulses to the skeletal muscles for contraction does not occur. Breathing and movement are impaired and can cause death if not continually managed.

Autoimmunity can also develop against a specific tissue component or multiple components that are present in many organs or tissues resulting in widespread problems or symptoms. An example of this type of autoimmunity is systemic lupus erythematosus (SLE) in which autoantibodies are produced against many cellular proteins and almost all organs are affected to some degree. Common autoimmune diseases include psoriasis, rheumatoid arthritis, polyarteritis nodosa, and Hashimoto thyroiditis. Other diseases, such as type 1 diabetes mellitus, may have multiple causes, one of which is autoimmune.

Management of autoimmunities depends on the organ or organs affected. For example, in type 1 diabetes, the person uses insulin to manage the disease and its complications, not drugs that alter the immune system. For other autoimmune diseases in which controlling the immune response is the best way to manage the disorder (e.g., rheumatoid arthritis, psoriasis), anti-inflammatory drugs and immunosuppressive drugs are commonly used to suppress the excess immune responses.

 Memory Jogger

Autoimmunity represents a failure of the immune system to recognize a person's normal cells as "self" and treats these cells as if they were foreign invaders.

Transplantation Immunology

For many decades it has been possible to remove a diseased or nonfunctioning organ from one patient (recipient) and surgically replace it with a healthy organ from another person (donor). The success of this type of therapy was limited because the recipient's immune system recognized the newly transplanted organ as "foreign" even though the new organ's function could save the recipient's life. The T cells and some other leukocytes were mainly responsible for attacking and destroying transplanted organs. Successful transplantation required that the recipient's immune system be suppressed to prevent his or her body from rejecting and destroying the transplanted organ. Some of the original drugs used to prevent transplant rejection caused such profound immunosuppression that recipients often died from infection. Newer antirejection drugs now work on *selective immunosuppression*, suppressing only the immune system cells most responsible for transplant rejection, placing the recipient at less risk for developing overwhelming infection.

Acute rejection is the most common type of rejection in transplanted organs. It first usually occurs within 1 to 12 weeks after transplantation and may recur intermittently for years. Two pathologic mechanisms are responsible. The first mechanism is antibody mediated and results in vasculitis and blood vessel necrosis within the transplanted organ and leads to organ destruction. In the second mechanism, certain types of the recipient's T cells enter the new organ and start inflammatory responses that eventually destroy the organ cells.

An episode of acute rejection after solid organ transplantation does not automatically mean that the patient will lose the new organ. Drug management of the recipient's immune responses at this time may limit the damage to the organ and allow it to continue to function.

General drug therapy to prevent solid organ rejection is lifelong and uses combination drug therapy. These drugs do suppress the immune system to some degree,

Memory Jogger

The four types of immunosuppressant drugs are:
- Corticosteroids
- Disease-modifying antirheumatic drugs
- Cytotoxic drugs
- Selective immunosuppressants

and the dosage must be adjusted to the immune response of each patient. **Antirejection drugs** are used to suppress the components of the immune system responsible for rejection of transplanted tissues and organs.

TYPES OF IMMUNOSUPPRESSANT DRUGS

Corticosteroids

Corticosteroids are drugs similar to natural cortisol that suppress bone marrow production of all white blood cells (WBCs) and inhibit immune responses as well as inflammation. Because the corticosteroids cause such a general immunosuppression and can greatly increase the patient's risk for infection, they now are used more sparingly than in years past. Although listed in this chapter, see Chapter 6 for a full discussion of the actions, side effects, and other issues related to immunosuppressive therapy with corticosteroids.

Disease-Modifying Antirheumatic Drugs

Disease-modifying antirheumatic drugs (DMARDs) are drugs that reduce the progression and tissue destruction of the inflammatory disease process by inhibiting tumor necrosis factor (TNF). Although sometimes considered general immunosuppressant agents, they most specifically target the immune cellular product TNF. This product is made by inflammatory cells and by some lymphocytes. DMARDs are used to treat many different types of autoimmune disorders, such as rheumatoid arthritis, ankylosing spondylitis, psoriasis, psoriatic arthritis, Crohn disease, and ulcerative colitis. See Chapter 6 for a full discussion of the actions, side effects, and other issues related to immunosuppressive therapy with DMARDs.

Cytotoxic Drugs

Cytotoxic drugs are those with actions that purposely destroy cells. They are used most commonly as cancer chemotherapy with the intent of killing off cancer cells. Because any dividing cells are more sensitive to the killing effects of these drugs, normal cells such as bone marrow cells are suppressed. For this action, cytotoxic drugs such as methotrexate and cyclophosphamide have been used to suppress the excess immunity experienced by patients with various autoimmune diseases. However, even when given at lower doses than those used for cancer chemotherapy, these drugs have many harmful side effects and can lead to profound general immunosuppression. With the development of more specific immunosuppressant drugs, cytotoxic therapy now has a much smaller role in immunosuppressive therapy. See Chapter 12 for more discussion of the actions, side effects, and other issues related to cytotoxic drug therapy.

Selective Immunosuppressants

Selective immunosuppressants are drugs that more selectively target the immune system cells and products responsible for autoimmune diseases and transplant rejection. They are less likely to cause profound generalized immune suppression. Drug categories for selective immunosuppressants include antiproliferatives, calcineurin inhibitors, monoclonal antibodies, and polyclonal antibodies. For autoimmune diseases, selective immunosuppressants may be used as single agent therapy. When used for transplant rejection, most selective immunosuppressants are given as combination therapy that includes a corticosteroid, an antiproliferative, and a calcineurin inhibitor. During acute episodes of transplant rejection, higher doses of the drugs in this combination are used. The monoclonal antibodies and the polyclonal antibodies are used only during acute rejection episodes. These drugs are not approved for use as therapy for autoimmune diseases.

How Selective Immunosuppressants Work. Antiproliferative drugs slow the growth of immune system cells responsible for autoimmune diseases and for transplant rejection in several ways. Azathioprine, although somewhat less selective than other antiproliferatives, inhibits the metabolism of purines, which are important in

Memory Jogger

The four categories of selective immunosuppressants are:
- Antiproliferatives
- Calcineurin inhibitors
- Monoclonal antibodies
- Polyclonal antibodies

DNA synthesis and cell division. It suppresses the actions of T cells, which are cytotoxic to transplanted organs and cause tissue damage in some autoimmune diseases.

Mycophenolate is more selective in suppressing lymphocyte activity, both T cells and B cells. This drug reversibly inhibits an enzyme needed for lymphocyte reproduction. It also prevents T cells already present from being active. Both actions selectively suppress the immune responses most associated with autoimmune tissue destruction and transplant rejection.

Sirolimus selectively inhibits T-cell activation and reproduction by blocking the signal transduction pathways, especially mTOR, that promote movement of T cells through the cell cycle for cell division. This drug also interferes with the ability of B cells to mature into antibody-producing cells. The overall amount of antibodies produced, including the ones that attack and destroy self-cells, is significantly reduced.

Everolimus acts in a similar way to sirolimus. It also inhibits the mTOR pathway important to cell division and proliferation in lymphocytes. This drug greatly reduces protein synthesis and cell division in immune system cells that attack self-cells and those that attack cells of transplanted organs. Like some of the other antiproliferatives, it does have some effect against certain cancer cells.

Calcineurin inhibitors work to prevent the first phase of T-cell activation by binding to protein and forming a complex that inhibits calcineurin present in some immune system cells. Calcineurin normally promotes the expression of genes that allow T cells both to divide and to be activated. With less calcineurin around, T-cell activation and cell division are significantly reduced, resulting in less damage to transplanted tissues and organs. The two drugs in this class are cyclosporine and tacrolimus.

Monoclonal antibodies are antibodies produced by mouse cells or a combination of mouse and human antibody-producing cells against a protein found on the surface of all human T cells. Once these antibodies have bound to their target, they stop all T-cell functions, including those that attack transplanted tissues and organs. These drugs do not have any effect on other types of immune system cells. They must be administered intravenously. One drug produced using only mouse cells, monomurab-CD3, is no longer manufactured, but facilities that have a supply of the drug are permitted to continue to use it. For the drugs that are made as a result of recombinant technology using mouse/human cell hybrids (basiliximab and daclizumab), the drug targets only a receptor on activated T cells. Thus these are the most specific immunosuppressants and are very effective at initially preventing acute transplant rejection.

Polyclonal antibodies are antibodies directed against human T cells. These antibodies are produced by other animals (horses and rabbits) in response to the administration of human white blood cells, especially T cells. They are very effective in attacking and eliminating human T cells and can lead to a profound immunosuppression. Their use is now confined to times when a person is having an acute rejection episode after kidney transplantation that does not respond to other types of immunosuppressive therapy.

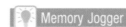 **Memory Jogger**

Monoclonal antibodies are used short term for prevention of transplant rejection, and polyclonal antibodies are used short term as treatment for an acute rejection episode that does not respond to other types of immunosuppressive therapy.

Dosages for Selective Immunosuppressant Drugs

Drug Class	Drug Examples	Dosage
Antiproliferatives	azathioprine (Azasan, Imuran)	*Adults:* 1-5 mg/kg orally once daily or 1-1.5 g intravenous (IV) *Children:* 1-2 mg/kg orally once daily
	mycophenolate (CellCept, Myfortic)	*For Autoimmune Disease:* *Adults:* 250 mg to 2 g orally daily *Children:* 15-25 mg/kg orally twice daily *For Transplant Rejection Prevention* *Adults:* 1.5 g orally twice daily or 1.5 g IV twice daily *Children:* 600 mg/m² orally twice daily

Continued

Dosages for Selective Immunosuppressant Drugs—cont'd

Drug Class	Drug Examples	Dosage
	sirolimus (Rapamune)	*For Transplant Rejection Prevention*
		Adults and children weighing more than 40 kg: 6 mg orally loading dose followed by 2 mg orally once daily for maintenance
		Children weighing less than 40 kg: 3 mg/m² orally as a loading dose followed by 1 mg/m² orally once daily for maintenance
	everolimus (Zortress)	*For Kidney Transplant Rejection Prevention*
		Adults: 0.75 mg orally every 12 hours initially. Dosages adjust according to patient responses.
		Children: Safety and efficacy have not been established.
		For Liver Transplant Rejection Prevention
		Adults: 1 mg orally twice daily initially
		Children: Safety and efficacy have not been established.
Calcineurin inhibitors	cyclosporine (Neoral, Gengraf, Sandimmune)	*For Autoimmune Disease*
		Adults: 1.25 mg/kg orally twice daily
		Children: 50 mg/m² orally twice daily
		For Transplant Rejection Prevention
		Adults and Children: 4-8 mg/kg orally twice daily initially
	tacrolimus (Astagraf XL, HECORIA, Prograf)	*Adults:* Immediate-release capsules, 0.1 mg/kg orally every 12 hours; extended-release capsules, 0.2 mg/kg orally once daily
Monoclonal antibodies	muromonab-CD3 (Orthoclone OKT3)	*Adults and children weighing 30 kg or more:* 5 mg IV once daily for 10-14 days
		Children weighing less than 30 kg: 2.5 mg IV once daily for 10-14 days
	basiliximab (Simulect)	*Adults and children weighing 35 kg or more:* 20 mg IV within 2 hours before transplant surgery and 20 mg IV 4 days after transplantation
		Children weighing less than 35 kg: 10 mg IV within 2 hours before transplant surgery and 10 mg IV 4 days after transplantation
	daclizumab (Zenapax)	*Adults and children older than 11 months:* 1 mg/kg IV within the 24 hours before transplantation, followed by 4 more doses of 1 mg/kg IV once every 2 weeks
Polyclonal antibodies	antithymocyte globulin-equine (Atgam)	*For Treatment of Acute Kidney or Heart Transplant Rejection*
		Adults: 10-15 mg/kg IV daily for 14 days
		Children: 5-25 mg/kg IV daily for 8-14 days
	antithymocyte globulin-rabbit (RATG, Thymoglobulin)	*For Treatment of Acute Kidney or Heart Transplant Rejection*
		Adults: 1.5 mg/kg IV daily for 7-14 days

Intended Responses
- Immune-mediated tissue damaging actions slow or stop
- Manifestations of autoimmune disease are reduced
- Transplanted organs continue normal function
- The patient retains enough immune function to prevent serious infections

Side Effects. All selective immunosuppressants cause some degree of immunosuppression and place the patient at increased risk for infection. Most of these drugs are not given to a patient who has a systemic infection. Because some immune system cell numbers are reduced, the symptoms of infection may not be obvious.

Side effects of the selective immunosuppressants drugs are varied. The most common side effects for all of these drugs are gastrointestinal disturbances of all types and a variety of skin rashes. Sirolimus and everolimus elevate serum cholesterol levels.

The most common side effects of the calcineurin inhibitors are hypertension, elevated serum cholesterol levels, and hyperglycemia. Cyclosporine also causes many patients to have gingival (gum) hyperplasia.

Adverse Effects. In addition to the risk for serious bacterial and fungal infections, all selective immunosuppressants increase the risk for cancer development. This problem is thought to be related to reduced immunosurveillance by loss of immune system cell recognition when normal cells transform to cancer cells. The risk is higher for the drugs that are taken long term, including the antiproliferatives and the calcineurin inhibitors.

Adverse effects of these drugs vary by their mechanism of action. The antiproliferatives and the calcineurin inhibitors can cause liver toxicity and liver failure. Intravenous antiproliferatives increase the risk for phlebitis and thrombosis at the administration site.

Most antiproliferatives, the calcineurin inhibitors, and basiliximab are associated with electrolyte imbalances, especially of potassium, phosphorus, and magnesium.

Although serious allergic responses and anaphylaxis are possible with the use of any selective immunosuppressants, the risk for these problems is much higher for patients receiving monoclonal antibodies and very high for patients receiving polyclonal antibodies. Proteins from other species (e.g., mouse, horse, rabbit) are present in these formulations and can trigger severe reactions.

What To Do Before Giving Selective Immunosuppressants. Precautions are needed when mixing or handling antiproliferative drugs. These drugs can be absorbed through skin and mucous membranes and exert effects on those preparing them. Use personal protective equipment (PPE) when preparing and administering these drugs to prevent accidental exposure. See Chapter 12 for more information on PPE.

Obtain a list of all other drugs that the patient takes because most selective immunosuppressants interact with many other drugs. Check with the pharmacist for possible interactions and the need to consult the prescriber about dosage or changing the patient's other drugs.

Because many selective immunosuppressants can lead to liver toxicity, make sure that the patient does not have a liver problem before starting these drugs. Check the patient's most recent laboratory values for liver problems (elevated liver enzyme levels). (See Table 1-3 in Chapter 1 for a listing of normal values.)

For all intravenous (IV) formulations, mix only with the manufacturer recommended diluent. Do not mix or administer with other IV medications, and do not administer other drugs through the same IV line used for immunosuppressant therapy.

Before giving monoclonal antibodies, ask patients whether they have any known allergies to mouse proteins. (Although these drugs contain more human antibody parts than mouse, mouse proteins are still present and can cause severe allergic reactions.)

Check to see whether any drugs for premedication have been ordered to be administered before giving either monoclonal antibodies or polyclonal antibodies. Ensure that emergency equipment is close at hand in case of severe allergic reactions or anaphylaxis.

What To Do After Giving Selective Immunosuppressants. All patients taking or receiving any selective immunosuppressant should have regular monitoring of blood cell counts with a complete blood cell count (CBC). Assess CBCs and report abnormalities to the prescriber.

Memory Jogger

Monoclonal antibodies and polyclonal antibodies are more likely, especially polyclonal antibodies, to trigger a serious hypersensitivity reaction and anaphylaxis.

Drug Alert!

Action/Intervention Alert

Always use personal protective equipment when mixing or administering selective immunosuppressants to prevent accidental exposure.

QSEN: Safety

Drug Alert!

Interaction Alert

Before giving selective immunosuppressants, ask the patient about all other drugs or supplements that he or she takes and then check with the pharmacist to avoid a possible drug interaction.

QSEN: Safety

Drug Alert!

Administration Alert

Check to see whether any drugs for premedication have been ordered to be administered before giving either monoclonal antibodies or polyclonal antibodies. Ensure that emergency equipment is close at hand in case of severe allergic reactions or anaphylaxis.

QSEN: Safety

Monitor patients closely during infusions of any parenteral selective immunosuppressant but especially the monoclonal antibodies and polyclonal antibodies for severe allergic (hypersensitivity) reactions and anaphylaxis. If signs or symptoms of hypersensitivity occur, stop the infusion immediately and notify the Rapid Response Team. Be sure to document the reaction because the patient should never receive the offending drug again.

Check the patient daily for yellowing of the skin or sclera *(jaundice)*, which is a symptom of liver problems. The best places to check are the whites of the eyes closest to the iris, the roof of the mouth, and the skin of the chest.

Monitor electrolyte values, especially potassium, phosphorus, and magnesium. Report abnormal electrolytes to the prescriber.

Assess the IV site during and after infusions for signs of phlebitis, thrombosis, or irritation.

What To Teach *Patients Receiving Selective Immunosuppressants.* Teach patients taking or receiving any selective immunosuppressants the common signs and symptoms of infection. Stress to them the importance of immediately reporting any indication of infection to the prescriber. Remind them to check with their prescriber for which types of vaccinations they should receive. Also remind them to keep all appointments for monitoring of blood counts and other laboratory tests.

Teach patients receiving selective immunosuppressant drugs the importance of taking their drugs exactly as prescribed to maintain the effectiveness in reducing symptoms of autoimmune disease or preventing transplant rejection. Even a few missed doses can lead to tissue damaging responses and transplant rejection episodes.

Tell patients to notify the prescriber if they develop yellowing of the skin or eyes, darkening of the urine, or lightening of the stools. These problems are signs of liver toxicity, a serious adverse effect of these drugs. Also warn patients to avoid drinking alcohol or using acetaminophen while taking these drugs.

Teach patients taking oral capsules not to crush or open the capsules and to drink a full glass of water with the drug.

For patients taking the oral suspensions of sirolimus or cyclosporine, teach them to mix the drug exactly as directed, using the recommended solution (milk, orange juice, apple juice), NOT WATER. After drinking the suspension, they must rinse the container with the same solution and drink the rinse for better drug effectiveness. In addition, cyclosporine must be mixed in a glass container, not a plastic one. When a patient is prescribed to take both sirolimus and cyclosporine, teach him or her to separate the drug dosages by at least 4 hours.

Teach patients taking oral sirolimus or tacrolimus not to take the drug with grapefruit juice.

Warn patients not to take other drugs or supplements without checking with the prescriber because the antiproliferatives and calcineurin inhibitors interact with so many other drugs.

Life Span Considerations for Selective Immunosuppressants

Considerations for Pregnancy and Lactation. All antiproliferatives are associated with poor pregnancy outcomes. Pregnancy is an absolute contraindication for the use of these drugs. It is recommended that sexually active women in childbearing years use two reliable methods of contraception during therapy with these drugs and for 12 weeks after they are discontinued. Breastfeeding while on these drugs is also contraindicated.

The calcineurin inhibitors, the monoclonal antibodies, and the polyclonal antibodies have a moderate to high likelihood of increasing the risk for birth defects or fetal damage. Therefore the use of any of these drugs during pregnancy and lactation is not recommended. For episodes of acute transplant rejection, their use during pregnancy must be assessed for each patient individually.

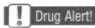

Drug Alert!

Teaching Alert

Teach patients the importance of taking their drugs exactly as prescribed to maintain the effectiveness of the drugs.

QSEN: Safety

Drug Alert!

Teaching Alert

Teach sexually active women in childbearing years taking antiproliferative drugs to use two reliable methods of contraception during therapy with these drugs and for 12 weeks after they are discontinued.

QSEN: Safety

Get Ready for Practice!

Key Points

- Inflammation helps protect the body from infection but cannot provide true immunity to any specific disease-causing microorganism.
- Antibody-mediated immunity (also known as *humoral immunity*) can be transferred from one person or animal to another.
- Antibodies transferred from one person into another person have a short-term effect.
- The four types of vaccines currently available are inactivated vaccines, attenuated vaccines, toxoids, and biosynthetic vaccines.
- Natural, active immunity is the most beneficial and long-lasting type of immunity.
- Vaccinations cause artificial active immunity and require "boosting" for best long-term effects.
- For some infectious organisms, such as influenza, there are many strains, each of which requires vaccination for immunologic protection.
- Artificially acquired passive immunity is indicated when people are known to have been exposed to deadly diseases and their vaccination status is not known or insufficient for protection.
- Urge pregnant women to receive seasonal influenza vaccination and the Tdap vaccination during every pregnancy.
- Reactivation of the virus that causes chickenpox (varicella zoster virus [VZV]) is responsible for shingles.
- Artificially acquired active immunity is used to help people develop immunity to a dangerous disease without the risk for becoming sick first.
- A person's normal membrane proteins would be antigens in another person.
- Autoimmunity represents a failure of the immune system to recognize a person's normal cells as "self" and treats these cells as if they were foreign invaders.
- Transplant rejection is a normal response of the immune system that can damage or destroy the transplanted organ.
- Patients who receive transplanted organs (unless from an identical sibling) need to take immunosuppressive drugs daily to prevent transplant rejection.
- Patients who take immunosuppressive drugs have an increased risk for infection and cancer development.
- Monoclonal and polyclonal antibodies contain some proteins from other animal species and are more likely to cause severe allergic reactions and anaphylaxis.
- Before giving any selective immunosuppressant drug, ask the patient about all other drugs or supplements that he or she takes and then check with the pharmacist to avoid a possible drug interaction.
- Always use personal protective equipment when mixing or administering selective immunosuppressants to prevent accidental exposure.
- Teach sexually active women in childbearing years taking antiproliferative drugs to use two reliable methods of contraception during therapy with these drugs and for 12 weeks after they are discontinued.

Additional Learning Resources

evolve Be sure to visit your Evolve website (http://evolve.elsevier.com/Workman/pharmacology/) for additional online resources.

SG Go to your Study Guide for additional learning activities to help you master this chapter content.

Review Questions

See the Answer Keys—In-text Review Questions for answers to these questions.

Test Yourself on the Basics

1. What does a sensitized B cell produce when it is stimulated with exposure to a foreign invader?
   A. Antigen
   B. Antibody
   C. Vaccine
   D. Toxin
2. What type of white blood cell (leukocyte) provides true immunity?
   A. Eosinophil
   B. Lymphocyte
   C. Macrophage
   D. Neutrophil
3. Which statement about artificially acquired passive immunity is true?
   A. It can be transferred from one person to another.
   B. It is the longest-lasting type of immunity.
   C. It requires "boosting" on a regular schedule.
   D. It is present in adults but not in children or teenagers.
4. Which vaccination uses a toxoid rather than a killed vaccine or an attenuated vaccine to stimulate immunity?
   A. Polio
   B. Measles
   C. Tetanus
   D. Hepatitis A
5. What is the desired response of successful vaccination?
   A. Inactivation of dangerous toxoids produced by certain disease-causing viruses
   B. Immunization with immune resistance to the substance in the vaccine
   C. B cells convert to T cells that are better able to recognize invading microorganisms
   D. Development of generalized protective inflammatory responses and innate immunity
6. Which antirejection drug belongs to the calcineurin inhibitor class?
   A. Azathioprine (Imuran)
   B. Basiliximab (Simulect)
   C. Cortisol (Prednisone)
   D. Tacrolimus (Prograf)

7. What category of selective immunosuppressant drugs is most likely to trigger a severe allergic reaction or anaphylaxis?
   A. Antiproliferatives
   B. Calcineurin inhibitors
   C. Monoclonal antibodies
   D. Polyclonal antibodies

8. What is the immunologic outcome of autoimmune disease?
   A. The person is more at risk for infection.
   B. The person is a risk for tissue damage from inappropriate immune responses.
   C. The person is unlikely to develop a fever even when serious infection is present.
   D. The person will be unable to generate specific antibodies in response to a vaccination.

Test Yourself on Advanced Concepts

9. A 75-year-old woman tells you that she is afraid she will get shingles if she visits her older sister who has shingles. What is your best response?
   A. "You can only get shingles from the virus left in your body from when you had the chickenpox."
   B. "Shingles and chickenpox are caused by the same virus. So if you have already had chickenpox, you are immune to shingles."
   C. "Yes, shingles is a highly contagious disease and is easily transmitted from one person to another by air droplets."
   D. "Have you ever had shingles? Because once you have shingles, you will never get sick with it again."

10. A patient who has many serious health problems has just been exposed heavily to hepatitis B. Because this person may not survive an infection at this time, he is given human immunoglobulin with a high concentration of antihepatitis antibodies. What type of immunity will result from this intervention?
    A. Artificially acquired active immunity
    B. Artificially acquired passive immunity
    C. Naturally acquired active immunity
    D. Naturally acquired passive immunity

11. Why is antibody-mediated immunity considered to be a type of "adaptive" immunity?
    A. The immune system adapts to the presence of specific invaders or antigens by making specific antibodies against those invaders or antigens.
    B. The antibody-making cells are more resistant to environmental attacks on the immune system than are the cells involved in innate immunity.
    C. The immune system is able to adapt to the severity of infection by matching the number of neutrophils and other white blood cells generated with the number of organisms causing the infection.
    D. After childhood, the immune system adapts the rate of leukocyte production with the rate of leukocyte destruction to maintain a "steady-state" or constant number of white blood cells for maximum infection protection.

12. Why does artificially acquired passive immunity have such a short duration of effectiveness?
    A. Because antibodies are made of protein, they are digested and excreted by the intestinal tract within a week to 10 days.
    B. Antibodies made by another person or animal are viewed as a foreign invader by the recipient's immune system.
    C. This type of immunity requires constant "boosting" to maintain normal levels of antibody production.
    D. It can be easily overwhelmed when invading microorganisms reproduce rapidly.

13. Which mother should receive RhoGAM?
    A. An Rh-positive mother who just delivered an Rh-negative infant
    B. An Rh-positive mother who just delivered an Rh-positive infant
    C. An Rh-negative mother who just delivered an Rh-negative infant
    D. An Rh-negative mother who just delivered an Rh-positive infant

14. Which immunizations are recommended for pregnant women to receive during each pregnancy? Select all that apply.
    A. Diphtheria
    B. Hepatitis B
    C. Human papilloma virus
    D. Pertussis
    E. Polio
    F. Measles
    G. Seasonal influenza
    H. Tetanus

15. The patient who received basiliximab (Simulect) just before and on the fourth day after his kidney transplant asks how long he will have to take the prescribed oral mycophenolate (CellCept). What is your best response?
    A. "Because acute rejection is most common during the first 12 weeks after transplantation, you can stop the drug after 3 months."
    B. "We will monitor your white blood cell count and when lymphocytes remain lower than normal for a year, we will discontinue the drug."
    C. "Because you will be at an increased risk for infection, you will need to continue taking this drug for the rest of your life."
    D. "Because this drug prevents rejection, you will need to take the drug as long as the new kidney continues to function."

16. A patient is prescribed a daily dose of azathioprine (Imuran) of 2 mg/kg orally daily. The patient weighs 165 lb.
    What is the patient's weight in kg?_____
    What is the correct dose?_____
    The drug is available in a 50-mg scored tablet. How many tablets will you give?_____

Critical Thinking Activities

See the Answer Keys—Critical Thinking Activities for answers to these activities.

Two months after a kidney transplant, a patient returns and has an acute rejection episode. He says, "I was doing so well with my new kidney and the thought of having to go back to getting hemodialysis treatments 3 days each week is depressing. I took my medicine every day, although I did have some trouble trying to remember to rinse the container of Neoral after I took it and then drink the rinse."

1. Is this patient correct in assuming that the transplanted kidney will not work anymore and that dialysis will again be necessary? Provide a rationale for your response.
2. What is the generic name of the drug Neoral?
3. What kind of drug is it?
4. What will you tell this patient about taking this drug the correct way and "drinking the rinse"?
5. What drug or drugs do you believe this patient will have to take during an acute rejection episode and why?

Objectives

After studying this chapter you should be able to:

1. Explain how normal cells become cancer cells and what features cancer cells have.
2. Explain the basis for combination chemotherapy for cancer.
3. List the common side effects of cancer chemotherapy.
4. Describe how to manage and document an episode of extravasation.
5. Explain the rationale for hormone manipulation therapy.
6. Discuss the uses of biological response modifiers as supportive therapy in the treatment of cancer.
7. Explain the basis of targeted therapy for cancer.

Key Terms

alkylating agents (ĂL-k-lā-tĭng Ā-jěnts) (p. 197) Cytotoxic drugs that cross-link DNA, making the two DNA strands bind tightly together, which prevents proper DNA and RNA synthesis and inhibits cell division.

angiogenesis inhibitors (ăn-jē-ō-JĔN-ĭ-sŭs ĭn-HĬB-ĭ-tŭrz) (p. 204) A type of targeted therapy that inhibits the activity of the mammalian target of rapamycin (mTOR), which then reduces blood vessel growth in cancer cells and disrupts many pro–cell division signal transduction pathways.

antimetabolites (ăn-tĭ-mĕ-TĂB-ō-līts) (p. 195) Cytotoxic drugs similar to normal metabolites needed for vital cell processes that act as counterfeit metabolites and impair cell division.

antimitotic agents (ăn-tĭ-mī-ŏ-tĭk Ā-jěnts) (p. 197) Cytotoxic drugs that interfere with the formation of tubules so cells cannot separate during cell division.

antitumor antibiotics (ăn-tĭ-TOO-měr) (p. 195) Cytotoxic drugs that damage the DNA of the cell and interrupt DNA or RNA synthesis.

cancer (KĂN-sŭr) (p. 193) Abnormal cell growth that serves no useful purpose, is invasive, and without intervention would lead to death. Also known as *malignancy*.

carcinogen (kăr-SĬN-ō-jěn) (p. 194) Any substance or event that can damage the DNA of a normal cell and cause cancer development.

cytotoxic effects (sī-tō-TŎKS-ĭk ĕf-FĔKTS) (p. 195) Cell-damaging and cell-killing effects.

epithelial growth factor receptor inhibitors (EGFRIs) (ĕ-pĭ-THĒL-ē-ăl GRŌTH FĂK-tŭr rē-SĔP-tŭr ĭn-HĬB-ĭ-tŭrz) (p. 204) A type of targeted therapy drugs that binds to and blocks the epidermal growth factor receptors on some types of cancer cells, slowing the growth of cancers that are dependent on the growth factor.

extravasation (ĕks-trăv-ĕ-SĀ-shŭn) (p. 198) Leakage of an irritating chemotherapy drug into the tissues surrounding the vein used to infuse the drug, leading to tissue damage.

miscellaneous chemotherapy drugs (kē-mō-THĔR-ă-pē DRŬGZ) (p. 197) Cytotoxic drugs with mechanisms of action that are either unknown or do not fit those of other chemotherapy drug categories.

multikinase inhibitors (MKIs) (măl-tĭk-ĭ-nās ĭn-HĬB-ĭ-tŭrz) (p. 204) A type of targeted therapy that inhibits the activity of specific kinase enzymes in cancer cells, preventing the activation of transcription factors.

proteasome inhibitors (PRŌ-tē-ă-sōm ĭn-HĬB-ĭ-tŭrz) (p. 204) A type of targeted therapy that prevents the formation of a large complex of proteins (a proteasome) in cancer cells, which slows or stops their growth.

targeted therapy (TĂR-gĕt-ĕd THĔR-ă-pē) (p. 202) A group of drugs for cancer treatment that takes advantage of one or more differences in cancer cell growth or metabolism that either are not present or are less common in normal cells.

topoisomerase inhibitors (tō-PŌ-ĭ-SŎM-ĕr-āz ĭn-HĬB-ĭ-tŭrz) (p. 197) Cytotoxic drugs that disrupt an enzyme (topoisomerase) needed for DNA synthesis and cell division, which causes DNA breakage and cell death.

tyrosine kinase inhibitor (TKI) (TĪ-rō-sēn KĪ-nāz ĭn-HĬB-ĭ-tŭr) (p. 204) A type of targeted therapy drug that inhibits the enzyme tyrosine kinase and slows or stops the cancer cell from dividing.

vascular endothelial growth factor receptor inhibitor (VEGFRI) (văs-KYOO-lăr ĕn-dō-THĒL-ē-ăl GRŌTH FĂK-tŭr ĭn-HĬB-ĭ-tŭr) (p. 204) A type of targeted therapy drug that binds to and blocks the vascular endothelial growth factor receptors, which results in a reduced blood supply to the tumor.

vesicants (p. 198) Drugs and chemicals that cause tissue damage on direct contact.

REVIEW OF RELATED PHYSIOLOGY AND PATHOPHYSIOLOGY

Cancer is abnormal cell growth that serves no useful purpose, is invasive, and without intervention would lead to death. Cancer is a common health problem in North America, with more than 1.8 million people being newly diagnosed each year.

Growth of cells and tissues is expected during infancy and childhood, and many body cells continue to grow to replace damaged or dead cells long after maturation is complete. This growth is well controlled, ensuring that the right number of cells is always present in any tissue or organ.

Neoplasia is any new or continued cell growth not needed for normal development or replacement of dead and damaged tissues. Whether the new cells form tumors that are benign (grow by expansion rather than invasion and do not spread) or cancerous, neoplastic cells develop from normal cells. Thus cancer cells were once normal cells but changed to no longer look, grow, or function normally. The strict genetic processes controlling normal growth and function have been lost. *All cells or tumors designated as cancer are malignant and, with the exception of two types of skin cancer, would eventually lead to death if left untreated.*

Normal cells divide *(undergo mitosis)* for only two reasons: to develop normal tissue or replace lost or damaged tissue. Cell division *(mitosis)* occurs in the well-recognized pattern described by the cell cycle (Figure 12-1).

- **G_1:** The cell prepares for division by taking on extra nutrients, making more energy, increasing fluid, and growing a larger membrane.
- **S:** Making one cell into two cells requires twice as much of everything, including DNA in the nucleus. In the S phase the cell must double its DNA content through DNA synthesis.
- **G_2:** The cell makes important proteins that will be used in actual cell division and in normal physiologic function after cell division is complete.
- **M:** The single cell splits apart into two cells (actual mitosis).

In mitosis one cell divides into two cells that are identical to each other and to the original cell that started the mitosis. The steps of entering and completing the cell cycle are tightly controlled by proteins produced by *suppressor genes*. These proteins are the "brakes" of the cell division process.

Control of whether a cell enters the cell cycle and completes the cycle to form two new cells depends on the presence and absence of specific proteins known as *cyclins*. When cyclins are activated, they first allow a cell to leave the G_0 state and enter the cycle. These activated cyclins then permit the cell to move through the different phases of the cell cycle and actually divide. The cyclins are the products of *oncogenes* and can be considered the "gas pedal" of the cell division process. Suppressor gene products regulate the amount of cyclins present in a cell and ensure that cell division occurs only when it is needed. So normal cell division represents a balance between the proteins that promote cell division (cyclins) and those that limit cell division (suppressor gene products).

CANCER CELLS

Body cells are exposed to internal and external conditions that can damage genes and change how the cells grow or function. When either cell growth or cell function is changed, the cells are abnormal. Table 12-1 compares features of normal cells and cancer cells.

Although cancer cells were once normal cells, they have undergone genetic changes that result in loss of control over cell division. These cells generally have continuous cell division and reenter the cell cycle for mitosis almost as soon as they leave it. They also may divide more quickly than normal cells and do not respond to signals for normal cell death. As a result, cancer cells have an unlimited life span (are "immortal"). Because these cells have poor growth control and do not respect tissue borders, they overgrow and spread *(metastasize)* into other body areas. This invasion can damage important organs, often leading to death. Cancer cells invade

 Memory Jogger

Cancer cells were once normal cells that lost the strict control processes for normal growth and function.

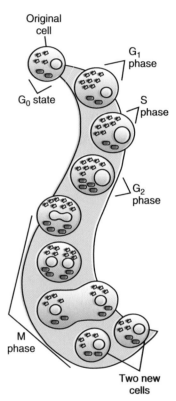

FIGURE 12-1 Activities inside the cell during different phases of the cell cycle. The yellow circle is the nucleus.

 Memory Jogger

Genes that make proteins to promote cell division are oncogenes. Genes that make proteins to control cell division are suppressor genes.

Table 12-1 Features of Normal and Cancer Cells

CHARACTERISTIC	NORMAL CELLS	CANCER CELLS
Cell division	None or slow	Rapid, continuous
Appearance	Specific features	Anaplastic, no identifying appearance, small and round
Differentiated functions	Many	Some or none
Adherence	Tight	Loose
Migratory	No	Yes
Growth	Well regulated	Unregulated, invasive

tissues both near and far away from the original tumor. Invasion and persistent growth make untreated cancer deadly.

CANCER DEVELOPMENT

The multistep process of changing a normal cell into a cancer cell is called *malignant transformation* or *carcinogenesis*. The first step in cancer development is damage to the genes controlling cell division *(suppressor genes)*, which then allows the genes promoting cell growth *(oncogenes)* to be activated. **Carcinogens** are substances or events that can damage normal cell genes and cause cancer development. They may be chemicals, physical agents, or viruses.

The original site in which normal cells develop into cancer is called the *primary tumor*. It is identified by the tissue from which it arose (parent tissue) such as breast or lung cancer. When primary tumors are located in vital organs such as the brain or lungs, they grow excessively and damage the vital organ so it cannot perform vital functions; death follows if left untreated. Metastasis occurs when cancer cells move from the primary location by breaking off from the original group and establishing new tumors in remote areas.

Tumors that have spread and formed new tumors elsewhere are called *metastatic* or *secondary tumors*. Even though the tumor is now in another organ, it is still a cancer from the original altered tissue. For example, when breast cancer spreads to the lung and bone, it is breast cancer in the lung and bone, not lung cancer and not bone cancer.

CANCER CAUSES

Cancer development takes years and depends on several tumor and patient factors. Three interacting factors influence cancer development: exposure to carcinogens, genetic predisposition, and immune function.

Oncogene activation resulting from suppressor gene inactivation is the main mechanism of carcinogenesis, regardless of the specific cause. When activated, these genes produce proteins (cyclins) that promote cell division. Oncogenes are controlled by the products of suppressor genes. When a normal cell is exposed to any carcinogen, the DNA in the genes controlling normal cell can be damaged or mutated, preventing them from controlling the activity of oncogenes. As a result, the oncogenes are overactive, and excessive growth occurs, causing the cells to change from normal to cancerous.

Personal and external factors increase the risk for cancer development. External factors, including environmental exposure, are responsible for about 80% of cancer development. Environmental carcinogens are chemical, physical, or viral agents that cause cancer. Carcinogens can be:

- Chemicals (including those in tobacco)
- Physical agents (radiation and chronic irritation of tissues)
- Certain viruses known as *oncoviruses* (e.g., human papilloma virus)

Personal factors, including immune function, age, and genetic risk, also affect whether a person is likely to develop cancer. These factors interact with external factors to affect any person's risk for cancer. Cancer is more likely to occur in older people,

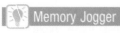
Memory Jogger

Suppressor gene inactivation leading to oncogene activation is the main mechanism of carcinogenesis.

those whose immune systems are not functioning at optimal levels, and those who have inherited a mutated gene that increases cancer risk.

CANCER CLASSIFICATION

Cancers are classified by the type of tissue from which they arise (for example, glandular, connective) and then divided into two major categories: solid and hematologic. Solid tumors develop from specific tissues (for example, breast and lung). Hematologic cancers (for example, leukemias and lymphomas) arise from blood cell–forming tissues. Cancers that arise from glandular tissue are *carcinomas* and are more common among adults. Glandular tissues include the linings of the gastrointestinal (GI) tract, the lungs, the ducts of the breast, prostate tissues, and any other glands that secrete substances. Cancers that arise from connective tissue are *sarcomas* and are more common among children. Connective tissues include bone, muscle, fibrous tissue, blood, glial cells of the brain, and other support tissues.

TYPES OF CANCER TREATMENT

Cancer therapies may be used alone or, more commonly, in combination to kill cancer cells. The types of therapy used depend on the specific type of cancer, whether or not the cancer has spread, and the health of the patient. Treatment regimens *(protocols)* have been established for most types of cancer based on experiments with cancer cells and experience with other patients with cancer. This chapter focuses on drugs used for cancer treatment, which include chemotherapy drugs, hormone manipulation, and targeted therapy.

CHEMOTHERAPY

Chemotherapy is the treatment of cancer with chemical agents, which can increase survival time and may cure the disease. The killing effect on cancer cells is related to the ability of chemotherapy to damage DNA and interfere with cell division

Patients with metastatic cancer will die unless treatment eliminates the metastatic cancer cells along with the original cancer cells. Chemotherapy is useful because its **cytotoxic effects** (cell-damaging and cell-killing effects) are systemic and can kill metastatic cancer cells that may have escaped local treatment

Chemotherapy drugs damage both normal cells and cancer cells. The normal cells most affected by these drugs are those that divide rapidly, including skin, hair, intestinal tissues, and blood-forming cells. The drugs are classified by the types of action they exert in the cancer cell. Table 12-2 lists chemotherapy drugs and their potential to induce nausea and vomiting and to damage surrounding tissue.

Chemotherapy Drug Categories

There are six categories of cancer chemotherapy drugs. The specific actions of each drug category are different, but the outcomes are the same: failure of cells to divide and promotion of cell death. All chemotherapy drugs are *high-alert drugs* that can cause serious harm if given at a dose that is too high or too low, if given to a patient for whom it was *not* prescribed, or if *not* given to a patient for whom it was prescribed.

How Chemotherapy Drugs Work

Antimetabolites are similar to normal metabolites needed for vital cell processes. Antimetabolite chemotherapy drugs act like "counterfeit" metabolites that fool cancer cells into using the antimetabolite in cellular reactions instead of the real metabolite. Because these drugs do not function as proper metabolites, their presence impairs cell division.

Antitumor antibiotics damage the DNA of the cell and interrupt DNA or RNA synthesis. Exactly how the interruptions occur varies with each agent.

Memory Jogger

Advancing age is the most important risk factor for cancer. Exposure to carcinogens adds up over a lifetime, and immune protection decreases with age.

Memory Jogger

Common cancer therapies include:
- Surgery
- Radiation
- Chemotherapy
- Hormone manipulation
- Targeted therapy

Memory Jogger

Unlike surgery and radiation, which are local therapies, chemotherapy is systemic, circulating to most body areas.

Memory Jogger

The six major chemotherapy drug categories are:
- Antimetabolites
- Antitumor antibiotics
- Antimitotics
- Alkylating agents
- Topoisomerase inhibitors
- Miscellaneous drugs

Table 12-2 Chemotherapy Drug Categories

DRUG	EMETOGENIC POTENTIAL	TISSUE DAMAGE POTENTIAL
Antimetabolites		
azacitidine (Vidaza)	Moderate	Irritant
capecitabine (Xeloda)	Low	None (oral drug)
cladribine (Leustatin)	Moderate	Bruising
cytarabine (Ara-C, Cytosar-U)	Moderate	Irritant
decitabine (Dacogen)	Moderate	Irritant
floxuridine (FUDR)	High	Bruising
fludarabine (Beneflur ♣, Fludara, FLAMP)	Low	Bruising
5-fluorouracil (Adrucil, Carac, Efudex, Fluoroplex)	Moderate	Irritant
gemcitabine (Gemzar)	Moderate	Bruising
6-mercaptopurine (Purinethol)	Low	None (oral drug)
methotrexate (Apo-Methotrexate ♣, Mexate, Folex)	Low-Moderate	Bruising
6-thioguanine (Lanvis)	Moderate-High	None (oral drug)
Antitumor Antibiotics		
bleomycin (Blenoxane)	Moderate	Irritant
dactinomycin (Cosmegen)	High	Vesicant
DAUNOrubicin (Cerubidine, DaunoXome)	High	Vesicant
DOXOrubicin (Adriamycin, Caekys ♣, Doxil, Rubex)	High	Vesicant
epirubicin (Ellence, Pharmorubicin ♣)	High	Vesicant
idarubicin (Idamycin)	Moderate-High	Vesicant
mitomycin C (Mutamycin)	Moderate	Vesicant
mitoxantrone (Novantrone)	Low	Irritant
pentostatin (Nipent)	Moderate-High	Bruising
plicamycin (Mithracin)	High	Irritant
valrubicin (Valstar)	None	None (intravesicular drug)
Antimitotics		
docetaxel (Taxotere)	Moderate	Bruising
etoposide (Etopophos, Toposar, VP-16, VePesid)	Low	Irritant
paclitaxel (Taxol)	Moderate	Irritant
vinBLAStine (Velban, Velbe, Velsar)	Low-Moderate	Vesicant
vinCRIStine (Oncovin, Vincasar PFS)	Low	Vesicant
vinorelbine (Navelbine)	Low	Vesicant
Alkylating Agents		
altretamine (Hexalen)	Moderate	None (oral drug)
busulfan (Busulfex, Myleran)	High	Bruising
carboplatin (Paraplatin, Paraplatin-AQ ♣)	High	Irritant
carmustine (BiCNU)	High	Irritant
chlorambucil (Leukeran)	High	None (oral drug)
cisplatin (Platinol)	High	Irritant
cyclophosphamide (Cytoxan, Procytox ♣)	High	Bruising
estramustine (Emcyt, Estracyt)	Moderate	Vesicant
ifosfamide (IFEX)	High	Bruising
lomustine (CCNU, CeeNU)	High	None (oral drug)
mechlorethamine (Mustargen)	High	Vesicant
melphalan (Alkeran)	High	None (oral drug)

Table 12-2 Chemotherapy Drug Categories—cont'd

DRUG	EMETOGENIC POTENTIAL	TISSUE DAMAGE POTENTIAL
oxaliplatin (Eloxatin)	Moderate-High	Vesicant
streptozocin (Zanosar)	High	Bruising
temozolomide (Temodal ♣, Temodar)	Moderate-High	None (oral drug)
thiotepa (Thioplex)	Low	Bruising
Topoisomerase Inhibitors		
irinotecan (Camptosar)	Moderate	Irritant
topotecan (Hycamtin)	Moderate	Irritant
Miscellaneous Agents		
arsenic trioxide (Trisenox)	Moderate	Not known
asparaginase (Elspar, Kidrolase ♣)	Low	Vesicant
dacarbazine (DTIC ♣)	Moderate-High	Irritant
hydroxyurea (Apo-Hydroxyurea ♣, Droxia, Hydrea)	Low	None (oral drug)
pegaspargase (Oncaspar)	Low	Bruising
procarbazine (Matulane, Natulan ♣)	High	None (oral drug)

Antimitotic agents interfere with the formation of tubules so cells cannot separate during cell division. As a result, the cancer cell either does not divide at all or divides only once.

Alkylating agents cross-link DNA, making the two DNA strands bind tightly together. This tight binding prevents proper DNA and RNA synthesis, inhibiting cell division.

Topoisomerase inhibitors disrupt an enzyme (topoisomerase) needed for DNA synthesis and cell division. This enzyme nicks and straightens the DNA helix, allowing the DNA to be copied, and then reattaches the DNA together. Topoisomerase inhibitor drugs prevent the actions needed for proper DNA maintenance, causing DNA breakage and cell death.

Miscellaneous chemotherapy drugs are those with mechanisms of action that are either unknown or do not fit those of other drug categories.

Combination Chemotherapy. Combination chemotherapy is the combination of two or more anticancer drugs given on a specific timed schedule called a *protocol*. These combinations are much more successful at controlling cancer and killing cancer cells than any single drug would be. However, the side effects and damage caused to normal tissues also increase with combination chemotherapy. The selection of drugs is based on known tumor sensitivity to the drugs and the degree of side effects expected.

Treatment Issues. Chemotherapy drugs are given on a regular basis and timed to maximize the number of cancer cells killed, as well as to minimize damage to normal cells. Most often chemotherapy is scheduled every 3 to 4 weeks for a specified number of times (usually 4 to 12 times). Giving higher doses of chemotherapy more often is called *dose-dense chemotherapy*. Dose-dense chemotherapy also results in more intense side effects than traditional schedules.

Chemotherapy has many unpleasant side effects. Patients and their families often need a great deal of education to understand why taking chemotherapy and maintaining the schedule are important for managing their cancer. Continuous support is needed to encourage patients to complete treatment protocols even when they feel tired and sick.

Most chemotherapy drugs are given intravenously, although other routes may be used for specific cancers. The standard of care designated by the Oncology Nursing

Memory Jogger

All chemotherapy drugs affect both normal cells and cancer cells.

Memory Jogger

Combination chemotherapy uses multiple drugs from different categories to kill more cancer cells.

Memory Jogger

Schedules for chemotherapy administration are timed to maximize the number of cancer cells killed, as well as to minimize damage to normal cells.

Drug Alert!

Administration Alert

Administration of IV cancer chemotherapy can only be performed
by a registered nurse who has
completed an approved chemotherapy course.

QSEN: Safety

Drug Alert!

Administration Alert

Because chemotherapy drugs are
dangerous and can be absorbed
through skin and mucous membranes, always use PPE when
mixing, handling, and giving these
drugs and when handling the
wastes and excretions of patients
receiving them.

QSEN: Safety

Society (ONS) and supported by the American Society of Clinical Oncologists (ASCO) for safe administration of intravenous (IV) chemotherapy is that administration of these drugs requires special education and competency. This does not mean that only an advanced practice nurse can perform this function; however, it does mean that the individual must be a registered nurse who has completed an approved chemo-therapy course.

All health care workers, including all licensed practical nurses/licensed voca-tional nurses and registered nurses, are responsible for providing care and comfort to patients during and after chemotherapy administration. Monitoring patient responses to therapy and managing side effects are important parts of care during this period.

A major complication of IV infusion is **extravasation**, a condition in which a che-motherapy drug leaks into tissues surrounding the infusion site, causing tissue damage. When the drugs given are **vesicants** (chemicals that cause tissue damage on direct contact), the results of extravasation can include pain, infection, and tissue loss (refer to Figure 5-5, *B* in Chapter 5). Surgical intervention is sometimes needed for severe tissue damage. See Table 12-2 for a list of known vesicant and irritant chemotherapy drugs.

Most chemotherapy drugs are absorbed through the skin and mucous mem-branes. As a result, health care workers who prepare or give these drugs (especially pharmacists, pharmacy technicians, and nurses) are at risk for absorbing them. Anyone preparing, giving, or disposing of chemotherapy drugs or handling the wastes or excretions from patients within 48 hours after receiving IV chemotherapy should use extreme caution and wear personal protective equipment (PPE), includ-ing eye protection, mask, double gloves, and gown.

Chemotherapy Preparation

Agents used for intravenous chemotherapy must be mixed under safe conditions. In addition to the PPE used by the person mixing the drugs, a biologic safety cabinet or vertical laminar flow hood is used to prevent the agents from aerosolizing and accidentally exposing others to their harmful effects. A vertical flow hood is used rather than a horizontal flow hood because although a horizontal flow hood can reduce the possibility of contaminants in the drugs, it actually vents outward, toward the person using the hood. This means that the person mixing the drugs would have increased exposure to the drugs. All equipment used for the preparation of chemo-therapy drugs is kept separate from that used to prepare nonhazardous drugs.

Most IV chemotherapy is administered in outpatient settings by certified chemo-therapy nurses. Because most chemotherapy drugs are highly toxic, precautions are needed to limit the exposure of these drugs to others and ensure patient safety. This is also true for those cytotoxic chemotherapies that are administered in oral formulations.

What To Do *Before* Intravenous Chemotherapy Is Given

Because many chemotherapy drugs are vesicants or irritants, make sure that the IV line is in a large vein and has an adequate blood return. Often the patient may have an implanted central catheter access with an internal or external port. These devices reduce the risk for extravasation but increase the risk for infection. Assess these devices before use and follow agency policy for preparing the skin and accessing these devices.

Doses for most chemotherapy drugs are calculated according to the type of cancer and the patient's size. Most commonly calculations are based on milligrams per square meter of body surface area (BSA), which includes first converting the patient's height in inches to centimeters and converting weight in pounds to kilograms. (An inch is equal to 2.54 centimeters and a kilogram is equal to 2.2 pounds.) So it is important to weigh the patient accurately each day that chemotherapy is to be administered before the dose is calculated. The formula for this calculation is the patient's height in centimeters multiplied by his or her weight in kilograms. The product of this multiplication is divided by 10,000. For example, a woman who is 68 inches tall (173 cm) and weighs 143 lb (65 kg) has a BSA of 11,245 cm^2, or 1.12 m^2.

The dose is usually calculated by the prescriber, and the drugs are prepared by a pharmacist or pharmacy technician. Check the dose on the label and recalculate it based on the patient's weight or total body surface area. Notify the pharmacist and the prescriber if there is a dose discrepancy.

Each chemotherapy dose is prepared individually for the patient. Use two identifiers, such as the patient's name, birthdate, or hospital identification number, to ensure that the correct patient receives the drugs.

Chemotherapy drugs are powerful, and the patient may have a reaction during administration. If the patient has had chemotherapy before, ask whether he or she had any problems or changes during or after the drugs were administered. Take the patient's vital signs (including temperature and blood pressure) and assess mental status before therapy starts. Use these findings as a baseline to determine patient responses to chemotherapy.

Administer any prescribed premedications before starting chemotherapy. Such drugs may include antiemetics to prevent nausea and vomiting, anti-inflammatories, antianxiety drugs, and pain medications. (Review information about these premedication drugs in the chapters relating to these types of drug therapy.)

What To Do *During* Intravenous Chemotherapy Administration

Although the actual infusion of chemotherapy drugs is the responsibility of the chemotherapy-certified nurse or oncologist, monitoring the patient during chemotherapy is the responsibility of all health care personnel. Instruct the patient to alert you immediately if he or she feels different in any way during the infusion.

Stay with the patient during the first 15 minutes of the infusion and retake vital signs. Thereafter check him or her every 15 minutes for any signs or symptoms of an allergic reaction: hives anywhere (especially at the IV site), low blood pressure, rapid and irregular pulse, swelling of the lips or lower face, the sensation of a "lump in the throat," or any other type of adverse reaction. If the patient is having an anaphylactic or adverse reaction, your first action is to prevent any more drug from entering him or her. Stop the drug from infusing but keep the IV access. If the drug is infusing high into the IV tubing, change the tubing after stopping the drug, and do not let any drug that remains in the tubing run into the patient.

The most important intervention for extravasation is prevention. Assess the IV flow rate and infusion site at least every 30 minutes. Check for swelling or redness at the site, which may indicate extravasation. Determine whether a blood return is present. Ask the patient about any pain or burning at the infusion site. Small extravasations resolve without extensive treatment if less than 0.5 mL of the drug has leaked into the tissues. If a larger amount has leaked, extensive tissue damage occurs, and surgical intervention may be needed. So close monitoring of the access site is critical during chemotherapy administration to prevent leakage of larger volumes. Immediate treatment depends on the specific drug. Coordinate with the oncologist and pharmacist to determine the specific antidote needed for the extravasated drug. Box 12-1 outlines how to document an extravasation event.

Take vital signs and assess mental status according to agency policy during IV chemotherapy administration. Document all assessments.

What To Do *After* Giving Intravenous Chemotherapy

When IV chemotherapy administration is complete, discontinue the infusion set using PPE. Dispose of the set according to agency policy, usually in a biohazard container. Assess the infusion site and document your findings. If the access site is a temporary peripheral line, discontinue it after all prescribed IV support drugs have been given. If the access is an indwelling central line, care for the access site according to agency policy.

Memory Jogger

The square meters for an average-size adult is not much over 1.4, and the square meters for a child or infant is considerably less than 1.

Drug Alert!

Administration Alert

Administer prescribed premedication on time to reduce unpleasant side effects.

QSEN: Safety

Drug Alert!

Action/Intervention Alert

When an allergic reaction or adverse event occurs, stop the drug from infusing but keep the IV access. If the drug is infusing high into the IV tubing, change the tubing after stopping the drug, and do not let any drug that remains in the tubing run into the patient.

QSEN: Safety

Drug Alert!

Action/Intervention Alert

Monitor the access site of any infusing vesicant at least every 30 minutes to prevent extravasation or limit damage by preventing leakage of larger volumes.

QSEN: Safety

Box 12-1	Documentation of Extravasation

- Document the date and time when extravasation was suspected or identified.
- Document the date and time when the infusion was started.
- Record the time when the infusion was stopped.
- Document the exact contents of the infusion fluid and the volume of fluid infused.
- Document the estimated amount of fluid extravasated.
- Document the needle type and size.
- Diagram the exact insertion site.
- Indicate on the diagram the location and number of venipuncture attempts.
- Record the time between the extravasation and the last full blood return.
- Identify all agents administered in the previous 24 hours through this site (list agent administered, dosage and volume, and order of administration).
- Take and record the patient's vital signs.
- Take a photograph of the site.
- Document the administration of neutralizing or antidote agents.
- Document the application of compresses.
- Document other interventions.
- Record the patient's responses to other interventions.
- Document the prescriber notification (including the time).
- Document the written and oral instructions given to the patient about follow-up care.
- Document any consultation request.
- Sign the documentation.

! Drug Alert!

Action/Intervention Alert

Compare assessment findings after chemotherapy with those obtained before administration.

QSEN: Safety

Assess the patient and compare the findings with those obtained before the chemotherapy session. Document all findings and notify the prescriber of any patient changes.

What To *Teach* Patients About Chemotherapy

Temporary and permanent physical damage can occur to normal tissues from chemotherapy because this treatment is systemic and exerts its effects on both normal and cancer cells. Serious short-term side effects occur with aggressive chemotherapy. Side effects that suppress bone marrow blood cell formation can be life threatening and are the most common reason for changing the dose or schedule. The suppressive effects on the bone marrow cause anemia, neutropenia, and thrombocytopenia. Less serious but common distressing side effects include nausea, vomiting, hair loss *(alopecia)*, open sores on mucous membranes *(mucositis)*, and changes in cognitive function. These side effects are referred to as cancer therapy *symptom distress*.

Patient teaching for cancer chemotherapy is extensive, continuous, and best accomplished with a team approach. A specialized oncology nurse is needed to assess patient learning needs and coordinate the highly complex patient education. Consult a cancer specialty textbook to learn about the extensive teaching needed to prevent complications and manage the numerous side effects of this therapy.

HORMONE MANIPULATION

Hormones are naturally occurring chemicals secreted by endocrine (ductless) glands and picked up by capillaries. Once in the bloodstream, hormones circulate to all body areas but exert their effects only on their specific target tissues. Some hormones make hormone-sensitive cancers grow more rapidly, and some cancers require specific hormones to divide. So decreasing the amount of hormones to hormone-sensitive tumors can slow cancer growth.

Hormone manipulation can control some types of cancer (for example, prostate cancer, breast cancer) for many years. Usually this therapy does not lead to a cure. As shown in Figure 12-2, prostate cancer is a hormone-sensitive cancer that grows faster when the hormone testosterone (an androgen) binds to its receptors. When an antiandrogen is given such as estrogen or flutamide (Eulexin), it binds to the

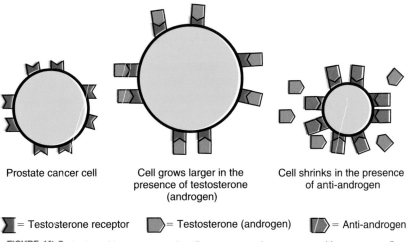

= Testosterone receptor   = Testosterone (androgen)   = Anti-androgen

FIGURE 12-2 Action of hormones and antihormones on hormone-sensitive cancer cells.

Table 12-3 Drugs Used for Hormone Manipulation of Cancer

TYPE OF AGENT	EXAMPLE
Hormone Agonists	
Androgen	fluoxymesterone (Androxy)
	methyltestosterone (Android, Methitest)
	testolactone (Teslac)
Estrogen	conjugated equine estrogen (Premarin)
	diethylstilbestrol (DES, Stilphostrol)
	ethinyl estradiol (Estinyl)
Progestin	medroxyPROGESTERone (Amen, Provera)
	megestrol (Apo-Megestrol ✤, Megace)
Luteinizing-hormone releasing hormone	leuprolide (Eligard, Lupron, Viadur)
	goserelin (Zoladex, Zoladex LA ✤)
Hormone Antagonists	
Antiandrogens	bicalutamide (Casodex)
	flutamide (Apo-Flutamide ✤, Eulexin, Novo-Flutamide ✤)
Antiestrogens	fulvestrant (Faslodex)
	tamoxifen (Apo-Tamox ✤, Nolvadex, Nolvadex D ✤, Soltamox, Tamofen ✤)
	toremifene (Fareston)
Hormone Inhibitors	
	aminoglutethimide (Cytadren, Elipten)
	anastrozole (Arimidex)
	exemestane (Aromasin)
	letrozole (Femara)

testosterone receptors, preventing the patient's testosterone from binding to those sites. When antiandrogens are present, they block testosterone from enhancing the growth of prostate cancer cells. This action does not kill the cancer cells but just slows their growth. When tumor growth is slowed, survival time increases. Table 12-3 lists drugs commonly used in hormone manipulation for cancer therapy.

Another class of drugs used for hormone therapy is the hormone inhibitors. These drugs inhibit production of specific hormones in the normal hormone-producing organs. For example, the aromatase inhibitor anastrozole (Arimidex) prevents production of estrogen in the adrenal gland and reduces blood estrogen levels. For breast cancer cells that need estrogen to grow, anastrozole limits the total amount of estrogen present and causes slower cancer cell growth.

 Memory Jogger

Hormone manipulation can control the growth of some cancers but usually does not cure the cancer.

Side Effects

Androgens and the antiestrogen receptor drugs cause masculinizing effects in women. Chest and facial hair may develop, menstrual periods stop, and breast tissue shrinks. Patients may have some fluid retention. For men and women receiving androgens, acne may develop, hypercalcemia is common, and liver dysfunction may occur with prolonged therapy. Women receiving estrogens or progestins have irregular but heavy menses, fluid retention, and breast tenderness. Men and women who take estrogen or progestins are at risk for deep vein thrombosis.

Feminine manifestations often appear in men who take estrogens, progestins, or anti-androgen receptor drugs. Facial hair thins, facial skin becomes smoother, body fat redistributes, and *gynecomastia* (breast development in men) can occur. Testicular and penile size decrease. Although sexual function may continue, achieving an erection is more difficult. Patients may benefit from professional counseling to manage problems with body image and sexual function.

TARGETED THERAPY

Targeted therapy for cancer treatment takes advantage of one or more differences in cancer cell growth or metabolism that either are not present or are less common in normal cells. These differences result from specific gene activation in cancer cells. Agents used as targeted therapies work to disrupt cancer cell division in one of several ways. Some of these drugs "target" and block growth factor receptors. Other agents for targeted therapy may be antibodies directed against a cellular substance needed by the cancer cell for growth or a substance in the signaling pathway of a cell that is important in turning on certain genes for cell growth. Figure 12-3 shows one type of signal transduction pathway in which events outside the cell and pathways inside the cell can be stimulated to turn on cell division. There are many such pathways, and each pathway has many steps. Targeted therapy drugs can block one or more steps in a pathway so that the signal for turning on cell division genes does not reach the cell nucleus and excessive cell division is stopped. Figure 12-3 provides an overview of places within a cancer cell pathway that can

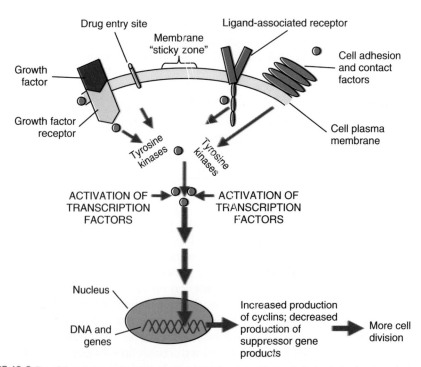

FIGURE 12-3 Possible cancer cell targets for targeted therapy. The red circles indicate areas for activity of targeted therapies.

| Table 12-4 | Common Agents Used for Targeted Therapy |

CLASSIFICATION	AGENT	CANCER TYPES
Tyrosine kinase inhibitors (TKIs)	Dasatinib (Sprycel)	Acute lymphocytic leukemia Chronic myelogenous leukemia
	Imatinib mesylate (Gleevec)	Chronic myelogenous leukemia
	Lapatinib (Tykerb)	Breast cancer (metastatic)
	Nilotinib (Tasigna)	Chronic myelogenous leukemia
Epidermal growth factor receptor inhibitors (EGFRIs)	Cetuximab (Erbitux)	Colorectal cancer Head and neck cancer
	Erlotinib (Tarceva)	Non–small cell lung cancer Pancreatic cancer
	Gefitinib (Iressa)	Non–small cell lung cancer
	Panitumumab (Vectibix)	Colorectal cancer
	Trastuzumab (Herceptin)	Her2 overexpressing breast cancer Gastric cancer
Vascular endothelial growth factor receptor inhibitors (VEGFRIs)	Bevacizumab (Avastin)	Cervical cancer Colorectal cancer Glioblastoma Non–small cell lung cancer Renal cell carcinoma
Multikinase inhibitors (MKIs)	Pazopanib (Votrient)	Renal cell carcinoma Soft tissue sarcoma
	Regorafenib (Stivarga)	Colorectal cancer Gastrointestinal stromal tumors (GIST)
	Sorafenib (Nexavar)	Hepatocellular cancer Renal cell carcinoma Thyroid cancer
Proteasome inhibitors	Bortezomib (Velcade)	Mantle cell lymphoma Multiple myeloma
Angiogenesis inhibitors	Everolimus (Afinitor)	Astrocytoma Breast cancer Renal cell carcinoma
	Lenalidomide (Revlimid)	Mantle cell lymphoma Multiple myeloma Myelodysplastic syndrome
	Temsirolimus (Torisel)	Renal cell carcinoma
Monoclonal antibodies	Alemtuzumab (Campath)	Chronic lymphocytic leukemia
	Ibritumomab tiuxetan (Zevalin)	Non-Hodgkins lymphoma
	Rituximab (Rituxan)	Chronic lymphocytic leukemia Non-Hodgkins lymphoma
	I^{131} tositumomab (Bexxar)	Non-Hodgkins lymphoma
	Gemtuzumab ozogamicin (Mylotarg)	Acute myelogenous leukemia

be targeted by different targeted therapy drugs to control or stop cancer cell growth. Table 12-4 lists common targeted therapy agents and the cancer types usually treated with them.

It is important to remember that targeted therapy drugs will not work unless the cancer cell overexpresses the actual target substance. Thus not all patients with the same cancer type would benefit from the use of targeted therapy. Each person's cancer cells must be tested in the laboratory to determine whether the cells have enough of a target to be affected by targeted therapy.

 Memory Jogger

Targeted therapies are effective only if the cancer cell has a target for the drug.

How Cancer Targeted Therapy Drugs Work

Tyrosine kinase inhibitors (TKIs) are drugs that inhibit the enzyme tyrosine kinase. Tyrosine kinases (TKs) are enzymes that activate some proteins in growth pathways. When there is less of this activated protein present in a cancer cell, its growth is slowed or stopped. There are many different TKs. Some are unique to the cell type; others may be present only in cancer cells that express a specific gene mutation. As a result, the different TKIs are effective in disrupting the growth of some cancer cell types and not others. All currently approved TKIs are oral agents.

Epithelial growth factor receptor inhibitors (EGFRIs) are drugs that bind to and block the epidermal growth factor receptors on some types of cancer cells. Certain cancer cells rely on growth factor binding to the receptor to promote its growth (see Figure 12-3). EGFRIs bind to the receptors and inhibit the growth promoting actions that these receptors have when they are bound to the growth factor itself. Some EGFRIs are antibodies, which must be given parenterally. Other EGFRIs are not antibodies and are given as oral drugs.

Vascular endothelial growth factor receptor inhibitors (VEGFRIs) are drugs that bind to and block the vascular endothelial growth factor receptors when they are overexpressed in some types of cancer cells. By preventing the growth factor from binding, new blood vessels cannot grow into the tumor, making it poorly nourished and unable to metastasize. Drugs from this class are given parenterally.

Multikinase inhibitors (MKIs) are drugs that inhibit the activity of specific kinase enzymes in cancer cells. They prevent the activation of transcription factors in some cancer cells and slow or prevent cancer cell growth. These drugs are most effective in cancers that have a specific gene mutation found most often in some renal cell carcinomas, GI stromal tumors, and pancreatic, colon, and non–small cell lung cancer cells.

Proteasome inhibitors work by preventing the formation of a large complex of proteins (a proteasome) in cells. The proteasome helps regulate the expression of genes that promote cell division and prevent cell death. Proteasome inhibitors limit the amount of proteasome present, making the cell less likely to divide and more likely to respond to signals for cell death.

Angiogenesis inhibitors target a specific protein kinase known as the *mammalian target of rapamycin (mTOR)*. When the drug binds to an intracellular protein, a protein-drug complex forms that inhibits the activity of mTOR. This action greatly reduces the concentrations of vascular endothelial growth factor (VEGF) and disrupts many pro–cell division signal transduction pathways.

Side Effects

Allergic reactions are an issue in patients receiving any targeted therapy that is an antibody. Most of these antibodies were developed in animals and may express some animal proteins. More recently much of the animal portion of these antibodies was removed, reducing but not eliminating the risk for allergic reactions. Patients receiving antibodies over time may develop their own antibodies to the drugs, making them less effective and possibly causing severe inflammatory or allergic reactions.

In addition, EGFRIs and VEGFRIs bind to those specific receptors when the receptors are on normal tissue. So side effects can occur in tissues that normally express these receptors, such as the skin, mucous membranes, and lining of the GI tract.

Common side effect of multikinase inhibitors include hypertension, nausea and vomiting, other GI disturbances, and mild bone marrow suppression. The most common side effects of the proteasome inhibitors are nausea, vomiting, anorexia, abdominal pain, bowel changes, and decreased taste sensation. Peripheral neuropathy is also common.

Hypersensitivity reactions to angiogenesis inhibitors is common. Hyperglycemia can occur and bone marrow suppression is moderate to severe with anemia, neutropenia, and thrombocytopenia. Other general side effects include headache, nausea and vomiting, back pain, muscle and joint pain, mucositis, diarrhea, and skin problems.

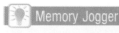 Memory Jogger

Because some normal cells have target receptors, targeted therapy drugs may cause side effects in skin and mucous membranes.

IMMUNOTHERAPY: BIOLOGICAL RESPONSE MODIFIERS

Biological response modifiers (BRMs) modify a patient's biologic responses to tumor cells. The BRMs in current use as cancer therapy are cytokines, which are small protein hormones made by white blood cells. Cytokines generally make the immune system work better.

Cytokines and other BRMs work as a cancer treatment by stimulating the immune system to recognize cancer cells and take actions to eliminate or destroy them. Some BRMs are also useful in a supporting role such as colony-stimulating factors that stimulate faster recovery of bone marrow function after treatment-induced suppression (see Chapter 20 for some examples).

BRMs as Cancer Therapy

Two common types of BRMs used as cancer therapy are the interleukins (ILs) and interferons (IFNs). Some agents can stimulate specific immune system cells to attack and destroy cancer cells; other agents block cancer cell access to an essential function or nutrient.

ILs are a group of substances that the body makes to help regulate inflammation and immune protection. Some are now synthesized as drugs. They help different immune system cells recognize and destroy abnormal body cells. In particular, IL-1, -2, and -6 appear to "charge up" the immune system and enhance attacks on cancer cells by macrophages, natural killer cells, and tumor-infiltrating lymphocytes.

Interferons are cell-produced proteins that can protect noninfected cells from viral infection and replication. Cancer-related functions of some interferons include:

- Slowing tumor cell division
- Stimulating growth and activation of natural killer cells (which attack cancer cells)
- Helping cancer cells resume a more normal appearance and function
- Inhibiting the expression of oncogenes

Interferons have been effective to some degree in the treatment of melanoma, hairy cell leukemia, renal cell carcinoma, ovarian cancer, and cutaneous T-cell lymphoma.

One drug classified as a BRM that has a somewhat different action is thalidomide (Thalomid), which reduces the formation of blood vessels in tumors. When tumor blood vessels are reduced, the tumor is poorly nourished, and cancer cells die.

BRMs as Supportive Therapy

BRMs used for supportive therapy during cancer treatment are the colony-stimulating factors. These factors induce more rapid recovery of the bone marrow after chemotherapy. When bone marrow suppression is shortened or less severe, patients are less at risk for life-threatening infections, anemia, and bleeding. Also, because the colony-stimulating factors allow more rapid bone marrow recovery, patients can receive their chemotherapy on time and may even be able to tolerate higher doses, improving the outcome of chemotherapy.

 Clinical Pitfall

Colony-stimulating factors may stimulate the growth of leukemia cells and are not used with leukemia.

QSEN: Safety

Side Effects

Patients receiving interleukins may have generalized and severe inflammatory reactions. Fluid shifts and capillary leak are widespread, with edema forming in most tissues. Tissue swelling affects the function of all organs and can be life threatening. Patients receiving high-dose BRM therapy should receive care in an intensive care or monitoring unit. The effects of BRM therapy are limited to the period of acute drug infusion and resolve when treatment stops.

Many BRMs induce symptoms of mild inflammation during and immediately after receiving the drug, including fever, chills, rigors, and flulike achiness. Problems are worse when higher doses are given but tend to become less severe over time.

Interferon therapy causes peripheral neuropathy. Some of the problems resulting from neuropathy include decreased sensory perception, visual disturbances, decreased hearing, unsteady balance and gait, and orthostatic hypotension. It is not known whether the neuropathy is temporary or permanent.

Rash and skin dryness, itching, and peeling occur with many types of BRM therapy. The skin problems are more severe at higher doses and when more than one type of BRM is used at the same time. These reactions are temporary but can cause much discomfort and distress to the patient.

Thalidomide is a powerful *teratogen* (can cause severe birth defects) and should never be given to pregnant women. Women of childbearing age who are sexually active are advised to use at least two forms of contraception to avoid the possibility of pregnancy.

 Clinical Pitfall

Never give thalidomide to a pregnant woman.

QSEN: Safety

Get Ready for Practice!

Key Points

- Normal cells divide only when needed, and their growth is strictly controlled.
- Transformation of a normal cell into a cancer cell involves mutation of the genes (DNA) of the normal cell.
- The actions of chemotherapy drugs on cancer cells are related to their ability to damage DNA and interfere with cell division.
- The normal cells most affected by these drugs are those that divide rapidly, including skin, hair, intestinal tissues, spermatocytes, and blood-forming cells.
- Regardless of the exact mechanism of action for cancer drugs, the overall results are failure of cancer cells to divide, leading to cancer cell death.
- Although administration of chemotherapy should be performed only by chemotherapy-certified registered nurses, monitoring the patient during chemotherapy administration is a responsibility of all licensed practical nurses/licensed vocational nurses and registered nurses.
- Extravasation of vesicants can lead to extensive tissue damage and tissue loss.
- The most important intervention for extravasation is prevention.
- The side effects of chemotherapy that suppresses bone marrow blood cell formation can be life threatening and are the most common reason for changing the dose or schedule.
- Hormone manipulation can help control the growth of hormone-sensitive cancers.
- Not all cancers of the same type have the right "targets" for targeted therapy.

Additional Learning Resources

evolve Be sure to visit your Evolve website (http://evolve.elsevier.com/Workman/pharmacology/) for additional online resources.

SG Go to your Study Guide for additional learning activities to help you master this chapter content.

Review Questions

See the Answer Keys—In-text Review Questions for answers to these questions.

Test Yourself on the Basics

1. Which personal factor is the most common cause of cancer development?
   A. Living in a geographic area with poor sanitation
   B. Having parents who died of cancer
   C. Eating a high-fat diet
   D. Advancing age
2. How do most cytotoxic chemotherapy drugs rid the body of cancer cells?
   A. Interfering with cancer cell division
   B. Preventing cancer cells from receiving needed vitamins
   C. Enhancing the immune system's ability to recognize and kill cancer cells
   D. Forcing cancer cells to undergo reverse transformation to become normal cells
3. Which chemotherapy drug has the highest potential to induce nausea and vomiting?
   A. azacitidine (Vidaza)
   B. fludarabine (Fludara)
   C. cyclophosphamide (Cytoxan)
   D. irinotecan (Camptosar)
4. Which agents for targeted therapy belong to the epidermal growth factor receptor inhibitor (EGRFI) class of drug? (Select all that apply.)
   A. bevacizumab (Avastin)
   B. cetuximab (Erbitux)
   C. gefitinib (Iressa)
   D. imatinib (Gleevec)
   E. lapatinib (Tykerb)
   F. rituximab (Rituxan)
   G. trastuzumab (Herceptin)
5. Which class of chemotherapy drugs exert their effects by preventing the actions needed for proper DNA maintenance so that DNA breakage occurs leading to cancer cell death?
   A. Antitumor antibiotics
   B. Hormone antagonists
   C. Multikinase inhibitors
   D. Topoisomerase inhibitors

6. Which of the following chemotherapy agents listed belong to the alkylating agent class? Select all that apply.
   A. azacitidine (Vidaza)
   B. bleomycin (Blenoxane)
   C. busulfan (Busulfex)
   D. cyclophosphamide (Cytoxan)
   E. docetaxel (Taxotere)
   F. irinotecan (Camptosar)
   G. methotrexate (Mexate)
   H. procarbazine (Matulane)
   I. oxaliplatin (Eloxatin)
   J. temozolomide (Temodar)

7. Which action is most important to prevent nausea and vomiting in the patient prescribed intravenous cytotoxic chemotherapy?
   A. Keeping the patient NPO (nothing by mouth) during the time the chemotherapy drugs are infusing
   B. Administering antiemetic medications before administering chemotherapy
   C. Ensuring that the chemotherapy is infused over a 4- to 6-hour period
   D. Assessing the patient's responses hourly during the infusion period

Test Yourself on Advanced Concepts

8. A patient asks why cancer cell growth is considered "uncontrolled." What is your best response?
   A. "Cancer cells always divide more rapidly than normal cells."
   B. "When each cancer cell divides, it usually produces more than two cells."
   C. "As you age, your immune system is less active, which allows cancer cells to grow faster."
   D. "Cancer cells divide almost continuously, and normal cells divide only when they are needed."

9. A patient with breast cancer asks why so many drugs are used together to treat her cancer. What is your best response?
   A. "Each drug works against cancer cells in different ways, and using several increases the likelihood that the cancer will be cured."
   B. "By using several drugs together, we can avoid using radiation therapy, which would cause many more permanent side effects."
   C. "Each drug goes to a separate body area. That way, because your cancer has spread to so many areas, all areas with cancer will receive the right drug."
   D. "The doctors are not sure which drug will work best against the cancer type that you have. Using several at the same time improves the chances that one will work."

10. You are monitoring a patient receiving IV chemotherapy that was started by a chemotherapy-certified nurse. After 2 hours the patient reports burning and pain at the IV site. Lowering the IV results in an observable brisk blood return. What is your best first action?

A. Stop the drug infusion and run at least 100 mL of normal saline into IV access.
B. Notify the chemotherapy-certified nurse who started the infusion.
C. Slow the rate of infusion but continue it because there is a good blood return.
D. Discontinue the infusion, remove the IV, and document the site condition.

11. A patient receiving tamoxifen (Nolvadex) asks how this therapy helps fight breast cancer. In addition to telling her that the breast cancer cells need estrogen to continue growing, what is your best response?
   A. "This agent reduces the availability of estrogen to your cancer cells."
   B. "This agent causes you to secrete testosterone instead of estrogen."
   C. "This agent kills off both the normal estrogen-secreting cells and the cancer cells."
   D. "This agent destroys circulating estrogen and all other female hormones."

12. A patient who has just been diagnosed with lymphoma asks why the treatment plan does not include the drug rituximab (Rituxan) about which he has read. What is your best response?
   A. "Your immune system is too weak to tolerate Rituxan."
   B. "This drug is experimental and too dangerous for you to take before trying other therapies."
   C. "Your lymphoma cells do not have the protein on which this drug works, so you would not benefit from this therapy."
   D. "You are young and can better tolerate the standard therapies for lymphoma that have been proven effective but have strong side effects."

13. A patient is prescribed tamoxifen (Nolvadex) 20 mg orally twice daily for a total daily dosage of 40 mg. The drug comes in 10-mg tablets. How many tablets does the patient take twice daily? _____tablet(s)

14. A child with cancer is to receive methotrexate 2.5 mg/kg intravenously. The child weighs 39.6 lb.
   a. What is the child's weight in kilograms?____kg
   b. What is the appropriate dose?____mg
   c. The drug is prepared at a concentration of 25 mg/mL. How many milliliters are the correct dose? _____mL
   The same drug is to be administered to an adult who weighs 165 lb.
   d. What is the adult's weight in kilograms?____kg
   e. What is the appropriate dose?____mg
   f. The drug is prepared at a concentration of 25 mg/mL. How many milliliters are the correct dose?_____mL

15. An adult with lung cancer is prescribed to receive cisplatin (Platinol) intravenously at a dosage of 79 mg per m^2. He is 6'4" tall and weighs 210 lb.
   What is his height in cm?_____cm
   What is his weight in kg?____kg
   What is his body surface area in m^2?_____
   What is the correct dose of cisplatin for this patient?_____mg

Critical Thinking Activities

See the Answer Keys—Critical Thinking Activities for answers to these activities.

A patient receiving cetuximab (Erbitux) as therapy for colorectal cancer reports that he must be allergic to the drug because he has developed a skin rash on his chest, back, and palms of the hands. He says that he guesses he will have to stop the therapy.

1. What type of anticancer therapy is cetuximab?
2. What are its expected side effects?
3. What will you tell this patient about stopping the cetuximab therapy?

chapter

13

Drug Therapy for Diabetes

http://evolve.elsevier.com/Workman/pharmacology/

Objectives

After studying this chapter you should be able to:

1. List the names, actions, usual dosages, possible side effects, and adverse effects of insulin.
2. Describe what to do before and after giving insulin.
3. Describe what to teach patients taking insulin, including what to do, what not to do, and when to call the prescriber.
4. List the names, actions, usual adult dosages, possible side effects, and adverse effects of noninsulin antidiabetic drugs.
5. Describe what to do before and after giving noninsulin antidiabetic drugs.
6. Explain what to teach patients taking noninsulin antidiabetic drugs, including what to do, what not to do, and when to call the prescriber.
7. Describe life span considerations for insulin therapy and for noninsulin antidiabetic drugs.

Key Terms

alpha-glucosidase inhibitors (ĂL-fă-glū-KŌ-sĭ-dās ĭn-HĬB-ĭ-tŭrz) (p. 220) A class of noninsulin antidiabetic drugs that work by slowing the digestion of dietary starches and other complex carbohydrates by inhibiting an enzyme that breaks them down into glucose.

amylin analogs (ĂM-ĭ-lĭn Ă-nă-lŏgs) (p. 220) A class of noninsulin antidiabetic drugs that are chemically similar to natural amylin, which delays gastric emptying and lowers after-meal blood glucose levels

diabetes mellitus (dī-ĕ-BĒ-tĕs MĔL-lĭ-tŭs) (p. 212) A metabolic disease that results from either the loss of the ability to make insulin or the loss of receptor sensitivity to the presence of insulin.

DPP-4 inhibitors (ĭn-HĬB-ĭ-tŭrz) (p. 220) A class of noninsulin antidiabetic drugs that work by inhibiting the enzyme DPP-IV, which normally breaks down and inactivates the incretin hormones, especially GLP-1. The result is an increase in the activity of normal incretin hormones.

glucagon (GLŪ-kă-gŏn) (p. 211) The hormone released by alpha cells of the pancreas and a synthetic drug that prevents hypoglycemia by breaking down glycogen from the liver into glucose.

glucose (GLŪ-kōs) (p. 210) The most common simple carbohydrate and the main fuel for the human body. Once inside cells, glucose is used to make the chemical energy substance adenosine triphosphate (ATP).

hyperglycemia (hī-pŭr-glī-SĒ-mē-ă) (p. 210) A blood glucose level above normal (higher than 110 mg/dL when fasting).

hypoglycemia (hī-pō-glī-SĒ-mē-ă) (p. 211) A blood glucose level below normal (lower than 70 mg/dL).

incretin mimetics (GLP1 agonists) (ĭn-krē-tĭn mĭ-MĔT-ĭk) (p. 220) A class of noninsulin antidiabetic drugs that work by acting like natural "gut" hormones that are secreted with meals at the same time insulin is secreted and help lower blood glucose by inhibiting glucagon secretion and reducing liver production of glucose.

insulin (ĬN-sŭl-ĭn) (p. 210) The hormone produced by the beta cells of the pancreas that prevents blood glucose levels from becoming too high.

insulin secretagogues (ĬN-sŭl-ĭn sĕ-KRĒ-tă-gŏgz) (p. 220) A class of noninsulin antidiabetic drugs known as *stimulators* that work by stimulating the beta cells of the pancreas to release preformed insulin.

insulin sensitizers (ĬN-sŭl-ĭn SĔN-sĭ-tī-zĕrs) (p. 220) A class of noninsulin antidiabetic drugs known as *sensitizers* that increase the sensitivity of the insulin receptor to the binding of naturally secreted insulin, which improves the movement of glucose from the blood into the cells the pancreas.

noninsulin antidiabetic drugs (nŏn-ĬN-sŭl-ĭn ăn-tĭ-dī-ă-BĔT-ĭk DRŬGZ) (p. 219) Oral and injectable drugs that use many actions to assist in lowering blood glucose levels.

sodium-glucose cotransport inhibitors (sō-de-um GLŪ-kōs kō-TRĂNS-pŏrt ĭn-HĬB-ĭ-tŭrz) (p. 220) The newest class of noninsulin antidiabetic drugs that lower blood glucose levels by preventing kidney reabsorption of glucose that was filtered from the blood into the urine.

209

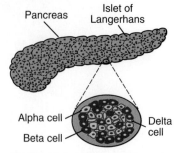

FIGURE 13-1 Close-up view of the pancreas showing the islets of Langerhans that contain the glucagon-secreting alpha cells and the insulin-secreting beta cells.

Memory Jogger

Body cells need glucose and oxygen to make enough adenosine triphosphate (ATP) to perform all bodily functions.

Memory Jogger

The trigger for insulin secretion is hyperglycemia, and its action is to restore normal blood glucose levels by allowing blood glucose to move into cells. Insulin *lowers* blood glucose levels.

OVERVIEW

The pancreas is an endocrine gland that makes two hormones, insulin and glucagon. These hormones are important for using the right "fuel" in the body and maintaining blood glucose balance. The beta cells of the pancreas make insulin, and the alpha cells of the pancreas make glucagon (Figure 13-1). Together insulin and glucagon ensure that the right amount of glucose is always present to provide enough energy for proper body *metabolism* (the energy use by each cell and amount of work performed within the body).

REVIEW OF RELATED PHYSIOLOGY AND PATHOPHYSIOLOGY

NORMAL PHYSIOLOGY

Glucose is the most common simple carbohydrate and the main source of fuel for the human body. Inside cells it is used to form *adenosine triphosphate (ATP)*, which is the main chemical energy substance that drives all of the cellular reactions of the body. The body makes its own ATP, mostly from glucose when adequate oxygen also is present. ATP is the "gasoline" that makes the body's "engine" run. For example, ATP provides the energy for skeletal muscle contraction for movement and maintenance of body temperature, heart muscle contraction for blood circulation, neuron excitation for thinking, and gastrointestinal work for food digestion. So for normal body function, people need a constant supply of glucose in the blood ready to enter cells and make sufficient amounts of ATP. However, too much glucose causes many problems. The right balance of insulin and glucagon, along with food intake, ensures that we always have the right amount of glucose in the blood.

Euglycemia is a normal fasting blood glucose level (between 70 and 110 mg/dL). Table 13-1 lists the laboratory values that indicate that control of glucose is adequate.

Insulin

Insulin is the hormone produced by the beta cells of the pancreas to prevent blood glucose levels from becoming too high. A blood glucose level above normal is called **hyperglycemia.** Insulin is made and released from the beta cells into the blood whenever blood glucose levels start to rise above normal levels. So the trigger for insulin secretion is hyperglycemia, and its action is to restore normal blood glucose levels by moving blood glucose into cells. The insulin binds to insulin receptors on the membranes of many cells. The result of having insulin bound to its receptor is that the cell membrane becomes more open to glucose, allowing the blood glucose to enter the cell (Figure 13-2). As glucose from the blood enters the cells, the blood glucose level returns to normal (euglycemia). The important thing to remember is that insulin lowers blood glucose levels.

Insulin is called the *hormone of plenty* because in the healthy person eating well makes blood levels of carbohydrates, proteins, and fats rise. When you have more than enough glucose to meet your energy needs, insulin allows the extra glucose to be converted to glycogen.

Table **13-1** Laboratory Indicators of Adequate Blood Glucose Control	
TEST	**VALUE**
Fasting blood glucose level	70 to 110 mg/dL
Hemoglobin A1c (A1C)	4% to 6%
Spot blood glucose level*	Less than 150 mg/dL
Blood ketone body level	Negative
Urine glucose level	Negative
Urine ketone body level	Negative

*Random, not fasting.

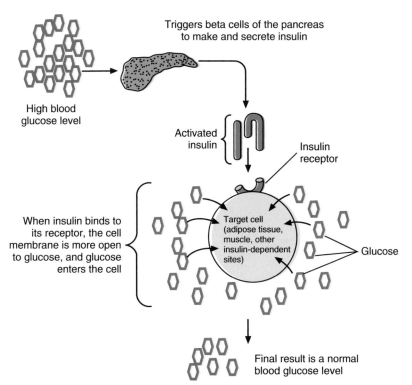

Triggers beta cells of the pancreas
to make and secrete insulin

High blood
glucose level

Activated
insulin

Insulin
receptor

When insulin binds to
its receptor, the cell
membrane is more open
to glucose, and glucose
enters the cell

Target cell
(adipose tissue,
muscle, other
insulin-dependent
sites)

Glucose

Final result is a normal
blood glucose level

FIGURE 13-2 Action of insulin.

Box 13-1   Effects of Insulin

- Prevents blood glucose levels from rising too high
- Prevents muscle breakdown
- Stores fats inside fat cells
- Builds glycogen (stored form of glucose) in the liver and muscle
- Improves protein digestion and use in the body
- Increases the amount of energy produced in the cells
- Induces cell division for growth and wound healing
- Maintains blood levels of cholesterol and other fats within normal limits

---

Glycogen is human starch that serves as the storage form of extra glucose. Molecules of glucose are linked together to form the trunk and branches of glycogen "trees" (Figure 13-3). Insulin also helps control protein and fat metabolism. Box 13-1 lists the effects of insulin.

Glucagon

If insulin were the only hormone controlling blood glucose levels, the body would be at risk for having blood glucose levels below normal, a condition called **hypoglycemia**. Low blood glucose levels reduce body metabolism because not enough glucose enters cells to make adequate amounts of ATP. If hypoglycemia is severe enough, it can quickly lead to death. So balancing blood glucose levels to avoid hypoglycemia involves the action of the hormone glucagon.

Glucagon is the hormone released by the alpha cells of the pancreas that prevents hypoglycemia by breaking down glycogen into glucose. It is released whenever blood glucose starts to fall below normal levels. The trigger for glucagon secretion is hypoglycemia, and its action is to raise the blood glucose level back up to normal. Glucagon starts actions that remove glucose from glycogen trees, resulting in release of free glucose into the blood (Figure 13-4), bringing the level back to normal (euglycemia). In addition to being a natural hormone, glucagon is also a drug used to treat severe hypoglycemia. Thanks to the action of glucagon, a person can go 10 to

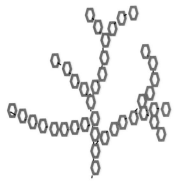

FIGURE 13-3 One glycogen "tree" with 40 molecules of glucose stored in it.

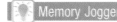 Memory Jogger

Hypoglycemia (low blood glucose levels) can rapidly lead to death.

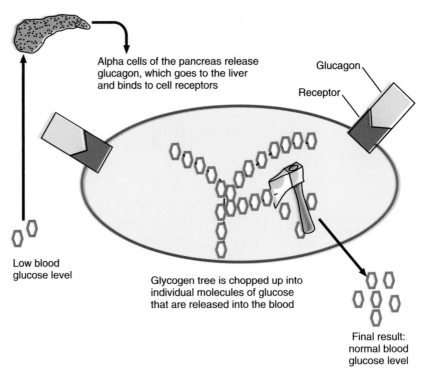

Alpha cells of the pancreas release glucagon, which goes to the liver and binds to cell receptors

Glucagon

Receptor

Low blood glucose level

Glycogen tree is chopped up into individual molecules of glucose that are released into the blood

Final result: normal blood glucose level

FIGURE 13-4 Action of glucagon.

 Memory Jogger

The trigger for glucagon secretion is hypoglycemia, and its action is to restore the blood glucose level back up to normal.

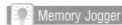 **Memory Jogger**

Blood glucose is controlled by insulin and glucagon. Insulin causes blood glucose levels to decrease, preventing hyperglycemia. Glucagon causes blood glucose levels to rise, preventing hypoglycemia.

 Memory Jogger

Patients with type 1 diabetes do not make their own insulin and must use insulin from other sources.

 Memory Jogger

Symptoms of untreated diabetes include excessive hunger, thirst, polydipsia, polyuria, weight loss, and fatigue.

12 hours without eating and not become so hypoglycemic that cells die. So glucagon and insulin have opposite actions.

The balance between insulin action and glucagon action keeps blood glucose levels in the normal range. Although the cell types for insulin and glucagon secretion are both in the pancreas, problems occur much more often with the cells that secrete insulin.

PATHOPHYSIOLOGY

Diabetes mellitus (DM) is a common metabolic disease that results from either the loss of the ability to make insulin or the loss of receptor sensitivity to the presence of insulin. The first result of either of these problems is increased blood glucose levels (hyperglycemia). The two most common forms of diabetes mellitus are type 1 and type 2. They differ in cause, usual age of onset, degree of insulin secretion remaining, and how they are treated. The two types have many of the same symptoms, and the long-term complications are the same. However, the drugs used to treat these disorders differ because people who have type 1 diabetes do not make any insulin and those with type 2 diabetes do continue to make some insulin.

Type 1 Diabetes

Type 1 diabetes (DM1) results when the beta cells of the pancreas no longer make and secrete any insulin. Without insulin the patient's blood glucose level becomes very high, but glucose cannot enter many cells. As a result, the body switches from using glucose to using fat to make ATP. Overall the body has less ATP available. Because insulin is no longer produced, patients who have DM1 must use insulin daily for the rest of their lives or receive a pancreas transplant.

Although DM1 can occur at any age, it most commonly begins in children and young adults. The first symptoms are caused by hyperglycemia. These include excessive hunger and eating (*polyphagia*), thirst, drinking more fluids than usual throughout the day (*polydipsia*), urinating more (*polyuria*), weight loss, and fatigue. The fasting blood glucose level is above 110 mg/dL, and often glucose is present in the urine.

If DM1 is not treated with insulin, hyperglycemia worsens, and the body uses more fat for fuel. When fat is used to make ATP, a by-product is the formation of ketoacids. If these ketoacids form faster than they are eliminated, the patient develops *diabetic ketoacidosis (DKA)*, a serious complication that can result in coma and death.

Type 2 Diabetes

Type 2 diabetes (DM2) is much more common than DM1. The cause of DM2 appears to be genetic, although not everyone with the known gene mutations develops the disease. The biggest nongenetic risk factors for developing the disease are obesity and a sedentary lifestyle. With DM2 the person still has beta cells that make some insulin; however, the insulin receptors are not very sensitive to insulin. As a result, insulin does not bind as tightly to its receptors as it should, and less glucose moves from the blood into the cells. So hyperglycemia is present with DM2.

Because some insulin is made and used with DM2, the symptoms are much more gradual in onset than those of DM1. In addition, because some glucose does get into the cells, fat is not used for fuel in DM2, and the person usually does not develop ketoacidosis.

Long-Term Complications of Diabetes

Insulin is important for all types of metabolism, not just for glucose control. Without adequate amounts of insulin the person with either type of diabetes has major changes in blood vessels that lead to organ damage, serious health problems, and early death. Box 13-2 lists many of the serious complications of untreated or poorly controlled diabetes. The long-term complications of the disease are the same for both DM1 and DM2.

TYPES OF DRUGS FOR DIABETES

Drug therapy for diabetes reduces the risks for many long-term complications and extends life. Patients who are able to control blood glucose levels with a combination of drug therapy, diet, and regular exercise also live longer, healthier lives.

The drug types used to manage diabetes are insulin and noninsulin antidiabetic drugs, which include oral agents and some injectable drugs that increase the amounts of other hormones (incretins and amylin) that work with insulin. All patients with DM1 must receive insulin therapy as hormone replacement for the rest of their lives. For the patient who has DM2 and still makes some insulin, other drugs can help maintain normal blood glucose levels in a variety of ways.

INSULIN THERAPY

The goals of insulin therapy for DM1 are to maintain blood glucose levels within the normal range, avoid ketoacidosis, and prevent or delay the blood vessel changes that lead to organ damage. Insulin is a small protein that is destroyed by stomach acids and intestinal enzymes and must be taken parenterally.

 Memory Jogger

Patients with DM2 make some of their own insulin, but the insulin receptors are resistant to binding with the insulin. This problem is most common among people who are overweight.

 Memory Jogger

Complications from untreated or poorly controlled diabetes include blindness; kidney failure; foot and leg amputations; hypertension; and increased risk for infection, heart attacks, and strokes.

 Memory Jogger

Insulin only controls diabetes; it does not cure the disease.

 Memory Jogger

Because insulin is destroyed by stomach acids and intestinal enzymes, it cannot be used as an oral drug. Most commonly it is injected subcutaneously, although an orally inhaled formulation is now available.

| Box 13-2 | Complications of Poorly Controlled Diabetes |

- Blindness
- Early death
- Erectile dysfunction
- High blood cholesterol levels
- High blood triglyceride levels
- Hypertension
- Increased risk for heart attack
- Increased risk for infection
- Increased risk for stroke
- Loss of touch sensation (peripheral neuropathy)
- Kidney failure
- Poor wound healing (especially on the feet and legs, leading to amputation)

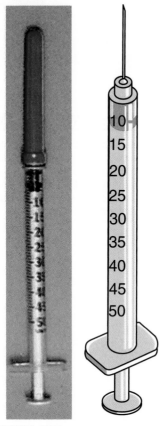

FIGURE 13-5 50-unit (U-50) insulin syringes. (From Lilley, L., Harrington, S., & Snyder, J. (2007). *Pharmacology and the Nursing Process* (5th ed.). St. Louis: Mosby.)

Types of Insulin

Although some insulin is obtained from animal sources, today most of it is synthetic. Regardless of insulin type, it is a *high-alert drug*, meaning that it can cause serious harm if the wrong dose is given, if a dose is given to a patient for whom it was *not* prescribed, or if a dose is *not* given to a patient for whom it was prescribed. For most patients with diabetes, insulin is injected subcutaneously using a special syringe with a short, thin needle (Figure 13-5). Special internal and external insulin pumps also can be used to deliver insulin either continuously as needed or hourly. Although both of these methods have advantages over regular injections, they are expensive and have some complications. Thus most patients with DM1 use either standard insulin syringes or prefilled automatic syringes or pens to inject insulin from once to as many as 8 or 10 times each day.

Many types of insulin are available as therapy for DM1, although all insulin works in the same way at the cellular level. Insulin types vary by how fast they work, how long the effects last (duration), and whether they are synthetic or come from animal sources. Table 13-2 lists the most common types of insulin for general injection and their features. Be sure to consult a drug reference for more information about a specific insulin.

Table 13-2 Types and Durations of Insulin

PREPARATION	TRADE NAME	ONSET (hr)	PEAK (hr)	DURATION (hr)
Rapid-Acting Insulin				
Insulin aspart	NovoLog	0.25	1-3	3-5
Insulin glulisine	Apidra	0.3	0.5-1.5	3-4
Insulin lispro injection	Humalog	0.25	0.5-1.5	5
Short-Acting Insulin				
Regular human insulin injection	Humulin R	0.5	2-4	5-7
	Novolin R	0.5	2.5-5	8
	ReliOn R	0.5	2.5-5	8
Intermediate-Acting Insulin				
Isophane insulin NPH injection	Humulin N	1.5	4-12	10-16 or longer
	Novolin N			
	ReliOn N			
70% human insulin isophane suspension/30% human regular insulin injection	Humulin 70/30	0.5	6-10	10-16
	Novolin 70/30	0.5	6-10	10-16
50% human insulin isophane suspension/50% human insulin injection	Humulin 50/50	0.5	3-5	10-16 or longer
70% insulin aspart protamine suspension/30% insulin aspart injection	NovoLog Mix 70/30	0.25	1-4	18-24
75% insulin lispro protamine suspension/25% insulin lispro injection	Humalog Mix 75/25	0.25	1-2	18-24
Long-Acting Insulin				
Insulin glargine injection	Lantus	2	None	24
Insulin detemir injection	Levemir	1	None	5.7-24

How Insulin Therapy Works

Just like the insulin the body makes, insulin injected into the body binds to insulin receptors on the membranes of many cells. The result of having the injected insulin bound to its receptor is that the cell membrane becomes more open to glucose, allowing glucose to leave the blood and enter cells (see Figure 13-2). As glucose from the blood enters the cells, the blood glucose level is reduced to normal (euglycemia).

Intended Responses

- Blood glucose levels are in the normal range.
- There is no glucose or acetone in the urine.
- Blood lipid levels are at or close to the normal range.

Side Effects. Insulin as a drug has few side effects. Side effects are usually related to having repeated subcutaneous injections at one site or body area. These problems include injection site infections and changes in the skin and subcutaneous tissue at injection sites.

Adverse Effects. The main adverse effect of insulin is the lowering of blood glucose levels *below* normal *(hypoglycemia)*. This action, sometimes called *insulin shock*, is dangerous because brain cells are very sensitive to low blood glucose levels and the patient can become nonresponsive very quickly. If the problem is not corrected quickly, the patient can die. The signs and symptoms of hypoglycemia are listed in Box 13-3.

Insulin Regimens

The goal of insulin therapy for patients with DM1 is to keep blood glucose levels within the normal range at all times. Better overall blood glucose control occurs with multiple injections of insulin each day.

An *insulin regimen* or program is the insulin injection schedule used to prevent hyperglycemia. The most effective regimens are those that provide insulin in a pattern that closely resembles the way insulin normally is released from the healthy pancreas. The normal pancreas releases a constant *(basal)* amount of insulin that keeps blood glucose levels normal between meals by balancing liver glucose production with whole-body glucose use. The normal pancreas is also stimulated by eating food to produce additional insulin to prevent blood glucose levels from rising too high after meals.

The total amount of insulin needed and how often it is needed for blood glucose control varies among patients. Usually the patient injects long-acting insulin at the beginning of the day for a basal dose. Shorter-acting insulin is taken before meals and snacks. The amount of insulin needed and injected is based on blood glucose levels. The patient checks his or her blood glucose level 2 to 12 times each day based on insulin regimen, activity level, age, total amount of calories needed in a day, and how his or her blood glucose level responds to the insulin. Some standard insulin regimens (injection programs) are shown in Figure 13-6.

Some patients who have DM1 inject insulin as a combination of more than one insulin type administered just once daily. However, control of blood glucose is managed better when insulin injections of smaller dosages are used more frequently.

Memory Jogger

Insulin injected into the body works in exactly the same way as insulin secreted by the pancreas.

Memory Jogger

Hypoglycemia is *always* a potential adverse effect of insulin therapy.

QSEN: Safety

Memory Jogger

Insulin side effects are:
- Injection site infections
- Skin and fatty tissue changes at injection sites

Box 13-3	Signs and Symptoms of Hypoglycemia

- Anxiety, confusion, loss of consciousness
- Cool, clammy skin
- Headache
- Hunger
- Increased sweating
- Rapid, pounding heart rate
- Shakiness, tremors

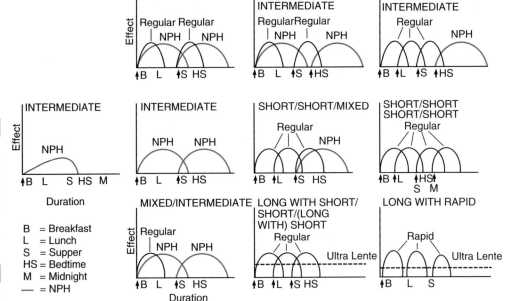

FIGURE 13-6 Examples of different insulin dosing schedules.

 Drug Alert!

Action/Interaction Alert

Whenever insulin is given *before* a meal, it is critical that the patient eat a meal of sufficient calories within 15 minutes of the insulin injection.

QSEN: Safety

 Memory Jogger

Intensified insulin regimens provide the best control over blood glucose levels but require many more "sticks" each day than other insulin injection regimens.

 Drug Alert!

Administration Alert

Insulin types are not interchangeable. Double check the order and your calculation with another licensed health care professional to ensure that you are giving the prescribed dose.

QSEN: Safety

 Drug Alert!

Administration Alert

Always use an insulin syringe that is calibrated and marked in the same unit concentration as the insulin you are giving.

QSEN: Safety

Clinical Pitfall

Never use any syringe other than an insulin syringe to give insulin.

QSEN: Safety

Clinical Pitfall

Do not use a rapid-acting insulin, short-acting insulin, insulin glargine, or insulin detemir if the liquid in the bottle is cloudy, if particles are present, or if the expiration date has passed.

QSEN: Safety

Regardless of the type of regimen, whenever short-acting insulin is given before a meal, the meal should be eaten within 15 minutes after receiving the injection to avoid hypoglycemia.

The most recommended insulin regimen for best control is the intensified regimen. These regimens include a basal dose of intermediate- or long-acting insulin and multiple-bolus doses of short- or rapid-acting insulin designed to bring the next blood glucose value into the target range. Insulin dosage is based on the patient's blood glucose patterns. Usually the patient must check the blood glucose levels at least eight times per day. Blood glucose testing 1 to 2 hours after meals and within 10 minutes before the next meal helps to determine how effective the bolus dose is.

What To Do *Before* Injecting Insulin

Insulin drug errors are common and have serious consequences, including death. The many different types of insulin increase the risk for errors. It is important not to interchange insulin types and to ensure that the dose prescribed is the one given.

Test the patient's blood glucose level before giving insulin and make sure that the patient can and will eat within 15 minutes of the insulin injection to prevent hypoglycemia. It is best to ensure that the meal is actually on the unit before giving the insulin.

Check the order carefully for the exact type and amount of insulin to be injected. Do not interchange insulin types. Insulin preparations are available in U-50, U-100, and U-500 concentrations. The most commonly used preparation is U-100 insulin (100 units per mL). When doses are less than 50 units, they are usually administered with a U-50 syringe (50 units per 0.5 mL). This drug is available in a concentration of 50 units on a 0.5-mL volume. U-100 insulin provides 100 units of insulin in 1 mL of drug. To give the correct amount of insulin, the syringe must be calibrated in the same units as the drug.

Check the insulin vial for color and clarity. Some insulin is supposed to be clear and colorless. This includes rapid-acting insulin, short-acting insulin, insulin glargine (Lantus), and insulin detemir (Levemir). If particles are present or if the liquid is cloudy, discard the insulin and open a new vial. All other insulin types have a cloudy appearance after they have been gently rotated.

Gently roll the insulin vial (or pen, cartridge, syringe, or other prefilled injection device) between your hands to mix and warm the insulin. Do not shake the vial because bubbles will form and the dose may not be accurate.

Needles on insulin syringes are small gauge (28 gauge, 29 gauge, and 30 gauge) and vary in length from ½ inch to 5⁄16 inch. Use shorter needles for thinner patients and longer needles for patients who have more subcutaneous tissue. Check and recheck that the amount and type of insulin you have drawn up into the syringe is the amount ordered. If possible, have another licensed health care professional also check the syringe volume and insulin type.

Select an appropriate site for the injection. Recommended sites are shown in Figure 13-7. Usually, the abdomen is the preferred site (except for a 2-inch circle around the umbilicus). Absorption of insulin after injection varies from site to site and can make the peak action of insulin less predictable.

Cleanse the site with an alcohol swab, and grasp a fold of skin in your nondominant hand. Insert the needle at a 90-degree angle (a 45-degree angle if the patient is very thin), and inject the insulin without pulling back on the plunger. (It is not necessary to check for a blood return, and pulling tissue back into the needle can cause bruising and other tissue damage.)

After the injection is complete, withdraw the needle rapidly while supporting the skin. Do not massage the site because doing so can change the rate that insulin is absorbed from the tissues.

If the patient is to receive two different types of insulin at the same time, it may be possible to mix the two types together in the same syringe so the patient is injected only once. Check with the pharmacist to be sure that the two prescribed types can be mixed together. Some insulin cannot be mixed with any other solution. For example, neither insulin glargine (Lantus) nor insulin detemir (Levemir) can be mixed with other insulin. If the prescribed types can be mixed, follow the directions in Box 13-4, which describes the correct technique to mix 10 units of regular insulin with 20 units of NPH insulin.

What To Do *After* Injecting Insulin

Check the patient hourly for signs and symptoms of hypoglycemia. These include confusion, cool and clammy skin, tremors, headache, hunger, and sweating (see Box 13-3). Keep a simple sugar (such as orange juice and sugar packets) on the unit. Ensure that the patient's meals or between-meal snacks are on time and that he or she eats them.

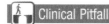
Clinical Pitfall

Do not shake an insulin container before drawing up the drug because bubbles will form and the dose may not be accurate.

QSEN: Safety

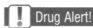
Drug Alert!

Administration Alert

After inserting the needle, inject the insulin without aspirating for blood and do not massage the site after removing the needle.

QSEN: Safety

Box 13-4   Guide for Mixing Two Types of Insulin

10 UNITS OF REGULAR INSULIN WITH 20 UNITS OF NPH INSULIN:
- After checking to make sure that you have the correct concentration and types of insulin, clean the rubber stoppers of each bottle with separate alcohol swabs.
- Draw up 20 units of air and inject it into the NPH bottle with the bottle in its normal, upright position. Always inject the air into the intermediate-acting insulin bottle first. The amount of air injected is the same amount as the insulin to be removed.
- Draw up 10 units of air and inject it into the regular insulin (short-acting insulin) bottle with the bottle in its normal, upright position. The amount of air injected is the same as the amount of insulin to be removed.
- Without removing the needle, turn the bottle upside down and withdraw 10 units of regular insulin; then withdraw the needle from the bottle. Always withdraw the shorter-acting insulin first. Make sure that the syringe is free from air bubbles.
- Now place the same needle with the syringe attached into the NPH bottle, invert the bottle, and withdraw 20 units of NPH insulin into the same syringe with the regular insulin. Take care not to inject any regular insulin into the NPH bottle.
- Check the syringe for the volume of insulin. For this example there should be 30 units in the syringe.

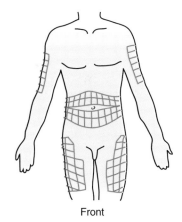
Front

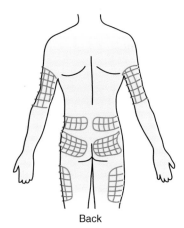
Back

FIGURE 13-7 Common insulin injection sites.

! Drug Alert!

Teaching Alert

Teach patients that it is important that at least one other family member, friend, companion, or neighbor also know how to inject insulin safely.

QSEN: Safety

Check the patient's response to insulin. Check blood glucose levels as often as ordered and whenever you suspect the patient may be hypoglycemic or hyperglycemic. Document the results.

The whole process of drawing up and injecting the correct amount of insulin without contaminating the drug or the needle may be frightening to a patient newly diagnosed with diabetes. A team approach to patient education, including a diabetes educator, can be very helpful. Usually teaching a patient how to self-inject insulin takes more than one teaching session and requires that he or she is alert enough to learn, can see well enough to ensure safe drug administration, and has good use of the arms, hands, and fingers to be able to perform the physical actions involved.

Teach patients to use the steps in Box 13-5 to self-administer insulin. To begin teaching, use normal saline solution and the same type of insulin syringe that the patient will use at home. Demonstrate how to correctly draw up insulin into the syringe and inject it. Have the patient, and whomever the patient designates as a helper, "teach back" the techniques to you, complete with explanations in his or her own words. Remind patients to always have a spare bottle of each type of insulin that they use. Using the manufacturer's recommendations, teach them about how to store insulin and any prefilled syringes, cartridges, or pens between uses.

Teach patients to check the injection site daily for any signs or symptoms of infection (warmth, redness, firmness to the touch, presence of drainage, pain in and around the area). The presence of any symptom indicating infection should be reported immediately to their prescriber.

Box 13-5   Patient Education Guide for Self-Injection of Insulin

- Wash your hands.
- Inspect the insulin container for the type of insulin and the expiration date.
- For rapid-acting insulin, short-acting insulin, insulin glargine, or insulin detemir, inspect the bottle for color and clarity. If particles are present or if the insulin is cloudy, discard the bottle and open a new one.
- For other insulin, gently rotate the bottle or container between the palms of your hands to mix the insulin.
- Clean the bottle stopper with an alcohol sponge (leave out this step if you are using a prefilled pen or cartridge).
- Remove the cover from the needle and pull back the plunger to draw in the same amount of air into the syringe as the amount of insulin you will be withdrawing from the bottle.
- Push the needle through the rubber stopper and inject the air into the insulin bottle with the bottle in the upright position (do not let the air bubble into the insulin).
- With the needle still in the bottle stopper, turn the bottle upside down and withdraw the same amount of insulin from the bottle as the air you put into the bottle.
- Make sure that the tip of the plunger is on the line of the syringe for your insulin dose.
- If air bubbles are present, tap the syringe while holding it upside down, letting the bubbles come to the top of the syringe where the needle is attached. Push out any air bubbles and recheck to ensure that the tip of the plunger is on the same line as your insulin dose.
- Remove the needle from the bottle stopper and recap the needle until you are ready to inject the insulin.
- Select an area within your usual injection site that has not been injected within the past 2 weeks.
- Cleanse the skin area with an alcohol swab.
- Remove the cap from the needle on the insulin syringe.
- Pinch up a fold of skin in the area you cleaned and push the needle in at a 90-degree angle.
- Push the plunger all the way down to ensure that the entire insulin dose is injected.
- Release the fold of skin and remove the needle straight out quickly.
- Do not rub or massage the spot where you injected the insulin.
- Place the syringe with the needle (without recapping it) into a puncture-proof container.

Teach patients the signs and symptoms of hypoglycemia (see Box 13-3). Urge them not to skip or delay meals. Tell them to always carry a carbohydrate source that contains at least 15 g of carbohydrate in a pocket or purse and to eat it at the first sign of hypoglycemia.

Stress to patients who are using insulin on a one-dose, two-dose, three-dose, or four-dose injection regimen the importance of keeping to the schedule for insulin injection and meals. For patients using insulin on an intensified injection regimen, there is more flexibility of meal timing because the injections are timed to the meals and blood glucose levels.

Life Span Considerations for Insulin

Pediatric Considerations. Many children have DM1 and require insulin injections and blood testing of glucose levels. A child may have daily differences in the amount or type of food eaten and the amount of exercise experienced. These differences can make having good control over blood glucose levels a real challenge.

Considerations for Pregnancy and Lactation. The disease is often more difficult to control during the physically stressful time of pregnancy. In addition, some patients who do not have diabetes may have problems with hyperglycemia only during pregnancy. This condition is called *gestational diabetes mellitus (GDM)*. Untreated diabetes during pregnancy increases health problems in the mother and can cause birth defects in the infant.

Insulin is the treatment of choice for diabetes during pregnancy. Insulin needs change during pregnancy and often increase during the last 6 months. Reassure patients who use additional insulin injections during pregnancy that the extra injections usually are not needed once the pregnancy is over.

Considerations for Older Adults. Type 1 diabetes is managed with insulin, and insulin use in an older adult can pose some special problems. Many older adults with DM1 have some degree of reduced vision and a decreased sense of touch as a result of the disease. These problems increase the risk for errors in insulin dosing, injection, and self-monitoring of blood glucose levels. Older patients may benefit from the use of prefilled insulin syringes, cartridges, or pens. Urge older adults with vision problems to use magnifying glasses and good light when testing blood glucose levels or withdrawing insulin.

The risk for hypoglycemia is increased in older adults, especially if they also take beta-adrenergic blocking drugs, warfarin (Coumadin), or other drugs that increase the hypoglycemic response. The older adult may eat less than a younger adult and must understand how to match insulin dosage and scheduling with food intake.

NONINSULIN ANTIDIABETIC DRUGS

Drugs for DM2 used to be called *hypoglycemic agents*. However, because the goal of therapy is to help the person become euglycemic rather than hypoglycemic, the correct term is *antidiabetic drug*. **Noninsulin antidiabetic drugs** are oral and injectable drugs that use many actions to assist in lowering blood glucose levels. Because they work in different ways to control blood glucose levels, two or more drugs may be used together for best control. Some patients with DM2 also require insulin therapy as temporary therapy or when the disease progresses.

The drugs for treating DM2 are classified by their chemical structures or their actions. The seven major classes of antidiabetic drugs are the insulin secretagogues ("stimulators"), the insulin sensitizers, the alpha-glucosidase inhibitors, the incretin mimetics (GLP-1 agonists), the amylin analogs, the DPP-4 inhibitors, and the sodium-glucose cotransport inhibitors. The mechanism of action for each class of drugs is different. The decision to use one type of drug with or instead of another type is based on how much beta cell function is left, how the patient responds to the drug, and the patient's overall health. Drug dosages are based on patient responses to therapy.

Teaching Alert

Teach patients the signs and symptoms of hypoglycemia (confusion, cool and clammy skin, tremors, headache, hunger, sweating). Urge patients not to skip or delay meals after taking insulin.

QSEN: Safety

Controlling DM1 in children is more difficult because of day-to-day variations in the amount and types of food eaten and in the amount of exercise experienced.

Insulin is the preferred drug to manage diabetes during pregnancy.

Interaction Alert

The risk for hypoglycemia with insulin is increased when patients also take beta-adrenergic blocking drugs, warfarin (Coumadin), or other drugs that increase the hypoglycemic response.

QSEN: Safety

The goal of drug therapy for DM2 is to have normal blood glucose levels, reduced blood fat levels, and normal body weight.

Memory Jogger

The seven classes of noninsulin antidiabetic drugs are:
- Insulin secretagogues (stimulators)
- Insulin sensitizers
- Alpha-glucosidase inhibitors
- Incretin mimetics (GLP-1 agonists)
- Amylin analogs
- DPP-4 inhibitors
- Sodium-glucose cotransport inhibitors

How Noninsulin Antidiabetic Drugs Work

Insulin secretagogues are noninsulin antidiabetic drugs known as "stimulators" that work by stimulating the beta cells of the pancreas to release preformed insulin. The increased insulin then lowers blood glucose levels. Types of drugs in this class are the second-generation sulfonylureas and the meglitinide analogs.

Insulin sensitizers are noninsulin antidiabetic drugs (biguanides and thiazolidine-diones) that do not act directly on the beta cells of the pancreas. Instead they increase the sensitivity of the insulin receptor to the binding of naturally secreted insulin, which improves the movement of glucose from the blood into the cells. These drugs also decrease liver glucose production and some help reduce the absorption of glucose from the intestinal tract into the blood. As a result, these drugs lower blood glucose levels to normal without causing hypoglycemia.

Alpha-glucosidase inhibitors are noninsulin antidiabetic drugs that work by slowing the digestion of dietary starches and other complex carbohydrates by inhibiting an enzyme that breaks them down into glucose. The result of this action is that blood glucose does not rise as far or as fast after a meal. Drugs from this class do not cause hypoglycemia when taken as the only therapy for diabetes.

Incretin mimetics (GLP1 agonists) are noninsulin antidiabetic drugs that work by acting like natural "gut" hormones that are secreted with meals at the same time insulin is secreted and help lower blood glucose levels in several ways. They inhibit glucagon secretion thus reducing liver production of glucose and they delay gastric emptying. This slows the rate of glucose absorption into the blood and makes the person feel full. The actions of these drugs rely on pancreatic insulin production and are not to be used for patients who have DM1.

Amylin analogs are noninsulin antidiabetic drugs that are chemically similar to natural amylin, which delays gastric emptying and lowers after-meal blood glucose levels; trigger satiety in the brain; and suppress glucagon action, which prevents liver release of glucose.

DPP-4 inhibitors are noninsulin antidiabetic drugs that work by inhibiting the enzyme DDP-IV, which normally breaks down and inactivates the incretin hormones, especially GLP-1. By inhibiting this enzyme, DPP-4 inhibitor drugs slow the inactivation of the natural incretin hormones. Thus it increases the active incretin hormone levels in the body, reducing both before- and after-meal blood glucose levels. These drugs work only when blood glucose is elevated.

Sodium-glucose cotransport inhibitors are the newest class of antidiabetic drugs. These drugs lower blood glucose levels by preventing kidney reabsorption of glucose that was filtered from the blood into the urine. Thus the filtered glucose is excreted in the urine rather than moved back into the blood.

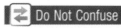

Do Not Confuse

glipiZIDE *with* **glyBURIDE**

An order for glipizide can be confused with glyburide. Although both drugs are oral antidiabetic drugs from the second-generation sulfonylurea class, the dosages are very different.

QSEN: Safety

Do Not Confuse

Micronase *with* **Microzide**

An order for Micronase can be confused with Microzide. Micronase is an oral antidiabetic drug, whereas Microzide is a diuretic.

QSEN: Safety

Do Not Confuse

Actos *with* **Actonel**

An order for Actos can be confused with Actonel. Actos is an oral antidiabetic drug from the thiazolidinedione class, whereas Actonel is a drug that prevents calcium loss from bones.

QSEN: Safety

Dosages for Common Oral Antidiabetic Drugs

Drug	Dosage (Adults Only)
Insulin Secretagogues	
Second-Generation Sulfonylureas	
glimepiride ❶ (Amaryl, Apo-Glimepiride ♣, Novo-Glimepiride ♣)	1-8 mg orally daily at breakfast or first meal of the day
glipiZIDE ❶ (Glucotrol) (Glucotrol XL)	Immediate-release: 5-40 mg orally once or 5-20 mg orally twice daily Extended-release: 5-20 mg orally once daily
glyBURIDE ❶ (Apo-Glyburide ♣, Diabeta, Gen-Glybe ♣, Euglucon ♣, Micronase) glyBURIDE, micronized ❶ (Glynase Pres-Tab)	1.25-20 mg orally daily in 1-2 divided doses 0.75-12 mg orally daily in 1-2 divided doses
Meglitinides	
nateglinide ❶ (Starlix)	60-120 mg orally within 15-30 min of every meal
repaglinide ❶ (GlucoNorm ♣, Prandin)	0.5-4 mg orally within 15-30 min of every meal

Dosages for Common Oral Antidiabetic Drugs—cont'd

Drug	Dosage (Adults Only)
Insulin Sensitizers	
Biguanides	
metformin ❶ (Apo-Metformin ✿, Fortamet, Glucophage, Glumetza ✿, Glycon ✿, Riomet) (Glucophage XR)	Immediate-release: 500-850 mg orally twice daily with meals Extended-release: 500-2000 mg orally once daily with evening meal
Thiazolidinediones ("glitazones," TZDs)	
pioglitazone ❶ (Actos, Apo-Pioglitazone ✿, Novo-Pioglitazone ✿)	15-45 mg orally daily
rosiglitazone ❶ (Avandia)	2-4 mg orally once or twice daily
Alpha-Glucosidase Inhibitors	
acarbose (Prandase ✿, Precose)	25-100 mg orally 3 times daily with first bite of a meal
miglitol (Glyset)	25-100 mg orally 3 times daily with first bite of a meal
Incretin Mimetics (GLp-1 agonists)	
exenatide ❶ (Byetta) exenatide extended release (Bydureon)	5-10 mcg subcutaneously twice daily before the two largest meals 2 mg subcutaneously once every 7 days
liraglutide ❶ (Victoza)	0.6 mg subcutaneously daily; gradually increase to 1.8 mg subcutaneously daily
Amylin Analogs	
pramlintide ❶ (Symlin)	DM1: 15-60 mcg subcutaneously with meal 3-4 times daily DM2: 60-120 mcg subcutaneously with meal 3-4 times daily
DPP-4 Inhibitors	
alogliptin ❶ (Nesina)	25 mg orally once daily
linagliptin ❶ (Tradjenta)	5 mg orally once daily
saxagliptin ❶ (Onglyza)	2.5-5 mg orally once daily
sitagliptin ❶ (Januvia)	100 mg orally once daily
Sodium-Glucose Cotransport Inhibitors	
canagliflozin ❶ (Invokana)	100-300 mg orally once daily
dapagliflozin ❶ (Farxiga)	5-10 mg orally once daily

❶ High-alert drug.

Intended Responses
- Blood glucose levels are in the normal range.
- There is no glucose in the urine.

Side Effects. Side effects common to most of the oral noninsulin antidiabetic drugs, amylin analogs, and incretin mimetics include nausea, vomiting, diarrhea, and rashes. *Exenatide, liraglutide,* and *pramlintide* may also cause irritation at the injection site. Additional side effects for the DPP-4 inhibitors include abdominal pain and increased incidence of respiratory infections.

Sulfonylureas also may cause increased sun sensitivity (photosensitivity), blurred vision, fluid retention, and anemia.

Meglitinides also may cause dizziness, back pain, upper respiratory infections, and flulike achiness.

Metformin (Glucophage) and the *alpha-glucosidase inhibitors* also may cause bloating, flatulence, indigestion, abdominal pain, and headache.

Common Side Effects

Noninsulin Antidiabetic Drugs

Nausea/Vomiting, Diarrhea

Rash

Thiazolidinedione drugs also may cause upper respiratory infections, headaches, muscle aches, fluid retention, weight gain, and anemia.

Adverse Effects. The most common adverse effect for many noninsulin antidiabetic drugs is severe hypoglycemia. The "stimulators," such as the sulfonylureas and the meglitinides, cause this effect individually because they force the beta cells to release more insulin anytime, even when the patient's blood glucose level is normal. The incretin mimetics, the amylin analogs, the DPP-4 inhibitors, and the sodium-glucose cotransport inhibitors also can cause hypoglycemia when used individually. For the insulin sensitizers and the alpha-glucosidase inhibitors the risk for hypoglycemia occurs only when the drugs are used in combination.

Metformin can cause lactic acidosis, which is the buildup of lactic acid in tissues when not enough oxygen is present to allow metabolism to occur normally. Signs and symptoms of lactic acidosis are muscle aches, fatigue, drowsiness, abdominal pain, hypotension, and a slow, irregular heartbeat. Drinking alcohol, having liver disease, or having kidney problems increases the risk for lactic acidosis.

Tests that involve the use of radio-opaque dye (such as urograms, angiograms, and other scans) can lead to kidney failure with metformin, usually within 48 hours. A patient who takes metformin may take the dose before receiving the dye but should not resume the drug again until 48 hours after testing with dye or surgery with anesthesia, or until good urine output has been reestablished.

Alpha-glucosidase inhibitors and *thiazolidinedione drugs* can cause liver problems, leading to jaundice, higher-than-normal liver enzymes, and difficulty digesting fatty meals. *Thiazolidinedione drugs,* especially rosiglitazone, may lead to heart failure as a result of water retention. Rosiglitazone (Avandia) has a black box warning indicating that it should not be prescribed for anyone who has or who is at risk for heart failure (see Chapter 1 for a discussion of black box warnings).

The *incretin mimetics* and *sodium-glucose cotransport inhibitors* are associated with an increased risk for pancreatitis. The *sodium-glucose cotransport inhibitors* can increase urine output to the extent that dehydration and electrolyte imbalances can occur.

The *DPP-4 inhibitors* are associated with a higher incidence of serious allergic reactions, including anaphylaxis, angioedema, and Stevens-Johnson syndrome.

What To Do *Before* Giving Noninsulin Antidiabetic Drugs

For all the noninsulin antidiabetic drugs that can cause hypoglycemia even when used alone, make sure that the patient's meal is actually on the unit before giving the drug and that he or she is able to eat the meal within a few minutes of taking the drug.

Check to see whether the patient is also taking any other drug that can make hypoglycemia worse. Observe the patient closely for hypoglycemia if he or she also is taking aspirin, nonsteroidal anti-inflammatory drugs (NSAIDs), warfarin (Coumadin), beta-adrenergic blockers, fluoroquinolone antibiotics, probenecid, or azole antifungal drugs.

For a patient who is just being started on a *sulfonylurea,* ask about any allergies to the sulfonamide type of antibacterial drugs. The sulfonylurea drugs are similar to the sulfonamides, and an allergy to one usually is associated with an allergy to the other.

Metformin (a biguanide) requires many actions before giving the drug. Check to see if the patient is scheduled for surgery or a scan test involving dye during the next 48 hours because the prescriber may hold the drug for 48 hours after the procedure to reduce the risk for kidney failure.

Check the patient's vital signs (including temperature, mental status, heart rate, and blood pressure) before starting metformin. Use this information as a baseline to determine whether any side effect or adverse effect is present.

Check the patient's daily urine output and current laboratory work, especially blood urea nitrogen (BUN) and serum creatinine levels because kidney problems increase the effects of the drug and the risk for lactic acidosis.

Memory Jogger

Noninsulin antidiabetic drugs that, when used alone, can cause hypoglycemia are the sulfonylureas, meglitinides, incretin mimetics, amylin analogs, DPP-4 inhibitors, and the sodium-glucose cotransport inhibitors.

Clinical Pitfall

Metformin (Glucophage) can cause lactic acidosis. Do not give this drug within 48 hours to anyone who has had testing with dye or surgery with anesthesia.

QSEN: Safety

Clinical Pitfall

Do not give the thiazolidinediones to a patient with severe heart failure.

QSEN: Safety

Drug Alert!

Action/Intervention Alert

Give noninsulin antidiabetic drugs with food (preferably with a meal) to reduce the risk for hypoglycemia.

QSEN: Safety

Clinical Pitfall

Do not give metformin to a patient with a serum creatinine higher than 1.4 mg/dL (females) or 1.5 mg/dL (males).

QSEN: Safety

If metformin (Glucophage XR) is prescribed, do not crush the tablet. Crushing the tablet destroys its time-release properties and may allow too much drug to enter the patient's bloodstream at one time.

With *alpha-glucosidase inhibitors* and *thiazolidinedione drugs,* check the patient's most recent laboratory tests, especially liver enzyme levels. These drugs are contraindicated for patients with liver disease.

With *thiazolidinedione drugs,* check the patient's vital signs (especially heart rate, blood pressure, and respiratory rate) and pulse oximetry. These vital signs serve as a baseline and can be used to help determine if a problem with heart failure is developing.

Check the patient's weight and indications of edema formation to use as a baseline to determine whether water retention occurs as a result of taking a thiazolidinedione.

What To Do *After* Giving Noninsulin Antidiabetic Drugs

Check the patient hourly for signs and symptoms of hypoglycemia (see Box 13-3). Keep a carbohydrate source that contains at least 15 g of carbohydrate on the unit. Ensure that the patient's meals are on time and that he or she is able to eat them.

With *alpha-glucosidase inhibitors* and *thiazolidinediones,* monitor liver function tests for elevations. Check the patient daily for jaundice by looking at the skin, roof of the mouth, or whites of the eyes. If these signs appear, notify the prescriber.

With *metformin,* check the patient's vital signs (including temperature, heart rate, and blood pressure) and mental status at least every 4 hours for symptoms of lactic acidosis. Urge him or her to drink plenty of water throughout the day and night to prevent dehydration.

With *thiazolidinediones,* weigh the patient daily and compare the results with his or her initial weight. Weight gain of more than $\frac{1}{2}$ lb in 1 day or 3 lb in 1 week is usually a result of water retention, which is an indication of heart failure. Check the patient's ankles for edema formation, which may indicate water retention or heart failure.

Check the patient's heart rate and blood pressure at least once each shift. Also listen to his or her lungs. Monitoring these vital signs can help identify a heart failure problem early.

With the *incretin mimetics* and the *amylin analogs,* check the injection sites for signs and symptoms of infection. Assess patients taking *incretin mimetics* or the *DPP-4 inhibitors* for signs and symptoms of pancreatitis (severe epigastric pain, vomiting). Also, with the *DPP-4 inhibitors,* observe the patient for any sign of an allergic reaction.

With the *sodium-glucose cotransport inhibitors,* assess the patient's fluid status for dehydration and his or her electrolytes for imbalances, especially of sodium and potassium. (See Table 1-4 in Chapter 1 for normal serum electrolyte values.)

What To *Teach* Patients About Noninsulin Antidiabetic Drugs

Teach patients the signs and symptoms of hypoglycemia (see Box 13-3). Urge them not to skip or delay meals. Tell them to always carry a carbohydrate containing at least 15 g of carbohydrate in a pocket or purse and to eat it at the first sign of hypoglycemia. Teach them to recheck their blood glucose level 15 minutes after eating the carbohydrate to determine whether additional carbohydrate is needed.

Instruct patients to avoid drinking alcohol because it is likely to induce hypoglycemia. If alcohol is used, it should be limited to one serving and taken either with food or right after a meal is completed.

Sulfonylureas increase sun sensitivity (photosensitivity) and greatly increase the risk for sunburn, even for people who have dark skin.

Meglitinides are given right before any meal or substantial snack. For most patients the drug is taken three times a day. If the patient has more than three meals in a day, the drug should also be taken with each of the extra meals. Teach patients to prevent hypoglycemia by taking the drug no sooner than 15 to 30 minutes before a meal.

 Clinical Pitfall

Do not crush metformin (Glucophage XR) tablets.

QSEN: Safety

 Drug Alert!

Action/Intervention Alert

Because thiazolidinediones (especially rosiglitazone [Avandia]) can cause or worsen cardiac complications, weigh the patient daily and monitor heart rate and rhythm, blood pressure, and lung sounds every 8 hours.

QSEN: Safety

 Drug Alert!

Teaching Alert

Teach patients the signs and symptoms of hypoglycemia: confusion, cool and clammy skin, tremors, headache, hunger, and sweating. Urge patients not to skip or delay meals.

QSEN: Safety

 Drug Alert!

Teaching Alert

Teach patients taking a sulfonylurea to avoid direct sunlight, use sunscreen, and wear protective clothing (including a hat) whenever sun exposure is likely to occur to prevent a severe sunburn.

QSEN: Safety

 Drug Alert!

Teaching Alert

Meglitinide drug doses are matched to meals. If a meal is missed, that drug dose must also be missed to prevent hypoglycemia.

QSEN: Safety

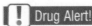

Teaching Alert

Exenatide (Byetta) and liraglutide doses are matched to the two main meals of the day. If a meal is missed, that drug dose must also be missed to prevent hypoglycemia. Pramlintide is taken before all meals. If a meal is missed, that drug dose must also be skipped.

QSEN: Safety

Drug Alert!

Teaching Alert

Teach patients taking an injectable noninsulin antidiabetic drug to check the injection site daily for symptoms of infection (warmth, redness, skin firm to the touch, presence of drainage, pain in and around the area) and to report any of these to their prescriber.

QSEN: Safety

Dosage Alert

The dose of metformin (Glucophage) for children over 10 years of age could be the same as for an adult because the dose is based on response, not size.

QSEN: Safety

Noninsulin antidiabetic drugs should not be taken by pregnant or breastfeeding women.

QSEN: Safety

Metformin should be taken with food. Teach patients not to chew or crush Glucophage XR tablets. Teach them that metformin can cause lactic acidosis, which can be avoided by drinking plenty of water (day and night), avoiding alcoholic beverages, and avoiding dehydration.

With *alpha-glucosidase inhibitors*, tell patients not to remove the drug from the foil wrapper until it is time to take it. The foil helps prevent the drug from deteriorating.

With *alpha-glucosidase inhibitors* or *thiazolidinediones*, teach patients the symptoms of liver impairment (jaundice of the skin and sclera, nausea and lack of appetite, dark urine, pale stools) and to report these to their prescriber.

With *thiazolidinediones*, teach patients to check for signs of water retention and heart failure. Patients should weigh themselves daily at the same time each day wearing the same amount of clothing. They should also check their pulse rates twice a day, noting the rate and the quality of the pulse. Instruct patients to keep a written record of daily weights and heart rates, and to report a weight gain of more than 3 pounds in 1 week, especially if the ankles are also swollen, to their prescriber. If the patient becomes increasingly short of breath over time, tell the patient to report this symptom to his or her prescriber.

The *incretin mimetics* and *amylin analogs* come in prefilled pens that contain a full 1-month supply of doses. Using the directions in Box 13-5 and the instructions on p. 218, teach patients how to activate the pen, attach the needle, and self-inject subcutaneously.

Instruct patients to store these drugs in the refrigerator and never to freeze them. Warm temperatures, freezing temperatures, and exposure to light can all make the drugs lose their effectiveness.

The *amylin analogs* (Pramlintide) slow stomach emptying and absorption of other drugs. Teach patients who are taking other oral drugs requiring a rapid onset of action (for example, analgesics) that it is important to take these drugs either 1 hour before or 2 hours after eating.

Teach patients taking a *DPP-4 inhibitor* to stop the drug and notify their prescriber as soon as possible if an allergic reaction occurs (rash, itching or hives, swelling of the face, lips, or tongue). Instruct them to go to the emergency department or call 911 immediately if breathing problems develop or if they should feel faint or light-headed.

Life Span Considerations for Noninsulin Antidiabetic Drugs
Pediatric Considerations. Noninsulin antidiabetic drugs from the sulfonylurea, alpha-glucosidase inhibitor, thiazolidinedione, incretin mimetics, amylin analog, DPP-4 inhibitors, and sodium-glucose cotransport inhibitor classes are not recommended for use in children who have DM2.

Metformin and meglitinides are prescribed for children with DM2 who are over 10 years of age. The dose for a child is based on how he or she responds to the drug rather than by size and weight.

Considerations for Pregnancy and Lactation. Diabetes is often more difficult to control during this physically stressful time. In addition, some patients who do not have diabetes may have problems with hyperglycemia only during pregnancy.

Insulin is the drug of choice for treating hyperglycemia during pregnancy. The noninsulin antidiabetic drugs are not approved for use during pregnancy and breastfeeding.

Considerations for Older Adults. Noninsulin antidiabetic drugs should be used with caution in older adults. The risk for hypoglycemia is increased in these patients, especially if they are also taking beta-adrenergic blocking drugs or warfarin (Coumadin). In addition, hypoglycemia may be harder to recognize in older adults. Often the dose prescribed for older adults, especially if they are malnourished, is *lower* than for younger adults.

Metformin must be used with caution in adults older than age 65. The older adult is more likely to have heart failure, poor circulation, kidney disease, or liver disease. All of these problems greatly increase the risk for the complication of lactic acidosis. If the drug is prescribed for an older adult, more careful monitoring of kidney and heart function is needed. Metformin is not recommended for patients older than age 80.

Alpha-glucosidase inhibitors should be used with caution in older adults and should not be used at all in those who are malnourished, have difficulty digesting or absorbing food, or have liver or intestinal tract problems. The intestinal side effects of the drugs may be worse in older adults.

Thiazolidinedione drugs are prescribed for older adults who have DM2 and do not have either liver impairment or cardiac problems. Because the cardiac status of older adults is likely to change more rapidly than younger adults, it is important to emphasize the signs and symptoms of heart failure.

Sodium-glucose cotransport inhibitor drugs cause diuresis and place the older adult at greater risk for dehydration and electrolyte imbalances. Teach older patients to ensure their fluid intake closely matches their urine output.

ORAL COMBINATION NONINSULIN ANTIDIABETIC DRUGS

Often DM2 is best controlled using more than one noninsulin antidiabetic drug. To simplify drug therapy, some oral drugs have been combined. The patient may not understand that a single tablet contains more than one drug. Be sure to teach the patient about the side effects, adverse effects, and issues that should be reported to their prescriber for both drugs contained in a combination tablet.

Common Oral Combination Noninsulin Antidiabetic Drugs for Type 2 Diabetes

Drug Name	Contains
Metaglip	glipiZIDE and metformin
Glucovance	glyBURIDE and metformin
Avandamet	metformin and rosiglitazone
Avandaryl	rosiglitazone and glimepiride

Get Ready for Practice!

Key Points

- Body cells use glucose and oxygen to make the chemical energy substance ATP to use as fuel for cellular work in the body.
- Hypoglycemia can lead to brain cell dysfunction and death.
- A patient with type 1 diabetes (DM1) does not make insulin and must take insulin for the rest of his or her life.
- A patient with type 2 diabetes (DM2) still makes some insulin. The insulin does not interact well with its receptor.
- Complications from untreated or poorly controlled diabetes include blindness; kidney failure; foot and leg amputations; hypertension; and increased risk for infection, heart attacks, and strokes.
- The goals of insulin therapy for DM1 are to maintain blood glucose levels within the normal range, avoid ketoacidosis, and prevent or delay the blood vessel changes that lead to organ damage.
- Check the order carefully for the exact type and amount of insulin to be injected. Do not interchange insulin types.

- Use an insulin syringe that is marked off in the same concentration units as the insulin you are injecting.
- Rotate the area for injection within one injection site.
- Administer insulin as a subcutaneous injection, not an intramuscular injection.
- Do not pull back on the plunger before injecting the insulin and do not rub or massage the injection site.
- When mixing two different types of insulin in the same syringe, inject both bottles with the amount of air equal to the dose of that insulin. Draw up the short-acting insulin first.
- Keep simple sugars (sugar packets, orange juice, glucose tables, glucose paste) and glucagon on the unit whenever a person with diabetes is a patient on the unit.
- Determine how well an older adult who is to self-inject insulin can see the markings on the syringe and reach the injection site.
- Because the different types of antidiabetic drugs work in different ways, a patient may be prescribed to take more than one type.

- After giving a noninsulin antidiabetic drug that can cause hypoglycemia, check the patient hourly for the signs and symptoms of hypoglycemia.
- Drugs that are likely to increase the effectiveness of antidiabetic drugs and increase the risk for hypoglycemia include aspirin, other nonsteroidal anti-inflammatory drugs (NSAIDs), warfarin (Coumadin), beta-adrenergic blockers, ciprofloxacin (Cipro), probenecid, and miconazole (Micatin).
- Remind patients to limit alcohol intake and drink only with or shortly after a full meal to prevent hypoglycemia.
- Meglitinide drugs should be taken right before a meal or a substantial snack. If a meal is skipped, that drug dose should also be skipped.
- Ensure that metformin (Glucophage) is not given to a patient within 48 hours after having a test involving dye or surgery requiring anesthesia (the drug increases the risk for lactic acidosis and can interact with dyes/anesthetic drugs, resulting in kidney damage).
- Signs and symptoms of lactic acidosis include muscle aches; fatigue; abdominal pain; hypotension; and a slow, irregular heartbeat.
- Do not crush Glucophage XR tablets.
- Alpha-glucosidase inhibitor drugs must be given with the first bite of food.
- Pramlintide is an injectable drug that should not be mixed with insulin, nor should it be injected within 2 inches of the site of an insulin injection.

Additional Learning Resources

evolve Be sure to visit your Evolve website (http://evolve.elsevier.com/Workman/pharmacology/) for additional online resources.

SG Go to your Study Guide for additional learning activities to help you master this chapter content.

Review Questions

See the Answer Keys—In-text Review Questions for answers to these questions.

Test Yourself on the Basics

1. What is the direct goal of drug therapy for diabetes mellitus?
   A. To cure diabetes
   B. To prevent blindness
   C. To keep blood glucose levels within the normal range
   D. To improve body weight and reduce the risk for hypoglycemia
2. How does the drug glucagon work to treat hypoglycemia?
   A. It acts on the liver to release stored glucose from glycogen.
   B. It is a concentrated form of glucose in which 1 mL is equal to 50 g of glucose.
   C. Glucagon inactivates circulating insulin, thus preventing blood glucose levels from decreasing.
   D. Glucagon prevents insulin from binding to insulin receptors, thus acting as an insulin antagonist.

3. Which signs and symptoms are associated with hypoglycemia or "insulin shock"? Select all that apply.
   A. Acute confusion
   B. Cool clammy skin
   C. Deep rapid respirations
   D. Fruity odor of the breath
   E. Headache
   F. Increased sweating
   G. Nausea
4. Which problem is a possible adverse effect of a drug from the sodium-glucose cotransport inhibitor class?
   A. Injection site irritation or infection
   B. Increased respiratory infections
   C. Congestive heart failure
   D. Dehydration
5. Which noninsulin antidiabetic drug can cause severe sunburn?
   A. metformin (Glucophage)
   B. rosiglitazone (Avandia)
   C. glyburide (Micronase)
   D. nateglinide (Starlix)

Test Yourself on Advanced Concepts

6. A patient with type 1 diabetes (DM1) asks why insulin must be injected instead of taken as a tablet. What is your best answer?
   A. "Injecting insulin increases how fast it can work to control your diabetes."
   B. "Insulin is a small protein that would be destroyed in the digestive system if swallowed."
   C. "The absorption of oral insulin is so slow that the dose cannot be controlled and the effects are unpredictable."
   D. "Injectable insulin more closely resembles the natural insulin that your pancreas makes compared with liquid oral insulin."
7. Why can people with type 2 diabetes (DM2) use noninsulin antidiabetic drugs to control the disease?
   A. In people with DM2, the liver is able to take over the endocrine functions of the nonfunctional pancreas.
   B. DM2 is a mild disease that does not have severe long-term complications.
   C. Ketoacidosis develops only rarely among people who have type 2 diabetes.
   D. People with DM2 continue to make pancreatic insulin.
8. When starting to draw up and administer a dose of NPH insulin, you find that the insulin in the vial is uniformly cloudy. What is your best action?
   A. Shake the vial vigorously.
   B. Draw up the medication.
   C. Add normal saline.
   D. Open a new vial.
9. What is the most important issue to teach a patient who uses short-acting insulin before meals?
   A. "Shake the bottle before drawing up the insulin so that it is well mixed."
   B. "Rotate the injection site to prevent the development of skin problems."
   C. "Rub the injection site for 1 minute to ensure best drug absorption."
   D. "Eat a meal within 15 minutes of injecting the drug."

10. A patient who uses insulin reports the area where he usually injects the drug is warm, red, and painful. What should you tell him to do?
    A. Apply ice to the site for 10 minutes 4 times daily.
    B. Immediately call the prescriber and report these symptoms.
    C. Discard the bottle of insulin you have been using and open a fresh one.
    D. Go immediately to the emergency department to have the insulin injected intravenously.

11. Which statement made by a patient newly diagnosed with DM1 indicates a need for more teaching?
    A. I will keep a syringe and insulin bottle in my pocket at all times.
    B. I will always eat within 5 to 10 minutes of taking my dose of regular insulin.
    C. I will rotate my insulin injections within one site rather than switching injection sites.
    D. I will not share my insulin syringes or needles with my brother who also has diabetes.

12. With which noninsulin antidiabetic drug should you remain alert for the possibility of hypoglycemia even when it is the only drug prescribed? (Select all that apply.)
    A. acarbose (Precose)
    B. canagliflozin (Invokana)
    C. glipizide (Glucotrol)
    D. miglitol (Glyset)
    E. pioglitazone (Actos)
    F. repaglinide (Prandin)
    G. Rosiglitazone (Avandia)
    H. sitagliptin (Januvia)

13. An older adult patient with type 2 diabetes who has been taking rosiglitazone (Avandia) for 1 month tells you that her urine is the color of coffee. What is your best action?
    A. Document this patient report as the only action.
    B. Encourage the patient to drink more water.
    C. Test the patient's urine for ketone bodies.
    D. Notify the prescriber immediately.

Critical Thinking Activities

See the Answer Keys—Critical Thinking Activities for answers to these activities.

Mrs. Sweet is a 44-year-old woman who has just been diagnosed with type 2 diabetes mellitus. She is 50 lb overweight and is hypertensive, for which she takes metoprolol (Lopressor). She is prescribed to take metformin (Glucophage) twice daily and alogliptin (Nesina) once daily. She asks why she isn't prescribed insulin like her grandmother, who also had "sugar."

1. What will you tell her about insulin therapy and why it isn't necessary for her at this time?
2. What class of drugs are metformin and alogliptin, and what are their possible side effects?
3. Is there any problem with taking these two different drugs for the same health problem? Why or why not?
4. Are there any problems or interactions that are likely with Mrs. Sweet's new drugs and her antihypertension therapy?
5. What will you teach this patient about her drug therapy?

14

Drug Therapy for Thyroid and Adrenal Gland Problems

http://evolve.elsevier.com/Workman/pharmacology/

Objectives

After studying this chapter you should be able to:

1. List the names, actions, usual adult dosages, possible side effects, and adverse effects of drugs for thyroid problems and for adrenal gland problems.
2. Describe what to do before and after giving drugs for thyroid problems and drugs for adrenal gland problems.
3. Explain what to teach patients taking drugs for thyroid problems or for adrenal gland problems, including what to do, what not to do, and when to call the prescriber.
4. Describe life span considerations for drugs for thyroid problems and drugs for adrenal gland problems.

Key Terms

aldosterone (ăl-DŎS-tĕ-rōn) (p. 234) A hormone secreted by the adrenal cortex that regulates sodium and water balance.

corticosteroids (kōr-tĭ-kō-STĔR-ōydz) (p. 234) Drugs similar to natural cortisol, a hormone secreted by the adrenal cortex that is essential for life.

thyroid hormone agonists (THĬ-rōyd HŎR-mōn Ă-gŏn-ĭsts) (p. 229) Drugs that mimic the effect of thyroid hormones, T3 and T4, helping to regulate metabolism.

OVERVIEW

An *endocrine gland* secretes one or more hormones into the blood, which then circulates everywhere until it reaches its target tissue(s). A *target tissue* is a tissue or organ that is affected or controlled by the hormone. For example, the target tissues of estrogen are the uterine lining and certain breast cells. Thyroid hormones and corticosteroids affect all body cells, so the entire body is their target tissue.

HYPOTHYROIDISM

REVIEW OF RELATED PHYSIOLOGY AND PATHOPHYSIOLOGY

? Did You Know?

The most common dietary sources of iodine are saltwater fish and table salt to which iodide is added.

The thyroid gland is located in the front of the neck just below the Adam's apple. It is one of the most important endocrine glands in the body and produces two thyroid hormones: thyroxine (T_4) and triiodothyronine (T_3). These two hormones are formed from the amino acid tyrosine and the mineral iodine.

When T_3 and T_4 leave the thyroid gland and enter other body cells, they bind to receptors inside the cell and activate the genes for metabolism. *Metabolism* is the energy use of each cell and the amount of work performed in the body. Thyroid hormones increase the rate of metabolism in any cell that they enter, speeding up the energy use and work output of each cell. Important functions controlled by thyroid hormones include:

- Assisting in brain development before birth and during early childhood
- Maintaining brain function throughout the life span
- Helping maintain the ability to think, remember, and learn
- Maintaining heart and skeletal muscle function
- Ensuring continued production of other hormones
- Maintaining effective respiratory function and cell uptake of oxygen

💡 Memory Jogger

Thyroid hormones regulate whole body metabolism.

Box 14-1	Signs and Symptoms of Hypothyroidism

ADULTS
- Constipation
- Decreased scalp hair, increased body hair
- Edema of the face, around the eyes, and on shins
- Feels cold all the time
- Lacks energy, sleeps excessively
- Lower than normal body temperature
- Menstrual irregularities
- No interest in sex
- Slow heart rate
- Slow respiratory rate
- Speaks slowly
- Thickened, waxy-feeling skin
- Thick tongue
- Thinks slowly
- Weight gain

INFANTS AND CHILDREN
- Constipation
- Excess facial and body hair
- Mental retardation
- Poor eater
- Protruding tongue
- Short stature
- Sleeps excessively

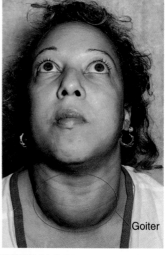

Goiter

FIGURE 14-1 Woman with a goiter. (From Ignatavicius, D. D., & Workman, M. L. (2016). *Medical-surgical nursing: Patient-centered collaborative care* (8th ed.). Philadelphia: Saunders.)

 Memory Jogger

A goiter can be present when the thyroid gland is overactive or underactive.

Hypothyroidism is a condition of low thyroid function, causing low blood levels of thyroid hormones (THs) and symptoms of slow metabolism. This very common health problem is also called an *underactive thyroid*. Thyroid cells may fail to produce enough thyroid hormones because they have been damaged and no longer function or because the person's diet does not include enough iodine or tyrosine to make thyroid hormones.

When the production of T_3 and T_4 is too low or absent, the blood levels of the hormones decline, and the patient's entire body metabolism is slowed, sometimes to dangerously low levels. In an effort to increase thyroid hormone production, the thyroid gland cells can divide, making the whole thyroid gland larger, forming a *goiter*, which is a distinct swelling in the neck. The presence of a goiter indicates that the patient has a thyroid problem but does not indicate whether the thyroid is underactive or overactive. Figure 14-1 shows a patient with a goiter. Box 14-1 lists other common symptoms of hypothyroidism.

If left untreated, hypothyroidism can slow metabolism to such a low level that the heart stops and death occurs. This severe type of hypothyroidism is called *myxedema* and requires immediate medical attention. Figure 14-2 shows a woman with severe hypothyroidism. Figure 14-3 shows an infant with hypothyroidism.

TYPES OF THYROID HORMONE REPLACEMENT DRUGS

LEVOTHYROXINE AND LIOTHYRONINE

How Thyroid Hormone Replacement Drugs Work
Keeping thyroid hormone function at the right level is essential for overall health. The goal of drug therapy is to ensure that the patient's whole body metabolism is as close to normal as possible. If the thyroid is not making these hormones at all or not making enough, replacement of thyroid hormones is needed to keep all cells, tissues, and organs functioning at the proper level. When a person has an underactive thyroid gland causing hypothyroidism, he or she generally must take thyroid hormone replacement drugs for the rest of his or her life.

Thyroid hormone replacement drugs are **thyroid hormone agonists**, which mimic the effect of the thyroid hormones T_3 and T_4, helping to regulate metabolism. They work just like the patient's own thyroid hormones by entering the blood and going into all cells. Once inside the cells, the drug binds to receptors on the DNA and activates the genes for metabolism. Just like T_3 and T_4, these drugs increase the rate of metabolism in any cell they enter, speeding up the energy use and work output of each cell.

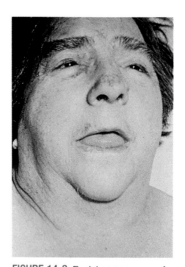

FIGURE 14-2 Facial appearance of a woman with severe hypothyroidism. (From Ignatavicius, D. D., & Workman, M. L. (2016). *Medical-surgical nursing: Patient-centered collaborative care* (8th ed.). Philadelphia: Saunders.)

 Memory Jogger

The goal of drug therapy for thyroid problems is to ensure that the patient's entire body metabolism is as close to normal as possible.

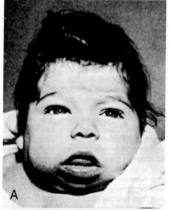

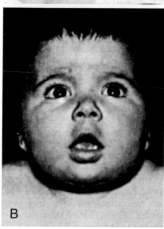

FIGURE 14-3 Facial appearance of an infant with hypothyroidism before treatment (A) and after thyroid hormone replacement therapy (B). (From Behrman, R. E., Kliegman, R. M., & Jenson, H. B. (2004). *Nelson textbook of pediatrics* (17th ed.). Philadelphia: Saunders.)

Common Side Effects

Thyroid Hormone Agonist Drugs

Hypertension   Insomnia   Increased bowel movements

Clinical Pitfall

Never substitute one type or brand of thyroid hormone replacement drug with another. Drug strengths vary (for example, liothyronine is four times as potent as levothyroxine), and patient responses vary.

QSEN: Safety

The drugs listed in the following table are those most commonly prescribed for thyroid hormone replacement. Be sure to consult a drug reference for information about other thyroid hormone agonist drugs.

Dosages for Common Thyroid Hormone Agonist Drugs

Drug	Dosage
levothyroxine sodium [synthetic] (Estre, Eltroxin ✦, Levo-T, Levothroid, Levoxyl, Synthroid, Unithroid)	*Adults:* Oral—25-250 mcg daily; IV—12.5-150 mcg daily *Children:* Oral—2-15 mcg/kg daily; IV—1-7.5 mcg/kg daily
liothyronine sodium [synthetic] (Cytomel, Triostat)	*Adults:* 25-100 mcg orally daily *Children 1-3 years:* Oral or IV—5-50 mcg daily

Intended Responses

- Body temperature is normal.
- Level of activity is normal.
- Heart rate, blood pressure, and respiratory rate are normal for the patient's age and size.
- Body weight is maintained when the patient takes in the amount of calories needed for his or her age, size, and activity level.
- The patient is mentally alert; he or she is able to remember people, places, and events from the recent and distant past.
- Bowel movement pattern is normal for the patient's usual bowel habits.

Side Effects. Thyroid hormone agonist drugs have few side effects. In general, the side effects are really those of an overdose of the drug, and the symptoms are those of hyperthyroidism.

Adverse Effects. The most serious adverse effect of thyroid hormone agonists is an increase in the activity of the cardiac and nervous systems. The increase in cardiac activity can overwork the heart and lead to angina pain, a heart attack, and heart failure.

In the nervous system, the increased activity can lead to seizures. Seizures are rare and can occur in any patient taking high doses of thyroid hormone replacement drugs but are more likely to occur in the patient who already has a seizure disorder.

Thyroid hormone agonists enhance the action of drugs that reduce blood clotting (anticoagulants), especially warfarin (Coumadin). This action can lead to excessive bruising and bleeding.

What To Do *Before* Giving Thyroid Hormone Agonist Drugs

Before giving the first dose of a thyroid hormone agonist drug, check the patient's blood pressure and heart rate and rhythm. The side effects and adverse effects of thyroid hormone agonists increase metabolic rate and cardiac activity.

Check the dose and the specific drug name carefully. Thyroid hormone agonists are not interchangeable because the strength of each drug varies.

Food and fiber impair the absorption of thyroid hormone agonists from the intestinal tract. Ensure that the drug is given 2 hours before a meal or fiber supplement or at least 3 hours after a meal or fiber supplement.

What To Do *After* Giving Thyroid Hormone Agonist Drugs

Check the patient's blood pressure and heart rate and rhythm to determine whether the drug is working and if there are side effects. Ask the patient whether he or she has any chest pain or discomfort. This symptom may be the first indication of an adverse cardiac effect.

If the patient also takes a drug that affects blood clotting, especially warfarin (Coumadin), check at least once each shift for any sign of increased bleeding. Look for bleeding from the gums; unusual or excessive bruising anywhere on the skin; bleeding around intravenous (IV) sites or for more than 5 minutes after discontinuing an IV; and for the presence of blood in urine, stool, or vomitus.

What To *Teach* Patients About Thyroid Hormone Agonist Drugs

When a patient is diagnosed with hypothyroidism and is first prescribed a thyroid hormone replacement drug, the dose for the first several weeks is low. Usually it is increased slowly every 2 to 3 weeks until the patient has normal blood levels of TH and signs of normal metabolism. Teach patients not to increase the dose beyond what is prescribed for them. Increasing the drug too quickly can lead to adverse effects such as a heart attack or seizures. Teach them to check their own pulse each morning before taking the drug and again each evening before going to bed. If the pulse rate becomes 20 beats higher than the normal rate for 1 week or if it becomes consistently irregular, they should notify their prescriber. Tell them to go to the emergency department immediately if they start to have chest pain.

Teach patients that they need to take the drug daily to maintain normal body function. If the patient is ill and cannot take the drug orally, instruct him or her to contact the prescriber to get a parenteral dose of the drug. Remind patients not to stop the drug suddenly or to change the dose (up or down) without contacting their prescriber.

Taking the drug with food or with a fiber supplement reduces the absorption of the drug. Teach patients to take it 2 to 3 hours before a meal or taking a fiber supplement or at least 3 hours after a meal or taking the supplement.

Remind patients who also take warfarin (Coumadin) to keep all follow-up appointments and appointments for blood-clotting tests because these drugs increase the effectiveness of warfarin. Teach them to avoid situations that can lead to bleeding and other drugs (such as aspirin) that can make bleeding worse.

Life Span Considerations for Thyroid Hormone Replacement Drugs

Pediatric Considerations. Children may develop hypothyroidism or may have been born with the problem. They must take thyroid hormone replacement drugs for their entire life. During infancy and early childhood when the patient is going through periods of rapid growth, he or she actually needs a *higher* drug amount per kilogram of body weight than does an adult!

Considerations for Pregnancy and Lactation. Women with hypothyroidism usually have difficulty becoming pregnant. Once pregnant, however, thyroid hormone replacement drugs are safe to take during pregnancy. In fact, for a pregnant woman who has hypothyroidism, not taking the drug can lead to problems with the pregnancy and the fetus. Pregnant women often need a *higher* dose of the drug. Because thyroid hormone replacement drugs can enter breast milk and increase the infant's metabolism, the mother taking these drugs should not breastfeed.

Considerations for Older Adults. The metabolism of older adults is more sensitive to thyroid hormone replacement drugs, and they are more likely to have adverse cardiac and nervous system effects. For this reason older adults who need these drugs are usually prescribed a lower dose than younger adults. In addition, older adults are more likely to have diabetes. Thyroid hormone replacement drugs change the effectiveness of insulin and other drugs for diabetes, and often drugs for diabetes need to be increased to prevent high blood sugar levels *(hyperglycemia)*. Teach older adults with diabetes and hypothyroidism to check their blood glucose levels more frequently.

Interaction Alert

Drugs for thyroid hormone replacement increase the action of warfarin (Coumadin), increasing the risk for bleeding. Assess the patient for excessive bleeding.

QSEN: Safety

Teaching Alert

Teach patients to take thyroid drugs 2 to 3 hours before or at least 3 hours after eating a meal or taking a fiber supplement.

QSEN: Safety

 Memory Jogger

Remind pregnant women who have hypothyroidism to be sure to continue thyroid hormone replacement.

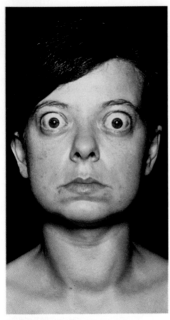

FIGURE 14-4 Facial appearance of a woman with hyperthyroidism from Graves disease. Note the bulging eyes, goiter, and lack of body fat. (From Ignatavicius, D. D., & Workman, M. L. (2016). *Medical-surgical nursing: Patient-centered collaborative care* (8th ed.). Philadelphia: Saunders.)

Memory Jogger

The effects of thyroid-suppressing drugs are usually not seen until 3 to 4 weeks after they have been taken daily.

Do Not Confuse

Methimazole *with* Metolazone

An order for methimazole can be confused with metolazone. Methimazole is a thyroid-suppressing drug, whereas metolazone is a diuretic.

QSEN: Safety

Do Not Confuse

Propylthiouracil *with* Purinethol

An order for propylthiouracil can be confused with Purinethol. Propylthiouracil is a thyroid-suppressing drug, whereas Purinethol is a cancer chemotherapy drug.

QSEN: Safety

| Box **14-2** | Signs and Symptoms of Hyperthyroidism |

GENERAL SYMPTOMS
- Diarrhea
- Difficulty sleeping
- Feeling too warm most of the time
- Fine tremors of the hands
- Heartbeat irregularities
- High blood pressure
- Higher than normal body temperature
- Menstrual irregularities
- Rapid heart rate
- Sweating
- Thinning of scalp hair
- Weight loss

ADDITIONAL SYMPTOMS SPECIFIC TO GRAVES DISEASE ONLY
- Blurred vision
- Bulging or protruding eyes (exophthalmia)

HYPERTHYROIDISM

REVIEW OF RELATED PHYSIOLOGY AND PATHOPHYSIOLOGY

Hyperthyroidism is an increase in thyroid gland activity causing high blood levels of thyroid hormones (T_3 and T_4) and symptoms of increased metabolism. This health problem is also called an *overactive thyroid*. Thyroid cells may produce excessive thyroid hormones for several reasons, but the most common type of hyperthyroidism is Graves disease. As a result of hyperthyroidism with excessive production of thyroid hormones, the patient's body metabolism is much faster than normal. With some types of hyperthyroidism, such as Graves disease, the patient also has a goiter.

Another name for hyperthyroidism is *thyrotoxicosis* because the side effects of excessive thyroid hormones can cause toxic side effects to some organs. Symptoms of hyperthyroidism from any cause are listed in Box 14-2. The excess thyroid hormones increase the metabolism of all cells above normal levels and make every organ work harder, especially the heart. Additional symptoms that occur only with hyperthyroidism caused by Graves disease include bulging or protruding eyes (*exophthalmos*) (Figure 14-4) and blurred vision.

When hyperthyroidism is severe, it is called *thyroid crisis* or *thyroid storm*. This condition is an extreme state of hyperthyroidism in which all symptoms are more severe and life threatening. The patient has a fever; dangerously high blood pressure; and a rapid, irregular heartbeat. Symptoms can develop quickly; if not treated, this problem can lead to seizures, heart failure, and death.

TYPES OF THYROID-SUPPRESSING DRUGS

METHIMAZOLE AND PROPYLTHIOURACIL

How Thyroid-Suppressing Drugs Work

Most of the time hyperthyroidism is a permanent health problem that is treated by destroying all or part of the thyroid gland by surgically removing either some or all of it (*thyroidectomy*) or using radiation to destroy thyroid cells. Drug therapy to reduce thyroid production of hormones is often used before surgery. If the patient is too ill for surgery or radiation, thyroid-suppressing drugs may be used long term in place of these treatments.

Thyroid-suppressing drugs enter the thyroid gland and combine with the enzyme responsible for connecting iodine (iodide) with tyrosine to make active T_3 and T_4. This action keeps the enzyme so busy working on the drug that it does not have the opportunity to make active thyroid hormones. These drugs do not affect the hormones already formed and stored in the thyroid gland, so it may take as long as 3 or 4 weeks for a person to use all of the thyroid hormones made and stored before the drug was started.

Dosages for Common Thyroid-Suppressing Drugs

Drug	Dosage
methimazole (Northyx, Tapazole)	*Adults:* Initial dose: 5-20 mg orally every 8 hours; maintenance dosage—5-10 mg orally every 8 hours *Children:* Initial dose—0.5-0.7 mg/kg orally in 1-3 divided doses at 8-hr intervals; maintenance dosage—usually one-half the initial dose
propylthiouracil (Propacil, Propyl-Thyracil ♣, PTU)	*Adults:* Initial dose—100-150 mg orally every 8 hr; maintenance dosage—50 mg orally every 8 hr *Children:* Initial dose—15-50 mg orally every 8 hr; maintenance dosage—determined by response

Intended Responses
- Body temperature is normal.
- Level of activity is normal.
- Heart rate, blood pressure, and respiratory rate are normal for the patient's age and size.
- Body weight is maintained when the patient takes in the amount of calories needed for his or her age, size, and activity level.
- Bowel movement pattern is normal for the patient's usual bowel habits.

Side Effects. Thyroid-suppressing drugs have many minor side effects. These include rash, loss of taste sensation, headache, muscle and joint aches, itchiness, drowsiness, nausea, vomiting, lymph node enlargement, and swelling of the feet and ankles.

Adverse Effects. A major adverse effect of thyroid-suppressing drugs is bone marrow suppression, which reduces the amount of blood cells. As a result, the patient is less resistant to infection and more likely to be anemic.

These drugs, especially propylthiouracil, can be hepatotoxic (liver toxic). Less often, these drugs can also damage the kidneys.

Thyroid-suppressing drugs enhance the action of drugs that reduce blood clotting (anticoagulants), especially warfarin (Coumadin). This action increases the risk for excessive bruising and bleeding.

What To Do *Before* Giving Thyroid-Suppressing Drugs
Check the patient's liver function tests before giving these drugs. Both thyroid-suppressing drugs are hepatotoxic. If a patient already has a liver problem, the effects of the drugs on the liver are worse and occur at lower doses.

Check the dose and the specific drug name carefully. Although methimazole and propylthiouracil work in the same way, they are not interchangeable because the strength of each drug varies.

What To Do *After* Giving Thyroid-Suppressing Drugs
Check patients who also take a drug that affects blood clotting, especially warfarin (Coumadin), at least once each shift for any sign of increased bleeding. Look for bleeding from the gums; unusual or excessive bruising anywhere on the skin; bleeding around IV sites or for more than 5 minutes after discontinuing an IV; and the presence of blood in urine, stool, or vomit.

Check the patient daily for yellowing of the skin or sclera (jaundice), which is a symptom of liver problems.

Check the patient's white blood cell count (WBC). Adverse effects of thyroid-suppressing drugs are bone marrow suppression, which reduces the WBC count and increases the risk for infection.

What To *Teach* Patients About Thyroid-Suppressing Drugs
Teach patients taking warfarin (Coumadin) to keep all follow-up appointments and appointments for blood-clotting tests because these drugs increase the effectiveness

Common Side Effects

Thyroid-Suppressing Drugs

Rash   Nausea   Headache

Muscle aches

 Clinical Pitfall

Do not substitute methimazole for propylthiouracil. Methimazole is 10 times stronger than propylthiouracil.

QSEN: Safety

of warfarin. Instruct them to avoid situations that can lead to bleeding and other drugs that can make bleeding worse.

Remind patients taking thyroid-suppressing drugs to avoid crowds and people who are ill because these drugs suppress the production of white blood cells in the bone marrow. This effect reduces the patient's immunity and resistance to infection.

Teach patients to check the color of the roof of the mouth and the whites of the eyes every day for the presence of a yellow tinge. Teach patients to report jaundice to their prescriber as soon as possible.

Life Span Considerations for Thyroid-Suppressing Drugs

Considerations for Pregnancy and Lactation. Thyroid-suppressing drugs have a high likelihood of increasing the risk for birth defects or fetal damage and can cause miscarriages. These drugs should not be given during pregnancy unless the benefits of treatment are thought to outweigh the risk in a life-threatening situation or when other treatments are not available. Women taking thyroid-suppressing drugs should not breastfeed because the drug could cause hypothyroidism in the infant.

Considerations for Older Adults. Older adults taking thyroid-suppressing drugs are more likely to have an adverse effect, and adverse effects are more likely to be severe. The older patient's resistance to infection is already lower than that of a younger adult because of age-related changes that occur in the immune system. Decreased bone marrow activity makes this problem worse. Many older adults also take warfarin (Coumadin). The effects of warfarin are increased when the patient also takes a thyroid-suppressing drug.

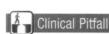 **Clinical Pitfall**

Thyroid-suppressing drugs should not be given to a woman who is pregnant or breastfeeding.

QSEN: Safety

ADRENAL GLAND HYPOFUNCTION

REVIEW OF RELATED PHYSIOLOGY AND PATHOPHYSIOLOGY

The adrenal glands are small triangular-shaped endocrine glands that sit on top of the kidneys (Figure 14-5). These two glands have two layers: the thick outermost layer, known as the *cortex*; and the inner layer known as the *medulla* (Figure 14-6). The cortex secretes two main types of steroid hormones, cortisol and aldosterone. Cortisol, a glucocorticoid, is essential for life and functions to regulate:

- The body's response to stress
- Carbohydrate, protein, and fat metabolism
- Emotional stability
- Immune function
- Sodium and water balance
- The normal excitability of heart muscle cells

Aldosterone is a mineral corticoid hormone secreted by the adrenal cortex that regulates sodium and water balance.

Adrenal gland hypofunction usually results in greatly reduced secretion of both cortisol and aldosterone. Common causes of adrenal gland hypofunction include autoimmune disease attacking and destroying the adrenal glands, adrenalectomy, abdominal radiation therapy, and disorders of the anterior pituitary gland. Signs and symptoms of adrenal gland hypofunction include hypoglycemia, salt craving, muscle weakness, hypotension, fatigue, low serum sodium levels, and high serum potassium levels. Depending on the cause, some people also have darkening of the skin. Without supplementation or replacement of cortisol and aldosterone, the person with adrenal gland hypofunction would eventually die.

TYPES OF ADRENAL HORMONE REPLACEMENT DRUGS

Cortisol and aldosterone deficiencies are corrected by replacement therapy. **Corticosteroids** are drugs similar to natural cortisol. These drugs, especially

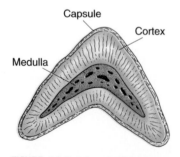

FIGURE 14-5 Location of adrenal gland on top of kidney.

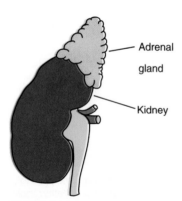

FIGURE 14-6 Adrenal gland layers. (From Ignatavicius, D. D., & Workman, M. L. (2016). *Medical-surgical nursing: Patient-centered collaborative care* (8th ed.). Philadelphia: Saunders.)

prednisone, correct cortisol deficiency or absence. Chapter 6 discusses corticosteroid therapy in detail.

Aldosterone deficiency is partially helped by corticosteroid therapy. Cortisol replacement may be supplemented with an additional mineralocorticoid hormone replacement, fludrocortisone (Florinef) to restore sodium and potassium balance. This drug acts in a similar manner to aldosterone and results in greater reabsorption of sodium with increased excretion of potassium. These actions help correct or prevent hyponatremia, hyperkalemia, and hypotension. The usual adult dosage is 0.1 to 0.2 mg orally once daily. Safety and efficacy have not been established for infants and children.

Side Effects. Side effects of fludrocortisone therapy are associated with the drugs action on fluid and electrolyte balance. Common problems include hypertension, edema formation, low blood potassium levels, and high blood sodium levels.

Adverse Effects. The most common adverse effect of fludrocortisone is congestive heart failure (CHF). If CHF develops, the drug dose is either reduced or stopped.

What To *Teach* Patients About Fludrocortisone

Teach patients to take fludrocortisone at the same time daily with food to prevent gastrointestinal problems.

Because the drug can cause fluid retention with weight gain, edema, and heart failure, teach patients to weigh themselves daily and keep a record of the weight. Instruct them to report a weight gain of 2 lb in a day or 3 lb in a week to the prescriber immediately.

Because the drug is typically used along with a corticosteroid, remind patients of the usual corticosteroid therapy precautions listed in Chapter 6.

Common Side Effects

Fludrocortisone

Hypertension   Edema   High sodium levels (Hypernatremia)

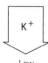

Low potassium levels (Hypokalemia)

ADRENAL GLAND HYPERFUNCTION

REVIEW OF RELATED PHYSIOLOGY AND PATHOPHYSIOLOGY

Unlike adrenal gland hypofunction in which all adrenal hormones are deficient, with adrenal gland hyperfunction, most commonly either cortisol is excessively secreted *(hypercortisolism* or *Cushing's disease)* or aldosterone is excessively secreted *(hyperaldosteronism).* Excessive secretion of both types of hormones is more rare. Adrenal gland hyperfunction can result in a problem within the adrenal gland, often an adrenal gland tumor, or it can be a result of problems in the pituitary gland that overproduces hormones that stimulate the adrenal gland to produce adrenal hormones in excess.

When adrenal gland hyperfunction is caused by a problem in the adrenal gland, surgery is the most common treatment. However, before surgery and for patients who are not able to have surgery, drug therapy can help manage the problems caused by adrenal gland hyperfunction.

TYPES OF DRUGS FOR ADRENAL GLAND HYPERFUNCTION

A variety of drugs are used to suppress adrenal hormones. Some drugs suppress cortisol production directly or indirectly. Others control the problems associated with hyperaldosteronism.

Dosages for Adrenal Hormone-Suppressing Drugs

Drug	Dosage
mitotane (Lysodren)	*Adults:* 1-2 g orally every 6-8 hours *Children:* Safety and efficacy have not been established
mifepristone (Korlym)	*Adults:* 300 mg orally once daily; can be increased to 1200 mg orally daily *Children:* Safety and efficacy have not been established

How Drugs to Suppress Adrenal Hormone Production Work

Mifepristone (Korlym) works by blocking corticosteroid receptors, which inhibits the action of cortisol. It is approved only for use in people who have type 2 diabetes and hyperglycemia along with hypercortisolism. Mitotane (Lysodren) works by directly inhibiting the adrenal gland production of cortisol. Additional drug therapy for hyperaldosteronism relies on spironolactone (Aldactone, Spironol, Novo-Spiroton ✦), a potassium-sparing diuretic that controls hypokalemia. See Chapter 15 for more information on spironolactone therapy.

Intended Responses
- Reduced blood levels of glucocorticoids and aldosterone
- Normal blood levels of sodium and potassium
- Normal blood levels of glucose
- Normal blood pressure

Side Effects. All drugs for suppression of adrenal hormone production are likely to cause nausea, vomiting, skin rashes, and dizziness. Mitotane can also cause bloody urine (hematuria). Mifepristone causes many side effects, including menstrual irregularities.

Adverse Effects. All drugs for suppression of adrenal production of cortisol can lead to problems of adrenal insufficiency. Mifepristone is also a drug used to induce abortion and can cause pregnancy loss.

What To *Teach* Patients About Drug Therapy to Suppress Adrenal Hormone Production

The most important point to teach patients taking any drug to suppress adrenal hormone production are the signs and symptoms of adrenal insufficiency. These include hypoglycemia, salt craving, muscle weakness, hypotension, and fatigue.

Because these drugs alter blood levels of sodium and potassium, remind patients to keep all appointments for laboratory blood work.

All of these drugs can cause nausea, vomiting, and other gastrointestinal upsets. Teach patients to take these drugs with food.

Instruct women of childbearing age who are sexually active to use two reliable forms of birth control while taking mifepristone.

Life Span Considerations for Drugs that Suppress Adrenal Hormone Production

None of the drugs used to suppress adrenal hormone production are approved for use in children or in women who are pregnant or breastfeeding.

Common Side Effects

Drugs That Suppress Adrenal Hormone Production

Nausea and   Skin rash   Dizziness
vomiting

Get Ready for Practice!

Key Points

- Proper thyroid function is essential for life. Both an underactive thyroid gland (causing hypothyroidism) and an overactive thyroid gland (causing hyperthyroidism) must be treated.
- Thyroid problems are very common.
- Side effects and adverse effects of thyroid hormone replacement drugs resemble hyperthyroidism.
- Infants and young children may need a *higher* dose (in terms of micrograms per kilogram of body weight) of thyroid hormone replacement drugs than adults and older adults need.
- Thyroid crisis (or thyroid storm) is an emergency situation. The death rate for thyroid crisis is about 30%, even when the patient is treated correctly.
- Teach patients taking thyroid hormone replacement drugs not to stop the drug suddenly or change the dose of the drug without consulting their prescriber.

- When thyroid hormone replacement drugs are first started, the dose is low and is increased slowly until the patient gets to the dose that keeps metabolism at a normal level.
- Thyroid hormone replacement drugs increase a patient's blood sugar level; patients with diabetes may need higher doses of insulin or other antidiabetic drugs.
- Both thyroid hormone replacement drugs and thyroid-suppressing drugs increase the effectiveness of warfarin (Coumadin), increasing a patient's risk for bleeding.
- The effects of thyroid-suppressing drugs may not be seen until 2 to 4 weeks after therapy has started because of the existing thyroid hormones stored in the gland.
- The adrenal cortex secretes hormones that are essential for life.
- Adrenal gland hypofunction results in low levels of glucocorticoids (corticosteroids) and aldosterone.
- Glucocorticoid deficiency is corrected with cortisol hormone replacement therapy, and aldosterone deficiency is corrected with fludrocortisone.
- Common problems and side effects of hormone replacement therapy for adrenal gland hypofunction are hypertension, weight gain, edema, low blood potassium levels, and high blood sodium levels.
- Drugs to suppress adrenal hormone production are not approved for use in children, pregnant women, or women who are breastfeeding.

Additional Learning Resources

evolve Be sure to visit your Evolve website (http://evolve.elsevier.com/Workman/pharmacology/) for additional online resources.

SG Go to your Study Guide for additional learning activities to help you master this chapter content.

Review Questions

See the Answer Keys—In-text Review Questions for answers to these questions.

Test Yourself on the Basics

1. What is the goal of therapy with thyroid hormone agonists?
   A. To cure hypothyroidism
   B. To reduce the size of the goiter
   C. To increase metabolism to normal levels
   D. To suppress natural thyroid hormone secretion from the thyroid gland
2. Which problem is an adverse effect of levothyroxine (Synthroid)?
   A. Obesity
   B. Heart failure
   C. Type 2 diabetes mellitus
   D. Venous thromboembolism

3. A patient taking levothyroxine sodium (Synthroid) reports all of the following changes. Which one should you report to the prescriber as an indication that the dose may be too high?
   A. An intended weight loss of 6 lb over a 3-week period
   B. Increased interest in sexual activity
   C. Increased thirst and urine output
   D. Nightly insomnia
4. Which electrolytes are most important to monitor for a patient who is taking fludrocortisone (Florinef) as hormone replacement therapy for aldosterone deficiency?
   A. Calcium and chloride
   B. Sodium and potassium
   C. Glucose and glucagon
   D. Magnesium and phosphorus
5. Which adrenal hormone-suppressing drug can cause pregnancy loss?
   A. aminoglutethimide (Cytadren)
   B. spironolactone (Aldactone)
   C. mifepristone (Korlym)
   D. mitotane (Lysodren)
6. Which drug used to treat adrenal gland problems can cause the side effect of bloody urine?
   A. aminoglutethimide (Cytadren)
   B. fludrocortisone (Florinef)
   C. mifepristone (Korlym)
   D. mitotane (Lysodren)

Test Yourself on Advanced Concepts

7. Which precaution is most important to teach a patient taking hormone replacement therapy for hypothyroidism?
   A. Report episodes of constipation or cold intolerance to the prescriber immediately.
   B. Be sure to take the drug with a full glass of water and drink at least 2 L daily.
   C. Call the prescriber if you are unable to take the drug dose orally.
   D. Do not drink alcoholic beverages while taking this drug.
8. A patient is newly pregnant and tells you that she has been taking levothyroxine (Synthroid) for the past 12 years for hypothyroidism. She asks you whether she should take this drug during pregnancy and while breastfeeding. What is your best response?
   A. "This drug should not be taken during pregnancy or while breastfeeding."
   B. "This drug can be taken during pregnancy but not while breastfeeding."
   C. "This drug can be taken during pregnancy and while breastfeeding."
   D. "This drug should not be taken during pregnancy but can be taken while breastfeeding."

9. A mother whose infant was born with hypothyroidism asks how long her baby girl will have to take thyroid hormone replacement therapy. What is your best response?
   A. "Because the thyroid gland will increase in size during puberty, she can stop taking the drug after she starts menstruating."
   B. "Most infants develop normal thyroid function by 1 year of age, so she will probably not have to take the drug after her first birthday."
   C. "It is too early in the therapy regimen to tell how long thyroid hormone replacement therapy will be needed."
   D. "Because she was born without a thyroid gland, she will have to take the drug for the rest of her life."

10. Which precaution is important to teach a patient taking propylthiouracil (Propacil) for hyperthyroidism before surgery?
    A. Avoid crowds and people who are ill.
    B. Expect your urine to become an orange-red color.
    C. Report a loss of taste sensation to the prescriber immediately.
    D. If you develop diarrhea, skip the drug until the diarrhea has resolved.

11. Which laboratory value indicates that drug therapy for adrenal hypofunction is effective?
    A. International normalized ratio (INR) is 0.9
    B. Serum potassium is 4.5 mEq/L
    C. Serum sodium is 131 mEq/L
    D. Hematocrit is 44%

12. Why are the effects of methimazole (Tapazole) delayed for the first 3 weeks?
    A. The metabolism of the patient with hyperthyroidism is so high that the drug is eliminated before it has a chance to work.
    B. The dose of the drug has to be increased slowly to reach an effective blood level without causing side effects.
    C. Time is needed for the drug to reduce the size of the thyroid gland.
    D. The drug has no effect on stored thyroid hormones.

13. A patient is prescribed mitotane (Lysodren) 1.5 g orally. The drug on hand is mitotane 500 mg tablets. How many tablets are needed for the 1.5 g dose? _____ tablets

14. A patient is prescribed levothyroxine 25 mcg by IV push. The drug on hand is levothyroxine sodium 100 mcg/mL. How many mL should be administered? _____ mL

Critical Thinking Activities

See the Answer Keys—Critical Thinking Activities for answers to these activities.

The patient is a 43-year-old woman who is scheduled to have a hysterectomy later today. During her preadmission testing, her vital signs are T = 100, P = 88 with several "skipped" beats, R = 20, BP = 160/148. She is 5'6" and weighs 110 lb. Her current drugs are metoprolol (Toprol 50 mg) for hypertension, levothyroxine (Synthroid) 200 mcg daily, and aspirin 81 mg daily. When you ask her about her hypertension, she shouts that her blood pressure problem is being managed and that you should focus on her impending surgery. Then she apologizes for her behavior and says that she has not been sleeping well lately, probably because of worrying about the scheduled surgery.

1. What type of drug is levothyroxine?
2. What are the side effects of this drug?
3. Which, if any, vital sign abnormalities, patient-reported signs or symptoms, and observed physical attributes and behavior(s) could be attributed to this drug? Provide rationales for your selections.
4. What should you do with this information?

Drugs That Affect Urine Output

Objectives

After studying this chapter you should be able to:

1. List the common names, actions, usual adult dosages, possible side effects, and adverse effects of diuretic drugs.
2. Describe what to do before and after giving diuretic drugs.
3. Explain what to teach patients taking diuretic drugs, including what to do, what not to do, and when to call the prescriber.
4. Describe life span considerations for diuretic drugs.
5. List the common names, actions, usual adult dosages, possible side effects, and adverse effects of drugs for overactive bladder.

6. Describe what to do before and after giving drugs for overactive bladder.
7. Explain what to teach patients taking drugs for overactive bladder, including what to do, what not to do, and when to call the prescriber.
8. Describe life span considerations for drugs for overactive bladder.

Key Terms

detrusor muscle (dē-TRŪ-zŭr MŬS-ŭl) (p. 248) The layer of involuntary muscle in the bladder wall; during urination it contracts to squeeze urine out of the bladder into the urethra.

diuretics (dī-ŭr-ĔT-ĭks) (p. 239) Drugs that help rid the body of excess water and salt (sodium).

loop diuretic (LŪP dī-ŭr-ĔT-ĭk) (p. 244) Powerful diuretic class of drugs that act on the ascending loop of Henle in the kidney. It is used primarily to treat hypertension and edema often caused by heart failure or renal insufficiency.

natriuretic diuretic (nā-trē-yū-RĔ-tĭk dī-ŭr-ĔT-ĭk) (p. 242) Diuretic that causes the excretion of sodium and water in the urine.

overactive bladder (OAB) (ŏ-vŭr-ĂK-tĭv BLĂ-dŭr) (p. 248) A problem with bladder function that causes a sudden urge to

urinate and can even lead to the involuntary loss of urine (incontinence).

potassium-sparing diuretic (pō-TĂS-ē-ŭm SPĂR-ĭng dī-ŭr-ĔT-ĭk) (p. 246) A drug that blocks exchange of sodium for potassium and hydrogen ions in the distal tubule, leading to increased sodium and chloride excretion without increased potassium excretion.

thiazide diuretic (THĪ-ŭ-zīd dī-ŭr-ĔT-ĭk) (p. 242) A diuretic drug class that slows down or turns off the salt pumps in the nephron tube furthest away from the capillaries and causes more sodium, potassium, and water to stay in the urine and leave the body through urination. It is used primarily in the treatment of hypertension.

DIURETICS

People often call these drugs "water pills" because they cause the body to lose water. **Diuretics** are drugs that help rid the body of excess water and sodium by increasing a person's urine output. They may work on the kidneys directly, or they may increase blood flow to the kidney. Either way, these drugs cause a person to urinate more and lose water from the body.

REVIEW OF RELATED PHYSIOLOGY AND PATHOPHYSIOLOGY

Urine is made from the blood. Blood travels to the kidneys where there are millions of small tubes called *nephrons*, which are the filtering units of the kidneys

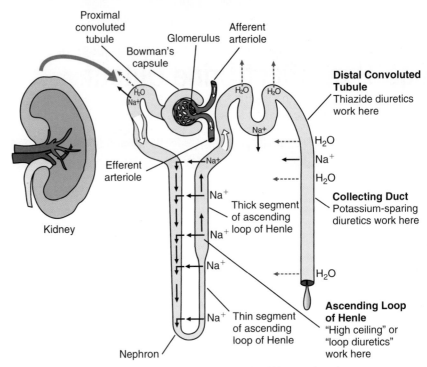

FIGURE 15-1 Sites of diuretic action on the kidney and nephrons.

(Figure 15-1). Each nephron has a collection of capillaries at the beginning of the nephron. Whole blood flows into these capillaries, which are leaky to water and small particles such as sugar, salt (sodium), potassium, and chloride but do not leak cells, proteins, and large particles. When whole blood goes through capillaries, the water and small particles leave the capillaries and go into the nephrons. The blood cells, proteins, and large particles go directly back into the blood.

The purpose of the nephrons is to act like a "washing machine" and take out all the waste products (such as urea and ammonia) and extra water, sodium, and potassium, keeping the blood "clean." In healthy kidneys, about 100 mL (3 to 4 oz) of water (and small particles) enters the nephron tubules each minute. If nothing happened to this 100 mL of water, everyone would have a urine output of 6000 mL (6 qt or 6 L) every hour, which is too much water for the body to lose and leads to dehydration. To prevent this much water from being lost along with the waste products, places along the nephron tubes *(renal tubules)* draw out most of the water and the helpful particles but keep the waste products in the urine. The cleaned water and helpful particles are put back into the blood by *reabsorption*. The waste products and excess sodium and potassium stay in the urine along with just enough water to allow them to be urinated out from the body *(excretion)*. In this way, a person loses waste products and excess particles without losing too much water.

The places in the nephron tubes that allow water, sodium, and potassium to be pulled out from the urine and put back into the blood have special "pumps" that remove the sodium and potassium. Because of the rule "where sodium goes, water follows," the pulling of sodium from the urine pulls water along with it. This process allows us to make only about 1 mL of urine each minute. The urine collects in the bladder until it is ready to be eliminated through urination. Most people have a urine output of about 2400 mL (nearly 2.5 quarts) each day. The amount of urine output increases when a person's fluid intake increases and decreases when fluid intake decreases.

Because the action of diuretics leads to increased urine output, patients taking these drugs are at increased risk for *dehydration*, a condition caused by the loss

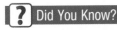

Did You Know?

Most people have a urine output of about 2400 mL/day.

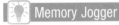

Memory Jogger

The rule "where sodium goes, water follows" works with sodium-excreting diuretics in the kidney. When sodium moves into the nephron tubules, water follows and is excreted in the urine.

of too much water from the body. Signs and symptoms of dehydration to watch for include:

- Increased pulse rate with a "thready" pulse that may be hard to feel
- Low blood pressure (hypotension)
- Thirst
- Sunken appearance to the eyeballs
- Dry mouth with thick, sticky coating on tongue
- Skin "tenting" on the forehead or chest (gently pinch up a section of skin on the forehead or chest, release it, and see how long it takes for the "tent" you made to go away)
- Constipation
- Decreased urine output (less than 30 mL/hr) with urine that is dark and strong smelling

Diuretics are used most often to treat problems when the body is retaining too much water, too much sodium, or too much potassium. They are often prescribed for people who have the following health problems:

- High blood pressure (hypertension)
- Heart failure
- Kidney disease
- Liver disease (cirrhosis)

Memory Jogger

Diuretics do not cure health problems, and the drugs may need to be taken daily for the rest of a patient's life.

GENERAL ISSUES IN DIURETIC THERAPY

There are several classes of diuretic drugs that have different, as well as common, actions and effects. In addition to the practices listed for drug administration in Chapter 2, general responsibilities for safe administration of diuretic drugs are listed in the following paragraphs. Specific responsibilities are listed with each individual class of diuretics.

Responsibilities before administering any diuretic drug include: always obtain a complete list of drugs that the patient is currently taking, including over-the-counter and herbal preparations. Obtain baselines for weight, blood pressure, and heart rate for comparison after giving a diuretic drug. If blood pressure is low (less than 90/60 mm Hg), ask the prescriber if the patient should receive the drug. Also check the latest set of blood electrolyte levels and notify the prescriber of any abnormal values. Ask patients about their usual urine output pattern.

Make certain that the patient does not have a problem with blockage in any area of the urinary system (for example, an enlarged prostate that interferes with urine flow). Giving diuretics to a person with a blockage can cause backflow of urine into the kidney and damage it.

Give scheduled doses in the morning to avoid loss of sleep because of the patient's need to urinate. Make sure that the patient has a urinal or other collection device to measure urine output.

Responsibilities after administering any diuretic drug include: make sure to recheck and continue to monitor blood pressure and heart rate at least once every 8 hours because rapid water loss decreases blood volume and lowers blood pressure. Monitor for signs of orthostatic hypotension such as dizziness or light-headedness. Ensure that the call light is within easy reach and instruct patients to call for help getting out of bed. Assist patients to change positions slowly. Have them sit on the side of the bed for 1 to 2 minutes before getting up and then stand up slowly.

Keep a record of urine output because increased urine output is an expected response to all diuretic drugs. Obtain daily weights at the same time each day, using the same scale and with the patient wearing the same or similar clothing.

Continue to monitor blood electrolyte levels for any changes that may result from the diuretic drug. The most important electrolytes to monitor are potassium and sodium.

Teach patients taking a diuretic drug to take it exactly as ordered by the prescriber. Tell them to take these drugs according to a schedule that will least affect daily

Drug Alert!

Monitoring Alert

After giving any diuretic drug, monitor blood pressure at least once every 8 hours. Rapid water loss decreases blood volume and lowers blood pressure.

QSEN: Safety

activities. For example, they should take single doses of diuretics early in the day to avoid having to awaken during the night to urinate. If a patient is taking more than one dose per day, the last dose should be taken no later than 6:00 pm to avoid frequent nighttime urination and disruption of sleep and rest. Tell them *never* to double the dose the next day if a dose is missed.

Teach patients about the signs of hypotension (for example, dizziness or lightheadedness). Because of the risk for hypotension, remind them to change positions slowly. Instruct patients on the proper techniques for checking their blood pressure and heart rate. Tell them to notify the prescriber if their heart rate is lower than 60 or higher than 100 beats per minute. If blood pressure is less than 90/60 mm Hg or they experience the symptoms of hypotension, they should notify their prescriber.

Teach patients to weigh themselves every day using the same scale and wearing the same or similar clothing after discharge. Instruct them to keep a record of their daily weights. Remind them to drink the same amount of fluid as they urinate each day.

TYPES OF DIURETICS

 Memory Jogger

The three major types of natriuretic diuretics are thiazide, loop, and potassium sparing.

There are two types of diuretics. The most commonly used diuretics are called **natriuretic diuretics**. They slow down or turn off the sodium (salt) pumps in the nephrons and make a person excrete more sodium. They include:

- Thiazide diuretics
- Loop diuretics
- Potassium-sparing diuretics

The second type of diuretics is osmotic diuretics such as mannitol (Osmitrol), which increase the blood flow to the kidneys. These drugs are used only in critical situations. Consult a critical care resource for a discussion of the use of osmotic diuretics.

Carbonic anhydrase inhibitors are another class of drugs that are sometimes used for diuresis. These drugs are primarily used for treatment of glaucoma and are discussed in Chapter 29.

THIAZIDE DIURETICS

How Thiazide Diuretics Work

Thiazide diuretics slow down or turn off the salt pumps in the nephron tubes furthest away from the capillaries (see Figure 15-1). They cause more sodium, potassium, and water to stay in the urine and leave the body through urination. This action reduces blood volume and lowers blood pressure. Commonly prescribed thiazide diuretics are listed in the following table. Be sure to consult a drug handbook for more information about a specific thiazide diuretic.

Dosages for Common Thiazide Diuretics

Drug	Dosage
chlorothiazide (Diuril)	*Adults:* PO—250 mg orally every 6-12 hr to decrease body water; 250-1000 mg orally daily to reduce blood pressure *Adults:* IV—250 mg every 6-12 hr to decrease body water; 500-1000 mg IV in single or 2 divided doses per day to lower blood pressure *Children:* Dose based on weight and determined by prescriber
hydrochlorothiazide (Apo-Hydro ♣, Microzide, Novo-Hydrazide ♣, Oretic)	*Adults:* 25-100 mg orally once or twice daily *Children:* Dose based on weight and determined by prescriber
metolazone (Zaroxolyn)	*Adults:* 5-20 mg orally once daily to decrease body water; 2.5-5 mg orally once daily to decrease blood pressure *Children:* Dose determined by prescriber

Intended Responses
- Urine output is increased.
- Urine is lighter in color.
- Blood pressure is lower.

Side Effects. The side effects of thiazide diuretics increase with higher blood levels of these drugs. At lower doses, side effects are less common. Potential side effects of thiazide diuretics include fluid and electrolyte imbalances such as decreased blood volume, potassium (hypokalemia), sodium (hyponatremia), chloride (hypochloremia), and magnesium (hypomagnesemia) and increased calcium (hypercalcemia) and urea (hyperuremia). Because of decreased blood volume, blood pressure drops faster when the patient moves from a sitting or lying position to a standing position, causing some dizziness or light-headedness *(postural hypotension)*. When postural hypotension is severe, the patient could faint and fall.

A decreased potassium level may result in dry mouth, increased thirst, irregular heartbeat, mood changes, muscle cramps, nausea, vomiting, fatigue or weakness, and weak pulses.

Decreased sodium level may lead to confusion, convulsions, decreased mental activity, irritability, muscle cramps, and unusual fatigue or weakness.

Adverse Effects. Adverse effects of thiazide diuretics include "passing out" or falling when changing positions, muscle weakness, and blurred vision. Metalazone can cause impaired glucose tolerance, glucosuria, and hyperglycemia in diabetic patients

What To Do *Before* Giving Thiazide Diuretics
In addition to the general responsibilities related to diuretic drug therapy (p. 241), check the most recent serum potassium level. If it is below 3.5 mEq/L or 3.5 mmol/L, inform the prescriber. Patients who have low blood potassium levels may develop life-threatening abnormal heart rhythms.

Ask patients about prior allergic reactions to thiazide diuretics. Ask women in their childbearing years if they are pregnant, plan to become pregnant, or are breastfeeding because thiazide diuretics should not be used during pregnancy or breastfeeding.

What To Do *After* Giving Thiazide Diuretics
In addition to the general nursing responsibilities related to diuretic drug therapy (p. 241), keep track of the patient's blood electrolyte levels, including potassium. Watch for signs of decreased potassium, including abnormal heart rhythms, muscle cramps, constipation, and changes in reflexes. Table 1-4 in Chapter 1 provides a summary of normal electrolyte values.

What To *Teach* Patients About Thiazide Diuretics
In addition to the general precautions related to diuretic drug therapy (pp. 241-242), teach patients the signs of decreased body potassium levels. Remind them to report side effects such as muscle weakness or cramps, sudden decrease in urination, and irregular heartbeat to the prescriber. Tell them to take all prescribed potassium pills or liquid. Instruct them to take the drug with food if stomach upset occurs.

Life Span Considerations for Thiazide Diuretics
Pediatric Considerations. Dosage of diuretic drugs is based on weight in children. Side effects in children are the same as in adults. Thiazide diuretics should be used with caution when infants have jaundice because the drugs worsen the condition.

Considerations for Pregnancy and Lactation. Thiazide diuretics have a moderate likelihood of increasing the risk for birth defects or fetal damage and should be avoided during pregnancy because they may cause side effects in the newborn,

Common Side Effects
Thiazide Diuretics
   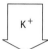
Dizziness Hypotension Hypokalemia
Hyponatremia

Drug Alert!
Administration Alert
Check the apical pulse of patients receiving a thiazide diuretic for a full minute to determine whether the rhythm is regular.
QSEN: Safety

 Clinical Pitfall
If a patient forgets to take a thiazide diuretic, a double dose should not be taken the next day.
QSEN: Safety

Clinical Pitfall

Thiazide diuretics should not be given during pregnancy or to breastfeeding mothers because they cause side effects, pass into breast milk, and may cause a decrease in the flow of breast milk.

QSEN: Safety

Do Not Confuse

Lasix *with* **Luvox**

An order for Lasix can be mistaken for Luvox. Lasix is a loop diuretic; Luvox is an antidepressant.

QSEN: Safety

including jaundice and low potassium levels. These drugs have been shown to cause birth defects (are teratogenic) in animals. They should also be avoided during breast-feeding because they pass into breast milk. Their action may decrease the flow of breast milk.

Considerations for Older Adults. Dizziness or light-headedness and signs of low potassium levels may be more likely in older adults because they are more sensitive to the effects of thiazide diuretics. This greatly increases the older adult's risk for falls. Teach these patients to change positions slowly and to always use the handrails when going up or down stairs.

LOOP DIURETICS

How Loop Diuretics Work

Loop diuretics (also called "high-ceiling" diuretics) slow down or turn off the sodium pumps in the nephron tube in a place different from thiazide diuretic action. They cause more sodium, potassium, and water to stay in the urine and leave the body through urination (see Figure 15-1). Loop diuretics are the most powerful diuretics. Although this power can be helpful, it also means that the *side effects are more severe* because there is greater water, sodium, and potassium loss. Another difference between loop diuretics and thiazide diuretics is that loop diuretics cause patients to lose calcium in the urine.

Commonly prescribed loop diuretics are listed in the following table. Be sure to consult a drug handbook for more information about a specific loop diuretic.

Dosages for Common Loop Diuretics

Drug	Dosage
furosemide (Furoside ♣, Lasix, Lasix Special ♣, Novosemide ♣, Urotrol ♣)	*Adults:* PO—20-80 mg daily; prescriber may increase dose as needed *Adults:* IV or IM—20-40 mg; prescriber may increase dose every 2 hours as needed; after dose is working, it is injected IV or IM 1 to 2 times daily *Children:* PO—2 mg/kg daily; prescriber may increase dose every 6-8 hr as needed *Children:* IV or IM—1 mg/kg; prescriber may increase dose every 2 hr as needed *Special Considerations:* Can be given IV slowly, no more than 4 mg/min For very high blood pressure in adults, 40-200 mg may be given IV
bumetanide (Bumex)	*Adults:* PO—0.5-2 mg daily; prescriber may increase dose as needed *Adults:* IM or IV—0.5-1 mg every 2-3 hr as needed *Children:* Dose must be determined by prescriber
ethacrynic acid (Edecrin)	*Adults:* PO—50-200 mg daily; single or divided doses *Adults:* IV—50 mg every 2-6 hr as needed *Children:* PO—25 mg daily; prescriber may increase dose as needed *Children:* IV—1 mg/kg
torsemide (Demadex)	*Adults:* 10-20 mg orally or IV once daily; may increase up to 200 mg daily as needed

Intended Responses
- Urine output is increased.
- Urine is lighter in color.
- Blood pressure is lower.

Side Effects. Among the more common side effects of loop diuretics is dizziness or light-headedness when the patient moves from a sitting or lying position to a standing position. This occurs because blood pressure drops in response to the loss of fluid from the blood vessels *(postural hypotension).*

Blood levels of potassium and sodium decrease *(hypokalemia, hyponatremia)* with loop diuretics. Signs and symptoms of low potassium include dry mouth, increased thirst, irregular heartbeat, mental and mood changes, muscle cramps or muscle pain, nausea, vomiting, fatigue, weakness, and weak pulses. Signs and symptoms of low sodium include confusion, convulsions, decreased mental activity, irritability, muscle cramps, and unusual fatigue or weakness.

An additional side effect of furosemide is increased sensitivity of skin to sunlight *(photosensitivity)*, possibly with skin rash, itching, redness, or severe sunburn. Ethacrynic acid may cause confusion, diarrhea, loss of appetite, and nervousness. Blurred vision, chest pain, and premature ejaculation or difficulty maintaining an erection may occur with bumetanide.

Adverse Effects. Fainting or falling when changing positions, muscle weakness, and irregular heart rhythms can occur.

Loop diuretics can be *ototoxic* (cause hearing loss from damage to the auditory [ear] tissues). Ototoxicity is reversible when the drug is discontinued, and it becomes worse when the patient is taking other ototoxic drugs such as aminoglycoside antibiotics (for example, gentamicin) while taking a loop diuretic. Hearing loss can occur when these drugs are given too rapidly by intravenous (IV) and/or in very high doses. The hearing loss is usually temporary.

High blood glucose (hyperglycemia) levels can also occur. Patients with diabetes must check their blood sugar (glucose) levels regularly.

What To Do **Before** ***Giving Loop Diuretics.*** In addition to the general responsibilities related to diuretic therapy (p. 241), check the most recent serum potassium level. If it is below 3.5 mEq/L or 3.5 mmol/L, be sure to inform the prescriber. Check to see whether the patient is scheduled to receive a potassium supplement. If the potassium level is low, the prescriber may want to order an extra dose of potassium. Check the serum sodium level. If it is below 135 mEq/L or 135 mmol/L, inform the prescriber.

Check the patient's prescribed drugs to determine whether another drug is also ototoxic. If you find that the patient is taking two or more ototoxic drugs, inform the prescriber.

If the drug is to be given intravenously, always check the IV site for patency and signs of inflammation or infection.

What To Do *After* Giving Loop Diuretics

In addition to the general responsibilities related to diuretic therapy (p. 241), monitor serum potassium levels and report low values (less than 3.5 mEq/L or 3.5 mmol/L) to the prescriber. Give prescribed potassium supplements as ordered. Continue to monitor patients for any signs of hearing loss.

Frequently check and record urine output. Regularly empty urine collection devices. Check IV sites for patency at least every 8 hours and monitor for signs of phlebitis or infection (for example, redness, swelling, warmth).

What To *Teach* Patients About Loop Diuretics

In addition to the general precautions related to diuretic therapy (pp. 241-242), remind patients that increased urine output can occur rapidly after an IV injection of loop diuretics. Make sure that the patient understands that urine output can increase dramatically within an hour of taking a loop diuretic, increasing the risk for unexpected or uncontrolled urination (incontinence).

Instruct patients to limit alcohol intake while taking loop diuretics. Alcohol increases the chance of dizziness, light-headedness, and fainting.

Instruct patients to report any decrease in hearing or "ringing" in the ears *(tinnitus)* to the prescriber because this may be the first indication of damage to the ear or hearing.

Tell patients who develop skin sensitivity with furosemide to stay out of direct sunlight, wear protective clothing, and use sun block products with a skin protection factor (SPF) of at least 15. Remind them not to use sunlamps or tanning beds.

Because loop diuretics cause loss of potassium, the prescriber may want the patient to eat foods that contain potassium. Tell patients to be sure to take any

Common Side Effects

Loop Diuretics

Dizziness

Hypotension

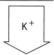
Hypokalemia

Hyponatremia

 Drug Alert!

Administration Alert

Give IV doses of furosemide (Lasix) slowly at a rate of 20 mg per minute to avoid ototoxicity.

QSEN: Safety

Drug Alert!

Teaching Alert

Teach patients that diuresis (increased urine output) can occur rapidly after IV administration of a loop diuretic and may lead to incontinence.

QSEN: Safety

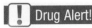 **Drug Alert!**

Teaching Alert

Teach patients taking loop diuretics about foods that contain potassium such as bananas and oranges or to drink citrus fruit juices.

QSEN: Safety

 Drug Alert!

Teaching Alert

Instruct older adults to report indicators of difficulty with hearing, including the need to increase the volume setting on the radio or television.

QSEN: Safety

prescribed potassium pills or liquid. Teach them to take it with food or drink to prevent stomach irritation.

Life Span Considerations for Loop Diuretics

Pediatric Considerations. Side effects of these drugs in children are expected to be the same as in adults. The dosage of furosemide is based on weight; however, some loop diuretic dosages must be determined individually by the prescriber.

Considerations for Pregnancy and Lactation. Loop diuretics have a moderate level of increased risk for birth defects or fetal damage and should not be given to women who are pregnant or breastfeeding. Animal studies have shown these drugs to cause fetal harm (are teratogenic). Furosemide passes into breast milk and should not be used while breastfeeding.

Considerations for Older Adults. Older adults are more sensitive to the effects of loop diuretics and are more likely to develop dizziness and light-headedness, which increases their risk for falls. They are also more likely to develop blood clots and signs of low blood potassium. Teach them to report new-onset muscle weakness to the prescriber. Older adults are more likely to have tinnitus and hearing loss with these drugs. Teach them to note whether they are having more difficulty hearing what is said and whether they need to set the volume higher on the radio or television.

POTASSIUM-SPARING DIURETICS

How Potassium-Sparing Diuretics Work

Potassium-sparing diuretics slow the sodium pumps so more sodium and water are excreted as urine, but these drugs do not increase the loss of potassium. In fact, they prevent potassium loss in the urine and cause more potassium to be returned to the blood. These drugs work in a place in the nephron tubes that is different from other diuretics (see Figure 15-1).

Commonly prescribed potassium-sparing diuretics are listed in the following table. Be sure to consult a drug handbook for more information on a specific potassium-sparing diuretic.

Dosages for Common Potassium-Sparing Diuretics

Drug	Dosage
spironolactone (Aldactone, Novospiroton ✦)	*Adults:* 25-200 mg orally daily divided into 2-4 doses to decrease body water, prescriber may increase dose as needed; 50-100 mg orally daily in a single dose or 2-4 divided doses to decrease blood pressure; 25-100 mg orally daily in single doses or 2-4 divided doses to treat low potassium levels *Children:* 1-3 mg/kg orally daily in a single dose or 2-4 divided doses
triamterene (Dyrenium)	*Adults:* 100 mg orally twice daily; prescriber may gradually increase dose *Children:* 2-4 mg/kg daily or every other day, divided into equal small doses; prescriber may increase dose as needed
amiloride (Midamor)	*Adults:* 5-10 mg orally once daily *Children:* Dose must be determined by prescriber

Intended Responses
- Urine output is increased.
- Urine is lighter in color.
- Blood pressure is lower.
- Serum potassium level stays within the normal range (3.5 to 5 mEq/L).

Side Effects. Blood pressure drops faster when the patient who is taking potassium-sparing diuretics moves from a sitting or lying position to a standing position, causing some dizziness or light-headedness (postural hypotension). Patient falls are more likely.

Blood levels of sodium decrease (hyponatremia). Symptoms of low sodium level include drowsiness, dry mouth, increased thirst, lack of energy, and muscle weakness.

Other common side effects of potassium-sparing diuretics include nausea, vomiting, stomach cramps, and diarrhea.

Women may develop *hirsutism* (facial hair), irregular menstrual cycles, and deepening of the voice. Men may have trouble getting or keeping an erection. Both men and women may develop breast enlargement (*gynecomastia* in men).

Triamterene may cause the skin to become more sensitive to sunlight (*photosensitivity*), possibly with skin rash, itching, redness, or severe sunburn.

Adverse Effects. Fainting or falling when changing positions may occur because of the decrease in blood volume and blood pressure.

Because these drugs "spare" potassium, the patient is at risk for increased potassium levels (hyperkalemia). A life-threatening side effect of high potassium level is development of an irregular heartbeat (*dysrhythmia*). Symptoms of a high potassium level include confusion; irregular heartbeat; nervousness; numbness or tingling in hands, feet, or lips; shortness of breath or difficulty breathing; unusual fatigue or weakness; and weakness or a heavy feeling in the legs.

What To Do Before Giving Potassium-Sparing Diuretics
In addition to the general responsibilities related to diuretic therapy (p. 241), check the most recent serum electrolyte levels. If the potassium level is greater than 5 mEq/L or 5 mmol/L or the sodium level is less than 135 mEq/L or 135 mmol/L, inform the prescriber.

What To Do *After* Giving Potassium-Sparing Diuretics
In addition to the general responsibilities related to diuretic therapy (p. 241), monitor the patient for signs and symptoms of high potassium. These include dry mouth, increased thirst, irregular heartbeat, mood changes, muscle cramps, nausea, vomiting, fatigue or weakness, and weak pulses. Also monitor for signs and symptoms of low sodium levels, including confusion, convulsions, decreased mental activity, irritability, muscle cramps, and unusual fatigue or weakness.

What To *Teach* Patients About Potassium-Sparing Diuretics
In addition to the general precautions related to diuretic therapy (pp. 241-242), teach patients to avoid eating excessive amounts of high-potassium foods such as meats, dairy products, dried fruits, bananas, cantaloupe, kiwi, oranges, avocados, broccoli, dried beans or peas, lima beans, soybeans, or spinach. Remind them to avoid using salt substitutes because these products contain potassium instead of sodium.

Life Span Considerations for Potassium-Sparing Diuretics
Pediatric Considerations. Safe use of these drugs has not been established or researched in children, but side effects are expected to be the same as in adults.

Considerations for Pregnancy and Lactation. Safe use of potassium-sparing diuretics during pregnancy and breastfeeding has not been established. All of these drugs pass into breast milk, but no problems have been noted in breastfeeding infants. Spironolactone has a high likelihood of increasing the risk of birth defects or fetal damage and should be avoided during pregnancy. Triamterene and amiloride have a low likelihood of increasing the risk for birth defects or fetal damage.

Considerations for Older Adults. Older adults are more sensitive to the action of potassium-sparing diuretics and more likely to experience side effects.

Common Side Effects

Potassium-Sparing Diuretics

Hypotension   Hyponatremia   Vomiting, Diarrhea

K^+K^+
K^+K^+
K^+K^+

Hyperkalemia

 Clinical Pitfall

Do not give potassium supplements, salt substitutes, or angiotensin-converting enzyme inhibitors to patients taking potassium-sparing diuretics because these drugs can increase the risk of developing high to extremely high blood potassium levels.

QSEN: Safety

? Did You Know?

Most salt substitutes are made by replacing sodium with potassium. Therefore, salt substitutes should be avoided while taking a potassium-sparing diuretic.

Normal Bladder
Detrusor muscle
contracts when
bladder is full

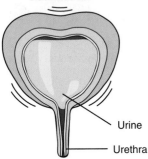

Urine

Urethra

Overactive Bladder
Detrusor muscle
contracts before
bladder is full

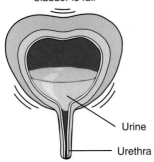

Urine

Urethra

FIGURE 15-2 Pathophysiology of overactive bladder.

OVERACTIVE BLADDER

An **overactive bladder (OAB)** is caused by sudden, involuntary contraction of the muscle in the bladder wall, which leads to a sudden, unstoppable need to urinate. Drugs for OAB are used to treat the symptoms of this disorder.

REVIEW OF RELATED PHYSIOLOGY AND PATHOPHYSIOLOGY

In people with OAB the layered, smooth muscle that surrounds the bladder (**detrusor muscle**) contracts spastically, sometimes without a known cause. This results in continuous high bladder pressure and the urgent need to urinate, also known as *urgency* (Figure 15-2). Normally the detrusor muscle contracts and relaxes in response to the amount of urine in the bladder and the initiation of urination.

People with OAB often have urgency at inconvenient and unpredictable times and sometimes lose control before reaching a toilet (*incontinence*). Thus OAB interferes with work, daily routine, intimacy, and sexual function; causes embarrassment; and can diminish self-esteem and quality of life. OAB is fairly common in older adults.

TYPES OF DRUGS FOR OVERACTIVE BLADDER

URINARY ANTISPASMODICS

How Urinary Antispasmodics Work

Drugs for OAB (urinary antispasmodics) are prescribed to treat and improve symptoms, including frequent urination, urgency of urination, and urinary incontinence. These drugs decrease the spasms of the detrusor muscle.

Commonly prescribed drugs for OAB are listed in the following table. Be sure to consult a drug handbook for more information about a specific drug for OAB.

Dosages for Common Urinary Antispasmodics

Drug	Dosage
oxybutynin (Ditropan)	*Adults/adolescents:* 5 mg orally 2-3 times daily (do not exceed 20 mg/day); extended release (XL)—5 mg daily (do not exceed 30 mg/day) *Children over 5 years:* 5 mg orally 2-3 times daily (do not exceed 15 mg/day)
oxybutynin transdermal system patch (Oxytrol; Gelnique)	*Adults:* 3.9 mg/day applied transdermally every 3-4 days; remove old patch before applying a new one; Gelnique—topical packet 100 mg daily; apply to abdomen, upper arms, shoulders, or thighs
tolterodine (Detrol, Detrol LA)	*Adults:* 2 mg orally twice daily; 4 mg orally once daily (Detrol LA)
solifenacin (VESIcare)	*Adults:* 5 mg orally once daily
darifenacin (Enablex)	*Adults:* 7.5 mg orally once daily; may increase to 15 mg once daily after 2 weeks
trospium chloride (Sanctura, Sanctura XR)	*Adults:* 20 mg orally twice daily 1 hr before meals; 60 mg once daily 1 hr before breakfast (Sanctura XR)

Intended Responses
- Urinary frequency is decreased.
- Urinary urgency is decreased.
- Urinary incontinence is decreased.

Side Effects. Frequent side effects of drugs for OAB include dry mouth, dry eyes, headache, dizziness, and constipation.

Adverse Effects. Adverse effects of these drugs include chest pain, fast or irregular heart rate, shortness of breath, swelling (edema) and rapid weight gain, confusion, and hallucinations. In addition, these drugs may cause decreased urination or no urine output and painful or difficult urination.

Signs of an allergic reaction include rash (hives); difficulty breathing; and swelling of face, lips, tongue, or throat.

Patients may be at increased risk for heatstroke during exercise or hot weather because these drugs decrease perspiration (sweating).

What To *Teach* Patients About Urinary Antispasmodics

Because most of these drugs are prescribed for outpatients, patient teaching is an essential part of your role. Teach patients to take these drugs on an empty stomach with water. If they experience stomach upset, the drugs may be given with milk or food.

Instruct patients not to crush, chew, break, or open extended-release or long-acting capsules. Tell them to swallow the capsule whole because these drugs are made to release the medication slowly into the body. When the capsules are opened in any way, the drug is released all at once. This may cause an initial overdose with more side effects and prevent the drug from being effective throughout the day.

If a dose is missed, teach patients to take it as soon as possible. If it is almost time for the next dose, they should skip the missed dose and take the drug at the next scheduled time. Tell them not to take extra pills to make up for the missed dose.

Remind patients to avoid becoming overheated or dehydrated during exercise or hot weather. These drugs may decrease sweating, placing patients at risk for heatstroke.

Teach patients to weigh themselves and report weight gain (more than 2 pounds per day) or increased swelling to the prescriber. Give instructions on how to take blood pressure and check heart rate. Tell them to report irregular heart rates to the prescriber.

Instruct patients to report urinary urgency, frequency, difficulty urinating or incontinence to the prescriber. Teach them to keep track of their fluid intake and output. Tell patients to contact their prescriber if urinary symptoms do not improve or if they become worse while taking these drugs.

Because of the visual side effects of OAB drugs, teach patients to avoid driving or any other activities that require clear vision and mental alertness until they know how the drugs will affect them.

Teach patients to avoid consuming alcohol within 2 hours of these drugs because side effects such as drowsiness are increased. They should drink alcohol only when they do not plan to drive or operate dangerous equipment.

Instruct patients using the transdermal patch system to apply a new patch to their skin every 3 to 4 days (as prescribed). The patch should be applied to a different clean, dry, and smooth area and pressed firmly to ensure that it stays in place. Teach patients to report skin redness, itchiness, or irritation to the prescriber.

Life Span Considerations for Urinary Antispasmodics

Considerations for Pregnancy and Lactation. Oxybutynin has a low likelihood of increasing the risk for birth defects or fetal damage. Other OAB drugs have a moderate likelihood of increasing the risk for birth defects or fetal damage. They are not recommended for use with pregnant or breastfeeding women.

Considerations for Older Adults. Older adults may be more sensitive to the effects of these drugs and may need to be prescribed lower drug doses.

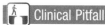

Common Side Effects

Urinary Antispasmodics

Headache   Dizziness   Constipation

Dry mouth   Dry eyes

 Clinical Pitfall

Patients taking drugs for OAB are at risk for heatstroke during exercise or hot weather.

QSEN: Safety

Drug Alert!

Teaching Alert

Teach patients using the transdermal patch system to remove the old patch before applying a new one.

QSEN: Safety

Get Ready for Practice!

Key Points

- Most diuretics work on the nephrons in the kidneys to increase urine output.
- Diuretics are prescribed to treat hypertension, heart failure, kidney disease, and liver disease.
- The two major types of diuretics are natriuretic diuretics (thiazide, loop, and potassium-sparing), and osmotic diuretics.
- The most common side effects of diuretics are dizziness and light-headedness related to hypotension.
- Patients taking potassium-sparing diuretics should be taught to avoid use of salt substitutes because these substitutes are made with potassium instead of sodium.
- Unless a patient is on a fluid restriction, be sure that fluid intake closely matches the urine output in a patient taking diuretics.
- Monitor patients taking diuretics for signs and symptoms of dehydration.
- Monitor electrolytes carefully when a patient is taking a diuretic.
- Check the blood pressure of a patient who is taking diuretics at least once per shift, even if it is not ordered.
- OAB is caused by spastic contractions of the detrusor muscle.
- People with OAB often experience urgency and leakage of urine (incontinence).
- Drugs for OAB decrease detrusor muscle spasms and relieve symptoms.
- Patients taking OAB drugs are at risk for heatstroke.

Additional Learning Resources

evolve Be sure to visit your Evolve website (http://evolve.elsevier.com/Workman/pharmacology/) for additional online resources.

SG Go to your Study Guide for additional learning activities to help you master this chapter content.

Review Questions

See the Answer Keys—In-text Review Questions for answers to these questions.

Test Yourself on the Basics

1. Which drug is a potassium-sparing diuretic?
   - A. Spironolactone
   - B. Bumetanide
   - C. Metolazone
   - D. Torsemide
2. Which two blood electrolyte levels must you check before giving a patient a loop diuretic such as furosemide (Lasix)?
   - A. Potassium and calcium
   - B. Calcium and sodium
   - C. Magnesium and potassium
   - D. Sodium and potassium

3. Which foods would you teach a patient prescribed hydrochlorothiazide (Oretic) to consume?
   - A. Grapefruit and carrots
   - B. Corn and squash
   - C. Bananas and broccoli
   - D. Chicken and beef
4. Which consideration applies to older adults prescribed loop diuretic therapy?
   - A. Depression
   - B. Increased risk for falls
   - C. Dosage varies with patient weight
   - D. Risk for increased potassium level
5. Which side effect is common when a patient is prescribed a drug for overactive bladder?
   - A. Dry mouth
   - B. Confusion
   - C. Nausea
   - D. Blurred vision

Test Yourself on Advanced Concepts

6. A patient prescribed furosemide (Lasix) has a potassium level of 3.4 mEq/L. What is your best action?
   - A. Document the finding as a normal level.
   - B. Hold the drug and notify the prescriber.
   - C. Instruct the patient to eat a banana and orange.
   - D. Repeat the lab test to ensure that it is correct.
7. Before giving a thiazide diuretic such as hydrochlorothiazide (Hydrodiuril), the patient's potassium level is 3.2 mEq/L. Which assessment takes priority at this time?
   - A. Blood pressure
   - B. Heart rate and rhythm
   - C. Respiratory rate
   - D. Body temperature
8. A patient is prescribed a daily IV dose of furosemide (Lasix). To ensure the safety of the patient, what action do you take before and after administering this drug?
   - A. Ensure that the IV flow rate is set for at least 125 mL/hr.
   - B. Check to be sure that the serum potassium level is 5 or higher.
   - C. Assess the IV site for patency.
   - D. Instruct the patient to call for help before getting out of bed.
9. A 50-year-old patient prescribed furosemide (Lasix) is preparing for discharge. Which teaching points will you include with discharge teaching? (Select all that apply.)
   - A. Urine output can increase dramatically.
   - B. There is no need to limit alcohol intake.
   - C. You may develop skin sensitivity, so wear protective clothing and stay out of direct sunlight.
   - D. Avoid potassium-rich foods such as bananas, avocadoes, and dried apricots.
   - E. Report any decrease in hearing or ringing in the ears.
   - F. This drug can cause you to have a very high blood potassium level.

10. A patient prescribed oxybutynin (Ditropan) asks you why his mouth and eyes are dry. What is your best response?
    A. "These are common side effects of drugs used to treat overactive bladder (OAB)."
    B. "I will notify your prescriber because you may need to be prescribed a different drug."
    C. "These are signs of an allergic reaction and you must avoid taking this drug again."
    D. "Let me check your vital signs and then I will notify your prescriber."

11. What must you teach an older adult being discharged with a prescription for a loop diuretic? (Select all that apply.)
    A. "Be sure to get up slowly."
    B. "You are at less risk for falls with these drugs than with thiazide diuretics."
    C. "Be sure to eat foods that are rich in potassium, like broccoli and bananas."
    D. "If you experience any new muscle weakness, make sure to report it to your prescriber."
    E. "You may need to set the volume of your radio or television at a higher level."
    F. "If you are to take the drug once a day, be sure to take it in the evening before bedtime."

12. A patient is to be given furosemide (Lasix) 80-mg IV push. The drug comes in a 10-mL vial with a concentration of 10 mg/mL. How many milliliters will be drawn up in a syringe to give this patient? _____ mL

13. A patient is prescribed hydrochlorothiazide (Microzide) 50 mg daily. The drug comes in 25-mg tablets. How many tablets will you teach the patient to take for each dose?
    _____ tablets

14. A patient with overactive bladder is prescribed darifenacin (Enablex) 15 mg once daily. The drug is available as 7.5-mg tablets. How many tablets will you give for each dose?
    _____ tablets

Critical Thinking Activities

See the Answer Keys—Critical Thinking Activities for answers to these activities.

Mrs. Smith is a 36-year-old woman with newly diagnosed hypertension. She is prescribed metolazone (Zaroxolyn) 2.5 mg daily. She tells you that she was recently married and wants to start a family within the next 2 years.

1. Which side effects will you teach the patient to report to the prescriber?
2. What precautions will you stress with regard to this drug and a potential pregnancy?
3. What dietary teaching will you provide associated with this drug?
4. When should you teach Mrs. Smith to take this drug and why?

Objectives

After studying this chapter you should be able to:

1. Explain how antihypertensive drugs lower blood pressure.
2. List the common names, actions, usual adult dosages, possible side effects, and adverse effects of angiotensin-converting enzyme (ACE) inhibitors and angiotensin II receptor blockers (ARBs).
3. Describe what to do before and after giving ACE inhibitors and angiotensin II receptor blockers.
4. Explain what to teach patients taking ACE inhibitors and angiotensin II receptor blockers, including what to do, what not to do, and when to call the prescriber.
5. List the common names, actions, usual adult dosages, possible side effects, and adverse effects for calcium channel blockers, beta blockers, alpha blockers, alpha-beta blockers, central-acting adrenergic drugs, and direct vasodilators.
6. Describe what to do before and after giving calcium channel blockers, beta blockers, alpha blockers, alpha-beta blockers, central-acting adrenergic drugs, and direct vasodilators.
7. Explain what to teach patients taking calcium channel blockers, beta blockers, alpha blockers, alpha-beta blockers, central-acting adrenergic drugs, and direct vasodilators, including what to do, what not to do, and when to call the prescriber.
8. Describe life span considerations for drugs used to treat hypertension.

Key Terms

ACE inhibitor (ĀS ĭn-HĬB-ĭ-tŭr) (p. 256) A drug that lowers blood pressure; ACE stands for angiotensin-converting enzyme.

alpha blocker (ĂL-fĕ BLŎ-kŭr) (p. 264) A drug that opposes the excitatory effects of norepinephrine released from sympathetic nerve endings at alpha receptors and causes vasodilation and a decrease in blood pressure. Also called alpha-adrenergic blocking agents.

alpha-beta blocker (ĂL-fĕ BĀ-tĕ BLŎ-kŭr) (p. 265) Drugs that combine the effects of alpha blockers and beta blockers.

angiotensin II receptor blocker (ăn-jē-ō-TĔN-sĭn TŪ rĕ-SĔP-tŭr BLŎ-kŭr) (p. 259) Angiotensin II receptor blockers (ARBs), also called angiotensin II receptor antagonists, are a group of drugs that modulate the renin-angiotensin-aldosterone system and lower blood pressure.

antihypertensive (ăn-tē-hī-pŭr-TĔN-sĭv) (p. 253) A substance or drug that lowers blood pressure.

beta blocker (beta adrenergic blocker) (BĀ-tĕ BLŎ-kŭr [BĀ-tĕ ăd-rĕn-ŬR-jĭk BLŎ-kŭr]) (p. 262) A drug that limits the activity of epinephrine (a hormone that increases blood pressure); beta blockers reduce the heart rate and the force of muscle contraction, thereby reducing the oxygen demand of the heart muscle.

calcium channel blocker (KĂL-sē-ŭm CHĂ-nĕl BLŎ-kŭr) (p. 260) A drug that slows the movement of calcium into the cells of the heart and blood vessels, relaxing blood vessels and reducing the workload of the heart.

central-acting adrenergic agents (SĔN-trŭl ĂK-tĭng ăd-rĕn-ŬR-jĭk Ā-jĕnts) (p. 267) Drugs that lower blood pressure by stimulating alpha receptors in the brain, which open peripheral arteries and ease blood flow.

diastolic blood pressure (dī-ĕ-STŎL-ĭk BLŪD PRĔSH-ŭr) (p. 253) Blood pressure when the heart is resting between beats.

direct vasodilators (dī-RĔKT văz-ō-DĪ-lā-tŭrz) (p. 268) Drugs that act directly on the smooth muscle of small arteries, causing these arteries to expand (dilate).

diuretic (dī-ŭr-ĔT-ĭk) (p. 256) See Chapter 15.

hypertension (hī-pŭr-TĔN-shŭn) (p. 253) Arterial disease in which chronic high blood pressure is the primary symptom. Abnormally elevated blood pressure.

hypertensive crisis (hī-pŭr-TĔN-sĭv KRĪ-sĭs) (p. 253) Dangerously high and life-threatening blood pressure of acute onset.

primary (essential) hypertension (PRĪ-mär-ē ĕs-SĔN-chŭl hī-pŭr-TĔN-shŭn) (p. 254) Hypertension for which there is no known cause but that is associated with risk factors; 85% to 90% of cases of hypertension are of this type.

secondary hypertension (SĔK-ŭn-dār-ē hī-pŭr-TĔN-shŭn) (p. 254) Hypertension caused by specific disease states and drugs.

systolic blood pressure (sĭs-STŎL-ĭk BLŪD PRĔSH-ŭr) (p. 253) Blood pressure when the heart contracts.

Table **16-1**   American Heart Association Blood Pressure Categories

BLOOD PRESSURE CATEGORY	SYSTOLIC (mm Hg)*	DIASTOLIC (mm Hg)*
Normal	Less than 120 mm Hg	Less than 80 mm Hg
Prehypertension	120-139 mm Hg	80-89 mm Hg
Stage 1 hypertension	140-159 mm Hg	90-99 mm Hg
Stage 2 hypertension	160 mm/Hg or higher	100 mm Hg or higher
Hypertensive Crisis Emergency Care Needed	Higher than 180 mm Hg	Higher than 110 mm Hg

Blood Pressure Categories defined by the American Heart Association, May 2014 (http://www.heart.org/HEARTORG/Conditions/HighBloodPressure/AboutHighBloodPressure/Understanding-Blood-Pressure-Readings_UCM_301764_Article.jsp. Reprinted with permission © 2015, American Heart Association, Inc.)
*Systolic blood pressure is the upper number; diastolic is the lower number.

Box **16-1**   Lifestyle Changes for Treating Hypertension

- Decrease salt (sodium) intake
- Decrease fat intake
- Lose weight
- Exercise regularly
- Quit smoking
- Decrease alcohol intake (not more than two alcohol drinks per day)
- Decrease and manage stress

OVERVIEW

Everyone's blood pressure goes up and down during a 24-hour period. Blood pressure goes up when you are active and down when you are resting or sleeping. Blood pressure is the force of blood pushing against the walls of the arteries as the blood flows through them. Low blood pressure is called *hypotension*. When blood pressure remains abnormally high, it is called **hypertension**. Often people are unaware of having high blood pressure because there are no specific symptoms. Sudden, dangerously high, and life-threatening blood pressure is called **hypertensive crisis**.

A sphygmomanometer and stethoscope are used to measure blood pressure. In some settings automatic blood pressure monitoring machines are used. Blood pressure measurements include two numbers. The higher number is called the **systolic blood pressure**. It represents pressure of blood against the artery walls when the heart contracts. The lower number is called the **diastolic blood pressure**. It represents pressure of blood against the artery walls when the heart relaxes.

As people age, they are more likely to develop hypertension. *Hypertension* is defined by the American Heart Association as a systolic blood pressure (SBP) of 140 to 159 mm Hg and/or a diastolic blood pressure (DBP) of 90 to 99 mm Hg. There are five classifications for blood pressure: normal, prehypertension, stage 1 hypertension, stage 2 hypertension, and hypertensive crisis (Table 16-1). According to the Centers for Disease Control and Prevention (CDC), in the United States alone, there are around 67 million people (one in every three adults) with hypertension.

Several risk factors have been associated with developing high blood pressure. Some, such as smoking, being overweight, and being physically inactive can be changed. Others, such as age, gender, family history, and race cannot be changed. Yet other risk factors (for example, diabetes and hyperlipidemia) can be controlled with drugs. Use of oral contraceptives (birth control pills) increases the risk for hypertension in younger women, whereas being postmenopausal increases the risk for older women. Treatment of hypertension includes lifestyle changes (Box 16-1) and drugs that lower blood pressure (**antihypertensives**).

REVIEW OF RELATED PHYSIOLOGY AND PATHOPHYSIOLOGY

ARTERIOSCLEROSIS AND ATHEROSCLEROSIS

Arteriosclerosis is the hardening of the arterial walls. High blood pressure causes arterial walls to thicken and harden. With *atherosclerosis* plaques are formed inside

Memory Jogger

Hypertension is a systolic blood pressure greater than 140-159 mm Hg and/or a diastolic blood pressure greater than 90 to 99 mm Hg.

Clinical Pitfall

When hypertension is not treated, the following health problems may result:
- Arteriosclerosis (atherosclerosis)
- Heart attack (myocardial infarction)
- Stroke (cerebrovascular accident, brain attack)
- Enlarged heart (cardiomyopathy)
- Kidney damage (may lead to end-stage kidney disease)
- Blindness

QSEN: Safety

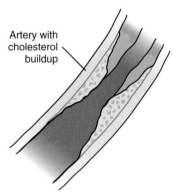

Artery with
cholesterol
buildup

FIGURE 16-1 Atherosclerosis.

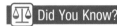

Did You Know?

About 25% of patients who are on kidney dialysis have kidney failure that was caused by hypertension.

Memory Jogger

The 2 main types of hypertension are primary (essential) and secondary.

the walls of arteries (Figure 16-1). As arterial walls harden and thicken, the arteries become narrow. Narrowed arteries decrease blood flow so body organs and tissues may not receive enough blood. Narrowed arteries can also result in the formation of clots that block the flow of blood. Reduced or blocked blood flow to the heart can cause a heart attack, whereas reduced or blocked blood flow to the brain can cause a stroke.

High blood pressure also makes the heart work much harder to pump blood to the lungs and body. Over time the extra work can cause the heart muscle to thicken and stretch. This can lead to an enlarged heart (*cardiomyopathy*) and heart failure.

High blood pressure can affect the ability of the kidneys to remove body wastes from the blood by hardening, thickening, and narrowing the arteries to the kidneys. This causes less blood flow to the kidneys and less filtering of waste products, which then build up in the blood. As kidney function becomes worse, kidney failure, including end-stage kidney disease (ESKD), can occur. When the kidneys fail, a patient needs either dialysis or a kidney transplant.

The two main types of hypertension are primary (essential) hypertension and secondary hypertension. *Primary hypertension* has no known cause. *Secondary hypertension* is caused by other diseases and drugs that raise blood pressure.

PRIMARY (ESSENTIAL) HYPERTENSION

Primary hypertension is the most common form of high blood pressure, accounting for 85% to 90% of cases. Although it has no known cause, it is associated with certain risk factors (Table 16-2). A contributing factor may be the changes that occur in the arteries as people age. With increasing age blood pressure rises, large arteries become stiffer, and smaller arteries may become partly blocked. Examples of other factors that play a part in developing high blood pressure include smoking, an unhealthy diet (too much fat, salt, and alcohol), stress, obesity, and changes in the kidneys.

SECONDARY HYPERTENSION

Secondary hypertension, the less common form of high blood pressure, is the result of other health problems or drugs. Examples of disorders that can cause this type of hypertension include partial blockages of the arteries to the kidneys (atherosclerosis)

Table 16-2	Causes of Hypertension	
TYPE OF HYPERTENSION	**CAUSES**	
Primary (essential) hypertension	Cause is unknown Associated risk factors: 　Family history 　High sodium intake 　High calorie intake 　Physical inactivity 　Excessive alcohol intake 　Low potassium intake	
Secondary hypertension	Specific diseases: 　Renal vascular disease 　Primary aldosteronism 　Pheochromocytoma 　Cushing's disease 　Coarctation of the aorta 　Brain tumors 　Encephalitis 　Psychiatric disturbances 　Pregnancy 　Sleep apnea	Medications: 　Estrogen (oral contraceptives) 　Glucocorticoids 　Mineralocorticoids 　Sympathomimetics

From Ignatavicius, D., & Workman L. (2013): *Medical-surgical nursing: Patient-centered collaborative care,* 7th edition, 2013, Elsevier.

and diseases that damage the kidneys such as infections and diabetes. Tumors of the adrenal glands, which sit on top of the kidneys, and sleep apnea may cause secondary hypertension (see Table 16-2).

Drugs that cause secondary hypertension include nonsteroidal anti-inflammatory drugs (NSAIDs) and corticosteroids. Other drugs that may result in high blood pressure include over-the-counter allergy and cold drugs that contain phenylephrine. Drugs that contain pseudoephedrine also cause elevated blood pressure. They do not require a prescription but are kept behind the counter at pharmacies and require photo identification and a signature for purchase due to the Combat Methamphetamine Act.

GENERAL ISSUES FOR ANTIHYPERTENSIVE THERAPY

Antihypertensive drugs are prescribed to control and manage high blood pressure. Awareness and treatment of hypertension are very important because, when left untreated, it can cause diseases that damage the heart and arteries, kidneys, and brain. Untreated hypertension also decreases life expectancy in adults. Treating the cause of secondary hypertension can cure the problem. Managing primary hypertension is a lifelong process and usually requires that patients continue with lifestyle changes and drugs for the rest of their lives.

In addition to the practices listed for drug administration in Chapter 2, general responsibilities for safe administration of antihypertensive drugs are listed in the following paragraphs. Specific responsibilities are discussed with each individual class of drugs.

Responsibilities before administering any antihypertensive drug include always getting a complete list of drugs that the patient is currently using, including herbal and over-the-counter drugs.

Obtain a baseline set of vital signs. If the patient's blood pressure is low (less than 90/60 mm Hg) or the heart rate is low (less than 60 beats per minute), notify the prescriber and ask if the patient should receive the drug. Ask the patient about signs and symptoms such as dizziness, light-headedness, or headaches.

Ask women of childbearing years if they are pregnant, planning to become pregnant, or breastfeeding because some of these drugs can harm the fetus directly or reduce blood pressure in the fetus.

Responsibilities after administering any antihypertensive drug include rechecking and continuing to monitor the patient's vital signs every 4 to 8 hours. Ask the patient about dizziness or light-headedness because these are signs of hypotension. If these symptoms occur, check the patient's blood pressure and heart rate while lying down, sitting, and standing (orthostatic vital signs). Notify the prescriber of positive orthostatic vital signs. *Orthostatic hypotension* is said to occur if, within 3 minutes of standing, systolic pressure drops by at least 20 mm Hg, diastolic pressure drops by at least 10 mm Hg, or heart rate increases more than 20 beats per minute. Instruct the patient to call for help when getting out of bed and make sure the call light is within easy reach. Help the patient change positions slowly.

Teach patients taking an antihypertensive drug the proper techniques for checking their blood pressure and heart rates. Tell them to keep a daily record. Remind patients about the symptoms of hypotension and tell them to change positions slowly. Patients experiencing these symptoms should be instructed not to drive, operate machines, or do anything that is dangerous until they know how the drug will affect them.

Instruct patients to keep all follow-up appointments with their prescriber to monitor blood pressure and side effects of antihypertensive drugs. Tell them to take all prescribed doses as directed. If a dose is missed and the next dose is not due for more than 4 hours, instruct patients to take the dose as soon as possible. If the next dose is due in less than 4 hours, tell patients to skip the missed dose and return to the regular dosing schedule. Remind patients never to take double doses of antihypertensive drugs.

Clinical Pitfall

A patient with high blood pressure should not take over-the-counter allergy and cold drugs that contain phenylephrine.

QSEN: Safety

Memory Jogger

Orthostatic hypotension criteria:
- Decreased SBP of 20 mm Hg or more
- Decreased DBP of 10 mm Hg or more
- Increased heart rate of 20 beats per minute or more

Drug Alert!

Teaching Alert

Teach patients to take missed doses as soon as possible; but if it is almost time for the next dose, skip the missed dose and return to the regular dosing schedule.

QSEN: Safety

Drug Alert!

Administration Alert

Patients with hypertension should not take over-the-counter drugs (such as drugs for appetite control, asthma, colds, and hay fever) without asking their prescriber.

QSEN: Safety

Did You Know?

Antihypertensive drugs will help control but will not cure hypertension. Patients may need to take these drugs for the rest of their lives.

Remind patients to notify the prescriber for any signs of hypotension or chest pain. Tell them to consult with their prescriber before taking over-the-counter drugs.

Discuss with patients lifestyle changes that will help manage hypertension including weight loss, exercise, stress reduction, smoking cessation, and a low-salt, low-fat diet.

Remind patients that these drugs will help to control, *not* cure, high blood pressure and that they may take these drugs for the rest of their lives. Stress the importance of controlling high blood pressure to prevent other serious health problems such as heart failure, kidney disease, and vascular diseases.

Instruct patients taking antihypertensive drugs to obtain and wear a medical alert bracelet that states the drug, dose, and diagnosis.

TYPES OF ANTIHYPERTENSIVE DRUGS

Several types of drugs are used to control hypertension. They may be used alone or in combination with other drugs. Antihypertensive drugs have several classes:

- **Diuretics**—drugs that eliminate excess water and salt from the body (see Chapter 15).
- **Angiotensin-converting enzyme (ACE) inhibitors**—drugs that lower blood pressure. For people with diabetes, especially those with protein (albumin) in their urine, ACE inhibitors also help slow kidney damage.
- **Angiotensin II receptor blockers (ARBs)**—drugs that change the action of the renin-angiotensin-aldosterone system. These drugs block the activation of angiotensin II type 1 receptors. Angiotensin II receptor blockers are mainly used in the treatment of hypertension when the patient is intolerant of ACE inhibitor therapy. These drugs are also called *angiotensin receptor antagonists.*
- **Calcium channel blockers**—drugs that slow the movement of calcium into the cells of the heart and blood vessels. This in turn relaxes the blood vessels, increases the supply of oxygen-rich blood to the heart, and reduces the work-load of the heart.
- **Beta blockers** (beta-adrenergic blockers)—drugs that limit the activity of epi-nephrine (a hormone that increases blood pressure). Beta blockers reduce the heart rate and force of contraction, leading to decreased oxygen demand by the heart muscle.
- **Alpha blockers**—drugs that oppose the excitatory effects of norepinephrine released from sympathetic nerve endings at alpha receptors and cause blood vessel relaxation and vasodilation, leading to a decrease in blood pressure. These drugs are also called alpha-adrenergic blocking agents.
- **Alpha-beta blockers**—drugs that combine the effects of alpha and beta blockers.
- **Central-acting adrenergic agents**—drugs that lower blood pressure by stimulat-ing alpha receptors in the brain, which widen (dilate) peripheral arteries and ease blood flow. Central-acting adrenergic agents such as clonidine are usually pre-scribed when all other antihypertensive medications have failed. For treating hypertension, these drugs are usually administered in combination with a diuretic.
- **Direct vasodilators**—drugs that act directly on the smooth muscle of small arteries, causing these arteries to expand (dilate).

DIURETICS

Diuretics control blood pressure by eliminating excess salt and water from the body. Those most commonly used include loop, thiazide, and potassium-sparing diuretics. See Chapter 15 for additional information on diuretic drugs.

ANGIOTENSIN-CONVERTING ENZYME (ACE) INHIBITORS

How ACE Inhibitors Work

ACE inhibitors block production of substances that constrict (narrow) blood vessels. They also help decrease the buildup of water and salt in the blood and body tissues.

The exact way that these drugs work is not known. They block an enzyme in the body that is necessary for production of angiotensin II (a substance that causes blood vessels to tighten or constrict). The result is that blood vessels relax and blood pressure is decreased. This also decreases heart workload and increases the blood flow and oxygen to the heart and other organs.

These drugs are often given to patients with health problems such as heart failure, kidney disease, and diabetes. ACE inhibitors are often prescribed *along with* diuretics to control hypertension, and combined ACE inhibitor/diuretic drug forms are available. For example, lisinopril/hydrochlorothiazide (Prinzide, Zestoretic) is often prescribed for the management of hypertension; lisinopril is an ACE inhibitor, and hydrochlorothiazide is a diuretic.

Usually the first doses of an ACE inhibitor are lower when the patient is also taking a diuretic or has renal (kidney) impairment. Be sure to consult a drug reference book for information on any specific ACE inhibitor.

Dosages for Common ACE Inhibitors

Drug	Dosage
captopril (Capoten, Novo-Captopril ♣)	*Adults:* 12.5-50 mg orally 2-3 times daily
enalapril (Vasotec)	*Adults:* 2.5-40 mg orally daily as single dose or 2 divided doses
lisinopril (Prinivil, Zestril)	*Adults:* 10-40 mg orally once daily
perindopril (Aceon)	*Adults:* 4-16 mg orally daily as single dose or 2 divided doses
quinapril (Accupril)	*Adults:* 10-80 mg orally daily as single dose or 2 divided doses
ramipril (Altace)	*Adults:* 2.5-20 mg orally once daily as single dose or 2 divided doses
trandolapril (Mavik)	*Adults:* 1-4 mg orally once daily; in African-American patients begin with 2 mg daily
benazepril (Lotensin)	*Adults:* 20-40 mg orally once daily as a single dose or in 2 divided doses
fosinopril (Monopril)	*Adults:* 20-40 mg orally once daily as a single dose or in 2 divided doses

Intended Responses
- Production of angiotensin II is decreased.
- Vasodilation of blood vessels is increased.
- Excess tissue water and salt are decreased.
- Blood pressure is lowered.
- Workload on the heart is decreased.

Side Effects. The more common side effects of ACE inhibitors include hypotension; protein in the urine; taste disturbances; increased blood potassium level (*hyperkalemia*); headache; and persistent, dry cough. If one ACE inhibitor causes a cough, it is likely that others will as well, and the patient will need to be prescribed another type of antihypertensive drug.

Adverse Effects. Adverse effects include fever and chills; hoarseness; swelling in the face, hands, or feet; trouble swallowing or breathing; stomach pain; chest pain; rashes and itching skin; and yellow eyes or skin. Some patients also develop dizziness, light-headedness, or fainting.

Allergic reactions and kidney failure are serious but rare adverse effects with ACE inhibitors.

 Memory Jogger

The generic names for ACE inhibitors end in "-pril" (for example, enalapril).

 Do Not Confuse

Accupril *with* Aciphex

An order for Accupril may be confused with Aciphex. Accupril is an ACE inhibitor, whereas Aciphex is a proton pump inhibitor used for healing gastrointestinal ulcers.

QSEN: Safety

 Do Not Confuse

Zestril *with* Zetia

An order for Zestril may be confused with Zetia. Zestril is an ACE inhibitor, whereas Zetia is a cholesterol-lowering drug.

QSEN: Safety

 Do Not Confuse

Benazepril *with* Benadryl

An order for benazepril may be confused with Benadryl. Benazepril is an ACE inhibitor, whereas Benadryl is an antihistamine.

QSEN: Safety

Common Side Effects

ACE Inhibitors

 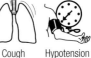

Cough   Hypotension   Taste disturbances

Hyperkalemia   Headache

 Drug Alert!

Administration Alert

If a patient taking an ACE inhibitor develops a persistent, dry cough, the prescriber should be notified, and the drug discontinued.

QSEN: Safety

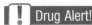

Drug Alert!

Action/Intervention Alert

Monitor patients for angioedema, which is a serious adverse effect of ACE inhibitors.

QSEN: Safety

Drug Alert!

Interaction Alert

ACE inhibitors may increase the effect of decreased blood pressure in patients who are also taking diuretics. ACE inhibitors and potassium-sparing diuretics cause much higher increases in blood potassium levels.

QSEN: Safety

Drug Alert!

Teaching Alert

Tell patients who are taking ACE inhibitors that drinking alcohol can increase the low blood pressure effect and the risk for dizziness or fainting.

QSEN: Safety

Angioedema. Angioedema is a diffuse swelling of the eyes, lips, and tongue (see Figure 1-6). It may occur with allergic reactions to these drugs and may be life threatening. Swelling of the trachea (windpipe/airway) can interfere with breathing, a life-threatening event. Angioedema can occur months or even years after ACE inhibitor therapy is started.

Neutropenia (decreased leukocytes in the blood) may occur, increasing the risk for infections. Infections may develop in the throat, intestinal tract, other mucous membranes, or the skin. Symptoms of neutropenia include any signs of infection such as chills, fever, or sore throat.

Some ACE inhibitors (for example, enalapril, quinapril, and ramipril) cause increased sun sensitivity (photosensitivity).

What To Do *Before* Giving ACE Inhibitors

In addition to the general responsibilities related to antihypertensive therapy (p. 255), ask about any allergies to drugs, foods, preservatives, or dyes because more people develop allergies with ACE inhibitors than with any other drugs for blood pressure. Ask patients if they are also taking diuretics to control blood pressure because ACE inhibitors enhance the blood pressure–lowering effects of diuretics.

What To Do *After* Giving ACE Inhibitors

In addition to the general responsibilities related to antihypertensive therapy (p. 255), check patients' blood potassium levels because these drugs reduce the excretion of potassium. This is even more important if the patient is also prescribed a potassium-sparing diuretic. Keep track of urine output and weight. Kidney failure is a rare but serious adverse effect of these drugs.

Check for any signs or symptoms of allergic reactions or infections.

What To *Teach* Patients About ACE Inhibitors

In addition to the general precautions related to antihypertensive therapy (pp. 255-256), tell patients to take this drug at the same time every day. Captopril (Capoten) should be taken 1 hour before eating or on an empty stomach.

Tell patients not to drink alcohol until they talk with their prescriber because ACE inhibitors can increase the low blood pressure effect and the risk for dizziness or fainting.

Teach patients to avoid salt substitutes. Salt substitutes contain potassium, and a side effect of ACE inhibitors is increased blood potassium level (hyperkalemia).

Instruct patients to report any side effects of ACE inhibitors to their prescriber. Tell patients to go to the emergency room immediately to report any facial swelling because this is a sign of angioedema, a life-threatening adverse reaction. Remind patients that angioedema can occur even months to years after beginning to take these drugs.

Teach patients taking enalapril (Vasotec), quinapril (Accupril), or ramipril (Altace) to limit direct sunlight, wear protective clothing, and use sunscreens because sun sensitivity (photosensitivity) is a side effect of these drugs.

Life Span Considerations for ACE Inhibitors

Pediatric Considerations. Children are more sensitive to the effects of ACE inhibitors for blood pressure. They are at higher risk of having severe side effects from the drugs. Before giving these drugs to children, parents should discuss the benefits and risks with their pediatric cardiologist.

Considerations for Pregnancy and Lactation. ACE inhibitors have a high likelihood of increasing the risk for birth defects or fetal damage. They are not prescribed for women who are pregnant or are thinking about becoming pregnant. Lisinopril has a moderate likelihood of increasing the risk for birth defects or fetal damage during the first trimester and a high likelihood of increasing the risk for birth defects or fetal damage during the second and third trimesters. These drugs pass into breast milk and should not be used while breastfeeding because they can lower blood pressure and lead to kidney damage in the infant.

Considerations for Older Adults. Older adults are at greater risk for postural hypotension when taking ACE inhibitors because of the cardiovascular changes associated with aging. Teach patients to not stand or sit up quickly because this may lower blood pressure rapidly, causing dizziness and an increased risk for falls. Also instruct them to hold on to railings when going up or down steps.

ANGIOTENSIN II RECEPTOR BLOCKERS (ARBs)

How ARBs Work

Angiotensin II receptor blockers (ARBs) block the effects of angiotensin II (vasoconstriction, sodium and water retention) by directly blocking the binding of angiotensin II to angiotensin II type 1 receptors.

These drugs may be given in combination with diuretics. Losartan combined with the thiazide diuretic hydrochlorothiazide (Hyzaar) is often prescribed to control high blood pressure. Lower doses of ARBs are used when a patient is taking a diuretic or has renal (kidney) or hepatic (liver) impairment. These drugs are inactivated by the liver and excreted from the body by the kidney. Patients who have impairment of either of these organs may have higher blood levels of the drugs and are at greater risk for side effects or adverse effects. Be sure to consult a drug reference book for additional information on any angiotensin II receptor blocker.

Dosages for Common Angiotensin-II Receptor Blockers

Drug	Dosage
losartan (Cozaar)	*Adults:* 25-100 mg orally daily as a single dose or in 2 divided doses
valsartan (Diovan)	*Adults:* 80-320 mg orally once daily
irbesartan (Avapro)	*Adults:* 150-300 mg orally once daily
candesartan (Atacand)	*Adults:* 16-32 mg orally once daily
telmisartan (Micardis)	*Adults:* 20-80 mg orally once daily
eprosartan (Teveten)	*Adults:* 400-800 mg orally once daily or in 2 divided doses
olmesartan (Benicar)	*Adults:* 20-40 mg orally once daily

Intended Responses
- Vasodilation of blood vessels is increased.
- Excess body water and salt are decreased.
- Blood pressure is lowered.
- Workload on the heart is decreased.

Side Effects. There are few documented side effects from ARBs. Side effects include dizziness, fatigue, headache, hypotension, diarrhea, and high blood potassium levels (hyperkalemia).

Adverse Effects. Adverse effects are rare but include kidney failure and life-threatening angioedema (swelling of the face, eyes, lips, tongue, and trachea that can interfere with breathing) (see Figure 1-6).

An additional rare adverse effect is liver toxicity or drug-induced hepatitis. These drugs should not be given to patients who have known liver problems.

What To Do *Before* Giving ARBs

In addition to the general responsibilities related to antihypertensive therapy (p. 255), check blood urea nitrogen (BUN) and creatinine levels for preexisting kidney disease

 Clinical Pitfall

ACE inhibitors should not be prescribed for women who are pregnant. They can cause low blood pressure, severe kidney failure, increased potassium, and even death in a newborn when used after the first trimester of pregnancy.

QSEN: Safety

 Memory Jogger

The generic names for ARBs end in "-sartan" (for example, valsartan, losartan, candesartan).

 Do Not Confuse

Cozaar *with* Colace or Zocor

An order for Cozaar may be confused with Colace or Zocor. Cozaar is an angiotensin II receptor blocker used to decrease blood pressure. Colace is a stool softener, and Zocor is a drug used to decrease blood lipids (fats).

QSEN: Safety

Do Not Confuse

Benicar *with* Mevacor

An order for Benicar may be confused with Mevacor. Benicar is an ARB used to treat hypertension, and Mevacor (lovastatin) is a cholesterol-lowering drug.

QSEN: Safety

Common Side Effects

Angiotensin II Receptor Blockers

Dizziness   Headache   Hypotension

Diarrhea   Hyperkalemia

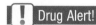

Drug Alert!

Action Alert

Report any swelling of the face, eyes, lips, or tongue to the prescriber immediately. These are signs of life-threatening angioedema. Do not administer the drug to the patient again because this is a life-threatening adverse reaction.

QSEN: Safety

Do Not Confuse

niCARdipine *with* NIFEdipine

An order for niCARdipine may be confused with NIFEdipine. Both are calcium channel blockers.

QSEN: Safety

Do Not Confuse

Norvasc *with* Navane

An order for Norvasc may be confused with Navane. Norvasc is a calcium channel blocker, whereas Navane is an antipsychotic drug used for schizophrenia and other psychotic disorders.

QSEN: Safety

because these drugs are excreted by the kidneys. Ask whether the patient has any kidney or liver problems because these drugs can worsen liver disease.

What To Do *After* Giving ARBs

In addition to the general responsibilities related to antihypertensive therapy (p. 255), look for any swelling of the face, including the eyes, lips, or tongue (signs of angioedema). Report this immediately to the prescriber. Do not administer the drug to the patient again because this is a life-threatening adverse reaction. Check the urine output and weight. Report decreased urine output or weight gain to the prescriber.

Check laboratory values for any changes in the blood potassium level because these drugs reduce potassium excretion by the kidneys. If the potassium level is higher than 5.5 mEq/L, notify the prescriber. Assess heart rate and rhythm, especially for a slow rate. If the patient has a heart monitor, assess for an increasing height of T waves—a sign of high potassium level. Check bowel sounds every shift. Increased bowel sounds and diarrhea are associated with high potassium levels.

What To *Teach* Patients About ARBs

In addition to the general precautions related to antihypertensive therapy (pp. 255-256), remind patients to get up slowly to prevent dizziness and falls. Alcohol use, standing for long periods, exercise, and hot weather may contribute to hypotension.

Instruct female patients to talk with their prescriber if they are taking an angiotensin II receptor blocker and plan to become pregnant. These drugs can cause harm to the fetus.

Tell patients to go to the emergency department immediately to report any facial swelling because this is a sign of angioedema, a life-threatening adverse reaction. Remind them that angioedema can occur months to years after beginning to take these drugs. Teach them that if this happens, they should avoid taking this drug ever again.

Life Span Considerations for ARBs

Pediatric Considerations. Safe use of these drugs in children under the age of 18 has not been researched or established.

Considerations for Pregnancy and Lactation. Angiotensin II receptor blockers have a moderate likelihood of increasing the risk for birth defects or fetal damage during the first trimester and a high likelihood during the second and third trimesters. They should not be taken during the second or third trimesters of pregnancy. Valsartan (Diovan) has a high likelihood of increasing the risk for birth defects or fetal damage during all trimesters. These drugs can interfere with fetal blood pressure control and kidney function. They have been associated with problems in fetal kidney and skull development. It is not known if they pass into breast milk; however, a woman who plans to breastfeed should not use these drugs because there is not enough evidence that infants will be safe when a mother is breastfeeding while taking ARBs.

CALCIUM CHANNEL BLOCKERS

How Calcium Channel Blockers Work

Calcium channel blockers block calcium from entering the muscle cells of the heart and arteries. Blocking calcium causes a decrease in the contraction of the heart and also dilates (widens) the arteries. Widening the arteries causes a decrease in blood pressure and reduces the workload of the heart.

When these drugs are prescribed for older patients or patients with hepatic (liver) or renal (kidney) impairment, initial lower doses are used. Amlodipine (Norvasc) may be combined with atorvastatin (Caduet), with an ACE inhibitor (Lotrel), or with an ARB (Exforge). Be sure to consult a drug reference book for information on any calcium channel blocker drug.

Dosages for Common Calcium Channel Blockers

Drug	Dosage
amlodipine (Norvasc)	*Adults:* 2.5-10 mg orally once daily
diltiazem (Cardizem)	*Adults:* 30-120 mg orally 3-4 times daily, or 60-120 mg twice daily as SR capsules, or 180-240 mg once daily as XR/CD capsules; do not exceed 360 mg/day IV: 0.25 mg/kg; may repeat after 15 min with dose of 0.35 mg/kg IV infusion: 5-15 mg/hr
felodipine (Plendil)	*Adults:* 2.5-10 mg orally daily
niCARdipine (Cardene)	*Adults:* 20 mg orally 3 times daily. May be given as 30-60 mg twice daily as SR capsules IV infusion: 5-15 mg/hr
NIFEdipine (Adalat, Novo-Nifedin ♣, Nu-Nifedin ♣, Procardia, Procardia XL)	*Adults:* 10-30/mg orally 3 times daily, do not exceed 180 mg daily; XL—initially 30-60 mg daily, titrate upward as necessary and do not exceed 90 mg daily *Note: Do **not** give immediate-release capsules sublingually*
verapamil (Calan, Isoptin, NovoVerapamil ♣, Nu-Verap ♣)	*Adults:* 80-120 mg orally 3 times daily *Children:* 4-8 mg/kg orally daily in 3 divided doses

Intended Responses
- Heart contraction is decreased.
- Artery dilation (widening) is increased.
- Heart workload is decreased.
- Blood pressure is lowered.
- Blood flow and oxygen to the heart are increased.
- Decreased episodes of supraventricular tachycardia.

Side Effects.   The most common side effects of these drugs are constipation, nausea, headache, flushing, rash, edema (legs), hypotension, drowsiness, and dizziness.

Adverse Effects.   Dysrhythmias may occur with calcium channel blockers, including irregular, rapid, pounding, or excessively slow heart rhythms (less than 50 beats per minute).

Patients with heart failure symptoms may worsen with verapamil and diltiazem because of the increased abilities of the drugs to reduce the strength and rate of heart contraction.

Stevens-Johnson syndrome (erythema multiforme) is a potentially lethal skin disorder resulting from an allergic reaction to drugs, infections, or illness. It causes damage to blood vessels of the skin. Symptoms include many different types of skin lesions (see Figure 1-5), itching, fever, joint aching, and generally feeling ill.

Rare but serious adverse effects include difficulty breathing; irregular, rapid, or pounding heart rhythm; slow heart rate (<50 beats per minute); bleeding; chest pain; and vision problems (difficulty seeing).

What To Do *Before* Giving Calcium Channel Blockers
In addition to the general responsibilities related to antihypertensive therapy (p. 255), find out if the patient has any health problems that may be affected by these drugs such as heart failure, blood vessel disease, and liver or kidney disease.

What To Do *After* Giving Calcium Channel Blockers
In addition to the general responsibilities related to antihypertensive therapy (p. 255), report irregular heart rhythms to the prescriber. Watch for side effects or adverse effects of these drugs. If a patient develops skin lesions, itching, fever, and achy joints, report this to the prescriber at once because these are signs of Stevens-Johnson syndrome and allergic reaction to the drug.

Common Side Effects

Calcium Channel Blockers

Hypotension   Constipation;   Headache
                    Nausea

Dizziness   Rash

⚠ Drug Alert!

Action/Intervention Alert

Calcium channel blockers can cause a severe skin disorder called Stevens-Johnson syndrome. Always check the patient for skin lesions, itching, fever, and achy joints.

QSEN: Safety

What To *Teach* Patients About Calcium Channel Blockers

In addition to the general precautions related to antihypertensive therapy (pp. 255-256), remind patients to get up and change positions slowly to decrease dizziness. Explain that exercising in hot weather can cause dizziness and low blood pressure.

Explain that if the patient should suddenly stop taking these drugs after taking them for several weeks, hypertension may return. The prescriber can advise the patient on how to gradually stop taking the drug.

Life Span Considerations for Calcium Channel Blockers

Pediatric Considerations. Safe use of calcium channel blockers in children has not been researched. Before using these drugs with children, parents should discuss risks and benefits with the prescriber.

Considerations for Pregnancy and Lactation. Calcium channel blockers have a moderate likelihood of increasing the risk for birth defects or fetal damage. Their effects have not been tested in human pregnancy. In studies of laboratory animals, birth defects and stillborns have occurred. Women should consult with their prescriber and pediatrician before using these drugs during pregnancy. Some calcium channel blockers pass into breast milk. Women who wish to breastfeed while taking these drugs should discuss this with their prescriber because the effects on the infant will be the same as for the mother who is taking the drug.

Considerations for Older Adults. Older adults may be especially sensitive to the effects of calcium channel blocking agents. This may increase the chance of side effects during treatment. A lower starting dose may be required.

BETA BLOCKERS

How Beta Blockers Work

Beta blockers (beta adrenergic blockers) block the effects of epinephrine (adrenaline) on the heart. They decrease the heart rate and force of heart contractions, which leads to decreased blood pressure. As a result, the heart does not work as hard and requires less oxygen.

Beta blockers are classified as cardioselective and noncardioselective. *Cardioselective* drugs work only on the cardiovascular system. *Noncardioselective* drugs have effects on all of the organs and systems of the body (systemic effects).

When beta blockers are prescribed for a patient with kidney damage, a lower dose of the drug is prescribed, or the time between doses is increased. An older adult may also be started on a lower drug dose. Be sure to consult a drug reference book for information about a specific beta blocker.

Memory Jogger

The generic names of beta blockers end with "-olol" (for example, metoprolol, atenolol).

Do Not Confuse

Inderal *with* Adderall

An order for Inderal may be confused with Adderall. Inderal is a noncardioselective beta blocker, whereas Adderall is a stimulant used for narcolepsy and attention-deficit/hyperactivity disorder in children.

QSEN: Safety

Do Not Confuse

Toprol XL *with* Topamax

An order for Toprol XL may be confused with Topamax. Toprol XL is an extended-release form of metoprolol, a cardioselective beta blocker. Topamax is a central nervous system anticonvulsant.

QSEN: Safety

Dosages for Common Beta Blockers for Hypertension

Drug	Dosage
Acebutolol ❶ (Monitan ✷, Sectral)—selective	*Adults:* 400-1200 mg orally daily in 2 divided doses
atenolol ❶ (Apo-Atenolol ✷, Novo-Atenol ✷, Tenormin)—selective	*Adults:* 25-200 mg orally once daily
betaxolol ❶ (Kerlone)—selective	*Adults:* 10-20 mg orally once daily
bisoprolol ❶ (Zebeta)—selective	*Adults:* 2.5-20 mg orally once daily
labetalol ❶ (Normodyne, Trandate)—nonselective	*Adults:* PO: 100-400 mg orally twice daily *Adults:* IV: 20 mg initially; additional doses of 40-80 mg may be given every 10 min as needed; do not exceed 300 mg total dosage
metoprolol ❶ (Betaloc ✷, Lopresor ✷, Lopressor, Nu-Metop ✷, Toprol XL)—selective	*Adults:* PO: 100-450 mg orally once daily or in 2 divided doses; extended-release forms should be given once daily *Adults:* IV: 5 mg every 2 min for 3 doses followed by oral dosing

Dosages for Common Beta Blockers for Hypertension—cont'd

Drug	Dosage
nadolol ❶ (Corgard)—nonselective	*Adults:* 40-320 mg orally once daily
propranolol ❶ (Detensol ♣, Inderal, NovoPranol ♣)—nonselective	*Adults:* 40-120 mg orally twice daily; extended action form, 80-120 mg once daily *Children:* 0.5-1 mg/kg orally daily in 2-4 divided doses; may increase as needed (usual range 2-4 mg/kg daily in 2 divided doses)
timolol ❶ (Apo-Timol ♣, Blocadren, Novo-Timol ♣)—nonselective	*Adults:* 10-30 mg orally twice daily

❶ High-alert drug.

Intended Responses
- Heart rate is decreased.
- Force of heart contraction is decreased.
- Work of heart is decreased.
- Blood pressure is lowered.

Side Effects. Fairly common side effects of beta blockers include decreased sexual ability, dizziness or light-headedness, drowsiness, trouble sleeping *(insomnia),* and fatigue or weakness.

Less common side effects that must be reported to the prescriber include difficulty breathing or wheezing; cold hands or feet; mental depression; shortness of breath; slow heart rate (less than 50 beats per minute); and swelling in the ankles, feet, or lower legs.

Depression is another side effect that has been associated with taking beta blockers. A patient with a history of depression may notice that it becomes worse while taking these drugs. Beta blockers may also cause depression for the first time.

Adverse Effects. Signs of drug overdose include very slow heart rate, chest pain, severe dizziness or fainting, fast or irregular heart rate, difficulty breathing, bluish-colored fingernails and palms, and seizures. Report these signs and symptoms to the prescriber at once.

Adverse effects may also include "passing out" or falling when changing positions related to orthostatic (postural) hypotension.

Other adverse effects include back or joint pain, dark urine, dizziness or fainting when getting up, fever or sore throat, hallucinations, irregular heart rate, skin rash, unusual bleeding or bruising, and yellow eyes or skin. These drugs can affect the blood glucose level of a patient with diabetes and may cause hypoglycemia or hyperglycemia.

What To Do *Before* Giving Beta Blockers
In addition to the general responsibilities related to antihypertensive therapy (p. 255), check blood glucose levels regularly for patients with diabetes. Beta blockers can mask signs of hypoglycemia such as rapid heart rate, making it difficult to recognize and treat. Ask patients about a history of depression.

What To Do After Giving Beta Blockers
In addition to the general responsibilities related to antihypertensive therapy (p. 255), assess heart rate and if it is less than 60 beats per minute, notify the prescriber. Continue to monitor blood glucose in patients with diabetes because these drugs can mask the signs of hypoglycemia. Watch for signs and symptoms of depression.

What To *Teach* Patients About Beta Blockers
In addition to the general precautions related to antihypertensive therapy (pp. 255-256), teach patients to stand or sit up slowly because these actions may lower blood

---

Common Side Effects

Beta Blockers

| Impotence | Dizziness | Insomnia, Lethargy, Drowsiness, Fatigue |

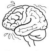

Depression

---

❶ **Drug Alert!**

Action/Intervention Alert

Beta blockers can decrease or increase blood glucose levels. Be sure to check blood glucose regularly in a patient with diabetes.

QSEN: Safety

Teaching Alert

Patients should never suddenly stop taking beta blockers. This may cause unpleasant and harmful effects such as increased risk for heart attack.

QSEN: Safety

Did You Know?

Beta blockers can affect the results of medical tests such as tests that raise heart rate and blood pressure.

Teaching Alert

Teach patients that beta blockers can cause new-onset depression or worsen existing depression.

QSEN: Safety

Monitoring Alert

Monitor older adults who have been prescribed beta blockers for mental confusion or changes in level of consciousness.

QSEN: Safety

pressure rapidly, causing dizziness and an increased risk for falls. Also instruct them to hold on to railings when going up or down steps.

Remind patients to check with the prescriber before stopping a beta blocker. It may be necessary to gradually decrease the daily dose of the drug. Suddenly stopping beta blockers can increase the risk of a heart attack.

Have patients notify their prescriber for any weight gain or increase in shortness of breath. These are signs of worsening heart failure.

Tell patients to always inform health care providers that they are taking a beta blocker before any form of surgical or emergency treatment. Remind patients to inform health care providers about beta blocker use before medical tests and allergy shots. These drugs can affect the results of medical tests and can cause serious reactions with allergy shots.

Tell patients that any chest pain experienced during activity should be reported to their prescriber so safe activity levels may be discussed.

Beta blockers can cause increased sensitivity to sunlight and cold. Tell patients to stay out of direct sunlight, use a sun block skin protector, and wear protective clothing. Advise patients to dress warmly during cold weather because decreased blood flow to the hands increases the risk for frostbite.

Teach patients that these drugs can cause new-onset depression or worsen existing depression.

Life Span Considerations for Beta Blockers
Pediatric Considerations. Use of beta blockers in children has not been researched. Although there is no evidence that risks from using beta blockers are different from those in adults, parents should discuss the risks and benefits with a pediatric cardiologist before a child begins taking these drugs.

Considerations for Pregnancy and Lactation. Most beta blockers have a moderate likelihood of increasing the risk for birth defects or fetal damage and should not be used during pregnancy unless absolutely necessary. Atenolol has a high likelihood of increasing risk and acebutolol has a low likelihood of increasing risk. These drugs are excreted in breast milk. No adverse effects on infants have been documented, but the possibility of slowed heart rate and lowered blood pressure exists. Women who are breastfeeding should consult with their prescriber about continued use of these drugs.

Considerations for Older Adults. Older adults are prescribed lower doses of beta blockers because they have a higher rate and intensity of side effects such as dizziness. A side effect of beta blockers that is more likely to occur in older adults is mental confusion. Teach family members to watch for this change and report it to the prescriber. These drugs may also decrease patients' ability to tolerate cool temperatures. Teach patients to dress warmly in cool weather and to wear hats and gloves when outdoors.

ALPHA BLOCKERS
How Alpha Blockers Work
Alpha blockers block receptors in arteries and smooth muscle. This relaxes the blood vessels and leads to an increase in blood flow and a lower blood pressure. Be sure to consult a drug reference book for information about any specific alpha blocker.

Dosages for Common Alpha Blockers

Drug	Dosage
doxazosin (Cardura)	*Adults:* 1-16 mg orally once daily
prazosin (Minipress)	*Adults:* 1-5 mg orally 2-3 times daily; do not exceed 20 mg daily *Children:* 20-400 mcg/kg orally daily in 2-3 divided doses; do not exceed 7 mg/dose or 15 mg daily
terazosin (Hytrin)	*Adults:* 1-10 mg orally daily in 1 or 2 divided doses

Intended Responses
- Artery relaxation and dilation (widening) are increased.
- Blood flow is increased.
- Blood pressure is lowered.

Side Effects. The most common side effects of alpha blockers are dizziness, drowsiness, fatigue, headache, nervousness, irritability, stuffy or runny nose, nausea, pain in the arms and legs, hypotension, and weakness.

A side effect of prazosin and terazosin is first-dose orthostatic hypotension because initially the patient is more sensitive to the blood pressure–lowering effects. As patients continue to take these drugs, they become less sensitive and have fewer problems with hypotension.

Adverse Effects. Alpha blockers can lower blood pressure more than is desired and cause side effects. Life-threatening effects are rare. Adverse effects to report to the prescriber include fainting; shortness of breath or difficulty breathing; fast, pounding, or irregular heart rhythm; chest pain; and swollen feet, ankles, or wrists.

What To Do *Before* Giving Alpha Blockers
In addition to the general responsibilities related to antihypertensive therapy (p. 255), ask male patients if they are taking any phosphodiesterase type 5 inhibitor erectile dysfunction drugs (e.g., sildenafil [Viagra], tadalafil [Cialis], or vardenafil [Levitra]).

What To Do *After* Giving Alpha Blockers
Be sure to review the general responsibilities related to care of patients after administering any antihypertensive drug (p. 255).

What To *Teach* Patients About Alpha Blockers
In addition to the general precautions related to antihypertensive therapy (pp. 255-256), tell patients not to drive or use machines for at least 24 hours after taking the first dose of an alpha blocker because a sudden drop in blood pressure can cause dizziness or confusion. Remind them to get up slowly, especially during the middle of the night.

Have patients weigh themselves twice a week and check their ankles for swelling. Weight gain and ankle swelling are signs that the body is holding onto extra fluid and should be reported to the prescriber.

Life Span Considerations for Alpha Blockers
Pediatric Considerations. Safe use of alpha blockers with children has not been established. Parents should discuss the risks and benefits of these drugs with a pediatric cardiologist.

Considerations for Pregnancy and Lactation. Alpha blockers have moderate likelihood of increasing the risk for birth defects or fetal harm. The effect of these drugs on pregnancy has not been researched or fully understood. Women who are pregnant or planning to become pregnant should inform their prescriber. Alpha blockers pass into breast milk; mothers who wish to breastfeed should discuss this with their prescriber and pediatrician. It may be necessary to avoid breastfeeding while taking these drugs.

Considerations for Older Adults. Older adults experience a higher frequency and stronger side effects of alpha blockers, especially hypotension, confusion, and increased risk for falling. They often need lower doses of these drugs.

ALPHA-BETA BLOCKERS
How Alpha-Beta Blockers Work
Alpha-beta blockers combine the effects of alpha blockers and beta blockers. They relax blood vessels like alpha blockers, and they slow the heart rate and decrease the

Common Side Effects
Alpha Blockers

Dizziness

Drowsiness

Headache

Hypotension

Runny nose

Pain in arms and legs

 Drug Alert!

Teaching Alert

Teach men that they should not be prescribed phosphodiesterase type 5 inhibitors (erectile dysfunction drugs) if they are also taking alpha blocker therapy because of the risk of severe hypotension.

QSEN: Safety

 Drug Alert!

Administration Alert

Give the first dose of prazosin and terazosin at bedtime and caution the patient not to get up without assistance. Orthostatic hypotension is a common side effect of the first doses.

QSEN: Safety

 Drug Alert!

Teaching Alert

Teach patients that weight gain and ankle swelling are signs that the body is holding extra fluid and should be reported immediately to the prescriber.

QSEN: Safety

 Drug Alert!

Teaching Alert

Alpha blockers pass into breast milk. Teach women who are breastfeeding or planning to breastfeed that it may be necessary to stop breastfeeding while on alpha blockers.

QSEN: Safety

force of heart contractions like beta blockers. These actions result in lower blood pressure. Be sure to consult a drug reference book for information on any specific alpha-beta blocker drug.

Dosages for Common Alpha-Beta Blockers

Drug	Dosage
carvedilol ❶ (Coreg)	*Adults:* 6.25-25 mg orally twice daily
labetalol HCL ❶ (Normodyne, Trandate)	*Adults:* PO: 100 mg orally twice daily (usual dosage range is 400-800 mg daily in 2-3 divided doses) *Adults:* IV: 20 mg (0.25 mg/kg) initially

❶ High-alert drug.

Common Side Effects
Alpha-Beta Blockers

Dizziness   Muscle weakness   Hypotension

Diarrhea   Hyperglycemia   Impotence

 Drug Alert!

Action/Intervention Alert

Because alpha-beta blockers can cause elevated blood glucose, be sure to monitor blood glucose levels regularly in patients with diabetes.

QSEN: Safety

Drug Alert!

Teaching Alert

Many blood pressure–lowering drugs can cause drowsiness or dizziness. Teach patients taking these drugs not to drive or operate machines.

QSEN: Safety

Intended Responses
- Artery relaxation and dilation (widening) are increased.
- Heart rate is decreased.
- Force of heart contraction is decreased.
- Heart workload is decreased.
- Blood pressure is lowered.
- Blood flow and oxygen to the heart are increased.

Side Effects. Common side effects of alpha-beta blockers include dizziness, fatigue, muscle weakness, orthostatic hypotension, diarrhea, impotence, and increased blood glucose levels (hyperglycemia).

Adverse Effects. Suddenly stopping alpha-beta blockers can cause life-threatening heart dysrhythmias, hypertension, or chest pain. Bradycardia, heart failure, and pulmonary edema can also occur.

Other adverse effects of these drugs may include yellow skin or eyes, swelling in the feet or ankles, weight gain, wheezing or trouble breathing, cold hands or feet, and difficulty sleeping.

What To Do *Before* Giving Alpha-Beta Blockers
In addition to the general responsibilities related to antihypertensive therapy (p. 255), obtain a baseline weight. Use this information to compare for changes after therapy is started and to determine whether an adverse reaction is occurring. Check the patient for swelling in the feet or ankles. If the patient has diabetes, check the blood glucose level.

What To Do *After* Giving Alpha-Beta Blockers
In addition to the general responsibilities related to antihypertensive therapy (p. 255), check blood glucose levels frequently for patients with diabetes, because these drugs may cause an increase in glucose levels.

Check intake and output and daily weights and look for any signs of fluid overload (swelling, difficulty breathing, crackles, and weight gain).

What To *Teach* Patients About Alpha-Beta Blockers
In addition to the general precautions related to antihypertensive therapy (pp. 255-256), explain that to suddenly stop taking these drugs can lead to life-threatening problems. Tell patients to contact the prescriber for irregular heart rate, heart rate less than 50 beats per minute, or blood pressure changes.

Tell patients not to drive or operate machines because the drug may cause dizziness or drowsiness. Remind them to change positions slowly.

Tell patients taking labetalol (Normodyne) that they may become more sensitive to cold and may need to dress warmly.

Remind patients with diabetes to carefully watch for signs of changes in blood sugar. These drugs may interfere with or mask some of the signs of low blood sugar. Patients may need to check their glucose levels more frequently and adjust the timing of their meals.

Life Span Considerations for Alpha-Beta Blockers
Considerations for Pregnancy and Lactation. Alpha-beta blockers have a moderate likelihood of increasing the risk for birth defects or fetal damage. Safe use in pregnancy or breastfeeding has not been researched and established. These drugs cross the placenta and into breast milk. They may cause slowed heart rate, hypotension, hypoglycemia, and respiratory depression in the newborn.

CENTRAL-ACTING ADRENERGIC AGENTS

How Central-Acting Adrenergic Agents Work
Central-acting adrenergic agents stimulate central nervous system receptors to decrease constriction of blood vessels, which leads to dilation (widening) of arteries, and to lower blood pressure. Be sure to consult a drug reference book for information about any specific central-acting adrenergic agent.

Dosages for Common Central-Acting Adrenergic Agents

Drug	Dosage
clonidine (Catapres, Dixarit ♣, Novo-Clonidine ♣)	*Adults:* 0.1 mg (100 mcg) orally twice daily; usual maintenance dosage range is 0.2-0.6 mg daily in 2-3 divided doses *Adults:* Transdermal: 0.1-0.3 mg (100-300 mcg) patch applied every 7 days *Children:* 0.05-0.4 mg (50-400 mcg) orally twice daily
methyldopa (Aldomet, Dopamet ♣, Nu-Medpa ♣)	*Adults:* PO: 250 mg orally 2-3 times daily; may increase up to 3 g daily in divided doses *Adults:* IV: 250-500 mg every 6 hr over 30-60 min; may increase up to 1 g every 6-8 hr *Children:* PO: 10-65 mg/kg orally daily in 2-4 divided doses; do not exceed 3 g daily *Children:* IV: 20-65 mg/kg daily in 4 divided doses

Intended Responses
- Vasodilation (widening) of arteries is increased.
- Blood pressure is lowered.
- Heart workload is decreased.

Side Effects. Central-acting adrenergic agents have a higher incidence of side effects than other blood pressure–lowering drugs. Common side effects include drowsiness, lethargy, dry mouth, and nasal congestion

Adverse Effects. Myocarditis associated with allergic type reactions to methyldopa are rare but have been known to cause death.

What To Do *Before* Giving Central-Acting Adrenergic Agents
In addition to the general responsibilities related to antihypertensive therapy (p. 255), obtain a baseline weight on the patient.

When administering a clonidine patch, be aware that it is packaged with two patches. The smaller patch contains the drug, and the larger patch is used to cover the drug patch. If the patch falls off, a new patch should be placed on the patient. Be sure to record the date and time and initial the patch before placing it on the patient.

What To Do *After* Giving Central-Acting Adrenergic Agents
In addition to the general responsibilities related to antihypertensive therapy (p. 255), keep track of the patient's intake and output. Check feet and ankles for swelling. Listen to the patient's lungs for crackles. Watch for signs of mental status

Common Side Effects

Central-Acting Adrenergic Agents

Drowsiness, Lethargy Dry mouth Nasal congestion

changes suggesting that blood pressure may be too low. Look for psychiatric signs of depression such as difficulty concentrating, sleep changes, or a loss of interest in daily activities.

What To *Teach* Patients About Central-Acting Adrenergic Agents

In addition to the general precautions related to antihypertensive therapy (pp. 255-256), teach patients that these drugs should be discontinued gradually. If the drugs are stopped suddenly, blood pressure could become dangerously high.

For dry mouth, encourage patients to perform frequent mouth care with rinses, tooth brushing, and the use of sugarless gum.

If the patient is using transdermal clonidine, teach that the patch can stay on during bathing or swimming. Teach patients that this medication is packaged with two patches. The smaller patch contains the actual drug; and the larger patch, which does not contain medication, is used to cover the drug patch. If the patch falls off, tell the patient to apply a new patch.

Life Span Considerations for Central-Acting Adrenergic Agents

Considerations for Pregnancy and Lactation. Clonidine has a moderate likelihood of increasing the risk of birth defects or fetal damage. Safe use of clonidine (Catapres) in pregnancy or breastfeeding has not been researched or established. This drug should be avoided during pregnancy and breastfeeding. Methyldopa (Aldomet) has a low likelihood of increasing the risk of birth defects or fetal damage when prescribed by mouth and a moderate likelihood when prescribed intravenously. Oral methyldopa has been used safely during both pregnancy and breastfeeding. It is also safely used to treat pregnancy-induced hypertension.

Considerations for Older Adults. Older adults are very sensitive to the actions of central-acting adrenergic agents and tend to have an increased risk of orthostatic hypotension. Teach older adults to change positions slowly and to ask for help getting up because of the increased risk for dizziness and falling. Lower doses of these drugs are recommended.

DIRECT VASODILATORS

How Direct Vasodilators Work

A *vasodilator* is any drug that relaxes blood vessel walls. **Direct vasodilators** act directly on the peripheral arteries, causing them to dilate (widen), which leads to lower blood pressure. Be sure to consult a drug reference book for information on any specific direct vasodilator.

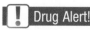

Drug Alert!

Action/Intervention Alert

Frequent mouth rinses, oral care, and chewing sugarless gum can relieve the dry-mouth side effect of central-acting adrenergic agents.

Drug Alert!

Administration Alert

Oral methyldopa (Aldomet) has been used safely during pregnancy and breastfeeding and to treat pregnancy-induced hypertension.

Dosages for Common Direct Vasodilators

Drug	Dosage
hydralazine (Apresoline, Novo-Hylazin ✦)	*Adults:* PO: 10 mg orally 4 times daily; may gradually increase up to 300 mg daily *Adults:* IV: 5-40 mg daily in 4 divided doses; may repeat as needed *Children:* PO: 0.75 mg/kg orally daily in 2-4 divided doses; may gradually increase to 7.5 mg/kg daily in 2-4 divided doses *Children:* IM, IV: 1.7 mg/kg daily in 4-6 divided doses
minoxidil (Loniten)	*Adults:* 5 mg orally daily may increase gradually up to 100 mg daily; do not exceed 100 mg daily *Children less than 12 years old:* 0.2 mg/kg orally daily (maximum 5 mg daily); may increase gradually to 0.25-1 mg/kg daily (maximum 50 mg daily)

Intended Responses
- Vasodilation (widening) of arteries is increased.
- Blood pressure is lowered.
- Heart workload is decreased.

Side Effects. Direct vasodilators, along with central-acting adrenergic agents, have a higher incidence of side effects. Common side effects include tachycardia and salt (sodium) retention (hypernatremia).

Adverse Effects. Stevens-Johnson syndrome may occur with minoxidil. This is a severe inflammatory eruption of the skin and mucous membranes (see Figure 1-5).

What To Do *Before* Giving Direct Vasodilators

In addition to the general responsibilities related to antihypertensive therapy (p. 255), be sure to get a baseline weight for the patient.

What To Do *After* Giving Direct Vasodilators

In addition to the general responsibilities related to antihypertensive therapy (p. 255), keep track of intake and output. Check the patient's feet and ankles for swelling. Listen to the patient's lungs for crackles. These drugs increase the risk for fluid retention and edema formation.

What To *Teach* Patients About Direct Vasodilators

In addition to general precautions related to antihypertensive therapy (pp. 255-256), instruct patients to contact the prescriber if more than two doses are missed. These drugs should be discontinued gradually because blood pressure can become dangerously high if they are stopped suddenly.

Tell patients to report any persistent heart rate increase of more than 20 beats per minute to the prescriber. This may be a sign of heart failure.

Teach patients to weigh themselves and check their feet and ankles for swelling twice a week. Tell them to report a weight gain of more than 3 pounds in 1 week to the prescriber because this may indicate heart failure.

Life Span Considerations for Direct Vasodilators

Pediatric Considerations. The same side effects that occur with adults may affect children. Doses for children are based on weight.

Considerations for Pregnancy and Lactation. Hydralazine (Apresoline) has a low likelihood of increasing the risk for birth defects or fetal damage and has been used safely during both pregnancy and breastfeeding to decrease high blood pressure in women. Small amounts of this drug pass into breast milk, putting infants at minimal risk for side effects. A woman who plans to breastfeed should discuss this with the prescriber.

Common Side Effects

Vasodilators

Tachycardia

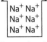

Hypernatremia

⚠ Drug Alert!

Action/Intervention Alert

With vasodilator drugs, report a sustained increase in heart rate of more than 20 beats per minute to the prescriber immediately.

QSEN: Safety

Get Ready for Practice!

Key Points

- Hypertension is defined as a systolic blood pressure greater than 140 to 159 mm Hg and/or a diastolic blood pressure greater than 90 to 99 mm Hg.
- Untreated hypertension can lead to many health problems, including heart attack, stroke, and kidney disease.
- Teach patients prescribed drugs to lower blood pressure to sit up and stand slowly because dizziness and hypotension are common side effects of these drugs.
- Beta blockers slow the heart rate and decrease the force of the contraction of the heart.
- ACE inhibitors slow the production of angiotensin II, a potent vasoconstrictor, by the body.

- Angiotensin II receptor blockers (ARBs) block the action of angiotensin II, leading to increased vasodilation (widening) of arteries.
- Angioedema (swelling of the face, eyes, lips, and tongue) is a life-threatening adverse effect of angiotensin II receptor blockers and ACE inhibitors.
- Calcium channel blockers decrease the force of the contractions of the heart and dilate the arteries.
- Alpha blockers relax blood vessels, leading to arterial widening and lower blood pressure.
- Alpha-beta blockers combine the effects of alpha blockers and beta blockers to lower blood pressure.
- Monitor patients with diabetes carefully when taking alpha-beta blockers because these drugs cause hyperglycemia (high blood sugar).

- Methyldopa (Aldomet), a central-acting adrenergic drug, is the drug of choice for controlling high blood pressure during pregnancy.
- A sustained heart rate increase of more than 20 beats per minute should be reported to the prescriber when a patient is taking a direct vasodilator drug.
- Always check blood pressure, heart rate, and weight and look for swelling of the ankles or feet before and after giving antihypertensive drugs.
- Encourage patients to adopt lifestyle changes that will help to control high blood pressure such as weight loss, regular exercise, and low-salt diets.
- Be sure that patients know how to check their heart rate and blood pressure and understand the importance of follow-up checks.

Additional Learning Resources

evolve Be sure to visit your Evolve website (http://evolve.elsevier.com/Workman/pharmacology/) for additional online resources.

SG Go to your Study Guide for additional learning activities to help you master this chapter content.

Review Questions

See the Answer Keys—In-text Review Questions for answers to these questions.

Test Yourself on the Basics

1. When a patient is prescribed an antihypertensive drug for blood pressure changes that occurred after chronic kidney disease, what is the alteration in blood pressure called?
   A. Diastolic blood pressure
   B. Systolic blood pressure
   C. Primary hypertension
   D. Secondary hypertension

2. A patient prescribed an angiotensin II receptor blocker (ARB) for hypertension now has a blood pressure of 90/68. What side effects do you expect the patient to experience? (Select all that apply.)
   A. Light-headedness
   B. Nausea
   C. Dizziness
   D. Diarrhea
   E. Cough
   F. Abnormal potassium level

3. Which action must you take before giving any antihypertensive drug?
   A. Weigh the patient.
   B. Get a list of all drugs the patient is taking.
   C. Determine whether the patient has an infection.
   D. Perform a complete physical assessment.

4. A patient with chronic uncontrolled hypertension is prescribed several antihypertensive drugs. The prescriber orders prazosin (Minipress). When should you administer the first dose?
   A. 9 AM after breakfast
   B. 12 noon with lunch
   C. 5 PM with dinner
   D. 10 PM at bedtime

5. An older adult patient with hypertension, chronic kidney disease, and liver failure is prescribed an ARB drug. What special precaution do you expect for this patient?
   A. The patient should be given this drug with food.
   B. The patient should be given a lower dose of this drug.
   C. The patient should be instructed to report diarrhea to the prescriber.
   D. The patient should be given this drug twice a day on an empty stomach.

Test Yourself on Advanced Concepts

6. A patient who is taking an ACE inhibitor for hypertension asks how this drug lowers blood pressure. What is your best response?
   A. "It eliminates excess water and salt from the body."
   B. "It blocks the conversion of angiotensin II."
   C. "It reduces the heart rate."
   D. "It dilates the arteries."

7. A patient who is taking captopril (Capoten) 25 mg twice daily develops dizziness. What is your priority action?
   A. Keep the patient on bed rest.
   B. Withhold the dose and notify the prescriber.
   C. Instruct the patient to call for help when getting out of bed.
   D. Place all four side rails in the upright position.

8. A patient prescribed hydralazine (Apresoline) develops a severe inflammatory eruption of the skin and mucous membranes. What is your best action?
   A. Apply an aloe-based lotion to the area.
   B. Reassure the patient that this is an expected side effect.
   C. Document these findings as the only action.
   D. Hold the drug and notify the prescriber.

9. Which statement by a patient who is prescribed metoprolol (Lopressor) indicates the need for additional teaching?
   A. "I will get out of bed slowly to avoid dizziness and decrease the risk of falling."
   B. "I will notify my prescriber if I experience any chest pains.
   C. "I will wear a sunscreen, long sleeves, and hat when I go outdoors."
   D. "I will stop taking this drug if my heart rate is less than 70 beats per minute."

10. A woman is prescribed oral methyldopa (Aldomet) to control pregnancy-induced hypertension. What must you teach the patient about this drug?
    A. Safe use of this drug during pregnancy has not been researched.
    B. This drug can be used safely during pregnancy and breastfeeding.
    C. This drug has fewer side effects than many other antihypertensive drugs.
    D. Research demonstrates that this drug causes birth defects in laboratory animal studies.

11. A patient takes enalapril (Vasotec) 5 mg once a day to control high blood pressure. For which life-threatening adverse effect do you assess the patient?
    A. Myocarditis
    B. Angioedema
    C. Liver failure
    D. Stevens-Johnson syndrome

12. Which signs/symptoms must you be sure to check for every 4 to 8 hours after giving a drug to treat high blood pressure? (Select all that apply.)
    A. Dizziness
    B. Decreased axillary temperature
    C. Hand grasp strength
    D. Crackles in lungs
    E. Blood pressure
    F. Heart rate
    G. Weight

13. Which points must you be sure to teach the patient who is going home and continuing to take prazosin (Minipres) 2 mg twice daily for blood pressure control? (Select all that apply.)
    A. Do not drive or operate machines.
    B. Avoid salt substitutes.
    C. Remember to change positions slowly.
    D. Weigh yourself twice a week.
    E. Take two pills of the drug in the evening if you miss your morning dose.
    F. Report any ankle swelling to your prescriber.
    G. Avoid aspirin or aspirin-containing products.

14. A 33-year-old female patient is currently taking captopril (Capoten) 12.5 mg daily to control her high blood pressure. She tells her prescriber that she plans to become pregnant. What drug will the prescriber most likely prescribe now?
    A. nadolol (Corgard)
    B. clonidine (Catapres)
    C. methyldopa (Aldomet)
    D. lisinopril (Prinivil, Zestril)

15. The prescriber orders losartan (Cozaar) 75 mg once daily. The pharmacy sends 25-mg tablets. How many tablets will you give the patient? _____ tablet(s)

16. The prescriber orders oral hydralazine (Apresoline) 0.375 mg/kg twice a day for an 8-year-old child. The child weighs 66 lb. How many milligrams of hydralazine will you give for each dose? _____ mg

17. A patient is to receive diltiazem (Cardizem) 0.25 mg/kg IV to control high blood pressure. The patient's weight is 70 kg. How many mg will you give? _____ mg

Critical Thinking Activities

See the Answer Keys—Critical Thinking Activities for answers to these activities.

Mr. Jones is a 65-year-old with primary hypertension for more than 25 years' duration. His mother and grandfather had high blood pressure. He does not exercise and admits that he is an alcoholic and smokes 1 to 2 packs of cigarettes every day. He lives alone, and his diet consists of mostly fast foods. Mr. Jones takes hydrochlorothiazide (Microzide) 50 mg twice a day and metoprolol (Lopressor) 100 mg twice a day. He tells you that he sometimes does not take his medications because he forgets.

1. What are Mr. Jones's risk factors for hypertension?
2. What should you teach Mr. Jones about his antihypertensive drugs?
3. What strategies could you suggest to Mr. Jones to help control his hypertension?

Objectives

After studying this chapter you should be able to:

1. List the common names, actions, usual adult dosages, possible side effects, and adverse effects of vasodilators and cardiac glycosides (digoxin).
2. Describe what to do before and after giving vasodilators and cardiac glycosides.
3. Explain what to teach patients taking vasodilators and cardiac glycosides, including what to do, what not to do, and when to call the prescriber.
4. Describe life span considerations for vasodilators and cardiac glycosides.
5. List the common names, actions, usual adult dosages, possible side effects, and adverse effects of human B-type

natriuretic peptides, positive inotropes, potassium, and magnesium.

6. Describe what to do before and after giving human B-type natriuretic peptides, positive inotropes, potassium, and magnesium.
7. Explain what to teach patients taking human B-type natriuretic peptides, positive inotropes, potassium, and magnesium, including what to do, what not to do, and when to call the prescriber.
8. Describe life span considerations for human B-type natriuretic peptides, positive inotropes, potassium, and magnesium.

Key Terms

cardiac glycosides (CAR-dē-ak GLĪ-kō-sīd) (p. 281) A class of drugs that improve heart failure by slowing down a heart rate that is too fast, allowing more time for the left ventricle to fill.

diastolic left heart failure (dī-ă-STŌL-ĭk LĔFT HĂRT FĀL-yŭr) (p. 276) Inadequate relaxation or "stiffening" of the ventricle that prevents the heart from filling enough before contraction.

heart failure (HĂRT FĀL-yŭr) (p. 272) Occurs when the heart cannot pump enough blood to meet the needs of the body. Also called pump failure.

human B-type natriuretic peptide (HŪ-măn B TĪP NĂ-trē-yū-RĔT-ik PĔP-tīd) (p. 284) A hormone that is produced by the heart ventricles and a synthetic drug with actions that include increased water elimination and blood vessel dilation.

magnesium (măg-NĒ-zē-ŭm) (p. 286) A major mineral that is the fourth most abundant in the human body. It helps the heart rhythm remain steady and keeps bones strong.

positive inotropes (PŎS-ĭh-tĭv ĬN-ō-trōp) (p. 285) Heart pump drugs that make the heart muscle contract more forcefully. They also relax blood vessels so blood can flow better.

potassium (pō-TĂS-ē-ŭm) (p. 286) A very important electrolyte that is essential for a healthy nervous system and a regular heart rhythm.

systolic left heart failure (sĭs-TŌL-ĭk LĔFT HĂRT FĀL-yŭr) (p. 275) Condition in which the heart is unable to contract forcefully enough to pump enough blood to meet the needs of the body.

vasodilators (VĂ-sō-dī-LĀ-tŏr) (p. 279) A class of drugs that act directly on the peripheral arteries to cause them to dilate (widen).

[?] Did You Know?

As many as 10% of adults over the age of 70 have heart failure. As much as 80% of hospital admissions for heart failure are for patients over age 65.

OVERVIEW

As the world population ages, the number of people diagnosed with heart failure is increasing. About 5 million people live with heart failure in the United States, and as many as 500,000 new cases occur each year. Heart failure can occur at any age; however, it is much more common in older people because they often have disorders that damage the heart muscle (for example, high blood pressure or heart attack), and age-related changes in the heart can make it pump less efficiently.

Heart failure occurs when the heart cannot pump enough blood to meet the needs of the body. Most heart failure is caused by hypertension. Many of the drugs used to treat hypertension are also used to treat heart failure. Other causes of heart failure include myocardial infarction, coronary artery disease, cardiomyopathy, substance abuse (alcohol and illicit or prescribed drugs), heart valve disease, congenital defects, cardiac infections and inflammations, and conditions that increase cardiac output and energy demands such as sepsis.

REVIEW OF RELATED PHYSIOLOGY AND PATHOPHYSIOLOGY

The heart is a muscular organ that is hollow and divided into four chambers: right atrium, right ventricle, left atrium, and left ventricle. The atrial and ventricular chambers are separated by one-way valves that open when the pressure in the first chamber is higher than that in the second chamber (Figure 17-1).

Blood enters the heart from the vena cava into the right atrium. This blood comes from the rest of the body; most of the oxygen has been used. From the right atrium, the blood moves through the tricuspid valve into the right ventricle. The muscle of the right ventricle contracts to make the pressure in this chamber higher than the pressure in the blood vessel known as the pulmonary artery. When right ventricular pressure is high enough, the pulmonary valve opens and allows blood to move from the right ventricle into the pulmonary artery. From there blood moves into the lungs, where it picks up oxygen. The oxygenated blood then moves into the left atrium. When the pressure in the left atrium is high enough, the blood moves through the mitral valve (also called the bicuspid valve) into the left ventricle. The muscles of the left ventricle are the strongest ones in the heart. They must contract and increase the pressure in the left ventricle to force the blood to leave the left ventricle through the aortic valve and into the aorta. Once oxygenated blood enters the aorta, it circulates throughout the entire body to deliver oxygen to every tissue and organ. So it is important that the muscles of the left ventricle have the best contraction to force blood into the aorta.

The muscles of the left ventricle are similar to other body muscles in that they contract best and strongest after a stretch. Think of a baseball pitcher winding up to throw a fastball. He or she first moves the arm back as far as possible to stretch the throwing muscles. This stretching before throwing allows the muscles to contract harder and faster, resulting in a better throw. When the muscles of the left ventricle are stretched to the best level, the result is a stronger contraction that moves more blood from the left ventricle into the aorta. Usually this stretch occurs naturally when

Memory Jogger

When the left ventricular muscle is stretched, a stronger heart contraction moves more blood from the left ventricle into the aorta and out to the body.

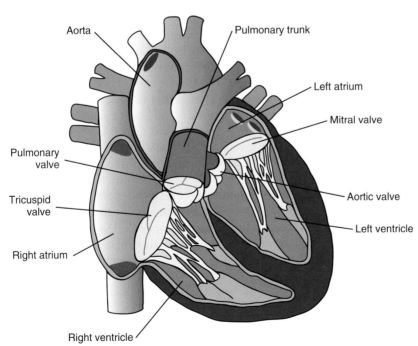

FIGURE 17-1 Heart chambers and valves.

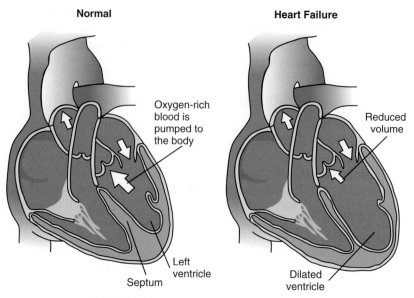

FIGURE 17-2 Normal heart and heart with heart failure.

Memory Jogger

Preload is the "stretching" of the muscle caused by blood filling the left ventricle.

Memory Jogger

Afterload is the pressure in the aorta that the left ventricle must overcome before blood can move from it into the aorta.

the right amount of blood fills the ventricle *(preload)*. If the muscle is not stretched enough, the resulting contraction is weak and moves only a small amount of blood into the aorta (just as a small windup before a pitch results in a weak and short throw).

One problem that can occur with the muscle of the left ventricle is that it can become *overstretched*. When any muscle is overstretched, its contraction is weaker. Think about a person with a rubber band. Not stretching the rubber band or stretching it only a little results in a weak snap. Stretching it more increases the snap. However, if the rubber band is overstretched, it becomes so flabby that it cannot "snap" back. When the muscles of the left ventricle are overstretched or flabby and the contraction is weak, too much blood remains in the left ventricle, and more blood arriving from the left atrium is added to it. This overstretches the muscle more and continues to weaken contractions, leading to heart failure (Figure 17-2). Blood then backs up into other heart chambers, leading to congestion in the lungs and the peripheral veins (Figure 17-3).

Some of the drugs used to treat heart failure work by actually making the muscles contract better. Others work by reducing the amount of blood in the left ventricle (preventing overstretching). Still others work by lowering the pressure in the aorta *(afterload)* so muscles of the left ventricle do not have to contract as hard or as strong to move blood out of the ventricle and into the aorta.

Heart function and blood pressure work together for good blood circulation and blood flow to ensure that oxygen is delivered to all body tissues and organs. Heart contractions must be strong enough to move blood into the arteries. Then arterial pressure must be high enough to move blood through the arteries and into the tissues and organs. *Mean arterial pressure (MAP)* is the average systolic blood pressure in the large arteries, including the aorta. For the average healthy adult the normal MAP range is between 70 and 100 mm Hg, which ensures good blood circulation to tissues. If MAP is too low (<60 mm Hg), tissues and organs will not receive enough blood to ensure oxygenation. MAP also is the pressure that the left ventricle must overcome to move blood from the left ventricle into the aorta during contraction (afterload). If MAP is higher than normal (>110 mm Hg), the heart, especially the left ventricle, has to work harder to move blood into the aorta. Heart attacks (myocardial infarction) and heart failure can occur when the heart has to work too hard for too long.

LEFT HEART FAILURE

When blood collects in the left side of the heart, it results in congestion in the lungs, decreased lung function, and difficulty breathing. Because the left ventricle pumps

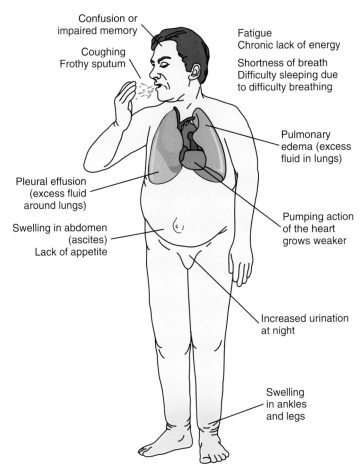

Confusion or
impaired memory

Coughing
Frothy sputum

Fatigue
Chronic lack of energy

Shortness of breath
Difficulty sleeping due
to difficulty breathing

Pulmonary
edema (excess
fluid in lungs)

Pleural effusion
(excess fluid
around lungs)

Swelling in abdomen
(ascites)
Lack of appetite

Pumping action
of the heart
grows weaker

Increased urination
at night

Swelling
in ankles
and legs

FIGURE 17-3 Signs and symptoms of heart failure and peripheral and pulmonary congestion.

Box **17-1**	**Signs and Symptoms of Left Heart Failure**

DECREASED CARDIAC OUTPUT
- Fatigue
- Weakness
- Oliguria (decreased urine output) during the day
- Angina
- Confusion, restlessness
- Dizziness
- Tachycardia, palpitations
- Paleness (pallor)

- Weak peripheral pulses
- Cool extremities

PULMONARY CONGESTION
- Hacking cough, worse at night
- Dyspnea/breathlessness
- Crackles or wheezes in lungs
- Frothy, pink-tinged sputum
- Tachypnea
- S_3/S_4 summation gallop (abnormal heart sounds)

Modified from Ignatavicius, D., & Workman, L. (2013). *Medical-surgical nursing: Patient-centered collaborative care* (7th ed.). Philadelphia: Saunders, p. 749.

---

blood to the body, symptoms include signs of decreased cardiac output (such as fatigue and weakness) and signs of pulmonary congestion (such as crackles and wheezes detected with a stethoscope). Box 17-1 lists the key signs and symptoms associated with left ventricular heart failure.

Left heart failure can be either systolic or diastolic. **Systolic left heart failure** is more common. It happens when the heart contractions are too weak to circulate enough blood to meet the needs of the body. The decrease in contractility causes a decrease in the amount of blood pumped out with each contraction, leaving more blood in the ventricle and causing an increase in preload. Afterload increases because of increased peripheral resistance usually as a result of high blood pressure. These two changes cause a decrease in *ejection fraction* (percentage of blood pumped with each

 Memory Jogger

Heart failure most commonly occurs in the left ventricle.

Memory Jogger

Normal ejection fraction is 50% to 70%. With systolic heart failure, the ejection fraction is less than 40%.

contraction) from a normal of 50% to 70% to less than 40%. The lower ejection fraction leads to less blood (cardiac output) for tissue perfusion. Blood collects in the pulmonary blood vessels, causing signs of lung congestion.

Diastolic left heart failure occurs when the left ventricle is not able to relax enough during diastole and causes a decrease in filling of the ventricles (preload) before contraction. A decrease in cardiac output results and not enough blood is pumped to meet the needs of the body. With diastolic failure the patient's ejection fraction may be very close to normal.

RIGHT HEART FAILURE

With right heart failure the right ventricle does not empty. This causes increased volume and pressure in the right side of the heart. When the right ventricle contracts poorly, signs and symptoms of peripheral congestion occur (Box 17-2) such as weight gain, swelling in the legs, *jugular vein distention* (Figure 17-4), and increased blood pressure. The pathophysiology of heart failure is summarized in Figure 17-5.

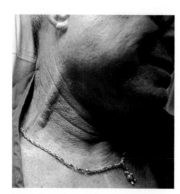

FIGURE 17-4 Jugular vein distention. (From Goldman, L., & Ausiello, D. (2007). *Cecil medicine* (23rd ed.). Philadelphia: Saunders.)

Box **17-2**   Signs and Symptoms of Right Heart Failure

SYSTEMIC CONGESTION
- Jugular (neck vein) distention
- Enlarged liver and spleen
- Anorexia and nausea
- Dependent edema (legs and sacrum)
- Distended abdomen

- Swollen hands and fingers
- Increased urine output (polyuria) at night
- Weight gain
- Increased blood pressure (from excess volume) or decreased blood pressure (from heart failure)

Modified from Ignatavicius, D., & Workman, L. (2013). *Medical-surgical nursing: Patient-centered collaborative care* (7th ed.). Philadelphia: Saunders, p. 749.

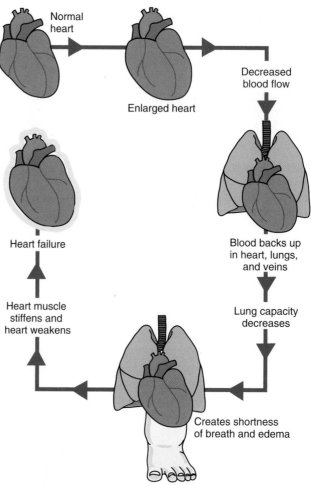

FIGURE 17-5 Pathophysiology of heart failure.

COMPENSATORY MECHANISMS FOR HEART FAILURE

The body has several ways to compensate for heart failure. In response to tissue hypoxia (not enough oxygen), the sympathetic nervous system is stimulated, and the hormones epinephrine and norepinephrine (catecholamines) are released. These hormones act on the heart in two ways. First, they increase the heart rate. Second, they increase the power of the heart muscle fibers to contract or shorten so the heart pumps more forcefully. The ability of the heart fibers to shorten is called *contractility*. These actions increase the amount of blood pumped by the heart in 1 minute, known as the *cardiac output*.

Sympathetic nervous system stimulation also causes arterial vasoconstriction (narrowing of the arteries). This helps the body to maintain blood pressure and improve blood flow to the tissues. The downside to this compensation is that narrowing of the arteries leads to increased afterload, more work for the heart, and increased oxygen needs. *Increased afterload can lead to worsening heart failure.*

When heart failure causes decreased blood flow to the kidneys, another compensation process called the *renin-angiotensin system (RAS)* is activated. This pathway causes release of two body chemicals: angiotensin II and aldosterone. *Angiotensin II* causes blood vessel constriction (increased afterload), whereas aldosterone leads to sodium and water retention (increased preload). Activation of the RAS leads to increased blood pressure.

A third way that the body can compensate for heart failure is by *myocardial hypertrophy* (enlargement) of the heart muscle. Increase in the heart muscle size can lead to more forceful contractions and increased cardiac output. But when the heart muscle becomes too big, it outgrows its blood supply. The thickened muscle also becomes "stiff," resulting in less effective contractions and diastolic heart failure.

TREATMENT FOR HEART FAILURE

Continuous heart function is needed for life. Unmanaged heart failure leads to death. Heart failure is usually a chronic disorder and can be "cured" only rarely. Goals for treatment include (1) making physical activity more comfortable, (2) improving quality of life, and (3) prolonging life. Interventions focus on:
- Treating the cause of heart failure.
- Controlling factors that can cause it to worsen.
- Treating its symptoms.

Lifestyle changes are an important part of a treatment plan. Suggested changes include weight loss, smoking cessation, and a low-salt and low-fat diet. Drug therapy only improves heart function; drugs do not cure heart failure. Because the damage to the heart muscle is not reversible, the only real cure for heart failure is a heart transplant.

GENERAL ISSUES IN HEART FAILURE THERAPY

There are several classes of drugs for heart failure that have both common and different actions and effects. Responsibilities for these common actions and effects are listed in the following discussion. Specific responsibilities are listed with each class of heart failure drugs.

Before administering any heart failure drug, obtain a complete list of drugs that the patient is currently taking, including over-the-counter and herbal drugs. Check the patient's blood pressure and heart rate. If the blood pressure is low (less than 90/60 mm Hg) or the heart rate is low (less than 60 beats per minute), check with the prescriber about whether the patient should receive the drug because many of these drugs lower heart rate further. Assess the apical pulse for a full minute because a patient with heart failure may have extra heart sounds and dysrhythmias causing irregular heartbeats. Check the drug order because some prescribers provide guidelines for when to administer and when to hold these drugs. Obtain a baseline weight for each patient because weight gain is a sign of worsening heart failure. Ask female

 Memory Jogger

Cardiac output (CO) is the product of heart rate (HR) and stroke volume (SV). The formula for this is $CO = HR \times SV$. An increase in heart rate and/or stroke volume results in an increase in cardiac output.

 Memory Jogger

The renin-angiotensin system causes vasoconstriction and body retention of sodium and water.

 Memory Jogger

The only real cure for heart failure is a heart transplant because the damage to the heart muscle is irreversible.

Memory Jogger

Remember that the apical pulse is displaced lateral to the midclavicular line with left heart failure.

? Did You Know?

Most over-the-counter cold and allergy medications constrict blood vessels and raise blood pressure.

Memory Jogger

The major classes of drugs to treat heart failure are:
- ACE inhibitors
- Beta blockers
- Vasodilators
- Cardiac glycosides
- Diuretics
- Human B-type natriuretic peptides
- Positive inotropes

patients of childbearing years if they are pregnant, breastfeeding, or planning to become pregnant.

After administering any heart failure drug, reassess and continue to monitor the patient's blood pressure and apical heart rate. Notify the prescriber if either measure is low. Ensure that the call light is within easy reach and tell the patient to call for assistance when getting out of bed because of the increased risk for dizziness, light-headedness, and hypotension with these drugs. Check for any signs or symptoms of allergic reactions or infections.

Teach patients receiving a heart failure drug to change positions slowly to prevent dizziness and falls. Instruct them to go from a lying position to sitting before standing. Tell patients that these drugs will help to control but will not cure heart failure; the drugs may be prescribed for life.

Talk with patients and their families about the importance of regular blood pressure and heart rate checks, at least once a week. Teach them proper techniques for checking blood pressure and heart rate. Teach the importance of regular follow-up visits to check and maintain control of their heart failure. Remind patients to check with their prescriber before taking any over-the-counter drugs, including cough or allergy remedies or herbal preparations. Tell patients to notify their prescriber for any weight gain or increase in shortness of breath because these are signs of worsening heart failure.

Instruct patients who experience dizziness, drowsiness, or light-headedness not to drive, use heavy equipment, or do anything that could be dangerous or require increased alertness until they know how the drug affects them. Encourage patients to get a medical alert bracelet identifying the use of any drug for heart failure.

TYPES OF DRUGS USED TO TREAT HEART FAILURE

Heart failure is a complex problem in which more than one normal action is disrupted. For this reason, usually a combination of drugs is used to manage symptoms and improve heart-pumping function. Some of these drugs have other uses. For example, antihypertensive drugs are commonly used in heart failure therapy for several reasons. First, hypertension is a common cause of heart failure. In addition, by lowering blood pressure these drugs allow the heart to pump more easily. Therefore drugs such as angiotensin-converting enzyme (ACE) inhibitors, angiotensin II receptor blockers (ARBs), and most beta-adrenergic blockers are part of drug therapy for heart failure. Diuretics help in the treatment of heart failure by reducing blood volume, relaxing arteries, and improving heart muscle pumping. Diuretic drugs are discussed in detail in Chapter 15. Chapter 16 discusses antihypertensive drugs. Other drugs used in the treatment of heart failure include anticoagulants (Chapter 20), which may be used to prevent clots from forming in the heart chambers; and antidysrhythmic drugs (Chapter 18), which may be prescribed for abnormal heart rhythms. This chapter focuses on the drugs with intended actions that are specific for the heart.

ACE INHIBITORS

ACE inhibitors are often among the first drugs prescribed to treat heart failure. Dosages for these drugs are different when used to treat heart failure rather than high blood pressure. The most common ACE inhibitors are listed in the following table. Be sure to consult a drug handbook for information about any specific ACE inhibitor. Refer to Chapter 16 for more general information about ACE inhibitors.

Dosages for Common ACE Inhibitors for Heart Failure

Drug	Dosage
captopril (Capoten)	*Adults:* 12.5-100 mg orally 2-3 times daily
enalapril (Vasotec)	*Adults:* 2.5-20 mg orally twice daily

Dosages for Common ACE Inhibitors for Heart Failure—cont'd

Drug	Dosage
fosinopril (Monopril)	*Adults:* 10-40 mg orally once daily
lisinopril (Zestril, Prinivil)	*Adults:* 2.5-40 mg orally once daily
quinapril (Accupril)	*Adults:* 5-20 mg orally once or twice daily
ramipril (Altace)	*Adults:* 1.25-5 mg orally once or twice daily
trandolapril (Mavik)	*Adults:* 1-4 mg orally once daily

BETA BLOCKERS

How Beta Blockers Work

Beta blockers block the effects of epinephrine (adrenaline) on the heart. They decrease the heart rate and the force of heart contractions, which results in a decrease in blood pressure. As a result the heart does not work as hard and requires less oxygen.

These drugs are often used with ACE inhibitors to treat heart failure. They may temporarily worsen heart failure symptoms but, when taken over a long period, they improve heart function.

Most dosages are the same as when used for high blood pressure. See Chapter 16 for the usual dosages and ranges. Those drugs with specific limits when used for heart failure are listed in the following table. Only the sustained-release form of metoprolol is used to treat heart failure. Be sure to consult a drug handbook for specific information about any specific beta blocker. Refer to Chapter 16 for more general information about beta blockers.

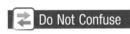

Do Not Confuse

Apresoline *with* Priscoline

An order for Apresoline may be confused with Priscoline. Apresoline is a vasodilator, whereas Priscoline is an alpha-adrenergic antagonist often used for persistent pulmonary hypertension in newborns.

QSEN: Safety

Dosages for Common Beta Blockers for Heart Failure

Drug	Dosage
carvedilol ❶ (Coreg, Coreg CR)	*Adults:* 3.125 mg orally twice daily (do not exceed 25-50 mg twice daily; weight-based dose); CR (controlled release)—10 mg daily (increase every 2 weeks; do not exceed 80 mg daily)
metoprolol ❶ (Toprol XL)	*Adults:* 12.5-25 mg orally once daily (do not exceed 200 mg/day)

❶ High-alert drug.

VASODILATORS

How Vasodilators Work

Vasodilators are a class of drugs that act directly on the peripheral arteries to cause them to dilate (widen). This leads to lowering of blood pressure and decreases the workload of the heart. Vasodilators are often given to patients who cannot take ACE inhibitors or angiotensin II receptor blockers. The vasodilator that is most commonly prescribed for heart failure is hydralazine (Apresoline).

Other vasodilators used for treating chronic heart failure include isosorbide dinitrate (Isordil) and nitroglycerin. Isosorbide dinitrate and nitroglycerin (NTG) produce greater venous vasodilation than arterial vasodilation. Nitroglycerin also increases coronary blood flow by dilating the coronary arteries. With vasodilation the heart is better able to pump blood out to meet the needs of the body. Be sure to consult a drug handbook for information about any specific vasodilator.

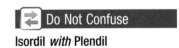

Do Not Confuse

Isordil *with* Plendil

An order for Isordil may be confused with Plendil. Isordil is a vasodilator, whereas Plendil is a calcium channel blocker.

QSEN: Safety

Dosages for Common Vasodilators for Heart Failure

Drug	Dosage
hydrALAZINE (Apresoline)	*Adults:* 25-50 mg orally 4 times daily; may increase to 300 mg daily in 3-4 divided doses
isosorbide dinitrate (Isordil, Imdur, Ismo, Isotrate ER, Monoket)	*Adults:* Ismo and Monoket: 20 mg orally twice daily 7 hours apart *Adults:* Imdur: 30-60 mg orally once daily (up to 240 mg/day)

Continued

Dosages for Common Vasodilators for Heart Failure—cont'd

Drug	Dosage
nitroglycerin (many brand names)	*Adults:* Sublingual or buccal: 0.3-0.6 mg; may repeat every 5 minutes 3 times *Adults:* Sublingual or lingual spray: 1-2 sprays; may repeat every 5 minutes 3 times *Adults:* Oral (sustained-release capsules): 2.5-9 mg every 6-8 hr *Adults:* IV: 5 mcg/min; may increase as needed *Adults:* Transdermal ointment: 1-2 inches every 6-8 hours *Adults:* Transdermal patch: 0.1-0.8 mg/hr up to 0.8 mg/hr; patch is worn 12-14 hr/day.

Common Side Effects

Vasodilators

Tachycardia   Hypernatremia   Headache

Dizziness   Hypotension

Administration Alert

Wear gloves to administer nitroglycerin ointment to prevent absorbing the drug through your skin.

QSEN: Safety

Administration Alert

Remove a patient's nitroglycerin ointment or patch during the time when he or she has his or her longest sleep period, usually at night before bedtime.

QSEN: Safety

Intended Responses

- Vasodilation of arteries (hydralazine) is increased.
- Venous vasodilation (nitroglycerin, isosorbide) is increased.
- Blood flow to coronary arteries (nitroglycerin) is increased.
- Blood pressure is lowered.
- Heart workload is decreased.

Side Effects. Common side effects of hydralazine include tachycardia and salt retention. Common side effects of nitroglycerin and isosorbide include hypotension, headache, dizziness, and tachycardia. Allergic reactions include skin rash, especially on the face.

Adverse Effects. Adverse effects are very rare with hydralazine. They include neutropenia and shock with overdose. Neutropenia is an acute disease marked by high fever and a sharp drop in circulating white blood cells. Decreased white blood cells can lead to life-threatening infections. Adverse effects of nitroglycerin and isosorbide are also very rare. Circulatory collapse and shock may occur with nitroglycerin overdose.

What To Do *Before* Giving Vasodilators

In addition to the general responsibilities related to heart failure therapy (pp. 277-278), wear gloves when administering nitroglycerin ointment. This drug can cause headaches if it is absorbed through the skin. Squeeze the ointment onto the special ruled paper. Choose an unused site on a hairless area of the patient's chest, back, or upper arm. Place the application paper on the skin drug side down. Gently press on the paper to evenly disperse the drug. Be careful not to spread ointment outside the borders of the paper. Put tape over the paper to keep it in place (Figure 17-6).

What To Do *After* Giving Vasodilators

In addition to the general responsibilities related to heart failure therapy (p. 278), for safe skin care, be sure to apply nitroglycerin drug patches or ointments to a different site with each dose. Remove the previous dose and use a tissue to clean off any ointment left on the patient's skin before applying the next dose. Avoid rubbing the skin too much because this can cause more ointment to be absorbed or could tear the skin. Note that leaving the ointment from the previous dose on a patient's skin is like giving a double dose of the drug.

Nitroglycerin (ointment or patch) loses its effectiveness when used continuously. This is why it is good to have some "drug-free" time during a 24-hour period. Be sure to remove the patches at night or when the patient has his or her longest sleeping period because the heart is less stressed during that time.

Monitor intake and output. Check the patient's feet and ankles for swelling. Listen with a stethoscope for crackles in the lungs. Ask the patient about headache or dizziness. A mild headache pain reliever such as acetaminophen (Tylenol) may be required for headaches related to nitroglycerin.

What To *Teach* Patients About Vasodilators

In addition to general precautions related to drugs for heart failure (p. 278), teach patients to contact the prescriber if more than two doses are missed because these drugs should be discontinued gradually. When the drugs are stopped suddenly, blood vessels constrict too much (known as a rebound response), causing less blood flow to the heart and a rapid rise in blood pressure.

Tell patients to report any heart rate increase of more than 20 beats per minute. An increase in headaches, dizziness, or light-headedness should also be reported to the prescriber.

Remind patients that sublingual and buccal nitroglycerin should be kept in place until dissolved. Nitroglycerin should cause a tingling sensation, which indicates that the drug is potent. Patients should not eat or drink until the tablet is dissolved. Note that if one tablet does not relieve chest pain, the patient should notify the prescriber.

Teach patients to store nitroglycerin tablets in the drug container distributed by the pharmacy. Remind them that the drug degrades (loses its strength or potency) quickly, especially when exposed to light or moisture. *A nitroglycerin tablet that has lost its potency will not have any helpful effect.* Also remind patients to make certain the drug container is labeled so that if another person is helping them during an attack of chest pain, the right drug will be given.

Instruct patients about the proper techniques for using nitroglycerin ointment or patches. Remind them to remove these drugs at night or during the period of their longest rest or sleep (e.g., a person who works nights should remove the drug while sleeping during the day).

Teach patients that although acetaminophen may be needed at first to relieve headaches, most people develop a tolerance for nitroglycerin and isosorbide, and the headaches decrease or disappear.

Tell patients to weigh themselves and check their feet and ankles for swelling at least twice a week. A weight gain of more than 3 pounds in 1 week is a result of water retention, which is an indicator of worsening heart failure and should be reported to the prescriber.

Life Span Considerations for Vasodilators

Pediatric Considerations. Safe use of isosorbide and nitroglycerin has not been established for children. Hydralazine dosage is based on weight and has been used safely with children.

Considerations for Pregnancy and Lactation. Isosorbide and nitroglycerin have a low to moderate likelihood of increasing the risk for birth defects or fetal damage. They may affect fetal circulation and should be used with caution during pregnancy. Hydralazine has been used safely for blood pressure control during pregnancy.

Considerations for Older Adults. Older adults may be more sensitive to the hypotensive effects of vasodilators. They may need to be started on lower doses. Older adults are more likely to develop orthostatic hypotension while taking vasodilators, and their risk of falls is increased. Stress the need to change positions slowly and use handrails when going up or down steps. In addition, warn older adults not to drive or operate heavy equipment until they know how vasodilators affect them.

CARDIAC GLYCOSIDES (DIGOXIN)

How Cardiac Glycosides Work

Cardiac glycosides are a class of drugs that improve heart failure by slowing down a heart rate that is too fast, allowing more time for the left ventricle to fill. They also work on the muscle fibers in the heart and increase the force of each heart beat (contractility). Both of these actions improve cardiac output. Digoxin is used for maintenance therapy with heart failure. It comes in oral (tablet, capsules, elixir) and IV forms. Prescribed doses are age and weight dependent. Digoxin doses also vary

Drug Alert!

Teaching Alert

Teach patients that a tingling sensation indicates a potent nitroglycerin tablet.

QSEN: Safety

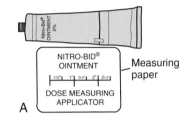

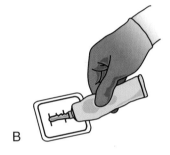

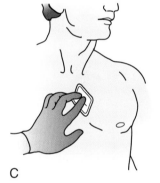

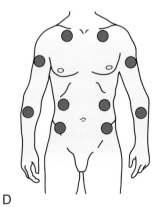

FIGURE 17-6 Application of nitroglycerin ointment. **A,** Check ointment dose and paper. **B,** Apply dose to the paper. **C,** Apply paper with the drug to the patient. **D,** Appropriate sites for drug application.

Drug Alert!

Teaching Alert

Sublingual and buccal nitroglycerin should not be swallowed. When swallowed, the liver destroys most of the drug so it is not effective.

QSEN: Safety

Memory Jogger

Intravenous (IV) hydralazine can also be used to treat high blood pressure associated with eclampsia (a serious condition that leads to seizures caused by high blood pressure) during pregnancy.

QSEN: Safety

Drug Alert!

Administration Alert

The dosages for digoxin are very low compared with those for most drugs. Be sure to calculate the correct dose carefully.

QSEN: Safety

Common Side Effects

Digoxin

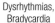

Dysrhythmias, Bradycardia   Fatigue   Anorexia, Nausea/Vomiting

Clinical Pitfall

Report common side effects of digoxin to the prescriber immediately because they are probably signs of digoxin toxicity, which can be life threatening.

QSEN: Safety

Drug Alert!

Action/Intervention Alert

Digoxin has a very narrow therapeutic range (0.8 to 2 ng/mL), and levels above 2 ng/mL are considered toxic. When a patient shows any signs of overdose (digoxin toxicity), a blood level for digoxin is drawn, and the dose is held.

QSEN: Safety

according to whether the dose is a loading or a maintenance dose. Be sure to consult a drug handbook for information about any specific cardiac glycoside.

Dosages for Common Cardiac Glycosides

Drug	Dosage
digoxin ❶ (Digitek, Lanoxicaps, Lanoxin, Digitaline ✚, Nativelle)	*Digitalizing (Loading) Doses* *Adults:* Oral tablets: 0.5-0.75 mg, then 0.125-0.375 mg every 6-8 hr (total of 0.75-1.25 mg in 24 hr) *Adults:* Oral capsules: 0.4-0.6 mg, then 0.1-0.3 mg every 6-8 hr (total of 0.6-1 mg in 24 hr) *Adults:* IV: 0.4-0.6 mg, then 0.1-0.3 mg every 6-8 hr (total of 0.6-1 mg in 24 hr) *Children over 10 years:* 10-15 mcg/kg orally or IV *Children 2-10 years:* 20-40 mcg/kg orally or IV *Children less than 2 years:* 40-60 mcg/kg orally or IV *Term neonate:* 25-35 mcg/kg orally or IV *Preterm neonate:* 20 mcg/kg orally or IV (Children and neonate digitalizing doses are divided into three or more doses, with the first dose one half of the total; give the second and third doses at 6- to 8-hour intervals.) *Maintenance Doses* *Adults:* 0.1-0.375 mg/day orally or IV *Children over 10 years:* 3-5 mcg/day orally or IV *Children 5-10 years:* 7.5-10 mcg/kg/day orally or IV *Children 2-5 years:* 10-15 mcg/kg/day orally or IV *Term neonate:* 8-10 mcg/kg/day orally or IV *Premature neonate:* 4-8 mcg/kg/day orally or IV (Dose varies depending on drug form and route ordered)

❶ High-alert drug.

Intended Responses
- Contractility is increased.
- Cardiac output is increased.
- Heart rate is decreased.

Side Effects. The most common side effects of digoxin (Lanoxin) are heart rhythm disturbances that are related to digoxin toxicity. Other common side effects to watch for include fatigue, bradycardia (slow heart rate less than 60 beats per minute), anorexia (loss of appetite), nausea, and vomiting.

Adverse Effects. Signs and symptoms of overdose include early signs such as loss of appetite, nausea, vomiting, diarrhea, or vision problems. Other signs include changes in heart rate or rhythm (irregular or slow), palpitations, or fainting. In infants and small children the earliest signs of overdose are changes in heart rate and rhythm. Children may not have the same symptoms as adults.

Dysrhythmias (abnormal and irregular heart rhythms) caused by digoxin can be life threatening.

What To Do *Before* Giving Cardiac Glycosides

In addition to the general responsibilities related to heart failure therapy (pp. 277-278), check the apical heart rate with a stethoscope for a full minute because these drugs can decrease heart rate and cause dysrhythmias. Note whether the heart rate is regular or irregular. If it is less than 60 beats per minute, greater than 100 beats per minute, or irregular, notify the prescriber. For a heart rate lower than 60 beats per minute, hold the dose, notify the prescriber, and ask whether the patient should receive this drug.

If the prescriber has ordered a cardiac monitor for the patient, make sure that the monitor is in place and ask the monitor watcher about the patient's baseline rhythm.

Ask female patients of childbearing years if they are pregnant, breastfeeding, or planning to become pregnant because digoxin passes from the mother to the fetus and also passes into breast milk.

Ask patients if they have a history of electrolyte disorders, heart rhythm problems, kidney or liver disease, or thyroid disease. Check the patient's serum potassium level and notify the prescriber if it is low (a low potassium level increases the risk for digoxin toxicity).

What To Do *After* Giving Cardiac Glycosides

In addition to the general responsibilities related to heart failure therapy (p. 278), check the apical heart rate for a full minute after giving each dose of this drug. After giving the drug, if the heart rate is less than 60 beats per minute or irregular, notify the prescriber.

If the patient is on a heart monitor, ask the monitor watcher whether his or her heart rate and rhythm have changed after each dose. Check the patient's current potassium, magnesium, and calcium laboratory values. Abnormal values may affect how this drug works. Monitor the patient for signs and symptoms of digoxin overdose such as loss of appetite, nausea, vomiting, and vision problems.

What To *Teach* Patients About Cardiac Glycosides

In addition to the general precautions related to drugs for heart failure (p. 278), explain that the heart rate should be checked every day before taking digoxin. Remind patients to tell the prescriber if their heart rate drops below 60 beats per minute, is greater than 100 beats per minute, or becomes irregular. Describe the signs and symptoms of overdose and instruct patients to report any of these to the prescriber.

Remind patients to weigh themselves every day and to report a weight gain of greater than 2 pounds per day to the prescriber.

Teach patients to take digoxin exactly as ordered by the prescriber. Digoxin should be taken every day at the same time, and a dose should not be skipped. A missed dose may be taken within 12 hours of its scheduled time. After that time, it should be skipped because a double dose can lead to toxicity.

Remind patients to avoid taking antacids within 2 hours of digoxin because antacids can affect the absorption of this drug.

Life Span Considerations for Cardiac Glycosides

Pediatric Considerations. Doses of digoxin are specific and age related. It has been used in newborns and children of all ages.

Considerations for Pregnancy and Lactation. Digoxin has a low to moderate likelihood of increasing the risk for birth defects or fetal damage. It passes from the mother to the fetus during pregnancy. It also passes to the baby through breast milk. Therefore breastfeeding is not recommended during digoxin therapy.

Considerations for Older Adults. Older adults are more sensitive to the effects of this drug and more likely to develop side effects, including digitalis toxicity. In addition, older adults may be taking diuretics that alter blood potassium levels, increasing the risk for changes in the activity of cardiac glycosides. Encourage older adults to take their medication exactly as prescribed and to keep all appointments for laboratory work to measure potassium and drug levels.

DIURETICS

Spironolactone (Aldactone), a potassium-sparing diuretic, is used to treat heart failure when systolic dysfunction is present. When prescribed in low doses, this drug

 Drug Alert!

Administration Alert

Always check the apical heart rate for a full minute before giving a cardiac glycoside.

QSEN: Safety

 Did You Know?

Foxglove is the name of a common garden plant that contains digitalis. Foxglove and its extract digitalis have been used as both a poison and a heart drug for hundreds of years.

 Drug Alert!

Administration Alert

Always check a patient's serum potassium level before giving a dose of digoxin. Prescribed diuretics can lead to low potassium, which increases the risk for digoxin toxicity.

QSEN: Safety

 Drug Alert!

Teaching Alert

Teach patients taking digoxin to check their pulse before taking the drug. Tell them to notify the prescriber if their heart rate is slower than 60 beats per minute, faster than 100 beats per minute, or irregular.

QSEN: Safety

 Drug Alert!

Teaching Alert

Remind patients to take the digoxin dose at the same time every day and to not take the drug with antacids.

QSEN: Safety

blocks the action of aldosterone, which causes the body to hold on to salt and water. When spironolactone is prescribed, another diuretic usually will also be prescribed at its regular dose to decrease the volume of fluid in the blood vessels and reduce the workload of the heart. Used together, these drugs help the body maintain a more normal blood potassium level.

For more information on diuretics and the usual doses of thiazide and loop diuretics, see Chapter 15. The doses of potassium-sparing diuretics when they are used to treat heart failure are listed in the following table. Be sure to consult a drug handbook for information about any specific diuretic.

Dosages for Common Potassium-Sparing Diuretics for Heart Failure

Drug	Dosage
amiloride (Midamor)	*Adults:* 5-10 mg orally daily
spironolactone (Aldactone)	*Adults:* 12.5-50 mg orally daily *Children:* 1-3 mg/kg orally daily
triamterene (Dyrenium)	*Adults:* 50-100 mg orally twice daily *Children:* 2-4 mg/kg orally once daily or once every other day

HUMAN B-TYPE NATRIURETIC PEPTIDES

How Natriuretic Peptides Work

Nesiritide (Natrecor) is **human B-type natriuretic peptide**, which is a hormone that is produced by the heart ventricles and a synthetic drug. The actions of this drug include increased water elimination and blood vessel dilation. Both are helpful when treating a patient with heart failure. This drug is given by the IV route and helps the body get rid of extra salt and water, thus lowering blood pressure. As a result, the patient is less short of breath and has less edema.

Dosages for Common Natriuretic Peptides for Heart Failure

Drug	Dosage
nesiritide ❶ (Natrecor)	*Adults:* 2 mcg/kg IV bolus followed by 0.01 mcg/kg/min continuous infusion

❶ High-alert drug.

Intended Responses
- Excess sodium and water in the body are decreased.
- Urine output is increased.
- Vasodilation is increased.
- Blood pressure is lowered
- Shortness of breath and swelling are decreased.

Side Effects. Side effects of natriuretic peptides include hypotension, dizziness, light-headedness, frequent urination, nausea, vomiting, nervousness, confusion, and palpitations.

Adverse Effects. Apnea (absence of breathing) is a life-threatening adverse effect of nesiritide.

What To Do *Before* Giving Nesiritide

In addition to the general responsibilities related to heart failure therapy (pp. 277-278), monitor for normal heart rate (60 to 100 beats per minute), blood pressure, and respiratory rate (12 to 20 breaths per minute). Remember that apnea is a life-threatening adverse effect of this drug.

? Did You Know?

Nesiritide is also a naturally occurring hormone that is produced by the ventricles of the heart.

Common Side Effects

Natriuretic Peptides

Hypotension Dizziness Frequent urination

Nausea Confusion Palpitations

Check the IV site for patency. Look for any signs of infection. This drug is given as an IV bolus followed by a continuous infusion.

What To Do *After* Giving Nesiritide

In addition to the general responsibilities related to heart failure therapy (p. 278), continue to monitor blood pressure, heart rate, and respiratory rate during nesiritide infusion. Continue to check the IV line for patency and signs of infection. Tell the patient to report any pain or discomfort at the IV site.

What To *Teach* Patients About Nesiritide

In addition to the general precautions related to drugs for heart failure (p. 278), explain to patients why this drug has been prescribed and how it will help them. Tell patients that frequent blood pressure checks are necessary to screen for hypotension and that you will be measuring urine output.

Life Span Considerations for Nesiritide

Nesiritide appears to have a low to moderate likelihood of increasing the risk for birth defects or fetal harm. However, it has not been tested during pregnancy or in children. Older adults have the same side effects as younger adults but are at greater risk for confusion. Teach family members to assess the level of alertness and thought processes of an older adult who has recently started taking prescribed nesiritide, especially during the first week of drug therapy.

POSITIVE INOTROPES (HEART PUMP DRUGS)

How Positive Inotropes Work

Positive inotropes are heart pump drugs that make the heart muscle contract more forcefully. They also relax blood vessels so blood can flow better. These drugs are used for people with severe heart failure symptoms. They are given intravenously to stimulate stronger heart contractions and keep blood circulating. Although some patients with heart failure receive these drugs while in the hospital, many also receive them at home using an infusion pump.

Do Not Confuse

DOPamine *with* DOBUTamine

An order for DOPamine can be confused with DOBUTamine. Both drugs are positive inotropes that increase the force of heart contractions.

QSEN: Safety

Drug Alert!

Administration Alert

The effects of DOPamine are dose related. Low-dose DOPamine (0.5-3 mcg/kg/min) causes renal vasodilation and increased urine output. Moderate-dose DOPamine (2-20 mcg/kg/min) causes increased force of heart contraction. High-dose DOPamine (more than 10 mcg/kg/min) causes peripheral vasoconstriction to increase blood pressure.

QSEN: Safety

Dosages for Common Positive Inotropes

Drug	IV Dosage
inamrinone ❶ (Inocor)	*Adults:* 0.75 mg/kg loading dose followed by 5-10 mcg/kg/min continuous infusion *Infants:* 3-4.5 mg/kg in divided doses followed by 5-10 mcg/kg/min infusion *Neonates:* 3-4.5 mg/kg in divided doses followed by 3-5 mcg/kg/min infusion
DOBUTamine ❶ (Dobutrex)	*Adults/Children:* Start low (0.5-1 mcg/kg/min) and titrate up as needed (usual range is 2-20 mcg/kg/min)
DOPamine ❶ (Intropin)	*Adults:* 2-50 mcg/kg/min *Children:* 2-30 mcg/kg/min
milrinone ❶ (Primacor)	*Adults:* Loading dose 50 mcg/kg followed by continuous infusion (0.375-0.75 mcg/kg/min)

❶ High-alert drug.

Intended Responses

- Contractility is increased.
- Cardiac output is increased.
- Blood vessel dilation is increased.
- Preload and afterload are decreased.
- Heart function and contractility are improved.
- Blood pressure is lowered.
- Circulation is improved.

Common Side Effects
Positive Inotropes

Hypertension   Tachycardia, Dysrhythmias

⚠ Drug Alert!
Administration Alert

Positive inotropic (heart-pump) drugs are given intravenously. Be sure that the IV line is patent so the drug does not go into the patient's tissues and cause damage.

QSEN: Safety

⚠ Drug Alert!
Teaching Alert

Positive inotropes are often given in the home setting because heart failure is a chronic disease. It is important to teach patients how to monitor the IV site and how to use the infusion pump.

QSEN: Safety

⚠ Drug Alert!
Administration Alert

Check and recheck the concentration of potassium to be sure it matches the prescriber's order before administering the drug. *Never* give potassium via IV push.

QSEN: Safety

Side Effects. Common side effects of positive inotrope drugs include hypertension, increased heart rate, premature ventricular contractions, and other dysrhythmias.

Inamrinone and milrinone can cause hypotension.

Adverse Effects. Ventricular dysrhythmias may occur with milrinone and may be life threatening. Rarely a patient may have allergic reactions to these drugs, including rash, fever, bronchospasm, and chest pain.

What To Do *Before* Giving Positive Inotropes

In addition to the general responsibilities related to heart failure therapy (pp. 277-278), during infusion of a heart-pump drug, frequently monitor the patient's heart rate and blood pressure (at least every 1 to 2 hours). Make sure that the patient's IV line is patent. Double check the IV rate by asking another nurse to check the calculation. These drugs cause vasoconstriction, so if infiltration occurs, reduced blood flow to the tissues can result in severe tissue damage and even tissue necrosis.

Ask whether the patient has a history of high blood pressure or heart dysrhythmias.

What To Do *After* Giving Positive Inotropes

In addition to the general responsibilities related to heart failure therapy (p. 278), watch the IV site for patency and any signs of infection such as pain, redness, swelling, and warmth. Remind the patient to immediately report any pain or discomfort at the IV site. Continue to check blood pressure and heart rate while a patient is receiving these drugs.

What To *Teach* Patients About Positive Inotropes

In addition to the general precautions related to drugs for heart failure (p. 278), teach patients about the signs and symptoms of IV lines that are no longer patent or that have developed an infection (for example, burning or pain, redness, swelling, warmth). Tell them to report any of these signs immediately.

For patients receiving these drugs at home, demonstrate how to use the infusion pump. Instruct them to report any problems with the pump immediately.

Tell patients why this drug has been ordered and give instructions not to stop the drug unless told to do so by the prescriber. Teach patients to inform the prescriber of any chest pain, dyspnea, numbness, or tingling or burning in the extremities.

Life Span Considerations for Positive Inotropes

Safe use of these drugs has not been determined during pregnancy or breastfeeding or with children. Positive inotrope drugs have a low to moderate likelihood of increasing the risk for birth defects or fetal harm.

Considerations for Older Adults. Older adults may be more likely to experience adverse effects of these drugs, especially chest pain and hypertension. Monitor the older adult receiving any positive inotropic drug at least every 2 hours for changes in blood pressure, heart rate, and heart rhythm.

POTASSIUM AND MAGNESIUM

How Potassium and Magnesium Work

Potassium is an important electrolyte that is essential for a healthy nervous system and a regular heart rhythm. **Magnesium** is a major mineral and is the fourth most abundant mineral in the human body. It helps the heart rhythm remain steady.

Patients taking diuretic drugs for heart failure can lose potassium and magnesium in their urine. To keep blood levels of potassium and magnesium within normal ranges, supplements are often prescribed.

Dosages for Common Potassium and Magnesium Supplements

Drug	Dosage
potassium ❶ (K-Dur, K-Lor, Kaon CL, K-Lyte, Slow-K, Klotrix, Kaochlor 10%)	*Adults:* PO: 20 mEq orally daily to prevent potassium deficit; 40-100 mEq orally daily to treat potassium deficit *Adults:* IV: Up to 200-400 mEq IV drip daily; do *not* exceed 10 mEq/hr *Children:* PO: 2-5 mEq/kg orally daily *Children:* IV: Up to 3 mEq/kg IV drip daily
magnesium ❶ (Max-Oxide, Uro-Mag)	Oral doses are age dependent: *Adults/Children older than 10 years:* 270-400 mg daily *Children:* 3-6 mg/kg daily in 3-4 divided doses.

❶ High alert drug.

Intended Responses

- Blood values for potassium and magnesium are normal (see Table 1-4 in Chapter 1).
- Low potassium and magnesium levels are prevented or corrected.
- Some abnormal heart rhythms are prevented.
- Heart muscle excitability is decreased.

Side Effects. Common side effects of potassium and magnesium include nausea, vomiting, diarrhea, gas, and abdominal discomfort.

When potassium is given intravenously, it can cause irritation at the IV site.

Adverse Effects. High potassium or magnesium levels can cause life-threatening electrocardiogram (ECG) changes and abnormal heart rhythms. *Potassium should never be given via IV push.*

Black, tarry, or bloody stools are signs of stomach bleeding and should be reported to the prescriber immediately.

Adverse effects with magnesium sulfate are rare and include complete heart block and respiratory arrest. With higher doses, muscle weakness and a loss of deep tendon reflexes can occur.

What To Do *Before* Giving Potassium or Magnesium

In addition to the general responsibilities related to heart failure therapy (pp. 277-278), check and recheck the dosage of potassium prescribed and the concentration of the drug in the vial. Concentrations vary considerably. An overdose of intravenous potassium can be lethal.

If the patient is on a heart monitor, check the heart rhythm or ask the monitor watcher about it. Check the patient's current laboratory values for potassium and magnesium. If these values are outside of the normal range, notify the prescriber. (See Table 1-4 for a listing of normal ranges.)

If the potassium level is low (less than 3.5 mEq/L), assess handgrip strength and bowel sounds at least every shift. Also assess respiratory rate and effort and oxygen saturation. Notify the prescriber if oxygen saturation drops below 90%.

What To Do *After* Giving Potassium or Magnesium

In addition to the general responsibilities related to heart failure therapy (p. 278), make sure that any follow-up laboratory values are drawn and sent to the laboratory.

If the patient has an IV site, recheck it for signs of irritation every 2 to 4 hours. Instruct the patient to report any pain or discomfort in the IV site immediately.

Watch for signs of potassium overdose *(hyperkalemia),* including slow and irregular heart rhythm, fatigue, muscle weakness, *paresthesia* (numbness and tingling), confusion, difficulty breathing, and ECG changes.

Common Side Effects

Potassium and Magnesium

Nausea/Vomiting, Diarrhea, Gas, Abdominal Discomfort

 Drug Alert!

Administration Alert

Monitor the IV site carefully when a patient is receiving IV potassium because this drug can be very irritating to peripheral IV sites. Give it with an infusion pump or controller to ensure safe administration. Do not ignore a patient's reports of pain or discomfort at the IV site.

QSEN: Safety

 Drug Alert!

Administration Alert

Potassium is a high-alert drug because it can lead to serious harm if given at too high a dose, given to a patient for whom it was not prescribed, or not given to a patient for whom it was prescribed.

QSEN: Safety

Box 17-3	Dietary Sources of Potassium

- Baked potato
- Bananas
- Beet greens
- Clams
- Halibut, tuna, cod fish
- Molasses
- Prune, carrot, tomato juice
- Soybeans
- Spinach
- Sweet potato
- Tomato paste, sauce, puree
- White, lima beans
- Winter squash
- Yogurt

Box 17-4	Dietary Sources of Magnesium

- Almonds
- Black beans
- Bran cereal
- Brazil nuts
- Buckwheat flour
- Cashews
- Halibut
- Mixed nuts
- Pumpkin and squash seed kernels
- Sesame seeds
- Soybeans
- Spinach
- Walnuts
- White beans
- Whole grain rice

Memory Jogger

Signs of increased blood potassium level include slow and irregular heart rhythm, fatigue, muscle weakness, paresthesia (numbness and tingling), confusion, difficulty breathing, and ECG changes.

Memory Jogger

Signs of increased blood magnesium level include muscle and generalized weakness, decreased reflexes (neuromuscular depression), hypotension, abnormal cardiac rhythm, drowsiness, decreased alertness and concentration, decreased rate of breathing/respiratory paralysis, CNS depression, and coma.

Also watch for signs of increased magnesium level such as muscle and generalized weakness, decreased reflexes (neuromuscular depression), hypotension, abnormal cardiac rhythm, drowsiness, decreased alertness and concentration, decreased rate of breathing/respiratory paralysis, central nervous system (CNS) depression, and coma.

Cardiac changes with high levels of magnesium include bradycardia, peripheral vasodilation, and hypotension. ECG changes show a prolonged PR interval and a widened QRS complex. Bradycardia can be severe and cardiac arrest is possible. Hypotension is also severe with a diastolic pressure lower than normal. *Patients with severe hypermagnesemia are in grave danger of cardiac arrest.*

What To *Teach* Patients About Potassium and Magnesium

In addition to the general precautions related to drugs for heart failure (p. 278), tell patients why a potassium or magnesium supplement has been ordered. If they miss a dose, it should be taken within 2 hours. *Patients should not take a double dose of either potassium or magnesium.* Instruct them to take potassium and magnesium supplements with food or right after meals with a full glass of water or fruit juice. Taking potassium on an empty stomach can cause nausea and vomiting.

Remind patients to avoid using salt substitutes that contain potassium. Provide a list of dietary sources of potassium (Box 17-3) and magnesium (Box 17-4).

Teach patients about the signs of too much potassium (such as palpitations, skipped heart beats, muscle twitching or weakness, or numbness and tingling) and tell them to report these signs to the prescriber immediately. Advise patients to have any laboratory values drawn as instructed to monitor responses to these supplements.

Life Span Considerations for Potassium and Magnesium

Considerations for Pregnancy and Lactation. Potassium has a low to moderate likelihood of increasing the risk for birth defects or fetal harm. Magnesium sulfate is safe to give during pregnancy. It is used during labor to lower the risk of seizures for patients with eclampsia. The infant may have decreased reflexes for the first 24 hours after birth when magnesium is used during labor.

OTHER DRUGS USED TO TREAT HEART FAILURE

Anticoagulants such as heparin and warfarin (Coumadin) prevent clots from forming or getting bigger and may be prescribed to treat heart failure (refer to Chapter 20).

The antidysrhythmic drug amiodarone (Cordarone) may be used to prevent or treat irregular heart rhythms that begin in the ventricles such as ventricular tachycardia (refer to Chapter 18). Irregular heart rhythms can be life threatening.

Get Ready for Practice!

Key Points

- Most heart failure is caused by high blood pressure.
- Most heart failure begins in the left ventricle and progresses to right heart failure.
- Left heart failure causes symptoms in the lungs, and right heart failure causes peripheral symptoms.
- Drugs for heart failure are prescribed to make physical activity more comfortable, improve quality of life, and prolong life.
- The only cure for heart failure is a heart transplant because the damage to the heart muscle is not reversible.
- Angiotensin-converting enzyme (ACE) inhibitors, angiotensin II receptor blockers (ARBs), vasodilators, and human B-type natriuretic peptides may be prescribed to decrease afterload.
- Diuretics may be prescribed to decrease preload by reducing the circulating blood volume.
- Digoxin and other positive inotropic drugs increase the force of heart contraction.
- Always check the heart rate for a full minute before giving a cardiac glycoside (digoxin).
- Digoxin (Lanoxin) has a narrow therapeutic range (0.8 to 2 ng/mL), and a value above 2 is considered toxic.
- Low-dose spironolactone (Aldactone) is used to block the action of aldosterone, a hormone that causes the body to hold on to salt and water.
- Instruct patients to report weight gain of more than 2 pounds in a day or 5 pounds in a week to the prescriber.
- Nesiritide (Natrecor) (a human B-type natriuretic peptide) causes water elimination and blood vessel dilation.
- Dopamine (Intropin), a positive inotropic drug, has effects that are dose related. At low doses, it increases kidney perfusion; at moderate doses, it increases contractility of the heart muscle; and at high doses, it causes constriction of the blood vessels.
- Rates of IV drugs for heart failure should always be controlled by an infusion controller device.

Additional Learning Resources

evolve Be sure to visit your Evolve website (http://evolve.elsevier.com/Workman/pharmacology/) for additional online resources.

SG Go to your Study Guide for additional learning activities to help you master this chapter content.

Review Questions

See the Answer Keys—In-text Review Questions for answers to these questions.

Test Yourself on the Basics
1. Which drug produces more venous vasodilation than arterial vasodilation?
   A. Digoxin
   B. Isosorbide
   C. Capoten
   D. Dobutamine
2. Before administering a dose of digoxin, which action is essential?
   A. Perform orthostatic vital signs.
   B. Place the patient on a cardiac monitor.
   C. Assess lungs for abnormal sounds such as crackles.
   D. Listen to the apical heart rate for a full minute.
3. What must you teach a patient about how to take sublingual nitroglycerine?
   A. Place the drug between your cheek and gums.
   B. Drink a full glass or water with the drug.
   C. Notify the prescriber every time you use this drug.
   D. A tingling sensation tells you that the drug is potent.
4. When you administer a vasodilator drug to an older adult, what is the primary risk?
   A. Severe headache
   B. Increased risk for falls
   C. Sudden increase in blood pressure
   D. Acute heart attack
5. Which foods will you teach patients are good sources of magnesium? (Select all that apply.)
   A. Bananas
   B. Almonds
   C. Black beans
   D. Sweet potatoes
   E. Soybeans
   F. Yogurt
   G. Molasses

Test Yourself on Advanced Concepts
6. A patient who has just been prescribed enalapril (Vasotec) for heart failure asks you how the drug will work. What is your best response?
   A. "It will cause your arteries and veins to dilate."
   B. "It will slow your heart rate."
   C. "It will decrease the fluid and sodium in your blood and tissues."
   D. "It will increase the contraction strength of your heart."

7. Which symptoms will you likely see in a patient with left heart failure? (Select all that apply.)
   A. Weak peripheral pulses
   B. Full jugular veins when sitting
   C. Pulmonary congestion
   D. Weight gain
   E. Hacking cough that is worse at night
   F. Crackles in the lungs

8. A patient was recently started on nitroglycerin ointment 1 inch every 6 hours. The patient asks you why the patch is removed at night. What is your best response?
   A. "I will contact the pharmacy and let you know the answer to this question."
   B. "This drug loses its effectiveness when it is used continuously."
   C. "A break in the use of this drug helps to protect your skin from irritation."
   D. "At night you will not need this drug because you have fewer heart failure symptoms."

9. Older adults are more sensitive to the effects of many heart failure drugs. Which drug is more likely to cause toxicity in older adults?
   A. digoxin (Lanoxin)
   B. isosorbide (Isordil)
   C. hydralazine (Apresoline)
   D. captopril (Capoten)

10. An adult patient prescribed magnesium (Max-Oxide) 400 mg by mouth daily tells you he has nausea after taking this drug. What should you teach the patient about taking this drug? (Select all that apply.)
    A. "Take your magnesium with a full glass of water."
    B. "Always take your magnesium on an empty stomach for better absorption."
    C. "You can take your magnesium right after a meal to decrease the nausea."
    D. "Over time you will develop a tolerance for magnesium, and the nausea will go away."
    E. "Always take your magnesium with food or a snack to avoid gastrointestinal symptoms."
    F. "Good food sources of magnesium include green leafy vegetables and almonds."

11. A patient is receiving dobutamine (Dobutrex) 0.5 mcg/kg/min by IV. Which manifestations indicate an infection at the IV site? (Select all that apply.)
    A. Pain at the IV site
    B. Blood in the catheter
    C. Redness at the site
    D. Hypotension
    E. Warmth at the site
    F. Swelling at the site

12. What are the most important teaching points for a patient who will go home with sublingual nitroglycerin to be used as needed for chest pains? (Select all that apply.)
    A. Keep the tablet in place under your tongue until it dissolves.
    B. Store the drug in the refrigerator to avoid exposing it to heat.
    C. You should experience a tingling sensation, which indicates that the drug is potent.
    D. If you experience a headache, acetaminophen can be taken for relief.
    E. Take the tablets with a full glass of water or juice.
    F. A decrease in blood pressure can be a side effect of this drug.

13. What should you teach the patient who has recently been prescribed nesiritide by IV infusion?
    A. Your blood pressure will be checked once a day.
    B. You may feel some burning at the IV site and that is to be expected.
    C. Monitoring your intake and output is important while you are receiving this drug.
    D. This drug rarely causes gastrointestinal side effects such as nausea.

14. A patient has been prescribed potassium bicarbonate (K-Lyte) 40 mEq to be given in 2 divided doses with a full glass of water or fruit juice. How much K-Lyte will you give with each dose? _____ mEq per dose

15. The prescriber has ordered dobutamine (Dobutrex) 0.5 mcg/kg/min for a patient who weighs 72 kg. What is the correct infusion rate for this patient? _____ mcg/min

16. A patient has been ordered digoxin (Lanoxin) 0.25 mg every morning. Digoxin is available in 0.125-mg tablets. How many tablets will you give the patient for each dose? _____ tablet(s)

Critical Thinking Activities

See the Answer Keys—Critical Thinking Activities for answers to these activities.

Mr. Lacey is a 72-year-old patient with heart failure that has been stable for the past 10 years. His signs and symptoms included: +1 bilateral lower leg swelling, visibly enlarged jugular neck veins, and crackles bilaterally in the lower lobes of his lungs. This morning he has a weight gain of 6 pounds over the past 2 days, as well as increased shortness of breath. His currently prescribed drugs include captopril (Capoten) 25 mg twice a day and furosemide (Lasix) 20 mg once a day.

1. What type of heart failure is indicated by Mr. Lacey's symptoms?
2. What does Mr. Lacey's weight gain and increased shortness of breath indicate?
3. What are the purposes of Mr. Lacey's prescribed medications?
4. What changes in Mr. Lacey's prescribed medications do you anticipate and why?
5. What are key teaching points for Mr. Lacey at this time?

Drug Therapy for Dysrhythmias

Objectives

After studying this chapter you should be able to:

1. Explain how different classes of drugs are used to treat abnormal heart rhythms.
2. List the common names, actions, usual adult dosages, possible side effects, and adverse effects of atropine, digoxin, adenosine, and magnesium sulfate.
3. Describe what to do before and after giving atropine, digoxin, adenosine, and magnesium sulfate.
4. Explain what to teach patients taking atropine, digoxin, adenosine, and magnesium sulfate, including what to do, what not to do, and when to call the prescriber.
5. Describe life span considerations for atropine, digoxin, adenosine, and magnesium sulfate.
6. List the common names, actions, usual adult dosages, possible side effects, and adverse effects of class I, II, III,

and IV antidysrhythmic drugs used to treat rapid abnormal heart rhythms.

7. Describe what to do before and after giving class I, II, III, and IV antidysrhythmic drugs used to treat rapid abnormal heart rhythms.
8. Explain what to teach patients taking class I, II, III, and IV antidysrhythmic drugs used to treat rapid abnormal heart rhythms, including what to do, what not to do, and when to call the prescriber.
9. Describe life span considerations for class I, II, III, and IV antidysrhythmic drugs used to treat rapid abnormal heart rhythms.

Key Terms

adenosine (ă-DĔN-ō-sēn) (p. 307) A drug administered intravenously for supraventricular tachycardia (SVT); adenosine can help identify SVT. Certain SVTs can be successfully terminated with adenosine.

antidysrhythmic drugs (ăn-tī-dĭs-RĬTH-Mĭk DRŬGZ) (p. 296) Drugs used to treat abnormal heart rhythms.

atropine (Ă-trō-pēn) (p. 296) A competitive muscarinic acetylcholine receptor antagonist used as a temporary treatment for abnormally slow heart rates.

beta blockers (BĚ-tă BLŎK-ěrz) (p. 304) (See Chapter 16.)

bradycardia (brā-dē-KĂR-dē-ă) (p. 293) Slow heart rate, usually considered to be less than 60 beats per minute.

bradydysrhythmia (brā-dē-dĭs-RĬTH-mē-ă) (p. 296) An abnormally slow heart rhythm.

calcium channel blockers (KĂL-sē-ŭm CHĂN-ŭl BLŎK-ěrz) (p. 307) (See Chapter 16.)

digoxin (dĭ-JŎK-sĭn) (p. 298) (See Chapter 17.)

dysrhythmia (dĭs-RĬTH-mē-ă) (p. 293) An abnormal heart rhythm.

magnesium sulfate (mă-NĒ-zē-ŭm SŬL-fāt) (p. 309) (See Chapter 17.)

potassium channel blockers (pō-TĂS-ē-ŭm BLŎK-ěrz) (p. 305) A class of drugs that act by inhibiting potassium movement through cell membranes. Blocking potassium channels lengthens the duration of action potentials.

premature contractions (prē-mă-CHŬR kŏn-TRĂK-shŭnz) (p. 294) Heart contractions that occur earlier than expected.

sodium channel blockers (SŌ-dē-ŭm CHĂN-ŭl BLŎK-ěrz) (p. 299) A class of drugs that act by inhibiting sodium movement through cell membranes. Results include slowing of the heart rate, reducing heart muscle cell excitability, and reducing speed of conduction.

tachycardia (tăk-ē-KĂR-dē-ă) (p. 293) Rapid heart rate, usually considered to be greater than 100 beats per minute.

tachydysrhythmia (tăk-ē-dĭs-RĬTH-mē-ă) (p. 298) An abnormally rapid heart rhythm.

REVIEW OF RELATED PHYSIOLOGY AND PATHOPHYSIOLOGY

Pumping blood to the body and the lungs is the basic function of the heart. The right side of the heart receives oxygen-poor blood from the body and sends it to the lungs. The left side of the heart receives oxygen-rich blood from the lungs and pumps it out to the body (Figure 18-1). To perform this function well, the heart must be strong

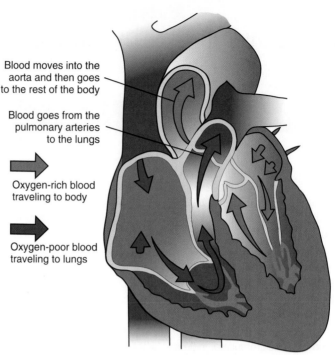

Blood moves into the aorta and then goes to the rest of the body

Blood goes from the pulmonary arteries to the lungs

Oxygen-rich blood traveling to body

Oxygen-poor blood traveling to lungs

FIGURE 18-1 Blood flow through the heart.

and have its own well-oxygenated blood supply. The blood supply to the heart muscle is delivered by the coronary arteries.

PACEMAKERS AND THE CARDIAC CONDUCTION SYSTEM

The heart has its own system of electrical impulses that travel through the heart muscle, causing the heart to contract and pump blood. It is this process, called the *electrical conduction system*, that controls the heart rate and rhythm. The part of the system that sets the heart rate and rhythm by generating impulses is called the *pacemaker*. Under normal circumstances, the *sinoatrial (SA) node*, composed of special muscle fibers capable of causing electrical impulses, is the pacemaker and controls the heart rate. The SA node initiates electrical impulses at a rate of 60 to 100 per minute. These impulses travel across pathways to the *atrioventricular (AV) node* and then down through the *His-Purkinje system* to cause the ventricles to contract and pump blood out of the heart (Figure 18-2).

When the SA node does not function, the AV node takes over as the second pacemaker of the heart. This secondary pacemaker usually causes 40 to 60 electrical impulses per minute, which results in a slower heart rate. If both the SA and the AV nodes are not working, the ventricular muscle cells become the third pacemaker of the heart, with a very slow rate of 20 to 40 impulses per minute. This slow rate of heart contractions is not enough to supply the body with the blood and oxygen it needs to function, and the patient may have symptoms such as confusion or a change in level of consciousness.

HEART RATE

Sometimes it is normal for the heart to beat faster or slower. Heart rate is related to a person's state of health and whether he or she is exercising or resting. For example, a young athlete may have a normal resting heart rate of 50 beats per minute with an exercising heart rate of 100, whereas an older adult may have a resting heart rate of 80 or 90 beats per minute and an exercising heart rate of 120 to 140. Normal heart rate ranges for adults and children are summarized in Table 18-1.

How fast the heart beats depends on how much oxygen-rich blood your body needs. During activity, excitement, fever, or shock, your body needs more

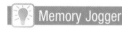

Memory Jogger

The normal pacemaker of the heart, the SA node, initiates 60 to 100 electrical impulses per minute.

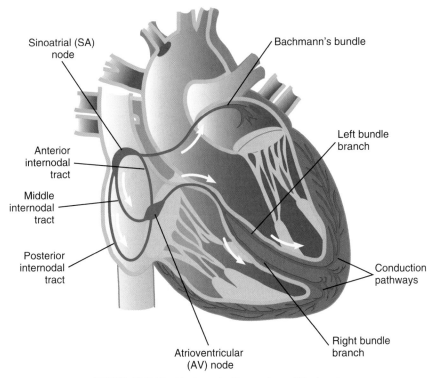

FIGURE 18-2 Electrical conduction system of the heart.

Table **18-1**	Normal Heart Rates
AGE-GROUP	**RANGE (BEATS/MIN)**
Adults	60-100
Children	70-120
Toddlers	90-150
Infants	120-160

oxygen-rich blood, so your heart rate may increase to 100 beats per minute or more. When you are resting or sleeping, your body needs less oxygen-rich blood, so your heart rate decreases sometimes to less than 60 beats per minute.

Normal Heart Rhythm

When the heart beats normally, each impulse that starts from the SA node causes the atria and ventricles to contract regularly and in sequence at a rate between 60 and 100 beats per minute. This normal rhythm of the heart is called *normal sinus rhythm* (Figure 18-3). This means that the impulse begins in the SA node and travels normally to cause the atria to contract and then to the ventricles to contract. A slow heart rhythm started by the SA node is called sinus **bradycardia** (less than 60 beats per minute). A rapid heart rhythm started by the SA node is called sinus **tachycardia** (more than 100 beats per minute).

Dysrhythmias

Dysrhythmias are abnormal heart rhythms (Box 18-1). They often begin with an abnormal unexpected impulse somewhere in the heart muscle tissue (but not from the SA node). Abnormal rhythms are often caused by problems with the electrical conduction system of the heart. Dysrhythmias may also be caused by heart muscle contractions that are irregular or faster or slower than normal. Most dysrhythmias have a negative effect on how well the heart works as a pump by decreasing *cardiac output* (the amount of blood the heart pumps in a minute).

 Memory Jogger

The electrical impulses that cause normal sinus rhythm begin in the SA node.

 Memory Jogger

A slow heart rate (less than 60 beats per minute) is bradycardia. A fast heart rate (more than 100 beats per minute) is tachycardia.

 Memory Jogger

Dysrhythmias decrease cardiac output, which leads to symptoms such as dizziness, light-headedness, fainting (syncope), and decreased peripheral pulses.

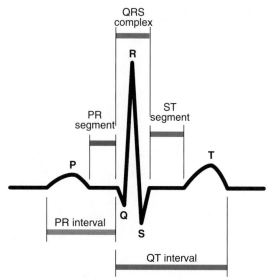

FIGURE 18-3 Normal sinus rhythm of the heart.

| Box 18-1 | List of Common Dysrhythmias |

ATRIAL
- Atrial fibrillation
- Atrial flutter
- Premature atrial contractions
- Sick sinus syndrome
- Supraventricular tachycardia

VENTRICULAR
- Asystole
- Premature ventricular contractions
- Pulseless electrical activity
- Ventricular fibrillation
- Ventricular tachycardia

JUNCTIONAL
- Junctional tachycardia
- Premature junctional contractions

HEART BLOCKS
- First-degree heart block
- Second-degree heart block
  - Mobitz type I/Wenckebach
  - Mobitz type II
- Third-degree heart block (complete heart block)

Dysrhythmias can be named according to where they begin. *Atrial dysrhythmias* begin in the atria, whereas *supraventricular dysrhythmias* originate above the ventricles and *ventricular dysrhythmias* begin within the ventricles.

Heartbeats that occur earlier than expected are called **premature contractions.** They can begin in the atria (premature atrial contractions [PACs]), in the AV node region (premature junctional contractions [PJCs]), or ventricles (premature ventricular contractions [PVCs]). A patient may notice the feeling of a skipped beat. An occasional premature beat is usually not serious; however, premature beats may lead to other serious dysrhythmias. When premature beats are frequent, cardiac output is decreased.

Other dysrhythmias cause the chambers of the heart (atria and ventricles) to quiver *(fibrillate)* instead of contracting normally and effectively. This fibrillation results from totally disorganized electrical activity and produces ineffective contraction and pumping of blood. When the atria fibrillate, it is called *atrial fibrillation.* Atrial fibrillation decreases cardiac output because the atrial portion of cardiac output is lost when the atria do not contract. *Ventricular fibrillation* is the name for the condition in which the ventricles fibrillate. Ventricular fibrillation is life threatening and can lead to death in minutes because no blood is pumped from the heart (cardiac output) when the ventricles quiver and do not contract.

Dysrhythmia Symptoms. Dysrhythmias may or may not cause symptoms in patients (Box 18-2). Often abnormal rhythms cause symptoms such as a fluttery feeling in the chest, racing heartbeats, slow heartbeats, chest pain, shortness of

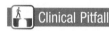
Clinical Pitfall

Without immediate intervention ventricular fibrillation leads to death within minutes.

QSEN: Safety

Box **18-2**   Common Symptoms of Dysrhythmias

- Chest pain
- Dizziness
- Fainting (syncope)
- Fluttering in the chest
- Light-headedness
- May have *no* symptoms
- Rapid heart rate
- Shortness of breath
- Slow heart rate

Box **18-3**   Risk Factors for Developing Dysrhythmias

- Age (older adults)
- Genetics (family history)
- Coronary artery disease
- Thyroid problems
  - Hypothyroidism—bradycardia
  - Hyperthyroidism—tachycardia
- Drugs and supplements
  - Cough/cold remedies with pseudoephedrine
- High blood pressure
- Obesity
- Diabetes
- Low blood sugar (hypoglycemia)
- Obstructive sleep apnea
- Electrolyte imbalance
  - Potassium
  - Sodium
  - Calcium
  - Magnesium
- Alcohol abuse
- Stimulant use
  - Caffeine
  - Nicotine
- Illicit drugs
  - Cocaine
  - Amphetamines

breath, light-headedness, dizziness, and fainting *(syncope)*. Having symptoms does not always mean having a serious dysrhythmia. Some people with symptoms do not have a serious dysrhythmia, whereas others with no symptoms may have a life-threatening dysrhythmia.

Risk Factors for Dysrhythmias. Several factors increase the risk for a person developing a heart dysrhythmia (Box 18-3). Older adults with age-related heart changes are more likely to have dysrhythmias. Genetics and family history increase the risk for them. For example, some people are born with an extra electrical impulse pathway and may develop *Wolff-Parkinson-White syndrome*, a type of dysrhythmia. Some disease processes may lead to dysrhythmias. Diabetes increases the risk for developing high blood pressure and coronary artery disease. High blood pressure and obesity increase the risk for developing coronary artery disease, with narrow arteries and heart damage that may cause abnormal heart rhythms. Thyroid problems may cause rapid or slow heart rates. *Obstructive sleep apnea* (a sleep disorder with pauses in breathing during sleep) can cause bradycardia and episodes of atrial fibrillation. Electrolyte imbalances can cause the heart to initiate abnormal electrical impulses. When electrolyte levels (such as potassium, sodium, calcium, and magnesium) are too high or too low, dysrhythmias may occur.

Drugs may also affect heart rhythm. Over-the-counter cold and cough drugs containing pseudoephedrine (for example, Sudafed) can cause tachycardia. Stimulants such as caffeine and nicotine can cause premature heartbeats and rapid (tachycardic) rhythms. Too much alcohol also can change the conduction of electrical impulses and increase the chance for atrial fibrillation. Illegal drugs such as cocaine and amphetamines can cause serious heart rhythm problems, including ventricular fibrillation, which can lead to sudden death.

Measuring the Heart Rate

The most accurate way to measure a patient's heart rate is to listen with a stethoscope over the apical region of the chest for a full minute. The apical heart rate is measured at the left fifth intercostal space in the midclavicular area (usually two fingers below the left nipple) (Figure 18-4). Listen with a stethoscope for a full minute. Count the number of heartbeats. Note any irregular rhythms.

 Clinical Pitfall

Some patients with symptoms do not have serious dysrhythmias, whereas others without symptoms may have life-threatening dysrhythmias.

QSEN: Safety

 Drug Alert!

Administration Alert

Over-the-counter cough and cold drugs that contain pseudoephedrine (Sudafed) can cause abnormal rapid heart rhythms.

QSEN: Safety

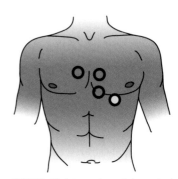

FIGURE 18-4 Location of the apical pulse.

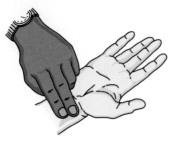

FIGURE 18-5 Checking the radial pulse.

An important part of teaching for a patient with an abnormal heart rate is how to count the heart rate. Tell the patient to obtain a watch or clock that has a second hand. Instruct him or her to place the index and middle finger of the dominant hand on the inner wrist of the opposite arm just below the base of the thumb (Figure 18-5). In this way the patient should feel the pulsing of the radial artery against the fingers. Have him or her count the number of pulse beats for a full minute. Also tell him or her to note whether the heart rhythm is regular or irregular when measuring the heart rate. A normal heart rhythm is regular.

GENERAL ISSUES RELATED TO ANTIDYSRHYTHMIC THERAPY

Antidysrhythmic drugs are used to treat abnormal heart rhythms and may be prescribed to increase or decrease the heart rate. The actions of drugs prescribed to treat rapid heart rates may be to decrease spontaneous contraction of myocardial cells, including pacemaker cells *(automaticity)*, slow ability of heart muscle cells to transmit electrical impulses *(conductivity)*, or prolong the refractory period of heart cells. The *refractory period* is the period of time after an impulse generation during which normal stimulation will not cause another impulse. During the absolute refractory period, an impulse *cannot* be conducted. During the relative refractory period, an impulse must be stronger than normal to be conducted.

Before giving any antidysrhythmic drug, be sure to get a complete list of the drugs that the patient is using, including over-the-counter and herbal drugs. Check the patient's heart rate and blood pressure. Watch for decreased or increased heart rate (less than 60 beats per minute or more than 100 beats per minute) and decreased blood pressure (less than 90/60 mm Hg), which may indicate decreased blood flow to the tissues. *Be sure to check the heart rate by listening to the apical pulse for a full minute.* If a cardiac monitor is being used, ask the monitor watcher, charge nurse, or prescriber about the patient's rhythm. Get a baseline weight for each patient because the dosage of many of these drugs is based on weight.

After giving any antidysrhythmic drug, be sure to recheck the patient's heart rate and blood pressure. Ask the monitor watcher about changes in the heart rhythm because all antidysrhythmic drugs can cause dysrhythmias. Ensure that the call light is within easy reach, and instruct the patient to call for help before getting out of bed. Instruct patients to get up and change positions slowly because of the possibility of decreased blood pressure, which can cause dizziness or fainting.

Teach patients receiving any antidysrhythmic drug proper techniques for how to check and record their heart rate and blood pressure daily. Remind patients to take these drugs exactly as instructed by the prescriber. *Patients should never take a double dose.* Tell them to talk with the prescriber before taking any over-the-counter drugs. Stress the importance of follow-up appointments with the prescriber to monitor the progress of dysrhythmia treatment. Advise them to wear a medical identification bracelet stating that an antidysrhythmic drug is being used and the reason for its use.

Warn patients to get up and change positions slowly because of the side effects of dizziness and drowsiness. Teach them to sit on the side of the bed for a few minutes before standing up. Caution them against driving or operating machines that require alertness until responses to the drugs are known.

TYPES OF ANTIDYSRHYTHMIC DRUGS

ATROPINE FOR BRADYDYSRHYTHMIAS

How Atropine Works on the Heart

Atropine is a competitive muscarinic acetylcholine receptor antagonist used to treat abnormally slow heart rhythms known as **bradydysrhythmias**. Atropine blocks the actions of the vagus nerve on the heart. The vagus nerve slows down the heart rate. By blocking the action of this nerve, atropine causes an increase in electrical impulse conduction and heart rate. This drug is used for a patient who has symptoms of bradycardia. Atropine may also be used in emergency situations when a patient's

---

⚠ Drug Alert!

Administration Alert

A patient with liver or kidney problems needs smaller doses of most antidysrhythmic drugs to avoid drug overdose and drug toxicity.

QSEN: Safety

⚠ Drug Alert!

Administration Alert

Monitor heart rate and rhythm after giving any antidysrhythmic drug because these drugs can also cause dysrhythmias.

QSEN: Safety

⚠ Drug Alert!

Teaching Alert

Teach patients who have been prescribed antidysrhythmic drugs to check and record their heart rate and blood pressure daily.

QSEN: Safety

heart rhythm is in asystole. *Asystole* is the absence of electrical or contraction activity within the heart. It appears on the electrocardiogram (ECG) monitor as a straight line or "flatline." In emergency settings atropine may also be given through the endotracheal (ET) tube of a patient who has been intubated. Usually twice the normal dose is used, and it is mixed with 5 to 10 mL of normal saline.

Atropine may also be given by the intraosseous (into the bone) route. Specially trained emergency care providers give drugs by endotracheal tube and intraosseous routes. Be sure to consult a drug handbook for specific information about atropine. Other uses for atropine include as a preoperative drug to decrease production of gastrointestinal and respiratory secretions and laryngospasm, bradycardia, and hypotension during anesthesia. This drug is also used topically to dilate pupils before eye examinations.

Dosage for Atropine

Drug	Dosage
atropine (Atropine Sulfate)	*Adults:* 0.5-1 mg IV every 5 min up to 3 mg or 0.04 mg/kg *Children:* 0.01-0.03 mg/kg IV every 5 min up to 1 mg in children and 2 mg in adolescents

Intended Responses
- Heart rate is increased.
- Cardiac output is increased.
- Symptoms such as dizziness and light-headedness are decreased.

Side Effects. Common side effects of atropine include tachycardia, drowsiness, blurred vision, dry mouth, and urinary hesitancy or retention.

Adverse Effects. A rare but serious and life-threatening effect of atropine is the occurrence of ventricular fibrillation. Because atropine increases heart rate and workload, it can also worsen heart ischemia (decreased blood flow to the heart muscle, causing chest pain) and heart blocks. Atropine can also cause PVCs or ventricular tachycardia.

Doses of atropine smaller than 0.5 mg may make bradycardia worse (paradoxical bradycardia).

What To Do *Before* Giving Atropine
In addition to the general responsibilities related to antidysrhythmic therapy (p. 296), check the patient's heart rate and blood pressure. Look for decreased heart rate and blood pressure, which may indicate decreased blood flow to the tissues.

Assess the intravenous (IV) site for patency and signs of infection and infiltration such as redness, swelling, warmth, or decreased IV flow. Ask the patient if the IV site is causing any discomfort.

Ask patients about eye problems such as glaucoma because atropine can make this problem worse.

What To Do *After* Giving Atropine
In addition to the general responsibilities related to antidysrhythmic therapy (p. 296), recheck the patient's heart rate and blood pressure because these should improve after atropine is given. Continue to monitor the IV site for patency. Check the patient's pulse for regularity and strength.

Bring the emergency cart to the patient's bedside because he or she may need to have the heart paced using a transthoracic temporary pacemaker.

Monitor urine output because urinary retention can be a side effect of atropine. Ask whether the patient is experiencing any problems with dry mouth, blurred vision, or drowsiness. Report serious side effects to the prescriber. Check for

 Drug Alert!

Administration Alert

Give twice the normal dose when atropine is given by ET tube. Mix the dose with 5 to 10 mL normal saline.

QSEN: Safety

 Memory Jogger

Use the acronym NAVEL to remember drugs that may be given by ET tube: Narcan, atropine, Valium, epinephrine, and lidocaine.

 Clinical Pitfall

Do not give large doses of atropine to older adults because they are more sensitive to its effects and may experience confusion.

QSEN: Safety

Common Side Effects

Atropine

Drowsiness   Blurred vision   Tachycardia

Dry mouth   Urinary retention

 Clinical Pitfall

Administering a dose of atropine less than 0.5 mg may make bradycardia worse (paradoxical bradycardia).

QSEN: Safety

bowel sounds and abdominal tenderness because atropine can also cause constipation.

What To *Teach* Patients About Atropine

In addition to the general precautions related to antidysrhythmic therapy (p. 296), teach patients that atropine is not prescribed for long-term use. It is usually given in a patient care setting and should be administered exactly as ordered by the prescriber. It may cause drowsiness, so caution patients about getting up without assistance.

Tell patients that atropine should increase heart rate and blood pressure. Improved blood flow to the tissues should lead to decreased symptoms such as dizziness. Atropine is used for short-term treatment for some patients with bradydysrhythmias; you will need to instruct them about more permanent solutions such as pacemakers.

Teach patients to use mouth rinses and frequent mouth hygiene to help relieve dry mouth and prevent tooth decay.

Remind patients to notify the prescriber or nurse for any vision problems. Atropine can affect the ability of the body to regulate heat, so caution patients to avoid strenuous activity in a hot setting.

Life Span Considerations for Atropine

Considerations for Pregnancy and Lactation. Atropine has a low to moderate likelihood of increasing the risk for birth defects or fetal harm. Intravenous atropine may cause tachycardia in the fetus and should be used with caution in pregnant women. However, it may be necessary when the mother's heart rate becomes too slow; otherwise the fetus may not receive enough oxygen and damage may occur.

Pediatric and Older Adult Considerations. Atropine should be used carefully in pediatric patients and older adults because they are more sensitive to its effects and more likely to have side effects. In addition, the risk for drug-induced myocardial infarction is greater in the older adult. Although all patients receiving atropine must be monitored, extra-close monitoring is needed when the drug is used for pediatric patients or older adults.

DIGOXIN

How Digoxin Works

Digoxin (Lanoxin) is a cardiac glycoside that may be used in small doses to increase contractility and slow conduction through the AV node, causing slowing of the heart rate. It is used for atrial fibrillation because it helps to slow the ventricular rate by blocking the number of electrical impulses that pass through the AV node to the heart ventricles. Digoxin also helps to strengthen the contractions in the ventricles so the heart is able to pump more blood with each heartbeat. Although listed in this chapter, see Chapter 17 for a full discussion of the actions, side effects, and other issues related to digoxin therapy.

DRUGS FOR TACHYDYSRHYTHMIAS

A **tachydysrhythmia** is an abnormally rapid heart rhythm. Drugs used to treat rapid abnormal heart rhythms work in one of three ways. They may reduce automaticity of the heart muscle cells, slow down conduction of electrical impulses through the heart, or prolong the refractory period of heart cells. Several classes of drugs are used to treat these dysrhythmias (Table 18-2). The drugs are classified by the way they work. Some drugs have characteristics of more than one classification.

Goals of treatment with these drugs include preventing and relieving symptoms, prolonging life, and suppressing the abnormal rhythms. Recent trends in the treatment of these heart rhythms include a decrease in the use of class I drugs and an

Drug Alert!

Teaching Alert

Teach patients to use mouth rinses and frequent hygiene to relieve dry mouth and prevent tooth decay.

QSEN: Safety

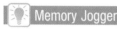

Memory Jogger

The three ways that drugs work to treat rapid abnormal heart rhythms are by:
- Reducing automaticity of the heart muscle cells
- Slowing down conduction of electrical impulses through the heart
- Prolonging the refractory period of heart cells

Table 18-2   **Classes of Common Antidysrhythmic Drugs for Tachydysrhythmias**

CLASS	PURPOSE
Class I: Sodium channel blockers	
Class Ia	Treat symptomatic PVCs, SVT, VT; prevent VF
Class Ib	Treat symptomatic PVCs, VT; prevent VF
Class Ic	Treat life-threatening VT or VF and SVT unresponsive to other drugs
Class I: Miscellaneous	Treat life-threatening ventricular dysrhythmias
Class II: Beta blockers	Treat SVT
Class III: Potassium channel blockers	Treat VT, VF; conversion of A fib and A flutter to sinus rhythm; maintain sinus rhythm
Class IV: Calcium channel blockers	Treat SVT
Unclassified	
Adenosine	Treat SVT
Magnesium sulfate	Treat torsades de pointes

A fib, Atrial fibrillation; *A flutter*, atrial flutter; *PVC*, premature ventricular contraction; *SVT*, supraventricular tachycardia; *VF*, ventricular fibrillation; *VT*, ventricular tachycardia.

increase in the use of class II and III drugs because there are more side effects with class I drugs.

CLASS I: SODIUM CHANNEL BLOCKERS

Sodium channel blockers are a class of drugs that act by inhibiting sodium movement through cell membranes. This results in slowing of the heart rate, reducing cell excitability, and reducing speed of conduction. There are three subclasses of sodium channel blocker drugs. Different subclasses are used to treat different tachydysrhythmias.

CLASS Ia DRUGS

How Class Ia Drugs Work

This group of drugs is used to treat patients who have symptoms associated with PVCs, supraventricular tachycardia (SVT), and ventricular tachycardia. Another use of these drugs is to prevent the occurrence of ventricular fibrillation.

Class Ia drugs decrease the excitability of the heart muscle cells and slow the conduction of electrical impulses through the heart. Together these actions slow the heart rate and make the rhythm more regular. Procainamide may also decrease the strength of heart contractions. Common doses of class Ia drugs are listed in the following table. Be sure to consult a drug handbook for information about any specific class Ia antidysrhythmic drug.

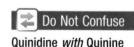 **Do Not Confuse**

Quinidine *with* **Quinine**

An order for quinidine may be confused with quinine. Quinidine is a class Ia antidysrhythmic drug, whereas quinine is an antimalarial drug.

QSEN: Safety

Dosages for Common Class Ia Antidysrhythmic Drugs

Drug	Dosage
quinidine (Quinidine sulfate, Quinaglute, Quinate ✦)	*Adults:* As sulfate—200-400 mg orally every 6-8 hr (immediate release); 300-600 mg every 8-12 hr (extended release) As gluconate (extended release)—324 mg orally every 8-12 hr *Children:* As sulfate, 6 mg/kg orally 5 times daily
procainamide (Pronestyl, Procanbid)	*Adults:* Up to 50 mg/kg orally daily in divided doses every 3-6 hr to maintain therapeutic blood levels (every 6-12 hr if extended release) IM—Up to 50 mg/kg daily in divided doses every 3-6 hr IV—1000 mg loading dose over 60 min and then 2-6 mg/min as a continuous infusion *Children:* 15-50 mg/kg orally daily in 3-6 divided doses
disopyramide (Norpace, Rythmodan ✦)	*Adults:* 300 mg orally loading dose followed by 150 mg every 6 hr (range 400-800 mg in 4 divided doses)

Common Side Effects

Class Ia Antidysrhythmic Drugs

Hypotension   Anorexia, Abdominal
cramping, Diarrhea,
Nausea

Intended Responses
- Heart rate is decreased.
- Abnormal supraventricular and ventricular rhythms are decreased.
- Heart rhythm is normal and regular.
- Cardiac output is increased.

Side Effects. Common side effects include hypotension, loss of appetite, abdominal cramping, diarrhea, and nausea. As many as 30% to 50% of patients develop gastrointestinal side effects while taking these drugs. Disopyramide also commonly causes constipation, dry mouth, urinary retention, and urinary hesitation.

Adverse Effects. Life-threatening adverse effects vary with the drug prescribed. Patients taking quinidine may become hypotensive or develop an abnormal life-threatening ventricular rhythm called *torsades de pointes.* The life-threatening effects of procainamide include seizures, heart block, asystole, and decreased white blood cell count with increased risk for infection. Disopyramide has been known to cause heart failure.

Allergic reactions to class Ia antidysrhythmic drugs are rare but serious. Signs of allergic reaction include fever, neutropenia, Raynaud's syndrome (ice-cold hands), muscle aches, skin rashes, and blood vessel inflammation in the fingers.

What To Do *Before* Giving Class Ia Drugs

In addition to the general responsibilities related to antidysrhythmic therapy (p. 296), although these drugs are best absorbed on an empty stomach with a full glass of water, if the patient develops gastrointestinal problems, you may need to give them with food.

If the patient being started on disopyramide has been taking quinidine, wait 6 to 12 hours after the last dose of quinidine to begin disopyramide. If immediate-release procainamide was being used, wait 6 hours after the last dose of procainamide to begin disopyramide.

What To Do *After* Giving Class Ia Drugs

In addition to the general responsibilities related to antidysrhythmic therapy (p. 296), monitor intake and output because these drugs may affect urine retention. Also monitor daily weights. For the patient taking disopyramide, watch for signs of heart failure such as ankle swelling or weight gain (Figure 18-6), shortness of breath, and crackles when you listen to the lungs with a stethoscope.

Ask the patient about stomach upset or diarrhea. Remind the patient taking quinidine to call for help before getting up and to change positions slowly because of the potential for hypotension (low blood pressure).

⚠ **Drug Alert!**

Administration Alert

When patients develop gastrointestinal symptoms, give class Ia drugs with food to help reduce the symptoms.

QSEN: Safety

⚠ **Drug Alert!**

Administration Alert

Monitor patient weight and intake and output because class Ia antidysrhythmic drugs can cause urinary retention.

QSEN: Safety

1+ Trace
A barely perceptible pit (2 mm)

2+ Mild
A deeper pit, with fairly normal contours, that rebounds in 10 to 15 seconds (4 mm)

3+ Moderate
A deep pit; may last for 30 seconds to more than 1 minute (6 mm)

4+ Severe
An even deeper pit, with severe edema that may last as long as 2 to 5 minutes before rebounding (8 mm)

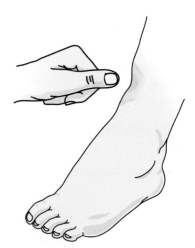

FIGURE **18-6** Pitting edema scale.

If he or she is also taking digoxin, watch for signs of digoxin toxicity because these drugs may lead to increased blood level of digoxin by as much as 50%. Indications of early digoxin toxicity include loss of appetite, nausea, vomiting, diarrhea, or vision problems. Other signs include changes in heart rate or rhythm (irregular or slow), palpitations, or fainting.

What To *Teach* Patients About Class Ia Drugs

In addition to the general precautions related to antidysrhythmic therapy (p. 296), remind patients to monitor urine output and to check and record daily weights. Instruct patients to report weight gain of more than 2 pounds a day to their prescriber. Demonstrate how to check ankles for swelling (see Figure 18-6), and tell patients to report any swelling or shortness of breath to their prescriber. Increased weight gain, ankle swelling, and shortness of breath are signs of worsening heart failure.

Remind patients that the blood level of these drugs must be maintained to achieve the expected actions. This is best achieved by taking the drug at the same time every day and exactly as prescribed.

Disopyramide can cause increased sun sensitivity (photosensitivity). Instruct patients to avoid exposure to sunlight and to wear protective sun block and clothing.

Teach patients taking quinidine to avoid high-alkaline ash foods (such as citrus fruits; milk; and vegetables such as broccoli, cabbage, and carrots). These foods can affect the excretion of quinidine and may lead to toxic levels of this drug.

Teach patients to avoid the herb St. John's wort while taking quinidine because it can cause a decreased blood level of this drug.

Life Span Considerations for Class Ia Drugs

Pediatric Considerations. Although some class Ia drugs (quinidine and procainamide) have been used for children with dysrhythmias, their safety has not been studied or established.

Considerations for Pregnancy and Lactation. Class Ia drugs have a low to moderate likelihood of increasing the risk for birth defects or fetal harm, and are generally not considered safe for use during pregnancy or breastfeeding.

Considerations for Older Adults. Older adults may eliminate class Ia drugs more slowly and are at higher risk for side effects and toxicity. Emphasize to older adults the importance of monitoring urine output and checking and recording daily weights. Instruct patients to report a weight gain of more than 2 pounds a day to their prescriber. Also demonstrate how to check ankles for swelling, and tell patients to report any swelling or shortness of breath to their prescriber because these are signs of heart failure.

CLASS Ib DRUGS

How Class Ib Drugs Work

Class Ib antidysrhythmic drugs are used to treat ventricular tachycardia and PVCs that cause patient symptoms. They are also used to prevent ventricular fibrillation, a life-threatening dysrhythmia.

Most of these drugs inhibit the ability of the ventricles to contract prematurely. This decreases the number of PVCs and episodes of ventricular tachycardia. In an emergency setting, amiodarone (Cordarone) is the first-line drug prescribed for ventricular tachycardia, followed by lidocaine (Xylocaine).

Lidocaine is only given intravenously or by airway inhalation (ET tube—remember "NAVEL") because, when given by mouth, the liver destroys most of the drug, making it ineffective. Lidocaine may be given intramuscularly in an emergency situation if an IV line is not available.

Common doses of class Ib drugs are listed in the following table. Be sure to consult a drug handbook for information about a specific class Ib antidysrhythmic drug.

 Drug Alert!

Teaching Alert

Teach patients taking quinidine to avoid large amounts of high-alkaline ash foods because they affect excretion of the drug and can lead to drug toxicity.

QSEN: Safety

 Drug Alert!

Interaction Alert

The herb St. John's wort can cause a decreased blood level of quinidine.

QSEN: Safety

 Clinical Pitfall

Lidocaine (Xylocaine) should never be used for patients with severe heart block dysrhythmias. Because the normal heart pacemaker is not functioning, this can lead to cardiac arrest.

QSEN: Safety

Dosages for Common Class Ib Antidysrhythmic Drugs

Drug	Dosage
lidocaine ❶ (Betacaine ✦, Xylocaine)	*Adults:* 50-100 mg IV bolus (may repeat once) followed by continuous infusion of 1-4 mg/min *Children:* 1 mg/kg IV bolus (up to 100 mg) followed by 20 mcg/kg/min continuous infusion (range 20-50 mcg/kg/min) *Adults/Children >50 kg:* 300 mg IM (4.5 mg/kg); may repeat in 60-90 min
mexiletine (Mexitil)	*Adults:* 200-300 mg orally every 8 hr (maximum 1200 mg daily) *Children:* 1.4-5 mg/kg orally every 8 hr
tocainide (Tonocard)	*Adults:* 400-600 mg orally every 8 hr (maximum 2400 mg daily)
phenytoin (Dilantin)	*Adults:* 50-100 mg IV every 10-15 min until dysrhythmia is gone (up to 15 mg/kg)

❶ High-alert drug.

Common Side Effects

Class Ib Antidysrhythmic Drugs

Confusion

Tremors

Drowsiness

Dizziness

Nausea

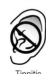
Tinnitis

Intended Responses
- Number of PVCs is decreased.
- Risk for ventricular tachycardia is decreased.
- Heart rhythm is regular and normal.
- Cardiac output is increased.

Side Effects. Common side effects include confusion and drowsiness. IV lidocaine may cause stinging at the IV site. Common side effects of mexiletine and tocainide include dizziness, tremors, nervousness, nausea, vomiting, and heartburn. A patient may also have visual disturbances, vertigo, or ringing in the ears (tinnitus). Dizziness and falls are more likely with older adults.

Adverse Effects. A life-threatening adverse effect of lidocaine is cardiac arrest. Dysrhythmias may worsen with mexiletine and tocainide. A patient may develop pneumonitis, pulmonary fibrosis, or pulmonary edema while taking tocainide. Decreased white blood cell count (*neutropenia*) with increased risk for infection is an adverse effect of both tocainide and phenytoin. Two additional adverse effects of phenytoin are aplastic anemia and Stevens-Johnson syndrome, a skin disorder resulting from an allergic reaction to drugs, infections, or illness. See Chapter 1 and Figure 1-5 for more information about this syndrome.

What To Do *Before* Giving Class Ib Drugs
In addition to the general responsibilities related to antidysrhythmic therapy (p. 296), ask specifically about herbal preparation use. St. John's wort may decrease the level of lidocaine in the blood.

To monitor for drug side effects, ask patients if they have ever had any problems with tremors, dizziness, light-headedness, visual problems, or ringing in the ears.

For IV drugs, be sure to check the IV site for patency and signs of infection. Ask the patient about stinging at the IV site.

What To Do *After* Giving Class Ib Drugs
In addition to the general responsibilities related to antidysrhythmic therapy (p. 296), tell the patient to report any chest pain or shortness of breath immediately. Watch for side effects, including confusion, tremors, dizziness, light-headedness, visual difficulties, and tinnitus (ringing in the ears).

Ask about any shortness of breath and listen to the patient's lungs with a stethoscope for crackles, a sign of heart failure. Watch the IV site for patency and any signs of infection. Ask whether the patient feels any stinging or burning at the IV site. Also ask him or her about numbness, which can be caused by lidocaine and may mask the signs of IV infiltration.

With older adults, check for signs of confusion and other side effects because they are more sensitive to the effects of these drugs. Confusion may be a sign of lidocaine

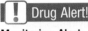

Drug Alert!

Monitoring Alert

Ask patients receiving IV lidocaine about any numbness at the IV site because this can mask signs of IV infiltration.

QSEN: Safety

toxicity in these patients. Heart rate changes include decreased heart rate and asystole with hypotension and shock.

What To *Teach* Patients About Class Ib Drugs

In addition to the general precautions related to antidysrhythmic therapy (p. 296), tell patients to report any of the following symptoms to the prescriber immediately:

- Irregular rhythms
- Heart rates less than 60 beats per minute or more than 100 beats per minute
- Chest pain
- Shortness of breath
- Wheezing

Life Span Considerations for Class Ib Drugs

Considerations for Pregnancy and Lactation. Class Ib drugs should not be used during pregnancy or breastfeeding because they cross the placenta and enter breast milk. All Class 1b drugs have a moderate likelihood of increasing the risk for birth defects or fetal harm. Phenytoin has a moderate to high likelihood of increasing the risk for birth defects or fetal harm.

Considerations for Older Adults. Older adults are more likely to experience dizziness and falls while taking Class Ib drugs. Instruct them to change positions slowly and to hold the handrails when using stairs to reduce the risk of falling. In addition, older adults are more likely to become confused. Instruct family members to assess them for confusion or any changes in level of cognition.

CLASS Ic DRUGS

How Class Ic Drugs Work

Class Ic antidysrhythmic drugs are used to treat life-threatening ventricular tachycardia or fibrillation and supraventricular tachycardia that does not go away when other drugs are used.

Flecainide (Tambocor) and propafenone (Rythmol) are oral drugs given to adults to slow the electrical impulse conduction of the heart. Common doses of class Ic drugs are listed in the following table. Be sure to consult a drug handbook for information about any specific class Ic antidysrhythmic drug.

Dosages for Common Class Ic Antidysrhythmic Drugs

Drug	Dosage
flecainide (Tambocor)	*Adults:* 100-200 mg orally every 12 hr
propafenone (Rythmol)	*Adults:* 150-300 mg orally every 8 hr; sustained-release (SR)—225-425 mg every 12 hr

Intended Responses

- Episodes of ventricular and supraventricular dysrhythmias are decreased.
- Cardiac output is increased.
- Symptoms are decreased.
- Heart rhythm is normal and regular.

Side Effects. Common side effects of class Ic antidysrhythmic drugs include dizziness, conduction system abnormalities leading to heart blocks, altered sense of taste, constipation, nausea, and vomiting. Patients taking flecainide may also have blurred vision and difficulty focusing. Side effects are more likely to occur with higher doses of these drugs.

 Drug Alert!

Administration Alert

Sudden changes in level of consciousness, confusion, and heart rate may be signs of lidocaine toxicity in older adults.

QSEN: Safety

Common Side Effects

Class Ic Antidysrhythmic Drugs

Dizziness   Constipation, Nausea/ Vomiting   Blurred vision

Altered taste

Drug Alert!

Administration Alert

Side effects of class Ic antidysrhythmic drugs are more likely to occur as the dosage increases.

QSEN: Safety

Adverse Effects. Adverse life-threatening effects of class Ic drugs include supraventricular and ventricular dysrhythmias such as heart blocks and ventricular tachycardia.

What To Do *Before* Giving Class Ic Drugs

In addition to the general responsibilities related to antidysrhythmic therapy (p. 296), check whether the patient has a history of bronchospasm because patients with this condition should not take propafenone.

What To Do *After* Giving Class Ic Drugs

In addition to the general responsibilities related to antidysrhythmic therapy (p. 296), ask the patient about dizziness, altered taste sensation, constipation, nausea, vomiting, and vision changes, which are indications of drug toxicity. Report any of these symptoms to the prescriber immediately.

What To *Teach* Patients About Class Ic Drugs

In addition to the general precautions related to antidysrhythmic therapy (p. 296), tell patients to report any visual disturbances or other symptoms, including fever, sore throat, chills, unusual bleeding or bruising, chest pain, shortness of breath, excessive sweating (diaphoresis), or palpitations, to the prescriber at once. These symptoms may indicate toxicity or life-threatening dysrhythmias.

Life Span Considerations for Class Ic Drugs

Pediatric Considerations. Class Ic antidysrhythmic drug use is not recommended for children because safety and effectiveness have not been established.

Considerations for Pregnancy and Lactation. Class Ic drugs have a low to moderate likelihood of increasing the risk for birth defects or fetal harm. They should be used during pregnancy only when the potential benefit outweighs the risk to the fetus. It is not known whether class Ic drugs are excreted in breast milk. Because of possible serious adverse reactions in nursing infants, a different method of infant feeding should be considered.

Considerations for Older Adults. A slight increase in the incidence of dizziness has been seen in older adults. Instruct them to change positions slowly and to hold handrails when using stairs to reduce the risk for falls. Because of the possible increased risk of liver and kidney problems in older adults, class Ic drugs should be used with caution in this group. The effective dose may be lower in these patients.

CLASS II: BETA BLOCKERS

How Beta Blockers Work

Beta blockers are used to treat supraventricular tachycardia. These drugs block the effects of epinephrine (adrenaline) on the heart. They decrease the heart rate and the force of heart contractions, which results in a decrease in blood pressure. Beta blockers are often used to slow the rate of ventricular contractions with supraventricular tachycardia, including rapid atrial fibrillation or flutter. As a result the heart does not work as hard and requires less oxygen. Cardioselective beta blockers work only on the cardiovascular system. Noncardioselective beta blockers have systemic effects. Although listed in this chapter, see Chapter 16 for a full discussion of the actions, side effects, and other issues related to beta blocker drug therapy.

When a beta blocker is prescribed for a patient with kidney damage, a lower dose of the drug is ordered, or the time between doses is increased. An older adult patient may also be started on a lower drug dose.

Common doses of class II beta blockers approved for use with dysrhythmias are listed in the following table. Be sure to consult a drug handbook for information about a specific class II beta blocker antidysrhythmic drug.

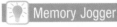

Administration Alert

Always ask older adults about liver or kidney problems because class Ic antidysrhythmic drug doses may be lower in these patients.

QSEN: Safety

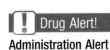

Beta blockers may work on the cardiovascular system (cardioselective) or have systemic effects (noncardioselective).

Dosages for Common Class II Beta Blocker Antidysrhythmic Drugs

Drug	Dosage
acebutolol ❶ (Monitan 🍁, Sectral)	*Adults:* 200 mg orally twice daily (usual therapeutic range 600-1200 mg daily)
esmolol ❶ (Brevibloc)	*Adults:* 500 mcg/kg/min IV as loading dose, followed by maintenance dose of 50 mcg/kg/min; may repeat loading and maintenance dose every 5-10 min until dysrhythmia is gone
propranolol ❶ (Detensol 🍁, Inderal, Novopranol 🍁)	*Adults:* 1-3 mg IV at a rate of 1 mg/min; 10-20 mg orally 3-4 times daily
sotalol ❶ (Betapace, Sotacar 🍁)	*Adults:* 80 mg orally every 12 hr; may increase (average dosage 150-320 mg/day)

❶ High-alert drug.

CLASS III: POTASSIUM CHANNEL BLOCKERS

How Potassium Channel Blockers Work

Class III antidysrhythmic drugs are **potassium channel blockers** (a class of drugs that act by inhibition of potassium movement through cell membranes). Blocking potassium channels lengthens the duration of action potentials. They are used to treat ventricular tachycardia and ventricular fibrillation, convert atrial fibrillation or flutter to normal sinus rhythm, and maintain normal sinus rhythm (amiodarone). Amiodarone (Cordarone) given intravenously is used to slow conduction through the AV node with atrial fibrillation and control ventricular tachycardia and fibrillation. Oral amiodarone is used to prevent recurrence of ventricular tachycardia and fibrillation and to maintain a normal sinus rhythm after conversion from atrial fibrillation or flutter. Dofetilide (Tikosyn) is given orally to keep a patient in normal sinus rhythm after conversion from atrial fibrillation. Ibutilide (Corvert) is given intravenously and makes cardioversion of a patient with atrial fibrillation or flutter to normal sinus rhythm more likely to be successful.

Common dosages of class III potassium channel blockers approved for use with dysrhythmias are listed in the following table. Be sure to consult a drug handbook for information about any specific class III potassium channel blocker antidysrhythmic drug.

Dosages for Common Class III Potassium Channel Blockers

Drug	Dosage
amiodarone (Cordarone)	*Adults:* IV loading dosage: 150 mg over 10 min, then 360 mg over the next 6 hr, then 540 mg over the next 18 hr IV maintenance dosage: 720 mg over 24 hr Oral loading dosage: 800-1600 mg daily for 1-3 wk Oral maintenance dosage: 200-400 mg daily
dofetilide (Tikosyn)	*Adults:* 125-500 mcg orally twice daily
ibutilide (Corvert)	*Adults:* IV weight based: More than 60 kg: 1 mg IV over 10 min Less than 60 kg: 0.01 mg/kg IV over 10 min Dose can be repeated once after 10 min if necessary
sotalol ❶ (Betapace, Sotacar 🍁)*	*Adults:* 80 mg orally every 12 hr; may increase (average dosage 150-320 mg daily)

❶ High-alert drug.

*Sotalol is a beta blocker but is considered a class III antidysrhythmic drug.

Common Side Effects

Class III Potassium Channel Blockers

Dizziness   Fatigue   Hypotension

Nausea,   Bradycardia   Tremor
Vomiting,
Anorexia,
Constipation

⚠ Drug Alert!

Administration Alert

Be sure to monitor the respiratory status of patients taking amiodarone.

QSEN: Safety

💡 Memory Jogger

Signs of IV patency include blood return and easy flushing. Signs of infection include swelling, redness, warmth, fever, and pain.

⚠ Drug Alert!

Administration Alert

Monitor for signs of thyroid problems such as changes in heart rate, which are more likely to occur during the first few weeks of treatment with amiodarone (Cordarone).

QSEN: Safety

Intended Responses

- Blood vessel constriction is decreased.
- Blood flow to coronary arteries and heart muscle is increased.
- Electrical impulse conduction in all heart muscle tissues is slowed.
- Heart rate is decreased.
- Strength of contractions in the left ventricle is decreased.
- Success of cardioversion to normal sinus rhythm (ibutilide) is increased.
- Normal heart rhythm and rate (oral amiodarone and dofetilide) are maintained.

Side Effects. Common side effects of class III potassium channel blockers include dizziness, fatigue, malaise, bradycardia, hypotension (especially for intravenous drugs), loss of appetite, constipation, nausea, vomiting, unsteady gait (ataxia), involuntary movement, numbness and tingling, poor coordination, and tremor. Side effects unique to amiodarone include photosensitivity, hypothyroidism, peripheral neuropathy, and microdeposits on the corneas.

Hyperthyroidism may occur with amiodarone. Thyroid problems are more likely to occur during the first few weeks of treatment. A patient who is taking amiodarone for a long period may develop blue discoloration of the face, neck, and arms.

Adverse Effects. Several potential life-threatening effects are associated with amiodarone, including adult respiratory distress syndrome (ARDS), pulmonary fibrosis, heart failure, worsening of heart dysrhythmias, decreased liver function, and toxic epidermal necrolysis. Toxic epidermal necrolysis is a rare but life-threatening skin disorder that is caused by an allergic reaction.

With dofetilide, patients also may experience chest pain or life-threatening ventricular dysrhythmias. It may also cause heart dysrhythmias.

What To Do *Before* Giving Potassium Channel Blockers

In addition to the general responsibilities related to antidysrhythmic therapy (p. 296), if the patient is to receive an IV drug, check the IV site for patency and signs of infection.

What To Do *After* Giving Potassium Channel Blockers

In addition to the general responsibilities related to antidysrhythmic therapy (p. 296), for IV drugs, continue to watch the IV line for patency and signs of infection. Be sure to monitor blood pressure when a patient is receiving IV amiodarone (Cordarone) because of the risk for hypotension.

Watch for signs of pulmonary problems such as ARDS (including crackles when you listen to the lungs with a stethoscope), difficulty breathing, fatigue, cough, and fever.

Look for signs of thyroid problems, including weight gain; lethargy; and swelling in the hands, feet, or around the eyes. Report any of these signs to the prescriber immediately.

Make sure that any follow-up laboratory tests (for example, liver and thyroid function tests) and ECGs are completed.

What To *Teach* Patients About Potassium Channel Blockers

In addition to the general precautions related to antidysrhythmic therapy (p. 296), tell patients taking amiodarone that they may need to wear dark glasses when going outside because of the potential for increased sensitivity to light. Also teach them to wear protective clothing and a sunscreen barrier for increased sun sensitivity (photosensitivity) while taking these drugs.

Remind patients that side effects may not appear for several days or weeks. Explain that long-term use of amiodarone may cause the development of a bluish discoloration of the face, neck, and arms. This side effect is reversible and will disappear over several months.

Tell patients that they will need eye examinations every 6 to 12 months to determine if corneal microdeposits or other eye changes have occurred. These changes would not necessarily be apparent to the patient during the early stages.

Be sure to advise male patients to tell the prescriber immediately about any pain or swelling in the scrotum. The prescriber may need to decrease the dosage of amiodarone.

Life Span Considerations for Potassium Channel Blockers
Considerations for Pregnancy and Lactation. Potassium channel blockers have a moderate to high likelihood of increasing the risk for birth defects or fetal harm. Pregnant women should not take amiodarone because it can harm the fetus. Women who are breastfeeding should not use these drugs; if the treatment is necessary, breastfeeding should be discontinued.

Pediatric and Older Adult Considerations. Potassium channel blockers should be used cautiously in pediatric patients and older adults.

CLASS IV: CALCIUM CHANNEL BLOCKERS

How Calcium Channel Blockers Work
Class IV antidysrhythmic drugs include the **calcium channel blockers** diltiazem (Cardizem) and verapamil (Calan, Isoptin). They are used primarily for the treatment of supraventricular tachycardia. As antidysrhythmic drugs, they act by slowing conduction through the SA and AV nodes of the conduction system of the heart, leading to a decreased heart rate. When these drugs are prescribed for older adults or patients with hepatic (liver) or renal (kidney) impairment, lower initial dosages are used.

Common dosages of class IV calcium channel blockers approved for use with dysrhythmias are listed in the following table. Be sure to consult a drug handbook for information about any specific class IV calcium channel blocker antidysrhythmic drug. Although listed in this chapter, see Chapter 16 for a full discussion of the actions, side effects, and other issues related to calcium channel blocker drug therapy.

Dosages for Common Class IV Calcium Channel Blockers

Drug	Dosage
diltiazem (Apo-Diltiaz ♣, Cardizem, Syn-Diltiazem ♣)	*Adults:* Oral: 30-120 mg 3-4 times daily; slow-release capsules 60-120 mg twice daily; extended-release capsules 240-360 mg once daily IV: 0.25 mg/kg over 2 min; second dose 0.35 mg/kg may be given after 15 min if needed; then follow with continuous infusion 5-15 mg/hr for up to 24 hr
verapamil (Calan, Isoptin, Novo-Veramil ♣, Nu-Verap ♣)	*Adults:* Oral: 40-120 mg every 6-8 hr IV: 5-10 mg; may give 10 mg after 30 min if needed *Children less than 1 year:* 0.1-0.2 mg/kg IV over 2 min *Children 1 to 15 years:* 0.1-0.3 mg/kg IV (maximum 5 mg) over 2 min; may repeat in 30 min if needed

UNCLASSIFIED ANTIDYSRHYTHMIC DRUGS

ADENOSINE

How Adenosine Works
Adenosine (Adenocard) is a drug administered intravenously for supraventricular tachycardia (SVT). Adenosine can to help identify the rhythm, and certain SVT rhythms can be successfully terminated with adenosine. Its action is similar to that of calcium channel blockers. It slows electrical impulse conduction through the AV node to help restore a patient to a normal sinus rhythm. Adenosine is an IV drug given as a rapid IV bolus injection. When given slowly, adenosine is eliminated from the body before

! Drug Alert!

Monitoring Alert

Male patients may experience pain or swelling in the scrotum while taking amiodarone (Cordarone), which should be reported to the prescriber immediately.

QSEN: Safety

it can reach the heart and act to slow the rhythm. After giving adenosine there will be a very brief period of asystole, then the heart will resume a normal rhythm. Be sure to consult a drug handbook for specific information about adenosine.

Dosages for Adenosine

Drug	Dosage
adenosine (Adenocard)	*Adults/Children over 50 kg:* 6 mg IV given rapidly over 1-2 seconds; flush with normal saline and elevate arm after giving drug IV push; second and third doses of 12 mg can be given if necessary *Children under 50 kg:* 0.05-0.1 mg/kg IV over 1-2 seconds; may repeat in 1-2 min if necessary

Drug Alert!

Administration Alert

Always give IV adenosine (Adenocard) rapidly over 1 to 2 seconds.

QSEN: Safety

Common Side Effects

Adenosine

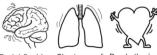

Facial flushing | Shortness of breath | Dysrhythmias

Drug Alert!

Administration Alert

Always have emergency equipment, including the crash cart and defibrillator, at the bedside before giving an IV dose of adenosine.

QSEN: Safety

Intended Responses
- Impulse conduction through the AV node is slower.
- Heart rate is decreased.
- Supraventricular tachycardia is eliminated.
- Heart rhythm is normal and regular.

Side Effects. Common side effects of adenosine include facial flushing, shortness of breath, and transient dysrhythmias such as atrial fibrillation and atrial flutter.

Adverse Effects. Allergic reactions are rare. Adenosine should not be used with heart block unless the patient has an artificial pacemaker in place because it may lead to asystole.

Fatal cardiac arrest, sustained ventricular tachycardia, and nonfatal myocardial infarction have been reported after giving injections of adenosine. Patients with unstable angina may be at greater risk. Emergency equipment must be available before this drug is given.

What To Do *Before* Giving Adenosine
In addition to the general responsibilities related to antidysrhythmic therapy (p. 296), tell the patient that there will be a brief period of asystole that may feel like a "mule kick" to the chest before the heart goes back into a normal rhythm.

Be sure that a physician is at the bedside. Bring emergency equipment to the bedside before giving this drug. Check the IV line for patency and any signs of infection. Draw the bolus up into a syringe and remember that it must be given by IV push *rapidly* over 1 to 2 seconds.

What To Do *After* Giving Adenosine
In addition to the general responsibilities related to antidysrhythmic therapy (p. 296), check blood pressure every 15 to 30 minutes immediately after adenosine has been given. Be sure to check the heart monitor for changes in heart rhythm.

What To *Teach* Patients About Adenosine
In addition to the general precautions related to antidysrhythmic therapy (p. 296), explain the purpose of giving adenosine. Warn patients that facial flushing may occur with this drug. Tell patients to call for help when getting up and to change positions slowly because doses of 12 mg or more can cause hypotension.

Instruct patients to report any facial flushing, shortness of breath, or dizziness immediately.

Life Span Considerations for Adenosine
Considerations for Pregnancy and Lactation. Adenosine has a low to moderate likelihood of increasing the risk for birth defects or fetal harm and should not be used during pregnancy because its safe use has not been studied or established.

Considerations for Older Adults. Older adults may be more sensitive to the effects of adenosine; however, these effects have not been studied.

MAGNESIUM SULFATE

How Magnesium Sulfate Works

Magnesium sulfate is a major mineral that the fourth most abundant in the human body. It helps the heart rhythm remain steady. Magnesium sulfate is used intravenously to prevent the ventricular dysrhythmia *torsades de pointes* from returning after a patient has been defibrillated (given an electric shock) to return into a normal rhythm. An IV magnesium sulfate bolus can sometimes eliminate torsades de pointes in a patient who is not symptomatic. A normal level of magnesium in the blood keeps the heart muscle from becoming overexcited and reduces the risk for this life-threatening dysrhythmia. The common dose of magnesium sulfate used is listed in the following table. Although listed in this chapter, see Chapter 17 for a full discussion of the actions, side effects, and other issues related to magnesium sulfate therapy. Be sure to consult a drug handbook for specific information about magnesium sulfate.

Dosages for IV Magnesium Sulfate for Dysrhythmias

Drug	Dosage
magnesium sulfate ❶	*Adults:* 1-2 g IV diluted with 10 mL of D₅W solution; give over 30 seconds (patient should be on cardiac monitor when receiving this drug) *Children:* Dosage not established

❶ High-alert drug.

OTHER DRUGS USED TO TREAT DYSRHYTHMIAS

Anticoagulants such as heparin and warfarin (Coumadin) are prescribed for rhythms when the patient is at increased risk for blood clots such as atrial fibrillation. For more information on these drugs, see Chapter 20.

Get Ready for Practice!

Key Points

- The normal pacemaker of the heart is the SA node, which initiates 60 to 100 electrical impulses per minute to the heart.
- Dysrhythmias are abnormal heart rhythms.
- Some patients with symptoms do *not* have serious dysrhythmias, whereas others with *no* symptoms may have life-threatening dysrhythmias.
- Ventricular fibrillation causes death within minutes if not treated.
- A watch or clock with a second hand is needed to check heart rate.
- Always check a patient's blood pressure, heart rate, and heart rhythm before and after giving an antidysrhythmic drug.
- Always check IV sites for patency and signs of infection before and after a patient is given an IV antidysrhythmic drug.
- Teach patients taking antidysrhythmic drugs to check and record their heart rate and rhythm every day and to report any abnormal findings to their prescriber.
- Check patients for signs of heart failure after receiving antidysrhythmic drugs. Check daily weights, listen for crackles in the lungs, and look for swelling.
- An older adult patient may need decreased doses of antidysrhythmic drugs because of increased sensitivity and age-related body changes.

- Adenosine must always be given by IV push rapidly over 1 to 2 seconds to be effective.
- Always have emergency equipment brought to the bedside before giving IV adenosine because of the risk of dysrhythmias and cardiac arrest.
- Magnesium sulfate is given to prevent the ventricular dysrhythmia torsades de pointes from returning after the patient's rhythm has been returned to a normal sinus rhythm.
- Anticoagulants are prescribed for abnormal heart rhythms with increased risk for clot formation such as atrial fibrillation or atrial flutter.

Additional Learning Resources

evolve Be sure to visit your Evolve website (http://evolve.elsevier.com/Workman/pharmacology/) for additional online resources.

SG Go to your Study Guide for additional learning activities to help you master this chapter content.

Review Questions

See the Answer Keys—In-text Review Questions for answers to these questions.

Test Yourself on the Basics

1. Which pulse site should you teach the patient to use to monitor his or her heart rate?
   A. Carotid
   B. Brachial
   C. Radial
   D. Femoral

2. What is a common side effect of atropine?
   A. Tachycardia
   B. Bradycardia
   C. Dizziness
   D. Confusion

3. What will you teach the patient to always do before taking his or her dose of digoxin?
   A. Check his or her oral temperature.
   B. Pour a full glass of fluid to drink when taking the drug.
   C. Take the drug with an antacid to prevent GI side effects.
   D. Take his or her radial pulse for a full minute.

4. What must you do before giving any antidysrhythmic drug by the IV route?
   A. Make sure that the IV is at least a 20-gauge catheter.
   B. Hang a bag of normal saline to infuse with the drug.
   C. Check the IV site for patency and signs of infection.
   D. Place a new IV catheter to be used only for the drug.

5. Which side effect of beta blockers may cause a younger male patient to not take his dose?
   A. Insomnia
   B. Erectile dysfunction
   C. Weakness
   D. Dizziness

Test Yourself on Advanced Concepts

6. A patient with an irregular and rapid heart rate is dizzy, light-headed, and short of breath. How will administration of digoxin (Lanoxin) treat this dysrhythmia? (Select all that apply.)
   A. Stimulates the heart to beat faster
   B. Blocks the number of electrical impulses passing through the AV node
   C. Increases the strength of heart contractions
   D. Increases the demand for blood supply to the heart
   E. Decreases excitability of heart muscle cells

7. For which dysrhythmia does the nurse anticipate administration of IV atropine (atropine sulfate)?
   A. Ventricular tachycardia
   B. Symptomatic bradycardia
   C. Atrial fibrillation
   D. Supraventricular tachycardia

8. What action must you take for a patient who is prescribed flecainide (Tambocor) 100 mg orally every 12 hours and whose heart rate is 72 beats per minute?
   A. Give the drug as prescribed.
   B. Give half the prescribed dosage.
   C. Hold the dose and notify the prescriber.
   D. Document the heart rate.

9. A patient asks you why amiodarone (Cordarone) has been prescribed for atrial fibrillation. What is your best response?
   A. "It will increase your heart rate."
   B. "It will slow your heart rate."
   C. "It will keep your heart in a normal rhythm."
   D. "It will increase the force of contraction in your heart."

10. What priority action do you take after giving a patient a dose of sotalol (Betapace) 80 mg orally every 12 hours?
    A. Monitor for changes in heart rate.
    B. Count the apical heart rate for 2 full minutes.
    C. Place the patient on a heart monitor.
    D. Check the dosage with another nurse or pharmacist.

11. Which side effect is commonly developed by patients taking the class Ia antidysrhythmic drug disopyramide (Norpace)?
    A. Gastrointestinal upset
    B. Hypotension
    C. Dizziness
    D. Constipation

12. For which symptom do you monitor for an older adult patient receiving intravenous lidocaine for frequent premature ventricular contractions?
    A. Hypotension
    B. Confusion
    C. Nausea and vomiting
    D. Constipation

13. What symptoms would you teach patients to report to the prescriber immediately for a prescription for tocainide (Tonocard)? (Select all that apply.)
    A. Irregular heart rhythm
    B. Abdominal pain
    C. Shortness of breath
    D. Heart rate less than 60 beats per minute
    E. Feeling tired and sleepy

14. For which side effect do you monitor after giving the class Ic antidysrhythmic drug propafenone (Rythmol)?
    A. Dizziness
    B. Confusion
    C. Tremors
    D. Nausea

15. A patient is to receive digoxin (Lanoxin) 0.25 mg once a day. The pharmacy sends digoxin 0.125-mg tablets. How many tablets will you give? _____ tablets

16. A child who weighs 21 kg is to be given an IV dose atropine 0.02 mg/kg. How many milligrams will you give? _____ mg

17. The prescriber has ordered adenosine (Adenocard) 6 mg IV rapidly over 1-2 seconds. Adenosine is available in vials containing 3 mg/1 mL. How many mL will you give? _____ mL

Critical Thinking Activities

See the Answer Keys—Critical Thinking Activities for answers to these activities.

Mrs. Smart is 78 years old and has a diagnosis of chronic atrial fibrillation. She has an irregular heart rate that ranges between 60 and 80 per minute. She is to be discharged with the following prescribed medications, including: digoxin (Lanoxin) 0.125 mg once daily and warfarin (Coumadin) 3 mg once daily. She asks you how these medications work.

1. What will you teach Mrs. Smart about the actions of these drugs?
2. Which important teaching points will you include about each drug?
3. What precautions will you teach Mrs. Smart about each of these drugs?

Drug Therapy for High Blood Lipids

Objectives

After studying this chapter you should be able to:

1. Explain how antihyperlipidemic drugs work to lower blood lipid levels.
2. List the common names, actions, usual adult dosages, possible side effects, and adverse effects of statins, bile acid sequestrants, cholesterol absorption inhibitors, and fibrate drugs.
3. Describe what to do before and after giving drugs to lower blood lipid levels.
4. Explain what to teach patients taking drugs to lower blood lipid levels, including what to do, what not to do, and when to call the prescriber.
5. Describe life span considerations for drugs to lower blood lipid levels.
6. List the common names, actions, usual adult dosages, possible side effects, and adverse effects of nicotinic acid.
7. Describe what to do before and after giving nicotinic acid.
8. Explain what to teach patients taking nicotinic acid, including what to do, what not to do, and when to call the prescriber.
9. Describe life span considerations for nicotinic acid.

Key Terms

antihyperlipidemics (ăn-tī-hī-pŭr-lĭp-DĒ-mĭks) (p. 311) Drugs that work against high levels of lipids (fats) in the blood.

bile acid sequestrants (BĪ-ŭl ĂS-ĭd sĕ-KWĔS-trĕnts) (p. 316) Cholesterol-lowering drugs that bind with cholesterol-containing bile acids in the intestines and remove them via bowel movements.

cholesterol (kō-LĔS-tŭr-ŏl) (p. 312) A fatty, waxy material that our bodies need to function. It is present in cell membranes everywhere in the body.

cholesterol absorption inhibitors (kō-LĔS-tŭr-ŏl ăb-SŌRP-shŭn ĭn-HĬB-ĭ-tŭrz) (p. 317) Cholesterol-lowering drugs that prevent the uptake of cholesterol from the small intestine into the circulatory system.

fibrates (FĪ-brāts) (p. 318) Lipid-lowering drugs that are used primarily to lower triglycerides and, to a lesser extent, LDL ("bad") cholesterol.

high-density lipoprotein (HDL) (HĪ DĔN-sĭ-tē lī-pō-PRŌ-tēn) (p. 313) The "good" cholesterol that exists in the body.

hyperlipidemia (hī-pŭr-lĭp-ĭ-DĒ-mē-ă) (p. 312) High levels of blood fats (plasma lipoproteins).

hypertriglyceridemia (hī-pŭr-trī-GLĬS-ŭr-ĭ-DĒ-mē-ă) (p. 312) High levels of triglycerides in the blood.

low-density lipoprotein (LDL) (LŌ DĔN-sĭ-tē lī-pō-PRŌ-tēn) (p. 311) The "bad" cholesterol that exists in the body.

nicotinic acid (nĭ-kō-TĬN-ĭk ĂS-ĭd) (p. 320) Special type of vitamin B that helps to decrease blood cholesterol levels.

statins (STĂ-tĭnz) (p. 314) A class of drugs used to lower LDL ("bad") cholesterol and triglycerides by inhibiting their production by the body.

triglyceride (trī-GLĬS-ŭr-īd) (p. 312) The chemical form of most fats in foods and the human body.

OVERVIEW

Lipid-lowering drugs are also called **antihyperlipidemics** because they work against high levels of lipids in the blood. These drugs are used with diet changes (for example, decreased intake of fat) to reduce the amount of certain fats and cholesterol in the blood. Some lipid-lowering drugs work to decrease the production of cholesterol in the body and increase the ability of the liver to remove the "bad" cholesterol **(low-density lipoprotein or LDL).** Others reduce the amount of fat from food that the body absorbs. Still others bind with cholesterol-containing bile acids in the intestines and promote cholesterol loss in the stool.

 Memory Jogger

Low-density lipoprotein (LDL) = "bad" cholesterol
High-density lipoprotein (HDL) = "good" cholesterol

Table 19-1	Lipid Profile Normal Values
TYPE OF LIPID	**NORMAL VALUE**
Total cholesterol	<200 mg/dL
Low-density lipoprotein (LDL)	60-180 mg/dL
Very low–density lipoprotein (VLDL)	25%-50%
High-density lipoprotein (HDL)	Male: >45 mg/dL Female: >55 mg/dL
Triglycerides	Male: 40-160 mg/dL Female: 35-135 mg/dL

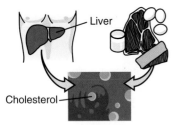

FIGURE 19-1 Cholesterol is produced by the liver, but it is also consumed in meat and dairy products.

REVIEW OF RELATED PHYSIOLOGY AND PATHOPHYSIOLOGY

Cholesterol is a fatty, waxy material that the body needs to function. It is present in cell membranes everywhere in the body. It is used to produce hormones, vitamin D, and bile acids that help digest fat. A person needs some cholesterol for important body functions. Cholesterol is produced by the liver, and it is in the foods that you eat (Figure 19-1). However, your body needs only a small amount of cholesterol; too much in the bloodstream contributes to the development of narrowed arteries such as atherosclerosis and coronary artery disease. The chemical form of most fats in foods and the human body is **triglycerides.** Both cholesterol and triglycerides are present in the blood, making up the plasma lipids.

A high level of blood fats (plasma lipoproteins) is called **hyperlipidemia.** Table 19-1 lists the normal values for a patient's lipid profile. A high level of triglycerides in the blood is called **hypertriglyceridemia.** Chronic hyperlipidemia can lead to many health problems, including:

- Atherosclerosis
- Coronary artery disease (angina, heart attack)
- Hypertension
- Pancreatitis
- Peripheral vascular disease, which leads to organ damage or impairment
- Stroke
- Xanthomas (skin atheromas—abnormal fat deposits)

CORONARY ARTERY DISEASE

The coronary arteries supply blood, oxygen, and nutrients to the heart muscle (myocardium). Atherosclerosis, a major contributor to development of coronary artery disease, begins by forming a fatty streak on an arterial wall, leading to fat buildup (plaques). Fat buildup in the walls of coronary arteries can result in partial or complete blockage of blood flow to the heart muscle (Figure 19-2). The main lipids involved are cholesterol and triglycerides. Partial blockage in the coronary arteries can result in chest pain *(angina)*; complete blockage can result in heart attack *(myocardial infarction)*. Table 19-2 summarizes lipid levels related to the risk of developing coronary artery disease (CAD).

FAMILIAL HYPERLIPIDEMIA

Some people develop high blood fat levels that are related to genetic or inherited factors. This is called *familial hyperlipidemia* or sometimes *familial hypercholesterolemia.* The liver makes too much cholesterol and other fats, which lead to increased levels of fats in the blood and the development of atherosclerosis. The reason for this condition is not completely clear; however, it tends to occur in families. For people who have a genetic factor leading to hyperlipidemia, simply reducing fatty foods does not help lower blood lipid levels. Antilipidemic drugs are prescribed to lower them.

 Memory Jogger

High blood lipid levels may result from genetic factors (familial hyperlipidemia).

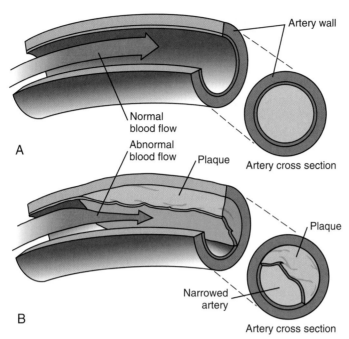

FIGURE 19-2 Cholesterol can form plaques that narrow arteries. **A,** Normal, clean artery. **B,** Artery with plaque formation.

Table 19-2 Lipid Values and Risk for Coronary Artery Disease

LIPID	VALUE (mg/dL)	RISK FOR CORONARY ARTERY DISEASE
Total cholesterol	<200	Low
	200-239	Borderline high
	>239	High
HDL ("good" cholesterol)	>35	Low
	<35	High
LDL ("bad" cholesterol)	<129	Low
	130-159	Borderline high
	>159	High
Triglycerides	<200	Low
	201-399	Borderline high
	400-1000	High
	>1000	Very high

HDL, High-density lipoprotein; *LDL,* low-density lipoprotein.

GENERAL ISSUES FOR ANTIHYPERLIPIDEMIC THERAPY

Lipid-lowering drugs are used most often to treat high blood lipid levels that fail to decrease with lifestyle changes such as reduced-fat diets, increased exercise, smoking cessation, and weight loss. When such changes do not result in lower blood lipid levels, the patient remains at risk for development of heart disease, especially in the presence of other risk factors such as high blood pressure (hypertension) and diabetes.

Lipid-lowering drugs may be prescribed for high total cholesterol or triglyceride levels, high levels of low-density lipoproteins (LDLs, or "bad" cholesterol), or low levels of **high-density lipoproteins (HDLs,** or "good" cholesterol). Some health problems for which these drugs are used include:
- Coronary artery disease (heart disease)
- Hypertension
- Stroke

Several classes of drugs affect blood lipid levels. Each class has both common and different actions and effects. Responsibilities for the common actions and effects are

Drug Alert!

Action/Intervention Alert

Be sure to monitor liver function blood test results because most antihyperlipidemic drugs can cause liver damage (hepatotoxicity).

QSEN: Safety

Drug Alert!

Teaching Alert

Instruct patients to fast (no eating or drinking) for at least 8 hours before a lipid profile blood test is obtained.

QSEN: Safety

Memory Jogger

All lipid-lowering drugs reduce high blood lipid levels, but they do not cure the problem; treatment is long term, and these drugs must be taken even after blood fat levels are normal.

Memory Jogger

There are five types of lipid-lowering drugs:
- Statins
- Bile acid sequestrants
- Cholesterol absorption inhibitors
- Fibrates
- Nicotinic acid

Memory Jogger

The generic names of HMG CoA reductase inhibitors ("statins") all end in "-statin" (for example, atorvastatin, rosuvastatin, simvastatin).

listed in the following paragraphs. Specific responsibilities are listed with each individual drug class.

Before giving any antihyperlipidemic drug, obtain a complete list of drugs that the patient is currently taking, including herbal and over-the-counter drugs. Ask women of childbearing age if they are pregnant, planning to become pregnant, or breastfeeding. Check patient histories for liver or muscle problems.

Before giving the first dose, be sure that the patient has baseline blood lipid and liver function tests drawn. Check his or her lipid blood tests *(lipid profile)* (see Table 19-1) and liver function tests (see Table 1-3). Notify the prescriber about any abnormal results.

After giving any antihyperlipidemic drug, be sure to notify the prescriber if liver function laboratory tests are elevated. Ask patients about symptoms of muscle damage such as soreness, pain, or weakness. Assess patients for signs of liver damage, including jaundice, dark urine, or light-colored stools.

Teach patients receiving any antihyperlipidemic drug to continue lifestyle changes that help lower cholesterol such as a low-fat diet, exercise, and weight control. Remind them to check with their prescriber before using any over-the-counter drugs.

Instruct patients not to eat or drink for 8 hours before having follow-up laboratory tests drawn (lipid profile, liver function tests) because these test results can be changed by substances in some foods and fluids. Remind them that these blood tests must be repeated every 3 to 6 months to monitor the effectiveness of lipid-lowering drugs.

Advise female patients to tell their prescriber if they plan to become pregnant or are at risk of becoming pregnant.

Teach that all lipid-lowering drugs reduce high blood lipid levels but that they do not cure the problem. Treatment is long term, and these drugs must be taken even after blood fat levels are normal. Remind patients to take the drug exactly as prescribed because this ensures the best result.

Tell patients to report signs and symptoms of decreased liver function, muscle problems, or changes in urine output to their prescriber.

TYPES OF LIPID-LOWERING DRUGS

There are five main types of lipid-lowering drugs. The group most commonly used is the "statins" (HMG CoA reductase inhibitors). They control the rate of cholesterol produced by the liver. The other drug types include bile acid sequestrants, cholesterol absorption inhibitors, fibrates, and nicotinic acid.

STATINS

How Statins Work

Statins inhibit HMG CoA reductase, an enzyme that controls cholesterol production in the body. They lower blood lipid levels by slowing the production of cholesterol and increasing the ability of the liver to remove LDL cholesterol from the blood. Statins are the most effective group of these drugs for lowering LDL cholesterol. Be sure to consult a drug reference book for information on any specific statin.

Dosages for Common Statins

Drug	Dosage
atorvastatin (Lipitor)	*Adults:* 10-80 mg orally once daily
fluvastatin (Lescol)	*Adults:* 20-40 mg orally once daily at bedtime or twice daily; extended-release (XL)—80 mg once daily
lovastatin (Mevacor, Altocor)	*Adults:* 20-80 mg orally once daily with evening meal
pitavastatin (Livalo)	*Adults:* 1-4 mg orally once daily
pravastatin (Pravachol)	*Adults:* 10-40 mg orally once daily
rosuvastatin (Crestor)	*Adults:* 5-40 mg orally once daily
simvastatin (Zocor)	*Adults:* 5-80 mg orally once daily in the evening

Intended Responses

- Total cholesterol is decreased.
- Triglycerides are decreased.
- LDL is decreased.

Side Effects. Side effects of statins are rare. Upset stomach, gas, constipation, abdominal pain, and cramps may occur. These symptoms are usually mild and disappear as the body adjusts to the drug. Other side effects include musculoskeletal discomfort and liver problems.

Adverse Effects. Patients may develop *rhabdomyolysis* (muscle breakdown). Signs and symptoms of rhabdomyolysis include general muscle soreness, muscle pain and weakness, vomiting, stomach pain, and brown urine. The urine turns brown because small reddish-brown pieces of broken-down muscle are removed from the body through the urine.

Statins may cause decreased liver function. Because of this danger, the prescriber should monitor liver function tests regularly (every 3 to 6 months). These tests are important because early, mild liver problems do not cause symptoms. Late symptoms of liver disease include yellowing *(jaundice)* of the skin, whites of the eyes, and roof of the mouth; pain over the liver on the right side just below the ribs; darkened urine; and pale gray-colored stools. The bile and bilirubin made by the liver normally leave the body in the stool, giving stool a medium-to-dark brown color. When the liver is not working well, these products do not reach the stool, so the stool becomes a light gray or green instead of brown. Bilirubin enters the urine, turning it dark, and gets into skin and mucous membranes, turning them yellow.

What To Do *Before* Giving Statins

In addition to the general responsibilities related to antihyperlipidemic therapy (p. 314), check the patient's baseline kidney function tests (blood urea nitrogen [BUN] and creatinine) because kidney failure can be a side effect of rhabdomyolysis. Normal values are listed in Table 1-4 in Chapter 1.

Ask patients about their alcohol consumption. Statins should not be given to patients who consume more than two alcoholic drinks per day because drinking alcohol puts even more stress on the liver.

What To Do *After* Giving Statins

In addition to the general responsibilities related to antihyperlipidemic therapy (p. 314), regularly assess the patient for signs and symptoms of decreased liver function or muscle breakdown, including constant fatigue, itchy skin, general weakness, and jaundice (yellowish color of the skin and sclera). Report these signs and symptoms to the prescriber immediately.

Be sure to monitor the patient's urine output. Renal failure can occur if rhabdomyolysis develops because protein released from broken-down muscle can block urine flow through the kidneys. Continue to check the patient's BUN and creatinine levels.

What To *Teach* Patients About Statins

In addition to the general precautions related to antihyperlipidemic therapy (p. 314), teach patients when to take their prescribed drug. Some statins should be taken in the evening, some once a day without regard for meals, and some may be taken twice a day.

Life Span Considerations for Statins

Pediatric Considerations. Safe use of statin drugs in children under 8 years of age has not been established. Statin use in older children is rare but may be prescribed for children with familial hypercholesterolemia.

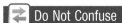

Do Not Confuse

Zocor *with* Cozaar

An order for Zocor may be confused with Cozaar. Zocor is a lipid-lowering statin, whereas Cozaar is a blood pressure–lowering angiotensin II receptor antagonist.

QSEN: Safety

Common Side Effects

Statins

 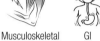

Musculoskeletal discomfort | GI discomfort | Liver problems

Drug Alert!

Action/Intervention Alert

After a patient begins taking a statin drug, be sure to monitor for signs of rhabdomyolysis.

QSEN: Safety

Clinical Pitfall

Women who are pregnant or breastfeeding should not take statin drugs.

QSEN: Safety

Considerations for Pregnancy and Lactation. Statins drugs have a high likelihood of increasing the risk for birth defects or fetal damage. They should not be given to women who are pregnant, plan to become pregnant, or are breastfeeding. Statins decrease the amount of fat in the body. Fat is essential to brain development in the fetus and infant. When there is not enough fat in the body during pregnancy and infancy, the fetus can suffer poor brain development and mental retardation.

Considerations for Older Adults. Statin drugs are safe for use in older adults if there is no history of muscle problems (*myopathy*) or liver disease. Remind older adults to contact their prescriber if they notice any new muscle weakness, muscle aches, or joint aches. Patients may think any muscle ache or weakness is related to aging, but this could be an indication of the adverse reaction rhabdomyolysis.

BILE ACID SEQUESTRANTS

How Bile Acid Sequestrants Work

The class of lipid-lowering drugs called **bile acid sequestrants** helps the body lose cholesterol. The drugs are taken by mouth and work directly on dietary fats in the intestine. They bind with cholesterol in the intestine, preventing the fats from being absorbed into the blood. This action then eliminates the cholesterol from the body through the stool. Be sure to check a drug reference book for information on any specific bile acid sequestrant drug.

? Did You Know?

Oat bran cereals such as oatmeal act the same way as bile acid sequestrants to lower blood lipids.

Dosages for Common Bile Acid Sequestrants

Drug	Dosage
cholestyramine (LoCHOLEST, Prevalite, Questran, Questran Light)	*Adults:* 4-24 g orally 1-6 times daily *Children:* 240 mg/kg orally daily in 3 divided doses (do not exceed 8 g day)
colesevelam (Welchol)	*Adults:* 3 oral tablets (625 mg each) twice daily or 6 tablets once daily; may increase to 7 tablets daily
colestipol (Colestid)	*Adults:* Granules: 5 g orally 1-2 times daily; may be increased monthly up to 30 g day in 1-2 doses Tablets: 2 g orally 1-2 times daily; may be increased monthly up to 16 g day in 1-2 doses

Common Side Effects

Bile Acid Sequestrants

GI discomfort, Nausea/Vomiting, Constipation, Gas

Intended Responses
- LDL cholesterol level is decreased.
- HDL cholesterol level is increased.

Side Effects. Side effects of bile acid sequestrants are rarely serious. The most common side effects are gastrointestinal symptoms, including constipation, bloating, nausea, vomiting, and gas.

Adverse Effects. Bile acid sequestrants decrease the ability of the body to absorb oral drugs. They also inhibit fat-soluble vitamins (A, D, E, and K), so patients may need to take a daily vitamin supplement. Bile acid sequestrants may change the action of the anticoagulant warfarin (Coumadin) in two ways. They can decrease the absorption of vitamin K, which would intensify the effects of warfarin and increase the risk for bleeding. Bile acid sequestrants can also directly bind warfarin in the intestinal tract and cause its rapid elimination. This action inactivates the activity of warfarin and increases the risk of clot formation. Therefore it is always important to monitor the international normalized ratio (INR) of a patient taking both warfarin and bile acid sequestrants.

! Drug Alert!

Administration Alert

If administering a bile acid sequestrant to a patient taking warfarin (Coumadin), be prepared to administer vitamin K, the antidote for warfarin.

QSEN: Safety

What To Do *Before* Giving Bile Acid Sequestrants

In addition to the general responsibilities related to antihyperlipidemic therapy (p. 314), do not give any bile acid sequestrants within 2 hours after giving any other oral drug because they can inhibit the absorption of other drugs.

Ask patients whether they are experiencing constipation. This is a very common side effect of the drug and can make the patient uncomfortable. Check whether the patient is prescribed warfarin (Coumadin).

What To Do *After* Giving Bile Acid Sequestrants

In addition to the general responsibilities related to antihyperlipidemic therapy (p. 314), after giving a bile acid sequestrant, assess the patient for gastrointestinal symptoms such as constipation, bloating, gas, nausea, or vomiting.

If the patient is taking warfarin, monitor for signs of bleeding such as easy bruising, clammy skin, pale skin, dizziness, increased heart rate, decreased blood pressure, shortness of breath, or confusion. Monitor INRs for changes that are higher or lower than the patient's prescribed therapeutic range. Give vitamin supplements if ordered.

Continue to monitor the patient for constipation.

What To *Teach* Patients About Bile Acid Sequestrants

In addition to the general precautions related to antihyperlipidemic therapy (p. 314), teach patients to take bile acid sequestrants with meals because they bind with cholesterol in the intestine. Remind them not to take other drugs for at least 2 hours before or 4 to 6 hours after bile acid sequestrants because bile acid sequestrants may interfere with absorption of other drugs. Tell patients to mix the powder forms of bile acid sequestrants with 4 to 6 ounces of fruit juice or water.

Tablet forms should be taken with large amounts of water (at least 12 to 16 ounces) to prevent stomach and intestinal problems such as bowel obstruction. Teach patients about the signs of bowel obstruction, including abdominal pain, bloating, vomiting, and diarrhea or constipation.

Tell patients that these drugs may be prescribed along with a statin drug to reduce cholesterol level further.

Life Span Considerations for Bile Acid Sequestrants

Pediatric Considerations. Cholestyramine (Questran) and colestipol (Colestid) should be avoided in children because they can cause intestinal obstructions. Safe use of colesevelam (Welchol) has not been established in children.

Considerations for Pregnancy and Lactation. Bile acid sequestrants have a low to moderate likelihood of increasing the risk for birth defects or fetal damage. Safe use of colesevelam (Welchol) has not been established for pregnancy or breastfeeding. The value of lowering cholesterol levels during pregnancy is controversial because the fetus needs a constant level of cholesterol for brain development.

CHOLESTEROL ABSORPTION INHIBITORS

How Cholesterol Absorption Inhibitors Work

Cholesterol absorption inhibitors are used when a low-fat, low-cholesterol diet does not control blood cholesterol levels. These drugs work to reduce the amount of cholesterol absorbed by the body. They are useful for patients who cannot take statin drugs because of side effects. They may also be used with statin drugs to increase the cholesterol-lowering effects. Be sure to consult a drug reference book for information on a specific cholesterol absorption inhibitor.

Dosage for Common Cholesterol Absorption Inhibitor

Drug	Dosage
ezetimibe (Zetia, Ezetrol ✦)	10 g orally once daily

Drug Alert!

Action/Intervention Alert

Always ask patients about constipation before administering bile acid sequestrants because these drugs can cause constipation.

QSEN: Safety

Drug Alert!

Action/Intervention Alert

When a patient is taking a bile acid sequestrant drug as well as warfarin, monitor for signs of bleeding.

QSEN: Safety

Drug Alert!

Administration Alert

Bile acid sequestrants should be taken 2 hours before or 2 hours after antacids.

QSEN: Safety

Common Side Effects

Cholesterol Absorption Inhibitors

GI discomfort,   Joint pain,   Rash
Diarrhea   Fatigue

Intended Responses
- Level of LDL cholesterol is decreased.
- Level of total cholesterol is decreased.

Side Effects. Common side effects of cholesterol absorption inhibitors include gastrointestinal discomforts such as stomach pain and diarrhea. Other common side effects include fatigue, back pain, joint pain, rash, and sinusitis.

Fenofibrate (Tricor), gemfibrozil (Lopid), and cyclosporine increase blood levels of ezetimibe (Zetia).

Adverse Effects. Angioedema is a rare adverse effect of ezetimibe. Angioedema is swelling beneath the skin, usually around the eyes, nose, and lips, caused by blood vessel dilation (see Figure 1-6). Swelling may be life threatening when it affects the airways.

What To Do *Before* Giving Cholesterol Absorption Inhibitors
In addition to the general responsibilities related to antihyperlipidemic therapy (p. 314), ask if the patient has a history of liver disease or muscle disorders. Also check his or her liver function tests because the use of this drug may worsen liver disease when prescribed with a statin drug.

What To Do *After* Giving Cholesterol Absorption Inhibitors
In addition to the general responsibilities related to antihyperlipidemic therapy (p. 314), check the patient for signs of decreased liver function such as decreased appetite, fatigue, jaundice, weakness, or muscle problems, including aches and pains. Monitor for fatigue or abdominal pain.

Monitor the patient for facial swelling, which may be an indicator of the adverse effect of angioedema. If this problem develops, hold the next dose and notify the prescriber immediately.

What To *Teach* Patients About Cholesterol Absorption Inhibitors
In addition to the general precautions related to antihyperlipidemic therapy (p. 314), tell patients to be sure to report any muscle pain, tenderness, or weakness to their prescriber. Teach them to take the drug once a day at the same time every day. Not only does this habit help the patient remember to take the drug, but it also can help make the timing of any intestinal symptoms from the drug more predictable. It can be taken at the same time as a statin drug but should be given at least 2 hours before or 4 hours after bile acid sequestrants.

Stress to the patient that they should go to the nearest emergency department if he or she develops swelling of the face or tongue or starts to have difficulty breathing or swallowing. These are signs of angioedema, a serious adverse reaction.

 Drug Alert!

Teaching Alert

Teach patients to go to the nearest emergency department if swelling of the face or tongue occurs.

QSEN: Safety

Life Span Considerations for Cholesterol Absorption Inhibitors
Pediatric Considerations. Safe use of these drugs in children under the age of 10 years has not been established.

Considerations for Pregnancy and Lactation. Ezetimibe has a moderate likelihood of increasing the risk for birth defects or fetal damage, and safe use of this drug during pregnancy has not been established. During breastfeeding, this drug should only be used if the benefits outweigh possible risks to the infant because it is not known if ezetimibe passes into breast milk.

FIBRATES

How Fibrates Work
Fibrates activate cell lipid receptors that bind to and collect cholesterol and other lipids from the blood and break them down for elimination. The main effects of fibrates are to decrease blood triglyceride levels and cause a mild increase in HDL

(or "good" cholesterol). These drugs decrease liver production of triglycerides and increase the use of triglycerides by the fat tissues for metabolism. Fibrates are the best group of these drugs for lowering triglyceride levels. They also increase cholesterol excretion in bile. Be sure to consult a drug reference book for information on a specific fibrate drug.

Dosages for Common Fibrates

Drug	Dosage
fenofibrate (Tricor)	*Adults:* 48-145 mg orally daily *Special Considerations:* May increase to maximum of 3 capsules (200 mg) daily
gemfibrozil (Lopid)	*Adults:* 600 mg orally twice daily *Special Considerations:* Give 30 min before morning and evening meal; may increase up to 1500 mg daily

Intended Responses
- Triglycerides are decreased.
- HDL cholesterol is mildly increased.

Side Effects. The side effects of fibrates are usually mild. The most common side effects are stomach upset and diarrhea. Other common side effects include gastrointestinal discomfort such as indigestion or heartburn (dyspepsia) and nausea. Patients may also experience muscle weakness, headache, pruritus, and rash.

Adverse Effects. In the patient with kidney disease, fibrates may cause increased creatinine levels. Fibrates increase cholesterol loss in bile, which may lead to the development of cholesterol-based gallstones. Bleeding can also occur in the patient taking fibrates.

Gemfibrozil (Lopid) interferes with the breakdown of statin drugs, causing higher levels of statins in the blood. This can lead to statin side effects, such as muscle damage, muscle weakness, rhabdomyolysis, or liver damage.

What To Do *Before* Giving Fibrates
In addition to the general responsibilities related to antihyperlipidemic therapy (p. 314), ask patients about a history of kidney, liver, or gallbladder disease.

What To Do *After* Giving Fibrates
In addition to the general responsibilities related to antihyperlipidemic therapy (p. 314), monitor the patient for indications of kidney, liver, or gallbladder disease such as changes in urine output, decreased appetite, fatigue, weakness, nausea, and vomiting.

If the patient is also taking warfarin (Coumadin), monitor for signs of bleeding such as easy bruising, clammy skin, paleness, dizziness, increased heart rate, decreased blood pressure, shortness of breath, and confusion.

Remind the patient that his or her prescriber will check liver and kidney function laboratory tests periodically.

What To *Teach* Patients About Fibrates
In addition to the general precautions related to antihyperlipidemic therapy (p. 314), teach patients to take fibrates 30 minutes before meals. Remind them that these drugs are usually given before the morning and evening meals. Instruct patients to avoid heavy alcohol use (more than two drinks per day). Tell patients *not* to drink grapefruit juice with fibrates.

Teach patients who are also taking warfarin to report any sign or symptom of bleeding such as easy bruising, clammy skin, pale skin, dizziness, increased heart rate, decreased blood pressure, shortness of breath, or confusion.

Common Side Effects

Fibrates

GI discomfort, Diarrhea   Musculoskeletal discomfort   Headache

Rash

! Drug Alert!

Interaction Alert

Fibrates can increase the effectiveness of warfarin (Coumadin) by causing a prolonged prothrombin time, which can lead to excessive bleeding.

QSEN: Safety

Clinical Pitfall

Patients should not drink grapefruit juice while taking fibrates because it interferes with the metabolism (breakdown) of fibrates in the body, making them less effective.

QSEN: Safety

Life Span Considerations for Fibrates

Considerations for Pregnancy and Lactation. Fibrates have a moderate likelihood of increasing the risk for birth defects or fetal damage. Safe use of these drugs during pregnancy or breastfeeding has not been established. Fibrates can cross the placenta and affect fetal brain development.

Considerations for Older Adults. Older adults are more likely to be taking the drug warfarin (Coumadin) and are at greater risk for bleeding problems. In addition to assessing themselves for signs and symptoms of bleeding, it is important that the INR be tested weekly. Remind the older adult to keep all appointments for INR testing.

NICOTINIC ACID AGENTS

How Nicotinic Acid Agents Work

Nicotinic acid (niacin) is a special type of vitamin B that helps to decrease triglyceride, total cholesterol, and LDL cholesterol levels. It also helps to increase HDL cholesterol. Nicotinic acid is given in doses much higher than the normal daily requirement. Although the effects of niacin are well known, the drug action leading to the lipid-lowering effect is not known. Be sure to consult a drug reference book for information about a specific form of niacin.

Dosages for Common Nicotinic Acid Agents

Drug	Dosage
niacin (immediate-release) (Niacor, Novo-Niacin ✦)	*Adults:* 1-2 g orally 2-3 times daily *Special Considerations:* Do not exceed 6 g daily Supplied in 500-mg tablets Start at low dose (500 mg) and increase slowly over several weeks
niacin (extended-release) (Niaspan, Slo-Niacin)	*Adults:* One 500-mg tablet (usual starting dose) *Special Considerations:* Every 4 weeks the prescriber may increase dosage by 500 mg up to maximum of 2000 mg taken once daily, depending on response to drug; maximum dose is 2000 mg daily

Common Side Effects
Nicotinic Acid Agents

Itching   GI discomfort   Headache

Tachycardia   Dizziness   Nasal inflammation

Intended Responses
- Total cholesterol level is decreased.
- Total triglyceride level is decreased.
- LDL cholesterol level is decreased.
- HDL cholesterol level is increased.

Side Effects. Nicotinic acid agents may cause many side effects. The most common are itching and nasal inflammation because the drug makes blood vessels dilate.

Other common side effects include gastrointestinal symptoms such as nausea, indigestion, gas, vomiting, diarrhea, and abdominal pain. The patient may also experience flushing (redness) and hot flashes, chills, dizziness, fainting, headaches, rapid heart rate (tachycardia), shortness of breath (dyspnea), sweating (diaphoresis), and swelling caused by fluid retention.

Adverse Effects. Liver problems, including toxicity, can occur, although liver failure is rare. Gout (painful swelling and redness of the toes, feet, or ankles) can occur because of a buildup of excess uric acid and calcium. Other adverse effects can include high blood sugar (hyperglycemia) and stomach ulcer flare-up. Nicotinic acid preparations are contraindicated for people who have hypertension, peptic ulcer disease, or any other active bleeding.

What To Do *Before* Giving Nicotinic Acid Agents

In addition to the general responsibilities related to antihyperlipidemic therapy (p. 314), obtain baseline vital signs, including blood pressure and heart rate. Also check a baseline blood sugar level for patients with diabetes. Be sure to check baseline liver function tests such as AST and ALT.

To prevent common side effects such as flushing and hot flashes, give aspirin 325 mg as prescribed, 15 to 60 minutes before administering nicotinic acid.

Find out whether patients have a history of liver disease or diabetes. Ask them about their usual alcohol intake. Also ask if they have ever had gout.

What To Do *After* Giving Nicotinic Acid Agents

In addition to the general responsibilities related to antihyperlipidemic therapy (p. 314), follow these specific responsibilities after giving nicotinic acid agents.

Notify the prescriber if liver function laboratory tests are elevated or if elevations of these tests are associated with nausea, vomiting, or weakness. Liver function tests that are three times the upper limits of normal indicate that the drug may need to be discontinued. (See Table 1-3 for normal liver function ranges.)

Check the patient's heart rate and blood pressure and notify the prescriber about any changes. Flushing or hot flashes can be reduced by the use of aspirin or nonsteroidal anti-inflammatory drugs (NSAIDs) 15 to 60 minutes before taking nicotinic acid or by taking nicotinic acid during or after meals.

Monitor blood glucose levels regularly for patients with diabetes because nicotinic acid can increase serum glucose levels.

What To *Teach* Patients About Nicotinic Acid Agents

In addition to the general precautions related to antihyperlipidemic therapy (p. 314), tell patients that nicotinic acid dosage is usually started low and gradually increased. Teach patients about side effects of nicotinic acid and the importance of notifying their prescriber for any side effects or adverse effects of these drugs. Instruct patients who are also taking a statin drug to notify their prescriber about any muscle pain, tenderness, or weakness.

To decrease gastrointestinal side effects, teach patients to take nicotinic acid agents with meals or snacks. Remind them to take bile acid sequestrants and nicotinic acid agents 4 to 6 hours apart. Teach patients to take a 325-mg aspirin tablet 15 to 60 minutes before the drug to prevent flushing or hot flashes.

Do not substitute a sustained-release form of the drug for an immediate-release form. Extended-release forms of the drug should be swallowed whole and never crushed or chewed.

Be sure to teach patients with diabetes that nicotinic acid may increase blood glucose levels. Doses of drugs used to control blood glucose may need to be increased.

Before any surgery or dental work, the surgeon or dentist should be notified that the patient is taking a nicotinic acid agent because this drug can slow the clotting process and excessive bleeding can occur. These problems are made worse if the patient also takes aspirin or an NSAID daily along with a nicotinic acid agent.

Life Span Considerations for Nicotinic Acid Agents

Considerations for Pregnancy and Lactation. Nicotinic acid has a moderate likelihood of increasing the risk for birth defects or fetal damage. It is secreted in breast milk. If a woman plans to breastfeed, she should avoid breastfeeding or discontinue the nicotinic acid agent to prevent the newborn from receiving large amounts of nicotinic acid.

Drug Alert!

Administration Alert

Give aspirin 325 mg 15 to 60 minutes before nicotinic acid to prevent flushing and hot flashes.

QSEN: Safety

Drug Alert!

Administration Alert

Gastrointestinal symptoms can be decreased by giving nicotinic acid with food.

QSEN: Safety

Clinical Pitfall

Extended-release forms of these drugs should never be crushed or mixed with water because crushing the drug causes immediate release of the entire drug dose and could lead to an overdose.

QSEN: Safety

Get Ready for Practice!

Key Points

- Low-density lipoproteins (LDLs) are the "bad" lipids.
- High-density lipoproteins (HDLs) are the "good" protective lipids.
- Hyperlipidemia (high level of fats in the blood) can lead to cardiovascular disease.
- Familial hyperlipidemia is a form of high blood fat that is related to genetic or inherited factors.
- Lipid-lowering drugs decrease the amount of fat in a patient's blood.
- The major types of lipid-lowering drugs include statins, bile acid sequestrants, cholesterol absorption inhibitors, nicotinic acid agents, and fibrates.
- Lipid-lowering drugs should not be given if a woman is pregnant or plans to become pregnant.
- Muscle breakdown (rhabdomyolysis) is a rare but serious adverse effect of statin drugs that can lead to kidney failure.
- Bile acid sequestrants can increase the action of warfarin (Coumadin) and cause excessive bleeding.
- Extended-release forms of lipid-lowering drugs (for example, niacin [Niaspan]) should not be crushed or given by feeding tube.
- Immediate-release forms of lipid-lowering drugs (for example, niacin [Niacor]) should not be substituted for extended-release drugs.
- Fibrates increase cholesterol excretion in bile, predisposing patients to gallstone formation.

Additional Learning Resources

evolve Be sure to visit your Evolve website (http:// evolve.elsevier.com/Workman/pharmacology/) for additional online resources.

SG Go to your Study Guide for additional learning activities to help you master this chapter content.

Review Questions

See the Answer Keys—In-text Review Questions for answers to these questions.

Test Yourself on the Basics

1. Which group of antihyperlipidemic drugs works best to lower triglycerides?
   A. Statins
   B. Fibrates
   C. Cholesterol absorption inhibitors
   D. Nicotinic acid
2. Which drug is a cholesterol absorption inhibitor?
   A. Ezetimibe
   B. Simvastatin
   C. Gemfibrozil
   D. Colestipol

3. When should you teach a patient to take a fibrate drug?
   A. At bedtime
   B. 1 hour after breakfast
   C. 30 minutes before meals
   D. 1 hour before lunch
4. What are the most common side effects of nicotinic acid drugs?
   A. Nausea and vomiting
   B. Dizziness and confusion
   C. Bleeding and bruising
   D. Itching and nasal inflammation
5. An older adult patient who is prescribed atorvastatin (Lipitor) tells you that she is experiencing more muscle aches and states, "I'm just getting old." What should you do?
   A. Give the drug because this is expected as a person ages.
   B. Offer the patient acetaminophen as needed.
   C. Suggest a physical therapy consult for an exercise program.
   D. Hold the drug and notify the prescribed immediately.

Test Yourself on Advanced Concepts

6. A patient asks you how ezetimibe (Zetia) lowers blood lipid levels. What is your best response?
   A. "They eliminate cholesterol in the stool."
   B. "They decrease production of cholesterol by the liver."
   C. "They bind with cholesterol bile acids."
   D. "They decrease the absorption of cholesterol by the body."
7. A patient taking a statin drug has elevated liver function tests. What is your best first action?
   A. Ask the patient if he or she has a history of kidney disease.
   B. Assess the patient for signs of liver failure.
   C. Ask the patient if he or she has experienced pale gray-colored stools.
   D. Hold the drug and notify the prescriber immediately.
8. Which question would you be sure to ask a patient before giving a bile acid sequestrant drug?
   A. "Have you experienced any constipation?"
   B. "Have you experienced any muscle soreness?"
   C. "Have you experienced any facial swelling?"
   D. "Have you experienced any difficulty breathing?"
9. A patient's LDL level is very high. Which drug and drug dosage would you teach the patient is best to correct the very high LDL level?
   A. simvastatin (Zocor) 5 mg by mouth every evening
   B. ezetimibe (Zetia) 10 mg by mouth every day
   C. gemfibrozil (Lopid) 600 mg twice a day
   D. nicotinic acid (Niacor) 1 g three times a day

10. An older adult prescribed atorvastatin (Lipitor) for familial hyperlipidemia tells you that he is having leg cramps. What is your best action?
    A. Administer acetaminophen (Tylenol) 650 mg as ordered.
    B. Instruct the patient to exercise his calf muscles to resolve the cramp.
    C. Suggest that he begin a regular walking exercise program.
    D. Hold the drug and notify the prescriber immediately.

11. The outpatient prescribed niacin 1 gram three times a day experiences flushing and hot flashes when taking this drug. What is your best action?
    A. Hold the drug and notify the prescriber.
    B. Ask the prescriber to order an antiemetic drug.
    C. Instruct the patient to take aspirin 325 mg 15 to 60 minutes before taking the drug.
    D. Reassure the patient that this is an expected side effect.

12. What action should you take for a patient prescribed niacin (Niacor) who needs dental surgery?
    A. Instruct the patient to take the niacin every day except the day of surgery.
    B. Notify the dental surgeon that the patient is taking niacin on a daily basis.
    C. Check the patient's blood pressure and heart rate.
    D. Monitor the patient for signs of rapid clotting.

13. You are providing teaching to a patient who has been prescribed nicotinic acid (Niacor). What information should you be sure to include in the teaching plan?
    A. "Nicotinic acid doses are usually started low and gradually increased."
    B. "Drink lots of water with Niacor to prevent upset stomach."
    C. "Avoid taking Niacor for at least 1 hour after antacids."
    D. "Mix Niacor with juice or water before taking your dose."

14. What do you teach a woman prescribed niacin (Niacor) who is planning to become pregnant and breastfeed her baby?
    A. This drug is safe for use during pregnancy.
    B. This drug is safe for use during breastfeeding.
    C. This drug should not be taken while breastfeeding.
    D. This drug has a low likelihood of increasing the risk for birth defects or fetal damage.

15. A child who weighs 25 kg is to receive cholestyramine (Questran) 240 mg/kg/day in three equally divided doses. What is the correct dose to administer to this child? _____ mg per dose

16. A patient is to be given Niacor 2 g orally. Niacor is supplied in 500-mg tablets. How many tablets will you administer? _____ tablet(s)

17. A patient is prescribed colestipol (Colestid) tablets 2 g per day in two divided doses. Tablets come in 500-mg tablets. How many tablets will you give for each dose? _____ tablet(s) per dose

Critical Thinking Activities

See the Answer Keys—Critical Thinking Activities for answers to these activities.

Mr. Peters is a 45-year-old who was diagnosed with hyperlipidemia during a routine physical examination. After following health care provider recommendations for a low fat diet and an exercise program, it was determined that treatment of his lipid levels would also require a prescription for a lipid-lowering drug. His prescriber ordered rosuvastatin (Crestor) 10 mg orally once a day. Mr. Peters returns to the prescriber's office a month after starting the drug stating that he is experiencing aches and pains in his legs.

1. What is the likely cause of Mr. Peters's discomforts?
2. What action do you anticipate from the prescriber and why?
3. What are key components of a teaching plan for Mr. Peters today?

Drugs That Affect Blood Clotting

Objectives

After studying this chapter you should be able to:

1. Explain how different classes of drugs affect blood clotting.
2. List the common names, actions, usual adult dosages, possible side effects, and adverse effects of thrombin inhibitors, clotting factor synthesis inhibitors, antiplatelet drugs, and thrombolytic (fibrinolytic) drugs.
3. Describe what to do before and after giving thrombin inhibitors, clotting factor synthesis inhibitors, antiplatelet drugs, and thrombolytic drugs.
4. Explain what to teach patients taking thrombin inhibitors, clotting factor synthesis inhibitors, antiplatelet drugs, and thrombolytic drugs, including what to do, what not to do, and when to call the prescriber.

5. Describe life span considerations for thrombin inhibitors, clotting factor synthesis inhibitors, antiplatelet drugs, and thrombolytic drugs.
6. List the common names, actions, usual adult dosages, possible side effects, and adverse effects of drugs that improve clotting.
7. Describe what to do before and after giving drugs that improve clotting.
8. Explain what to teach patients taking drugs that improve clotting, including what to do, what not to do, and when to call the prescriber.
9. Describe life span considerations for drugs that improve clotting.

Key Terms

anticoagulant (ăn-tē-kō-ĂG-yū-lĕnt) (p. 324) A drug used to prevent clot formation or to prevent a clot that has already formed from getting bigger.

antiplatelet drugs (ăn-tē-PLĂT-lĕt DRŬGZ) (p. 332) Drugs that interfere with blood clotting by either inhibiting cyclooxygenase (COX) formation of thromboxane A2 in platelets or by preventing the activation of platelets. Both types of actions prevent platelets from sticking together and clumping. Also known as platelet inhibitors.

clotting factor synthesis inhibitors (KLŎT-tĭng FĂK-tŭr SĬN-thĕ-sĭs ĭn-HĬB-ĭ-tŭrz) (p. 330) Drugs that decrease the production of clotting factors in the liver.

colony-stimulating factors (CSFs) (cŏl-ŏn-Ē STĬM-yū-lāt-ĭng FĂK-tŏrz) (p. 335) Drugs that increase the production of one or more types of blood cells within the bone marrow.

erythropoiesis-stimulating agents (ESAs) (ĕ-RĬTH-rō-poy-Ē-sis STĬM-yū-lāt-ĭng Ā-gĕntz) (p. 335) Drugs from the colony-

stimulating class that most specifically increase the production of red blood cells in the bone marrow. Also known as ESAs.

fibrinolytic (FĪ-brĭn-ō-LĬT-ĭk DRŬGZ) (p. 333) A drug from the thrombolytic class that breaks down fibrin in an already formed clot.

thrombin inhibitors (THRŎM-bĭn ĭn-HĬB-ĭ-tŭrz) (p. 328) Drugs that interfere with blood clotting by blocking the action of thrombin, which converts fibrinogen to fibrin to form clots.

thrombolytic (thrŏm-bō-LĬT-ĭk) (p. 333) A drug that breaks down a clot that has already formed.

thrombopoiesis-stimulating agents (TSAs) (THRŎM-bō-poy-Ē-sis STĬM-yū-lāt-ĭng FĂK-tŏrz) (p. 336) Drugs from the colony-stimulating factor class that specifically increase the production of platelets in the bone marrow.

OVERVIEW

The body of a normal, healthy person is able to prevent continuous bleeding by forming clots. A *blood clot* is blood that has been converted from a liquid to a solid state. Dangerous clots are called *thrombotic events,* which block blood flow and can cause extensive tissue damage from a lack of tissue oxygen.

To prevent these life- and limb-threatening events, prescribers often use drugs called **anticoagulants**. Anticoagulant drugs are used to reduce clot formation or to prevent an existing clot from becoming bigger. When a clot already exists, a throm-

Table 20-1	Normal and Therapeutic Coagulation Values	
TEST	**NORMAL RANGE**	**THERAPEUTIC RANGE**
Activated partial thromboplastin time (aPTT)	Mean normal range in seconds established by laboratory	1.5-2.5 times mean normal range in seconds established by laboratory*
International normalized ratio (INR)	0.8-1.2	2.0-3.0*

*Therapeutic ranges for an individual patient may be greater depending on the severity of the condition and other patient factors.

bolytic drug may be prescribed to dissolve it. Drug dosage and therapy with these drugs is guided by coagulation laboratory values (Table 20-1).

REVIEW OF RELATED PHYSIOLOGY AND PATHOPHYSIOLOGY

CLOT FORMATION

When a person is injured or wounded, the body protects itself from excessive bleeding (hemorrhage) by allowing the part of the blood called *platelets* and other proteins in the plasma to stick together and form a clot. This process begins with an enzyme called *thrombin* that, when activated, acts on the protein fibrinogen, converting it into fibrin which then creates threads that make the plasma sticky and able to form a clot. *Platelets* clump together to create the initial plug that helps to stop bleeding. This process of cellular reactions is called the *clotting cascade* (Figure 20-1) or *coagulation*. Ideally clot formation occurs only where it is needed to prevent hemorrhage.

THROMBOSIS

Thrombosis occurs when a clot (thrombus) forms in the vascular system. This process is often triggered by atherosclerotic plaques that narrow and damage blood vessels. When a thrombus develops in a coronary artery and blocks the blood supply to a part of the heart muscle, a heart attack *(myocardial infarction)* occurs. If a clot forms in an artery in the brain, a stroke can be the result. A clot in a deep vein such as a leg vein is a *venous thromboembolism,* or VTE (formerly called *deep vein thrombosis [DVT]*). A clot that forms a VTE may also break off, forming an *embolus* that travels through the bloodstream to another part of the body such as the brain or lungs.

 Memory Jogger

DVT (deep vein thrombosis) is now called a VTE (venous thromboembolism).

EMBOLUS

An *embolus* is a clot that travels through the bloodstream until it lodges in a blood vessel and blocks it. It can be a clump of bacteria, fat, or air; but it is most often a blood clot or portion of a clot. An embolus that travels to the brain can cause a stroke. An embolus in the lung is called a *pulmonary embolism,* which can cause severe, life-threatening problems in the respiratory system.

 Did You Know?

An embolus can be a clump of bacteria, fat, or an air bubble. Most often it is a clot or part of a clot.

GENERAL ISSUES FOR ANTICOAGULANT THERAPY

Anticoagulant drugs are prescribed to decrease the ability of the blood to form clots or to prevent an already-formed clot from becoming larger. These drugs are sometimes called *blood thinners,* but they do not actually thin the blood. They also do not dissolve clots that already exist. Drugs that dissolve existing clots are called *thrombolytics, fibrinolytics,* or sometimes *"clot busters."* Figure 20-1 shows where in the blood clotting cascade different types of anticoagulants and thrombolytics disrupt the clotting process.

Anticoagulant drugs may be prescribed to prevent clots from forming after a heart valve replacement, reduce the risk for stroke or heart attack, or prevent VTEs. They

 Memory Jogger

Anticoagulant drugs do not "thin" the blood or dissolve existing clots but will prevent new clots from forming and existing clots from becoming larger.

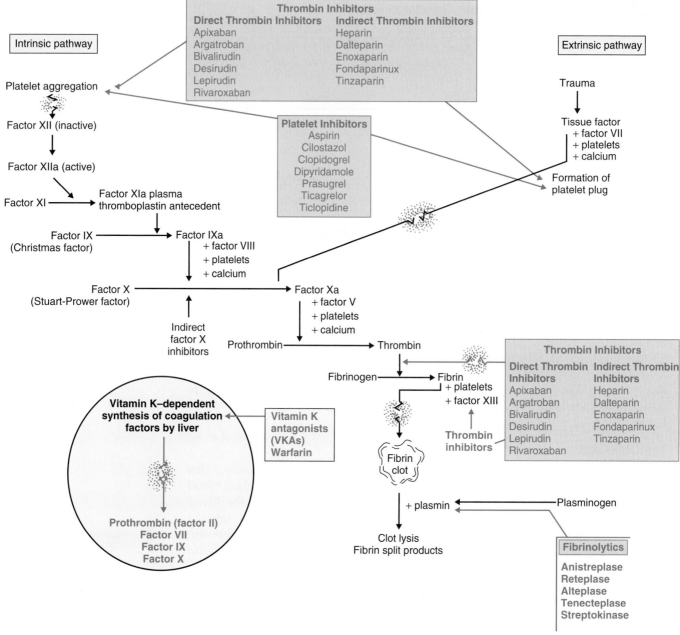

FIGURE 20-1 The clotting cascade. *RBC,* Red blood cell. (From Ignatavicius, D. D., & Workman, M. L. (2016). *Medical-surgical nursing: Patient-centered collaborative care* (8th ed.). Philadelphia: Saunders.)

are also used during open heart surgery to prevent clots from forming. These drugs may also be prescribed to prevent clots in patients who are on bed rest for a long period and for patients with heart dysrhythmias such as atrial fibrillation. Atrial fibrillation is an abnormal heart rhythm in which the atria do not contract effectively, leading to a high risk for clots forming in the atrial chambers of the heart. These clots may then break off and travel to other areas of the body as emboli.

When a clot already exists, thrombolytic drugs may be prescribed. Thrombolytic drugs break down clots that have already formed. They help to prevent death and additional tissue damage for patients with heart attack, stroke, pulmonary embolism, and other clot-related problems.

Intended responses for all anticoagulant drugs are:
- Clotting time is increased.
- Clot formation is decreased.

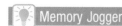 Memory Jogger

Thrombolytic drugs are used to dissolve clots that already exist in the body.

- Existing clots do not become larger.
- Thrombolytic events are prevented.
- Blood flow and oxygenation are maintained.

Several classes of drugs affect blood clotting. Each class has both different and common actions and effects. Responsibilities for these common actions and effects are listed in the following paragraphs. Specific responsibilities are listed with each individual class.

Before giving any drug that affects blood clotting, obtain a complete list of current drugs that the patient is taking, including over-the-counter and herbal preparations, especially aspirin or aspirin-containing products, gingko biloba, and St. John's wort. Check the heart rate and blood pressure. Also check the patient's baseline coagulation laboratory results.

Ask the patient whether he or she has ever had an allergic reaction to any kind of drugs, food, preservatives, or dyes.

When giving a drug that interferes with clotting and that has an antidote, be sure the antidote is available.

Ask female patients of childbearing age if they are pregnant, breastfeeding, or planning to become pregnant. Also determine whether the patient has had a baby, a miscarriage, or an abortion within the past 24 hours. These bleeding conditions are made worse by drugs that disrupt blood clotting, which can lead to serious hemorrhage.

Ask if the patient has a history of bleeding problems. Check the patient for any bruising and ask whether he or she bruises easily. Ask if he or she is currently taking any drugs by injection.

After giving any drug that affects blood clotting, check patients frequently for signs of bleeding or allergic reaction. Hemorrhage (excessive bleeding) is a risk of all anticoagulant drugs and may be life threatening. Signs of bleeding include abdominal swelling or pain, back pain, bloody urine, bloody stools (black and tarry), constipation, coughing up blood, dizziness, headaches, joint pain, and vomiting emesis that looks like coffee grounds.

Recheck the patient's blood pressure, heart rate, and pulse oximetry. Watch for changes that may indicate bleeding such as a decrease in blood pressure (less than 90/60 mm Hg), an increase in heart rate (more than 100 beats per minute), or a decrease in oxygen saturation 3% to 5% below the patient's baseline. Notify the prescriber immediately if the patient develops any signs or symptoms of bleeding.

Avoid giving intramuscular (IM) or intravenous (IV) injections. If you must give an IM or IV drug, hold pressure over the site for at least 5 minutes after administration. Use the smallest needle possible if you must give an IM injection.

Make sure that follow-up coagulation laboratory values are drawn and be sure to check these values because they determine the drug dose that is prescribed. Also check patients' total red blood cell counts and platelet counts to monitor for bleeding.

Teach patients receiving any drug that affects blood clotting about the importance of regular follow-up and blood tests that measure blood clotting. If a dose is missed, the patient should take it as soon as possible but should *never take a double dose because this could cause serious bleeding.* Teach patients to keep a record of each dose to prevent mistakes.

Teach about the side effects and signs of bleeding. These include bleeding from the gums while brushing teeth, bleeding or oozing from cuts or wounds, bruising, and nosebleeds that are excessive and hard to control. Signs of more serious bleeding include paleness around the mouth and nailbeds, rapid heart and respiratory rates, sensation of light-headedness or dizziness, and thirst.

Teach patients to use a soft toothbrush and electric shaver. Tell them to inform other prescribers, including dentists, about the use of these drugs before any surgery or dental work. Remind them to take the drug exactly as prescribed. Patients should

 Drug Alert!

Action/Intervention Alert

Hold pressure over an IM or IV site for at least 5 minutes when a patient is taking drugs that slow clotting.

QSEN: Safety

also be reminded to report any signs of bleeding or allergic reaction to the prescriber.

Tell patients to avoid contact sports and activities that may cause injuries because they can cause internal bleeding. Some activities that can cause internal bleeding (especially in the kidneys) and bleeding into the joints include running, jogging, jumping for any reason, and high-impact exercise.

Suggest that patients get and wear a medical alert bracelet that states they are taking an anticoagulant drug.

TYPES OF DRUGS THAT AFFECT BLOOD CLOTTING

ANTICOAGULANT DRUGS

Anticoagulant drugs come in three categories: direct and indirect thrombin inhibitors (for example, heparin), clotting factor synthesis inhibitors (for example, warfarin [Coumadin]), and antiplatelet drugs (for example, aspirin). These drugs prevent or slow the formation of clots. For this reason, their use is prohibited in people who have bleeding ulcers and those who have had surgery or have delivered a baby within the previous 24 hours.

THROMBIN INHIBITORS

How Thrombin Inhibitors Work

Thrombin inhibitors indirectly or directly interfere with blood clotting by blocking the action of thrombin, which converts fibrinogen into fibrin to form clots. Indirect thrombin inhibitors work by increasing the activity of a substance (antithrombin III) in the blood, which then inhibits thrombin. This class of drugs includes heparin, low-molecular weight heparin, dalteparin, fondaparinux (Arixtra), and tinzaparin. Direct thrombin inhibitors such as apixaban (Eliquis), Argatroban, bivalirudin (Angiomax), desirudin (Iprivask), lepirudin (Refludan), and rivaroxaban (Xarelto) block thrombin directly without affecting the action of antithrombin III.

Heparin may be given by IV or subcutaneous routes. IV heparin is usually given in the form of an IV push bolus followed by a continuous infusion. The bolus dose is usually based on the patient's weight; the infusion rate is based on and adjusted according to the patient's activated partial thromboplastin time (aPTT) laboratory results.

The goal of this therapy is to keep the aPTT (activated partial thromboplastin time) within a therapeutic range to prevent clots from forming. The therapeutic range for heparin is based on establishing a mean normal reference by the laboratory processing the tests. The therapeutic range should yield an aPTT that is 1.5 to 2.5 times greater than the mean normal range, also called the *control value*. Although the usual therapeutic range is 1.5 to 2.5 times the control, it may be extended to as high as 3.5 depending on why the patient's blood clotting is being controlled.

Subcutaneous heparin may be prescribed for therapeutic anticoagulation or prevention of clots and emboli. Subcutaneous injections are usually given every 8 to 12 hours.

Low-molecular-weight (LMW) heparin and fondaparinux are given by the subcutaneous route. Most commonly they are used to prevent VTE and pulmonary embolism. They are often given after surgeries that pose an increased risk for thrombotic events such as knee or hip replacement and abdominal surgeries.

The direct thrombin inhibitors are given intravenously to prevent clot formation or embolic complications. These drugs are used to treat patients who have developed a reaction to heparin *(heparin-induced thrombocytopenia [HIT])*. They may also be given with antiplatelet drugs to treat chest pain and some heart attacks. Oral direct thrombin inhibitors are often used long-term to prevent clotting events in people who have atrial fibrillation or other chronic conditions that promote clot formation. Be sure to consult a drug reference book for information about a specific thrombin inhibitor.

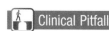

Clinical Pitfall

Anticoagulant drugs are generally not used in patients who are at risk for bleeding.

QSEN: Safety

Drug Alert!

Action/Intervention Alert

Always get a current and accurate weight for a patient who is to be placed on continuous-infusion heparin because the initial IV bolus dose is based on the patient's weight.

QSEN: Safety

Drug Alert!

Administration Alert

For continuous heparin infusion, the rate is based on the patient's aPTT laboratory results.

QSEN: Safety

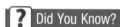

Did You Know?

A major advantage of using LMW heparin is that patients do not need to have laboratory work drawn to guide their therapy.

Dosages for Common Thrombin Inhibitors

Drug	Dosage
Indirect Thrombin Inhibitors	
heparin ❶ (Calcilean 🍁, Hepalean 🍁, heparin sodium)	*Adults:* IV bolus: weight-based (usual range 5000-10,000 units) followed by continuous infusion Subcutaneous: 8000-10,000 units every 8 hr or 5000-20,000 every 12 hr *Children:* IV bolus of 50-100 units/kg followed by continuous infusion of 100 units/kg every 4 hr
low-molecular-weight heparins ❶ dalteparin (Fragmin) enoxaparin (Lovenox) tinzaparin (Innohep)	*Adults:* Subcutaneous 100-200 units/kg per day 1 mg/kg every 12 hr or 1.5 mg/kg once daily 175 units/kg once daily
fondaparinux ❶ (Arixtra)	*Adults:* 5-10 mg daily
Direct Thrombin Inhibitors	
apixaban (Eliquis)	*Adults:* 2.5-5 mg orally twice daily
argatroban ❶ (Argatroban, Novastan)	*Adults:* IV infusion of 2 mcg/kg/min
bivalirudin ❶ (Angiomax)	*Adults:* IV bolus of 0.75 mg/kg followed by IV infusion of 1.75 mg/kg/hr (angioplasty)
desirudin (Iprivask)	*Adults:* 20-40 mg subcutaneously every 12 hrs
dabigatran (Pradaxa)	*Adults:* 150 mg orally twice daily
lepirudin ❶ (Refludan)	*Adults:* IV bolus of 0.4 mg/kg followed by continuous infusion of 0.15 mg/kg/hr
rivaroxaban (Xarelto)	*Adults:* 20 mg orally once daily or 15 mg orally twice daily

❶ High-alert drug.

Side Effects. A patient who is receiving anticoagulant therapy is always at increased risk for bleeding. Bleeding from the gums while brushing teeth, bleeding or oozing from cuts and wounds, bruising, and nosebleeds may occur. Female patients may develop heavy menstrual bleeding.

Other side effects include increased blood potassium (hyperkalemia), thinning of the bones (osteoporosis), decreased number of platelets (thrombocytopenia), decreased aldosterone, blood clots in the spinal cord, and hair loss (alopecia) with prolonged use.

Adverse Effects. Some patients develop allergic reactions (hypersensitivity) to these drugs. As described in Chapter 1, signs of allergic reaction include changes in skin color of the face, fast or irregular breathing, puffiness or swelling around the eyes, shortness of breath or difficulty breathing, chest tightness, wheezing, skin rash, hives, and itching.

Heparin-induced thrombocytopenia (HIT) is a low blood platelet count as a result of heparin use. It can lead to blood clots that can be mild or serious and fatal.

Heparin-induced skin necrosis is a rare but serious complication caused by subcutaneous heparin, most commonly seen on the abdomen where injection sites are located. In severe cases, surgery may be needed to remove necrotic skin.

What To Do *Before* Giving Thrombin Inhibitors
In addition to the general responsibilities related to anticoagulant therapy (p. 327), ensure that the antidote to heparin, protamine sulfate, is readily available whenever a patient is receiving heparin therapy.

LMW heparin should be given by deep subcutaneous injection with the patient lying down. To avoid losing any of the drug, do not expel the air bubble before

Common Side Effects
Thrombin Inhibitors

Bleeding   Dizziness   Hyperkalemia

 Drug Alert!
Action/Intervention Alert
The antidote to heparin is IV protamine sulfate.
QSEN: Safety

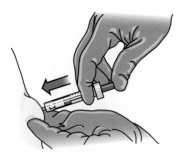

FIGURE 20-2 Injection technique for low-molecular-weight heparin.

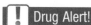 **Drug Alert!**

Action/Intervention Alert

To avoid losing any of the drug, do not expel the air bubble before injecting low-molecular-weight heparin.

QSEN: Safety

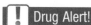 **Drug Alert!**

Teaching Alert

Teach patients to read labels of all over-the-counter and prescription drugs to determine whether they contain aspirin.

QSEN: Safety

 Did You Know?

Warfarin was originally developed as a rat poison and is still used for that purpose today.

 Memory Jogger

The normal INR range is 0.8 to 1.2; the therapeutic range is from 2.0 to 3.0 (or even up to 4.5), depending on the reason the person is prescribed to take this drug.

injection. The needle should be inserted into a skinfold held between the thumb and forefinger (Figure 20-2). *Remember not to aspirate before injection to avoid tissue damage.* The skinfold should be held until the injection is completed. To avoid bruising, do not rub the injection site.

What To Do *After* Giving Thrombin Inhibitors

In addition to the general responsibilities related to anticoagulant therapy (p. 327), for patients receiving continuous IV heparin, adjust the flow rate based on the prescriber's orders and the results of follow-up aPTT tests. Monitor the IV site for patency and signs of infection or phlebitis.

What To *Teach* Patients Taking Thrombin Inhibitors

In addition to teaching patients about the general care needs and precautions related to anticoagulant therapy (pp. 327-328), instruct patients not to take aspirin or aspirin-containing products while taking these drugs and to read the labels on both over-the-counter and prescription drugs to see if they contain aspirin. Patients should be taught not to take ibuprofen or any other nonsteroidal anti-inflammatory drug (NSAID) without asking their prescriber. Taking aspirin or NSAIDs while taking heparin increases the risk for bleeding.

Life Span Considerations for Thrombin Inhibitors

Considerations for Pregnancy and Lactation. Heparin has a low to moderate likelihood of increasing the risk for birth defects or fetal harm. It is the *drug of choice* when anticoagulation therapy is needed during pregnancy and breastfeeding. It may cause bleeding problems in the mother during the last trimester of pregnancy and during delivery of the baby. Heparin does not pass into breast milk, so it is safe while a mother is breastfeeding.

Considerations for Older Adults. Older adults are more sensitive to the effects of thrombin inhibitors and therefore more likely to experience side effects such as bleeding. Because of this, older adults may require lower drug doses. Bruising in general and at the injection site can be quite severe. Teach older adults to immediately apply cold compresses or ice packs to the injured area to reduce bruising and bleeding. Remind them to keep all appointments for blood-clotting tests.

CLOTTING FACTOR SYNTHESIS INHIBITORS

How Clotting Factor Synthesis Inhibitors Work

Clotting factor synthesis inhibitors decrease the production of clotting factors in the liver, specifically the vitamin K–dependent clotting factors (clotting factors II, VII, IX, and X). Because the only drugs in this class affect vitamin K–dependent clotting factors, they are known as *vitamin K antagonists (VKAs)*. VKAs decrease the synthesis of vitamin K in the intestinal tract, which then reduces the production of clotting factors II, VII, IX, and X, along with the anticoagulant proteins C and S. When the amounts of these critical clotting factors are reduced, anticoagulation results. The most commonly used VKA is warfarin (Coumadin, Jantoven), an oral agent. It is prescribed for adults and children to prevent forming of clots and emboli. Most patients are started on warfarin before being taken off of heparin. Patients may be prescribed heparin and warfarin together for a few days until the international normalized ratio (INR) is within the desired therapeutic range. Then the heparin is discontinued.

The *international normalized ratio (INR)* is a blood test used to monitor the effects of warfarin and determine an appropriate dose. Some patients may require higher or lower doses, depending on other medical conditions and personal genetic factors affecting the drug's metabolism. The normal range for the INR is 0.8 to 1.2; a therapeutic range is generally considered to be 2.0 to 3.0. If a patient has a mechanical heart valve, the therapeutic range is 2.5 to 3.5 because of the increased risk for clots forming on the valve.

Dosages for Common Clotting Factor Synthesis Inhibitors

Drug	Dosage
warfarin (Coumadin, Warfilone ♦)	*Adults:* Oral/IV—2-15 mg once daily for 2-4 days, then adjusted based on INR laboratory test results *Children:* Oral/IV—0.2 mg/kg once daily; maximum dosage is 10 mg; adjust based on INR laboratory test results

 High-alert drug.

Side Effects. Side effects of warfarin are uncommon but include excessive bleeding, blood in urine or stool, headache, upset stomach, diarrhea, fever, and skin rash.

Adverse Effects. Hemorrhage (excessive bleeding), although rare, can be life threatening. Symptoms include unusual bleeding or bruising, black or bloody stools, blood in the urine, fatigue, unexplained fever, chills, sore throat, stomach pain, or headaches that will not go away (often described as "the worst headache of my life"). Patients may also vomit emesis that resembles coffee grounds, indicating bleeding in the gastrointestinal system.

Warfarin-induced skin necrosis (Figure 20-3) is a rare but serious complication that typically happens in women who are obese and going through menopause. It is associated with large doses of warfarin and usually occurs within 1 to 10 days of starting the drug. Management involves using high doses of IM or IV vitamin K as an antidote for warfarin and heparin for anticoagulation. Vitamin K should be readily available when a patient in taking warfarin.

What To Do *Before* Giving Clotting Factor Synthesis Inhibitors

In addition to the general responsibilities related to anticoagulant therapy (p. 327), check the patient's INR laboratory results. Ensure that vitamin K, the antidote for warfarin, is readily available. A common brand of this antidote is phytonadione (AquaMEPHYTON).

Find out whether the patient is following a vegetarian diet or eats a lot of green salads because some vegetables are rich in vitamin K (for example, green leafy vegetables), which can decrease the action of warfarin. (Remember that vitamin K is the antidote for warfarin.)

Ask female patients of childbearing age if they are pregnant or planning to become pregnant because warfarin can cause birth defects and bleeding in an unborn baby.

Because many drugs and herbal supplements interfere with warfarin, be sure to check the patient's current drug list for interactions.

What To Do *After* Giving Clotting Factor Synthesis Inhibitors

In addition to the general responsibilities related to anticoagulant therapy (p. 327), tell the patient that an INR will be performed regularly to help adjust the dose of this drug.

Remind him or her to avoid intermittent large amounts of foods rich in vitamin K (especially leafy green vegetables) because they interfere with the action of warfarin.

What To *Teach* Patients About Clotting Factor Synthesis Inhibitors

In addition to the general care needs and precautions related to anticoagulant therapy (pp. 327-328), teach patients to maintain their current diet and to not attempt significant diet changes, such as an all-vegetarian or Atkins diet. Abrupt changes in a person's diet can alter the INR results. It is important for patients to tell their prescriber if they have recently or are currently including large amounts of foods that are rich in vitamin K (such as liver, green leafy vegetables, broccoli, and cauliflower) in their diet because vitamin K interferes with the action of warfarin. Warn that

Common Side Effects

Clotting Factor Synthesis Inhibitors

Bleeding   Headache   Upset stomach, Diarrhea

Fever   Rash

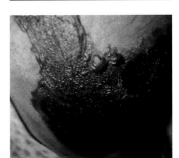

FIGURE 20-3 Warfarin-induced skin necrosis. (From Hoffman, R., et al. (2008). *Hematology: Basic principles and practice* (5th ed.). Philadelphia: Churchill Livingstone.)

Drug Alert!

Action/Intervention Alert

The antidote for warfarin is IM or IV vitamin K.

QSEN: Safety

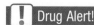

! Drug Alert!

Teaching Alert

Instruct patients not to take over-the-counter drugs (especially aspirin or aspirin-containing drugs) or herbal supplements without asking their prescriber first.

QSEN: Safety

! Drug Alert!

Teaching Alert

Remind patients that it takes several days after stopping warfarin for the body to recover its normal clotting ability.

QSEN: Safety

Clinical Pitfall

Warfarin should not be given during pregnancy.

QSEN: Safety

Did You Know?

Aspirin, the most commonly prescribed antiplatelet drug, comes in tablet, capsule, gum, and suppository forms.

Do Not Confuse

Aggrastat *with* **Argatroban**

An order for Aggrastat may be confused with Argatroban. Aggrastat is a platelet inhibitor, whereas argatroban is a thrombin inhibitor.

QSEN: Safety

alcohol can interfere with the action of warfarin, and advise patients to talk to their prescriber before drinking alcohol.

Life Span Considerations for Clotting Factor Synthesis Inhibitors

Pediatric Considerations. Although warfarin is rarely used in children, there are cases in which it is necessary. Side effects and risks are the same as for adults. Parents should be taught that their child should not receive IM injections, take aspirin-containing drugs, or participate in contact sports while taking this drug.

Considerations for Pregnancy and Lactation. Warfarin is a teratogen (can cause birth defects) and has a high likelihood of causing fetal harm. Women who are of childbearing age should use birth control while taking this drug.

Considerations for Older Adults. Older adults may require lower doses of warfarin because they are more sensitive to its effects and more likely to develop side effects such as bleeding and bruising. Older patients may need more frequent monitoring of the INR.

ANTIPLATELET DRUGS

How Antiplatelet Drugs Work

Antiplatelet drugs, also known as *platelet inhibitors,* use different mechanisms to prevent platelets from clumping together *(aggregating)* to form harmful clots. Antiplatelet drugs are prescribed for prevention of clots in the brain and cardiovascular system. They are used to treat patients with coronary artery disease, heart attack, angina, stroke, transient ischemic attacks (TIAs), and peripheral artery disease (PAD).

Aspirin is the most common antiplatelet drug. It works by irreversibly inhibiting the cyclooxygenase (COX) enzyme from making active thromboxane A_2 (TXA_2) in platelets. TXA_2 is critical for activating platelets, making them "sticky" and allowing them to clump together to form a platelet plug. After a single dose of aspirin, clotting is reduced for at least 36 hours until fresh platelets that have not been exposed to aspirin are released into circulation from the spleen. All other nonsteroidal anti-inflammatory drugs (NSAIDs) also inhibit the production of TXA_2 but to a lesser degree than aspirin. Platelets recover the ability to clump within 8 hours after an NSAID is taken.

Some antiplatelet drugs work by reversibly inhibiting a different enzyme in platelets that prevent them from becoming active and clumping. Drugs with this action include cilostazol and dipyridamole.

Other antiplatelet drugs reversibly or irreversibly block one or more receptors on platelet membranes that prevents their clumping together to form platelet plugs. Drugs with this action include clopidogrel, eptifibatide, prasugrel, ticagrelor, ticlopidine, and tirofiban. Be sure to consult a drug reference book for information about a specific antiplatelet drug.

Dosages for Common Antiplatelet Drugs

Drug	Dosage
aspirin (Acuprin, Arthrinol ♣, Ecotrin, Entrophen ♣, many other trade names)	*Adults:* 81-325 mg orally once daily
cilostazol (Pletal)	*Adults:* 100 mg orally twice daily
clopidogrel ❶ (Plavix)	*Adults:* 75 mg orally once daily
dipyridamole (Permole, Persantine)	*Adults:* 75-100 mg orally 4 times daily (in conjunction with warfarin therapy)
eptifibatide ❶ (Integrilin)	*Adults:* 180 mcg/kg IV bolus followed by continuous IV infusion of 2 mcg/kg/min
prasugrel (Effient)	*Adults:* 60 mg orally once as a loading dose followed by 10 mg orally once daily

Dosages for Common Antiplatelet Drugs—cont'd

Drug	Dosage
ticagrelor (Brilinta)	*Adults:* 180 mg orally once as a loading dose followed by 90 mg orally twice daily
ticlopidine ❶ (Ticlid)	*Adults:* 250 mg orally twice daily with food
tirofiban ❶ (Aggrastat)	*Adults:* 0.4 mcg/kg/min IV for 30 min, then 0.1 mcg/kg/min IV

❶ High-alert drug.

Side Effects. Common side effects of antiplatelet drugs include bleeding, headache, dizziness, and gastrointestinal disturbances.

Adverse Effects. As discussed in the general issues section, hemorrhage is the most common adverse effect and can be life threatening. Allergic reactions to these drugs have occurred but are not common. Adverse effects of salicylates (aspirin) are discussed in Chapter 6.

A decreased platelet count (thrombocytopenia) is the most common adverse effect of these drugs after bleeding. This problem is most common with the use of *cilostazol*, *clopidogrel*, *eptifibatide*, *ticlopidine*, and *tirofiban*.

What To Do *Before* Giving Antiplatelet Drugs

In addition to the general responsibilities related to anticoagulant therapy (p. 327), check the patient's platelet count.

Antacids interfere with the absorption of antiplatelet drugs. Give antiplatelet drugs 2 hours after or 1 hour before giving antacids. Also give antiplatelet drugs with meals or just after eating to decrease side effects such as nausea and upset stomach.

What To Do *After* Giving Antiplatelet Drugs and What To Teach Patients About Antiplatelet Drugs

Continue the general responsibilities related to anticoagulant therapy, and teach patients the general care needs and precautions related to anticoagulant therapy (pp. 327-328). To decrease the side effect of nausea, teach patients to take antiplatelet drugs with food.

Remind them that they may need to take these drugs for the rest of their lives to prevent clots from forming. Instruct them to continue taking antiplatelet drugs unless their prescriber stops the therapy.

Life Span Considerations for Antiplatelet Drugs

Considerations for Pregnancy and Lactation. Taking antiplatelet drugs during the last 2 weeks of pregnancy can cause bleeding problems in the baby before and after delivery. Antiplatelet drugs can be passed through breast milk to the baby. As discussed in Chapter 6, aspirin and other NSAIDs should not be taken during the last 3 months of pregnancy or while breastfeeding.

THROMBOLYTIC DRUGS

How Thrombolytic Drugs Work

Thrombolytic drugs, also called **fibrinolytic** drugs, are drugs that dissolve clots that have already formed. This is why these drugs have the nickname "clot busters." They are prescribed for patients who have had a heart attack, stroke, pulmonary embolism, or some other clot-related problem. All thrombolytic drugs activate plasminogen, an inactive form of plasmin found in body fluids and blood plasma. Plasminogen forms plasmin, an enzyme that dissolves the fibrin in blood clots. All thrombolytics are able to initiate the process of breaking down clots and can prevent new clots from forming.

Clot busters are IV drugs given in a setting with specially trained nurses (e.g., emergency department, cardiac catheterization lab, or intensive care unit). They may

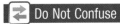
Do Not Confuse

Ticlid *with* Tequin

An order for Ticlid may be confused with Tequin. Ticlid is a platelet inhibitor, whereas Tequin is a quinolone antibiotic used to treat infections.

QSEN: Safety

Common Side Effects

Antiplatelet Drugs

Bleeding   Nausea, Upset   Headache
stomach

Drug Alert!

Teaching Alert

While taking an antiplatelet drug, teach patients to read labels of over-the-counter drugs to make sure that they are aspirin free and NSAID free.

QSEN: Safety

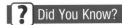
Did You Know?

The body makes its own naturally occurring clot busters such as tissue-type plasminogen activator.

be given by a peripheral IV line or through a long catheter that is guided to the clot. If started within 12 hours after the onset of symptoms for heart attack or 3 hours for stroke symptoms, thrombolytics can dissolve the clot that is blocking the artery and restore blood flow. This action may prevent or minimize tissue damage to the heart or brain. The sooner these drugs are begun, the more likely it is that they will achieve a positive result. About 12% of patients will have clots that form again, especially if the underlying problem that caused the clot has not been treated. In some situations (for example, a heart attack), thrombolytics are not used if more than 6 hours have passed since the symptoms began because tissue damage has already occurred, and at this point the drugs can cause more problems than they prevent.

The most commonly prescribed thrombolytic drugs are alteplase (Activase [t-PA]), tenecteplase (TNKase), and reteplase (Retavase). Urokinase (Abbokinase, Kinlytic), which had been removed from the market, is now approved only for treatment of massive, acute pulmonary embolism.

Drug Alert!

Administration Alert

The sooner thrombolytic drugs are started, the more likely it is that they will successfully dissolve a clot.

QSEN: Safety

Dosages for Common Thrombolytic Drugs

Drug	Dosage
alteplase (Activase [t-PA], Activase rt-PA ♦)	**Myocardial Infarction:** *Adults:* weight greater than 67 kg: 15 mg IV bolus, followed by 50 mg IV over 30 min, then 35 mg IV over 60 min; follow with heparin therapy **Pulmonary Embolism:** *Adults:* 100 mg IV over 2 hr followed by heparin therapy **Stroke:** *Adults:* 0.9 mg/kg (no more than 90 mg) IV over 1 hr (10% of dose given as bolus during first min)
reteplase ❶ (Retavase)	*Adults:* 10 units IV followed by additional 10 units in 30 min
tenecteplase ❶ (TNKase)	*Adults:* IV: weight-based (30-50 mg IV push)
urokinase (Abbokinase, Kinlytic)	**Indicated for use only for active lysis of a massive, acute pulmonary embolism** *Adults:* 4400 IU/kg IV infused over 10 min, followed by 4400 IU/kg/hr as a continuous infusion for 12 hours

❶ High-alert drug.

Do Not Confuse

t-PA (alteplase) *with* TNKase (tenecteplase)

An order for t-PA can be confused with TNKase. Both are thrombolytic drugs. t-PA is given by IV infusion, whereas TNKase is given by IV push. Dosages are also different.

QSEN: Safety

Common Side Effects

Thrombolytic Drugs

Bleeding   Fever   Hypotension

Intended Responses
- Clotting time is increased.
- Existing clot is dissolved.
- Blood flow is restored in a blocked artery.
- Tissue damage is prevented or minimized.

Side Effects. The most common side effects of thrombolytic drugs include bleeding or oozing from cuts, gums, and wounds and around injection sites. Other common side effects include fever and low blood pressure.

Adverse Effects. Patients who experience allergic reactions may have shortness of breath, fever, chills, chest tightness, swelling, wheezing, skin rash, hives, or itching.

Hemorrhage is a major risk when patients receive thrombolytic therapy because the action of these drugs is to break down clots. They increase the risk of hemorrhagic stroke because of the increased risk for bleeding, which includes bleeding into the brain.

What To Do *Before* Giving Thrombolytic Drugs

In addition to the general responsibilities related to anticoagulant therapy (p. 327), determine whether the patient has experienced any of the events listed in Box 20-1 because they are absolute contraindications for thrombolytic therapy. With absolute contraindications, the therapy should *not* be given. With some other high-risk

Box 20-1	Absolute Contraindications for Thrombolytic Drugs

- Active internal bleeding
- Cerebrovascular processes:
  - Cranial neoplasm
  - Recent spinal or cerebral surgery
  - Recent stroke (within 2 months)
- Increased blood pressure greater than 200/120 mm Hg
- Known bleeding disorders
- Pregnancy or recent delivery (24 hours)
- Prolonged cardiopulmonary resuscitation
- Recent head trauma
- Suspected aortic dissection

conditions, the prescriber weighs the pros and cons of the treatment before making a decision.

Check the patient's coagulation laboratory study results. Make sure that all ordered laboratory tests have been completed and that the patient has IV lines in place.

What To Do *After* Giving Thrombolytic Drugs

In addition to the general responsibilities related to anticoagulant therapy (p. 327), check the patient for any signs of bleeding at least every 2 hours and report these immediately. Ask the patient about headaches and monitor for changes in level of consciousness. Initially check the patient every 20 to 30 minutes, then every 1 to 2 hours, every 4 hours, every shift, and as needed.

Because of the risk for bleeding, do not give any injectable (intramuscular or subcutaneous) drugs to the patient. Do not start or remove IV lines. If a line must be removed, you will need to apply pressure to the site for at least 30 minutes.

Patients often also receive IV fluids, including anticoagulation with continuous heparin to prevent additional clots from forming. Make sure that these IV fluids are infusing at the correct rate and that the IV line is patent. Make sure that follow-up laboratory tests for coagulation are completed.

What To *Teach* Patients About Thrombolytic Drugs

Thrombolytic drugs are given in the hospital setting, so most patient teaching is done there. Instruct patients to report any problems with their IV access sites such as bleeding, swelling, pain, or numbness.

Instruct patients to report any unusual symptoms at once. Also tell them to report any arm or leg pain that seems to be getting worse.

Life Span Considerations for Thrombolytic Drugs

Considerations for Pregnancy and Lactation. Thrombolytic drugs have a moderate likelihood of increasing the risk for birth defects or fetal harm, especially during the first 5 months of pregnancy. Delivery of a baby within the past 24 hours is a contraindication to giving these drugs.

DRUGS THAT IMPROVE BLOOD CLOTTING

COLONY-STIMULATING FACTORS

How Colony-Stimulating Factors Work

Sometimes drugs are needed to *improve* the ability of the blood to clot rather than to decrease clotting. These drugs increase the number of red blood cells (RBCs) and platelets available to improve blood clotting and are known generally as **colony-stimulating factors (CSFs)**. The bone marrow normally makes these blood components in response to naturally occurring hormones. For example, when a person is *anemic* (has too few RBCs), the ability of the blood to carry oxygen is reduced, and tissues do not receive the normal amount of oxygen. When the kidney receives less oxygen, it secretes erythropoietin into the blood. This substance goes to the bone marrow and stimulates it to increase production of RBCs. Drugs that increase RBC levels are known as **erythropoiesis-stimulating agents (ESAs)**, and those that increase

 Clinical Pitfall

Thrombolytic drugs should not be given if there are absolute contraindications (see Box 20-1).

QSEN: Safety

 Clinical Pitfall

After a patient has received a thrombolytic drug, do not start or remove IV lines and do not give IM injections.

QSEN: Safety

 Drug Alert!

Teaching Alert

Instruct patients to report any problems with IV access sites such as bleeding, swelling, pain, or numbness.

QSEN: Safety

 Drug Alert!

Administration Alert

Bleeding is more likely to occur in children and older adults because they are more sensitive to the effects of thrombolytic drugs.

QSEN: Safety

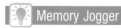

Memory Jogger

ESAs (erythropoiesis-stimulating agents) increase red blood cell (RBC) levels. TSAs (thrombopoiesis-stimulating agents) increase platelet levels.

platelet levels are known as **thrombopoiesis-stimulating agents (TSAs)**. ESAs and TSAs are similar to the naturally occurring hormones that trigger the bone marrow to produce more cells. ESAs make the bone marrow increase production of RBCs to the greatest extent, although they do increase all blood cell production to some degree. TSAs are more specific for stimulating the bone marrow to increase production of platelets, although the production of other cells also increases.

ESAs are most often used for patients who have chronic kidney disease, are anemic from cancer chemotherapy, or need to increase RBC counts before surgery. TSAs are most often used for patients who have low platelet counts from cancer chemotherapy. Both types of drugs reduce the need for transfusion of blood and blood products.

Dosages for Common Colony-Stimulating Factors

Drug	Dosage
Erythropoiesis-Stimulating Agents	
darbepoetin alfa (Aranesp)	*Adults/Children:* 0.45 mcg/kg IV or subcutaneously each week (can be given in divided doses 2 to 3 times per week until the hemoglobin level approaches 12 g/dL)
epoetin alfa (Epogen, Eprex ✦, Procrit)	*Adults/Children:* 50-100 units/kg IV or subcutaneously 3 times per week to maintain hemoglobin levels within the individualized target range
Thrombopoiesis-Stimulating Agents	
oprelvekin (Neumega)	*Adults/Children:* 50 mcg/kg subcutaneously once daily until the platelet count is greater than 50,000/mm³

Common Side Effects

Colony-Stimulating Factors

Hypertension

Headache

Fever, flushing

Pain at injection site

Intended Responses
- Blood cell levels are approaching normal.
- There is a reduced need for transfusion therapy.

Side Effects. Because these drugs increase blood cell production, the blood becomes more viscous (thicker). This effect raises blood pressure, increases clot formation, and slows blood movement through small vessels. Other side effects include headaches, general body aches, flushing, fever, chills, and pain at the injection site.

Adverse Effects. Because colony-stimulating factors increase blood viscosity and fluid retention, the patient is at risk for hypertension, blood clots, strokes, and heart attacks. In addition, certain types of cancer cells grow faster in the presence of these factors such as head and neck cancer cells, leukemias, and lymphomas. The basis of dosing for these drugs is to monitor individual patient hemoglobin or platelet levels to ensure that just enough cells are produced to avoid the need for transfusion.

What To Do *Before* Giving Colony-Stimulating Factors
If the patient is receiving a repeat dose of the drug, ask him or her if any allergic reactions or difficulty breathing occurred with a previous dose. If the patient has had such a response, notify the prescriber before giving the drug.

Check the patient's blood counts before therapy. If the platelet count is greater than 50,000/mm³ or if the hemoglobin level is at 12 g/dL (or higher), notify the prescriber before giving the drug.

Check the patient's blood pressure and use this value to monitor for drug-induced hypertension.

Follow the package directions for mixing and preparing the drug.

Ensure that oprelvekin (Neumega) is administered only by deep subcutaneous injection and not intravenously or intradermally.

What To Do *After* Giving Colony-Stimulating Factors

When giving the first IV dose of a colony-stimulating factor, check the patient every 20 minutes for any signs or symptoms of an allergic reaction (hives at the IV site, low blood pressure, rapid irregular pulse, swelling of the lips or lower face, the patient feeling a "lump in the throat"). If you suspect an allergic reaction, call the rapid response team and notify the prescriber.

Check the patient's blood pressure and complete blood count to determine the effectiveness of the drug and whether increased viscosity is occurring.

What To *Teach* Patients About Colony-Stimulating Factors

Teach patients to weigh themselves daily and report a weight gain of more than 2 lb in a 24-hour period or 4 lb in a week to their prescriber.

Teach them to report immediately any sign of a clot (swelling in one extremity, difference in skin color or temperature in one extremity, pain in one extremity) to their prescriber. Remind them to be sure to have blood tests done as often as prescribed.

Instruct them to go immediately to the emergency department for chest pain, shortness of breath, change in level of consciousness, difficulty speaking, numbness or drooping of one side of the face, or blurred vision. These are signs of a heart attack or stroke.

For patients who are self-administering the drug, teach them the proper technique for subcutaneous injection and how to monitor the site for problems.

Life Span Considerations for Colony-Stimulating Factors

Considerations for Pregnancy and Lactation. Colony-stimulating factors have a moderate likelihood of increasing the risk for birth defects or fetal harm. They should be avoided during pregnancy unless the benefits outweigh the possible risks. These drugs should not be used during breastfeeding.

Considerations for Older Adults. The increased viscosity of the blood is more likely to result in hypertension and increase the risk for congestive heart failure, pulmonary edema, heart attacks, and strokes. Older adults should be monitored more closely for blood cell responses, and the therapy should be stopped or decreased when hemoglobin levels approach 11 g/dL or if hypertension develops.

Drug Alert!

Teaching Alert

Teach patients to report signs of clot formation immediately (e.g., swelling in one extremity, pain in one extremity, a difference in temperature or color in one extremity).

QSEN: Safety

Get Ready for Practice!

Key Points

- Clot formation is a normal protective process that prevents blood loss.
- Dangerous forms of clots include thrombi and emboli.
- Anticoagulant drugs prevent clots from forming or existing clots from getting bigger.
- An initial IV bolus of heparin is based on the patient's weight; the rate of the continuous infusion is based on the aPTT laboratory results.
- LMW heparins such as enoxaparin (Lovenox) do not require laboratory tests to guide therapy.
- Protamine sulfate, the antidote to heparin, should be readily available when a patient is receiving heparin.
- Dose prescription for warfarin is guided by the INR laboratory test. A therapeutic INR is 2.0 to 3.0 (normal INR is 0.8 to 1.2).

- Vitamin K, the antidote for warfarin, should be available when a patient is receiving this drug.
- Antiplatelet drugs prevent platelets from clumping together (aggregating) to form clots.
- A patient taking warfarin and some other anticoagulant drugs should not take aspirin-containing drugs or NSAIDs at the same time because of the increased risk for bleeding.
- Thrombolytic (fibrinolytic) drugs dissolve existing clots. They are also called *clot busters*.
- Clot busters should be started as soon as possible after symptoms appear because the sooner they are started, the more likely it is that they will dissolve the clot and prevent tissue damage.
- A complete patient health history is very important before giving thrombolytic drugs because there are reasons the drugs may not be given (contraindications).
- Colony-stimulating factors are used to improve blood clotting.

Additional Learning Resources

evolve Be sure to visit your Evolve website (http://evolve.elsevier.com/Workman/pharmacology/) for additional online resources.

[SG] Go to your Study Guide for additional learning activities to help you master this chapter content.

Review Questions

See the Answer Keys—In-text Review Questions for answers to these questions.

Test Yourself on the Basics

1. What is the main purpose of anticoagulation therapy?
   A. To dissolve existing clots and improve blood flow
   B. To prevent a thrombus from becoming an embolus
   C. To prevent an embolus from becoming a thrombus
   D. To prevent clots from forming where they are not needed

2. Which condition is a common indication for the use of an anticoagulant drug?
   A. Pregnancy
   B. Brain surgery
   C. Atrial fibrillation
   D. Excessive bruising in an extremity after trauma

3. Which of the following drugs or supplements makes the risk for bleeding worse when a patient is also taking an anticoagulant drug? Select all that apply.
   A. Aspirin
   B. Caffeine
   C. Gingko biloba
   D. Nicotine
   E. Oral contraceptives
   F. St. John's wort
   G. Vitamin C
   H. Vitamin K

4. What agent is used as an antidote for a warfarin (Coumadin) overdose?
   A. Phytonadione
   B. Protamine sulfate
   C. Vitamin C
   D. Vitamin K

5. After bleeding, what is the most common adverse effect of most antiplatelet drugs?
   A. Decreased platelet count
   B. Lowered seizure threshold
   C. Pulmonary embolism
   D. Formation of stomach ulcers

6. What agent is used as an antidote for a heparin overdose?
   A. Phytonadione
   B. Protamine sulfate
   C. Vitamin C
   D. Vitamin K

Test Yourself on Advanced Concepts

7. Which action is essential before beginning continuous IV heparin therapy?
   A. Have the laboratory draw an INR blood test.
   B. Get an accurate baseline patient weight.
   C. Make a sign that states, "No IM or subcutaneous injections."
   D. Instruct the patient to remain on bed rest and use the call light.

8. Which anticoagulant drug must be avoided during pregnancy because it can cause birth defects in the fetus?
   A. Alteplase (Activase)
   B. Heparin (Hepalean)
   C. Warfarin (Coumadin)
   D. Rivaroxaban (Xarelto)

9. Which laboratory test result indicates that an antiplatelet drug is effective?
   A. International normalized ratio (INR) is increasing.
   B. Total red blood cell count is increasing.
   C. Platelet count is increasing.
   D. Platelet count is decreasing.

10. Which action is important to prevent losing any part of the drug dose when administering low molecular weight heparin?
    A. Not using dextrose in water to flush the IV line
    B. Not rubbing the injection site after injecting the drug
    C. Not expelling the air bubble before injecting the drug
    D. Not aspirating after inserting the needle into the injection site and before injecting the drug

11. Why is the antiplatelet effect of aspirin longer lasting than that of other nonsteroidal anti-inflammatory drugs (NSAIDs)?
    A. Aspirin irreversibly inhibits the production of TXA2, whereas NSAIDs cause reversible inhibition of this substance.
    B. Aspirin can be taken up to 6 times per day, and most NSAIDs can only be taken twice per day.
    C. Other NSAIDs have more effects on other tissues, but aspirin targets platelets specifically.
    D. Other NSAIDs are more rapidly metabolized and eliminated than is aspirin.

12. Why is it important to teach the patient starting on the anticoagulant warfarin (Coumadin) to limit his or her intake of leafy green vegetables?
    A. These foods contain vitamin K, which can increase the effects of warfarin.
    B. These foods contain vitamin K, which can reduce the effects of warfarin.
    C. These foods enhance aspirin activity and increase the risk for bleeding in the person who also takes warfarin.
    D. These foods reduce aspirin activity and increase the risk for pulmonary embolism in the person who also takes warfarin.

13. What is the major mechanism of action that allows thrombolytic drugs to dissolve clots?
    A. Increasing the blood level of the enzyme plasmin
    B. Decreasing the blood level of the enzyme plasmin
    C. Increasing the blood level of antithrombin III
    D. Decreasing the blood level of antithrombin III

14. Which problems, conditions, or drugs are absolute contraindications for thrombolytic therapy? Select all that apply.
    A. Previous heart attack 5 years before
    B. Chronic use of oral contraceptives
    C. Recent head trauma
    D. Undergoing cancer chemotherapy
    E. Delivering a baby within the past 24 hours
    F. Received a blood transfusion within the past 2 weeks
    G. Receiving low-molecular-weight heparin within the past 24 hours
    H. Taking aspirin 81 mg daily for the past 2 years
15. What is an intended response when a patient is prescribed epoetin alfa (Epogen)?
    A. Red blood cell levels normalize.
    B. New blood clots do not form.
    C. Clotting time is increased.
    D. Thrombolytic events are prevented.
16. A patient is to receive 3000 units of subcutaneous heparin. Heparin comes as 5000 units in 1 mL. How many milliliters will you give? _____ mL

Critical Thinking Activities

See the Answer Keys—Critical Thinking Activities for answers to these activities.

A 71-year-old man has been prescribed rivaroxaban (Xarelto) 20 mg orally every day for atrial fibrillation. He tells you that some of his friends are also taking "blood thinners" and that he is not looking forward to "all of those needle sticks" that his friends get every week. He also asks whether he needs to change his diet in any way while taking this drug.
1. What type of drug is rivaroxaban?
2. What is/are the major side effect(s) of this drug?
3. Will this patient need to have weekly blood tests with this drug? Why or why not?
4. What will you teach this patient about needed dietary changes?
5. What would you teach this patient to avoid excessive bleeding while taking this drug?

Drug Therapy for Asthma and Other Respiratory Problems

http://evolve.elsevier.com/Workman/pharmacology/

Objectives

After studying this chapter you should be able to:

1. Describe the names, actions, usual adult dosages, possible side effects, and adverse effects of bronchodilator drugs, anti-inflammatory drugs, and mucolytic drugs for respiratory problems.
2. Describe what to do before and after giving bronchodilator drugs, anti-inflammatory drugs, and mucolytic drugs.
3. Explain what to teach patients taking bronchodilator drugs, anti-inflammatory drugs, and mucolytic drugs, including what to do, what not to do, and when to call the prescriber.
4. Describe life span considerations for bronchodilator drugs, anti-inflammatory drugs, and mucolytic drugs.
5. List the names, actions, usual adult dosages, possible side effects, and adverse effects of drugs to treat pulmonary hypertension and pulmonary fibrosis.
6. Describe what to do before and after giving drugs to treat pulmonary hypertension and pulmonary fibrosis.
7. Explain what to teach patients taking drugs to treat pulmonary hypertension and pulmonary fibrosis.

Key Terms

anti-inflammatory drugs (ăn-tī-ĭn-FLĂM-ĕ-tōr-ē DRŬGZ) (p. 347) A class of drug that prevents or limits inflammatory responses to injury or invasion.

beta$_2$-adrenergic agonists (BE-tă TU ăd-rĕn-ĚRJ-ĭk ĂG-ō-nĭsts) (p. 343) Drugs that bind to the beta$_2$-adrenergic receptors and act like adrenalin, causing an increase in the production of a substance that triggers pulmonary smooth muscle relaxation.

bronchodilator (brŏn-kō-DĪ-lā-tŭr) (p. 343) A drug that relaxes the smooth muscle around airways, causing the center openings to enlarge.

cholinergic antagonists (kō-lĭn-ĚRJ-ĭk ăn-TĂG-ō-nĭsts) (p. 344) Drugs that block the parasympathetic nervous system allowing a person's natural epinephrine and norepinephrine to bind to smooth muscle receptors and cause bronchodilation.

corticosteroids (kōr-tĭ-kō-STĔR-ōydz) (p. 347) Drugs similar to natural cortisol that prevent or limit inflammation by slowing or stopping inflammatory mediator production.

endothelin-receptor antagonists (ĕn-dō-thē-lĭn rē-SĔP-tŏr ăn-TĂG-ō-nĭsts) (p. 350) Drugs that are able to block the endothelin-1 receptors on endothelial cells in blood vessels, resulting in blood vessel dilation.

mucolytic (myū-kō-LĬ-tĭk) (p. 349) A drug that reduces the thickness of mucus, making it easier to move out of the airways.

prostacyclin agents (prŏ-stă-SĪ-klĭnz) (p. 350) A drug group composed of naturally occurring and synthetic agents with the main effect of dilating pulmonary blood vessels.

OVERVIEW

All cells need oxygen (O_2) to live, grow, and perform their specific jobs. This oxygen comes from the air you breathe. Air with oxygen enters the nose and mouth and moves through the airways (trachea, bronchi, bronchioles) into air sacs located in the lungs. These air sacs are called *alveoli* and are the sites where oxygen from the air moves into the blood so it can be carried to all tissues and organs. The waste gas created in the tissues, *carbon dioxide (CO_2)*, moves from the blood into the alveoli so it can be exhaled.

The major health problems of the respiratory system are those that narrow the airways such as asthma or chronic bronchitis and diseases that destroy the alveoli

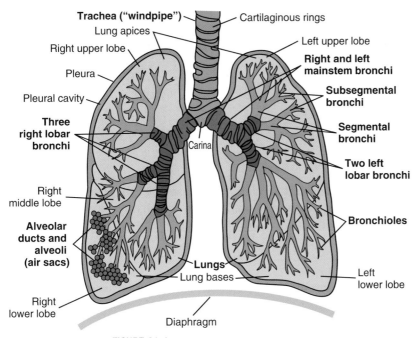

FIGURE 21-1 Normal anatomy of the lungs.

Trachea ("windpipe")
Lung apices
Right upper lobe
Pleura
Pleural cavity
Three right lobar bronchi
Right middle lobe
Alveolar ducts and alveoli (air sacs)
Right lower lobe

Cartilaginous rings
Left upper lobe
Right and left mainstem bronchi
Subsegmental bronchi
Segmental bronchi
Two left lobar bronchi
Bronchioles
Left lower lobe

Carina
Lungs
Lung bases
Diaphragm

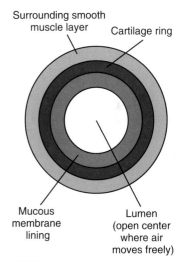

FIGURE 21-2 Close-up view of one small airway with attached alveoli.

Bands of smooth muscle
Alveoli

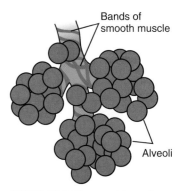

FIGURE 21-3 Cross section of a small airway showing the tissue layers.

Surrounding smooth muscle layer
Cartilage ring
Mucous membrane lining
Lumen (open center where air moves freely)

such as emphysema. *Chronic obstructive pulmonary disease (COPD)* is a respiratory disorder that is a combination of chronic bronchitis and emphysema. Other less common respiratory disorders that involve the lung tissue rather than the airways and result in impairment of gas exchange are pulmonary artery hypertension (PAH) and pulmonary fibrosis. This chapter is focused on drug therapy for asthma, COPD, PAH, and pulmonary fibrosis. Although any part of the lungs can become infected, infection is not a respiratory-related cause of disease. Drugs for infection, including respiratory infections, are discussed in Chapters 8 through 10.

REVIEW OF RELATED PHYSIOLOGY AND PATHOPHYSIOLOGY

Figure 21-1 shows the normal anatomy of the lungs, including the larger airways and the smaller airways leading to the alveoli. Figure 21-2 shows a close-up of one small airway with the alveoli attached. It is important for the airways to remain open for good airflow to and from the alveoli where oxygen and carbon dioxide are exchanged. As shown in Figure 21-3, the airways have several layers around a hollow middle section. It is also important that the membranes of the alveoli remain thin enough to permit oxygen and carbon dioxide to diffuse through them. In addition, blood vessels in the lungs must remain mostly dilated, relatively thin, and have lower pressures to allow good blood flow through the lungs for proper gas exchange.

The open center of the hollow part of the airway is called the *lumen.* Different health problems can affect the lumen in various ways, making it smaller or even closing it completely. The middle can be blocked by thick mucus and other substances. In addition, the mucous membrane lining of the tube can swell when it is inflamed and block off the open area. One of the layers around the tubes is made up of smooth muscle. If this smooth muscle constricts tightly, the center of the tube can be narrowed or even closed. This is called *bronchoconstriction.*

A common method to measure airway function is *peak expiratory rate flow (PERF).* It is the fastest airflow rate reached at any time during exhalation and measures how well the patient can exhale or blow out his or her breath. PERF is measured by blowing into a handheld meter during exhalation. It can indicate whether the airways are functioning properly or are narrowed. The normal range for PERF is

Memory Jogger

Keeping airways open is critical for air inhalation and ensuring that oxygen reaches the lungs.

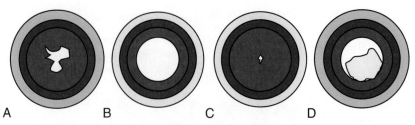

FIGURE 21-4 Different causes of narrowed airways. **A,** Mucosal swelling. **B,** Constriction of smooth muscle. **C,** Mucosal swelling and constriction of smooth muscle. **D,** Mucus plug.

established by age, size, and gender. A decrease in PERF of 15% to 20% below the expected value for a person may occur when the airways are narrowed. *When the PERF value drops below 50%, the patient has dangerously low airflow into and out of the airways.*

ASTHMA

Asthma is usually a chronic disorder in which airway obstruction occurs intermittently from constriction of the bronchial smooth muscles that surround the airways and from inflammation in the airways. It occurs in episodes or attacks. Between attacks the airways are open. Thus the problem is intermittent and reversible. Only the airways are affected, not the alveoli. Two problems can narrow the airways: bronchoconstriction (smooth muscle tightening) and inflammation, as shown in Figure 21-4. Bronchoconstriction blocks the airways from the outside of the airway, and inflammation causes swelling of the mucous membranes and obstructs the lumen, or the inside, of airways. This problem is worse when mucus plugs also form.

Inflammation of the mucous membranes lining the airways is a key event in triggering an asthma attack. It occurs in response to the presence of allergens; irritants such as cold air, dry air, or fine particles in the air; microorganisms; and aspirin. As described in Chapter 6, histamine and leukotrienes are released into the mucous membranes. When this happens, blood vessels dilate, the tissue swells, and mucus increases. These same factors may also cause the smooth muscles around the airways to tighten (constrict).

A patient with mild-to-moderate asthma has no symptoms between asthma attacks. Symptoms of an acute asthma attack are increased respiratory rate and a "wheeze," which is a squeaky or snorelike sound made when air moves through narrowed airways. With inflammation, the patient also has increased coughing. As breathing becomes less effective, blood oxygen levels decrease, and blood carbon dioxide levels increase. If the asthma attack is so severe that oxygen levels become too low, the patient can die.

CHRONIC OBSTRUCTIVE PULMONARY DISEASE

Chronic obstructive pulmonary disease (COPD) is a combination of chronic bronchitis and emphysema. *Chronic bronchitis* is a *persistent* inflammation of the airways. The mucous membranes of the airways are swollen, and the mucus-producing cells enlarge. This creates large amounts of thick, sticky mucus that narrow the airways. As a result, moving air into and out of the lungs is more difficult (see Figure 21-4). *Emphysema* is a problem in which the normal elastic tissue in the alveoli becomes loose and flabby. Because exhalation depends on recoil of the alveoli (just as the "stretch" of a full balloon helps it to deflate quickly), a loss of good elastic tissue makes moving air out of the lungs more difficult. Both chronic bronchitis and emphysema are progressive and become worse with time.

COPD is similar to asthma in terms of airway blockage. However, the symptoms of COPD *never* go away completely, even with drug therapy. The alveoli are damaged in COPD but not in asthma. Thick, sticky mucus is continuously produced in the patient with COPD.

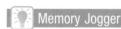

Memory Jogger

The two causes of airway obstruction with asthma are bronchoconstriction and inflammation.

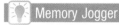

Memory Jogger

A severe asthma attack can lead to death.

TYPES OF DRUGS FOR ASTHMA AND COPD

When asthma is well controlled, the airway narrowing is temporary and reversible. With poor control attacks become worse, happen more often, and can become so severe that the person dies during an attack from lack of oxygen. The goals of drug therapy for asthma are to improve airflow, reduce symptoms, and prevent asthma attacks. The drugs used to help prevent airway closure from asthma come from several categories, depending on the exact problem that is triggering the airways to narrow.

Drug therapy for asthma in adults and children is based on disease severity. Some patients may need drug therapy with a *rescue drug (reliever drug)* only during an asthma episode. Others need daily drugs as *prevention* (known as *controller* drugs) to keep asthma attacks from happening. Total therapy involves the use of drugs that make the smooth muscle around the airways relax *(bronchodilators)* and anti-inflammatory drugs. Thus some drugs reduce the attack severity or stop the attack *(rescue* or *reliever* drugs), and other drugs actually prevent the attack *(controller* drugs).

Although COPD cannot be reversed, its progression can be slowed and the symptoms reduced with proper drug therapy. Drug therapy for COPD is based on disease severity and the patient's responses to the drugs. Because the chronic bronchitis airway problems of COPD are essentially the same as the airway changes occurring during an asthma attack, most of the drugs used to treat COPD are the same as those used to treat asthma. Sometimes the drug dosage or frequency differs, with the person who has COPD taking higher or more frequent doses.

The patient with asthma or chronic bronchitis can help manage his or her disease by assessing symptom severity at least twice daily with a peak flowmeter and adjusting prescribed drugs for inflammation and bronchospasms to prevent or relieve symptoms.

Because the airway narrowing associated with asthma and COPD have more than one cause, drug management usually requires the use of more than one drug type. The types of drugs usually prescribed for asthma and COPD are the bronchodilators, anti-inflammatories, and mucolytics. All of these drugs are used to manage asthma and COPD, although the doses, routes, and timing of the drugs may differ between the two disorders. More drugs for COPD are available as combination agents.

BRONCHODILATORS

Bronchodilators relax smooth muscles in the airways, causing the center openings to enlarge. They have no effect on inflammation. So when a patient's asthma or chronic bronchitis is caused by both bronchoconstriction and inflammation, at least two types of drug therapy are needed. These drugs types include beta$_2$-adrenergic agonists, cholinergic antagonists, and xanthines.

How Bronchodilators Work

Beta$_2$-adrenergic agonists bind to the beta$_2$-adrenergic receptors and act like adrenalin, causing an increase in the production of a substance that triggers pulmonary smooth muscle relaxation. The name of this substance is *cyclic adenosine monophosphate*, known as *cAMP*.

Short-acting beta$_2$-adrenergic agonists (SABAs) provide rapid but short-term relief. They are *rescue drugs* (or reliever drugs) because they are most useful when an asthma attack begins and when the patient is about to start an activity that is likely to induce an asthma attack. These drugs are used for COPD when the patient feels more breathless than usual. When inhaled, the drug is delivered directly to the lungs, and systemic effects are minimal (unless the agent is overused).

Long-acting beta$_2$-adrenergic agonists (LABAs) work in the same way as SABAs but need time to build up an effect. *Therefore LABAs are used to prevent an asthma attack because their effects last longer but have no value during an acute attack.* For COPD these drugs are taken daily to maintain open airways. The patient with COPD may use a nebulizer and mask for some of these drugs rather than a handheld inhaler.

Memory Jogger

Rescue or reliever drugs stop an asthma attack or reduce its severity; controller drugs prevent an attack from starting.

Memory Jogger

Types of drugs for asthma treatment and prevention and COPD maintenance include:
- Bronchodilators.
- Anti-inflammatories
- Mucolytics

Memory Jogger

Short-acting beta$_2$-adrenergic agonists (SABAs) are rescue drugs because they provide rapid but short-term relief.

Memory Jogger

Controller drugs for prevention, such as long-acting beta$_2$-adrenergic agonists (LABAs), must be taken daily and exactly as prescribed, even on days when no symptoms are present. They are NOT to be used as rescue drugs.

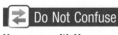

Do Not Confuse

Xopenex *with* **Xanax**

An order for Xopenex may be confused with Xanax. Xopenex is an inhaled short-acting bronchodilator, whereas Xanax is an oral benzodiazepine used to treat anxiety.

QSEN: Safety

Cholinergic antagonists, also known as anticholinergic drugs, block the parasympathetic nervous system. This blockade allows a person's natural epinephrine and norepinephrine to bind to smooth muscle receptors; bronchodilation results. These inhaled drugs also bind to mucous membrane receptors and decrease airway secretions. Like LABAs, they are *controller* (prevention) drugs and must be taken on a daily basis to prevent asthma attacks and reduce airway blockage in COPD. The patient with COPD is more likely to be prescribed a longer-acting cholinergic antagonist. *These controller drugs are used to prevent an asthma attack but have no value during an acute attack.*

Xanthines are powerful systemic drugs but have many side effects. For this reason, they are rarely used today. Check a drug handbook for information about xanthenes or methylxanthenes.

Dosages for Common Bronchodilators

Drug Category	Drug Name	Dosage
Short-acting beta$_2$-agonists (SABAs)	albuterol (Apo-Salvent ♣, PMS-Salbutamol ♣, Proventil HFA, Respirol, Ventolin HFA, VoSpire ER)	*Adults and Children:* 1-2 inhalations of 90 mcg every 4 to 6 hr
	levalbuterol (Xopenex)	*Adults:* 1-2 inhalations of 45 mcg every 4 to 6 hr *Children aged 4 to 12 years:* 1-2 inhalations of 45 mcg every 4 to 6 hr Safety and efficacy for children under age 4 years have not been established.
	pirbuterol (Maxair)	*Adults and children age 12 and older:* 1-2 puffs of 0.2 mg every 4 to 6 hr Safety and efficacy for children under age 12 years have not been established.
Long-acting beta$_2$-agonists (LABAs)	arformoterol (Brovana)	*Adults:* 15 mcg (contents of one 2-mL vial) every 12 hr via nebulization Safety and efficacy for children and adolescents have not been established.
	formoterol (Foradil, Oxeze ♣, Perforomist)	*Adults and children older than 5 years:* 12 mcg (content of one capsule) by DPI every 12 hr Safety and efficacy for children under age 5 years have not been established.
	salmeterol (Serevent)	*Adults and children older than 4 years:* 1 oral inhalation of 50 mcg every 12 hr Safety and efficacy for children under age 4 years have not been established.
Cholinergic antagonists	ipratropium (Apo-Ipravent ♣, Atrovent, Novo-Ipramide ♣, Nu-Ipratropium ♣)	*Adults and children aged 14 years and older:* 2-4 puffs of 17 mcg/puff 3-4 times daily by MDI
	tiotropium (Spiriva)	1 puff (18 mcg) daily (DPI)

DPI, Dry-powder inhaler.

Intended Responses

- Pulmonary smooth muscles relax.
- Airways widen, allowing air to move more freely into and out of the alveoli.
- Wheezing decreases or disappears.
- PERF increases compared with readings taken right before drug therapy.

Side Effects. Bronchodilators that are inhaled have few side effects unless the inhaler is heavily used. Using an inhaler too often allows the drug to be absorbed through the mucous membranes of the mouth, throat, or respiratory linings and enter the bloodstream. Once a drug has entered the bloodstream, it can have systemic effects. Some of the systemic effects of bronchodilators include rapid heart rate, increased blood pressure, a feeling of nervousness, tremors, and difficulty sleeping. The inhaled drugs can dry the mouth and throat and also may leave a bad taste in the mouth.

Cholinergic antagonists can cause some specific side effects if they reach the bloodstream. These effects include urinary retention, blurred vision, eye pain, nausea, and headache.

Adverse Effects. Some brands of inhaled bronchodilators contain preservatives that can cause minor-to-severe allergic reactions. Warn patients to check with their prescriber if a rash, chest pain, or lightheadedness occurs within a few minutes after using the inhaler. In addition, if a patient uses the inhaler more frequently than prescribed, enough drug can reach the blood to cause the blood vessels in the heart to constrict, leading to angina or a heart attack *(myocardial infarction)*.

What To Do *Before* Giving Bronchodilators

Many patients have never used an oral inhaler or a spacer (Figure 21-5) and may not know the correct technique. Ask whether the patient has ever used an inhaler. If the answer is yes, ask him or her to demonstrate or describe the technique used. If the patient has not used an inhaler or a spacer, teach the correct technique. Box 21-1 describes teaching tips for using an aerosol inhaler (also called a metered-dose inhaler) with a spacer; Box 21-2 describes teaching tips for using an aerosol inhaler without a spacer.

The powder used in a dry-powder inhaler may already be loaded in the inhaler or may have to be placed in the inhaler each time it is used. The technique used with dry-powder inhalers differs from that of standard aerosol inhalers (metered dose inhalers [MDIs]) because the powder must remain dry to be active. Box 21-3 describes teaching tips for how to use a dry-powder inhaler.

Use a stethoscope to listen to the lungs of the patient before administering an inhaled bronchodilator. This information can be used to determine drug effectiveness by comparing it with the patient's breath sounds after therapy.

What To Do *After* Giving Bronchodilators

Check the patient's breathing status after giving short-acting inhaler drugs to determine whether the drugs are effective. Breathing improvement as measured by a slower respiratory rate, decreased or absent wheezes, and pulse oximetry values of

Memory Jogger

An easy way to remember the side effects of cholinergic antagonists is the rhyme "can't see, can't spit, can't pee, can't … poop."

Common Side Effects

Bronchodilators

Tachycardia   Hypertension   Dry mouth

Tremors

Drug Alert!

Action/Intervention Alert

Assess for chest pain in the patient taking a bronchodilator.

QSEN: Safety

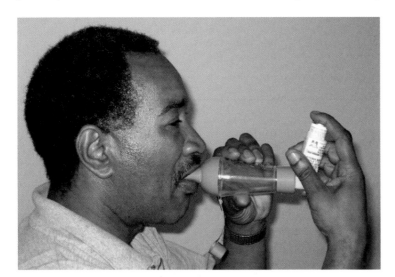

FIGURE 21-5 Patient using an aerosol inhaler with a spacer. (From Ignatavicius, D., & Workman, M. L. (2016). *Medical-surgical nursing: Patient-centered collaborative care* (8th ed.). St. Louis: Saunders.)

Box 21-1	Teaching Tips for Using an Aerosol Inhaler with a Spacer

- Before each use, remove the caps from the inhaler and the spacer.
- Insert the mouthpiece of the inhaler into the non-mouthpiece end of the spacer.
- Shake the whole unit three or four times vigorously to mix the drug in the inhaler.
- Place the mouthpiece of the spacer into your mouth, over your tongue. Seal your lips around the mouthpiece.
- Press down firmly on the canister to release one dose of the drug into the spacer.
- Breathe in slowly and deeply. If the spacer makes a whistling sound, you are breathing in too fast.
- Remove the mouthpiece from your mouth, closing your lips immediately.
- Keep your lips closed and hold your breath for at least 10 seconds, then slowly breathe out.
- If you are prescribed to take two puffs, wait at least 1 minute before taking the second puff.
- Use the same technique for the second puff as you did for the first.
- When finished, remove the inhaler canister from the spacer.
- Replace the caps on the inhaler and the spacer.
- At least once each day, clean the plastic mouthpiece and the cap of the inhaler by thoroughly rinsing them in warm, running tap water.
- Clean the spacer and its mouthpiece at least weekly by thoroughly rinsing them in warm, running tap water.

Box 21-2	Teaching Tips for Using an Aerosol Inhaler Without a Spacer*

1. Before each use, remove the cap and shake the inhaler according to the instructions in the package insert.
2. Tilt your head back slightly and breathe out fully.
3. Open your mouth and place the mouthpiece 1 to 2 inches away.
4. As you begin to breathe in deeply through your mouth, press down firmly on the canister of the inhaler to release one dose of the medication.
5. Continue to breathe in slowly and deeply (usually over 5 to 7 seconds).
6. Hold your breath for at least 10 seconds to allow the medication to reach deep into the lungs, then breathe out slowly.
7. Wait at least 1 minute between puffs.
8. Replace the cap on the inhaler.
9. At least once a day, remove the canister and clean the plastic case and cap of the inhaler by thoroughly rinsing in warm, running tap water.

*Avoid spraying in the direction of the eyes.

Box 21-3	Teaching Tips for Using a Dry-Powder Inhaler

For inhalers requiring loading:
- First load the drug by
  - Turning the device to the next dose of drug, *or*
  - Inserting the capsule into the device, *or*
  - Inserting the disk or compartment into the device.
  After loading the drug and for inhalers that do not require drug loading:
- Read your health care provider's instructions for how fast you should breathe for your particular inhaler.
- Place your lips over the mouthpiece and breathe in forcefully (there is no propellant in the inhaler; only your breath pulls the drug in).
- Remove the inhaler from your mouth as soon as you have inhaled (breathed in).
- Never exhale (breathe out) into your inhaler. Your breath will moisten the powder, causing it to clump and not be delivered accurately.
- Never wash or place the inhaler in water.
- Never shake your inhaler.
- Keep your inhaler in a dry place at room temperature.
- If the inhaler is preloaded, discard the inhaler after it is empty.
- Because the drug is a dry powder and there is no propellant, you may not feel, smell, or taste it as you inhale.

⚠ Drug Alert!

Administration Alert

When giving two or more inhalation drugs for asthma at the same time, give the bronchodilator first and wait at least 5 minutes before giving the second and third drugs.

QSEN: Safety

95% or higher usually occurs within 5 minutes of inhalation of short-acting bronchodilators. If a peak expiratory flowmeter is used to check breathing improvement, the peak flow should increase by at least 15% after using the drug.

Compare the patient's heart rate and blood pressure within 15 minutes after giving the drug to determine whether any systemic effects are present. Ask about any chest pain. Report severe tachycardia, a rapid rise in blood pressure, or chest pain immediately to the prescriber.

If a patient is to receive two or more drugs by inhaler for breathing problems, give the bronchodilator first and wait at least 5 minutes before giving the next drug. This action allows time for the bronchodilator to widen the airways so the next drug can be inhaled more deeply into the respiratory tract and be more effective.

What To *Teach* Patients About Bronchodilators

Inhaled bronchodilators can be very effective in controlling or preventing an asthma attack if used correctly. Teach patients to carry a short-acting beta agonist (SABA) inhaler with them at all times and to ensure that it contains enough drug to be effective. Teach patients that if the short-acting inhaler is needed increasingly more often as a "rescue" from asthma attacks, the prescriber should be notified and other therapy options discussed.

Long-acting beta-adrenergic agonists (LABAs) should be taken as prescribed even when symptoms of asthma are not present because these drugs are used to *prevent* an attack, not to stop an attack that has already started. *Therefore teach patients not to use LABAs to rescue them during an attack or when wheezing is getting worse but to use a SABA. Relying on LABAs during an attack can lead to worsening of symptoms and death.*

Life Span Considerations for Bronchodilators

Pediatric Considerations. Children under the age of 4 years often are not able to use an aerosol inhaler effectively. Usually nebulized forms of the drug with a tight-fitting facemask are required. With beta$_2$ adrenergic agonists, children taking the drugs close to bedtime have difficulty sleeping.

Considerations for Older Adults. Older adults may be more sensitive to the cardiac and nervous system side effects of bronchodilators. Teach older patients to check their pulse rates before and after taking a bronchodilator. Tell them to report any new development of tremors or sleep difficulties to their prescriber. Instruct them to call the life squad or go to the nearest emergency department if chest pain occurs.

Dry-powder inhalers that must be loaded by the patient can be difficult for older patients who have trouble with fine motor movements. Assess the older patient's ability to load and handle the inhaler. If he or she has difficulty, ask the prescriber to consider an inhaler type that does not require the patient to load the drug.

ANTI-INFLAMMATORY DRUGS

There are many **anti-inflammatory drugs** that prevent or limit inflammatory responses to injury or invasion. The drug types used as therapy for asthma and COPD are the corticosteroids, mast cell stabilizers, and leukotriene inhibitors. **Corticosteroids** work like natural cortisol to slow or stop production of inflammatory mediators. None of the anti-inflammatory drugs induce bronchodilation; therefore they are all *controller* drugs, not rescue drugs. Information about these drugs is presented in Chapter 6. Issues related to the aerosolized forms of these drugs delivered by inhalers are presented in the following sections.

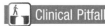 **Clinical Pitfall**

Do not use long-acting adrenergic inhalers for immediate relief of symptoms during an asthma attack. Only a short-acting adrenergic inhaler will be effective.

QSEN: Safety

 Memory Jogger

Anti-inflammatory drugs reduce inflammation but do not cause bronchodilation. They should never be used as rescue inhalers.

QSEN: Safety

Dosages for Common Inhaled Anti-inflammatory Drugs for Asthma and COPD

Drug	Dosage
Inhaled Corticosteroids	
beclomethasone (QVAR)	*Adults and children 4 years or older:* 1-2 puffs of 40 mcg twice daily Safety and efficacy for children under age 4 years have not been established.
budesonide (Pulmicort)	*Adults:* 2 puffs of 180 mcg twice daily *Children 6 years and older:* 1 puff of 180 mcg twice daily Safety and efficacy for children under age 6 years have not been established.
flunisolide (Aerospan HFA)	*Adults and Children 15 years and older:* 2 puffs of 80 mcg twice daily *Children 6-11 years:* 1 puff of 80 mcg twice daily Safety and efficacy for children under age 6 years have not been established.
fluticasone (Flovent HFA, Flovent Diskus)	*Adults:* 88-220 mcg twice daily by MDI (dosages per MDI vary-44 mcg, 110 mcg, 220 mcg) *Children:* 44-88 mcg twice daily by MDI

Continued

Dosages for Common Inhaled Anti-inflammatory Drugs for Asthma and COPD—cont'd

Drug	Dosage
mometasone (Asmanex)	*Adults and children 12 years and older:* 1 puff of 220 mcg once or twice daily *Children 4 to 11 years:* 1 puff of 110 mcg once or twice daily Safety and efficacy for children under age 4 years have not been established.
triamcinolone (Azmacort)	*Adults and Children 12 years or older:* 2-4 puffs of 75 mcg Children 6-11 years: 1-2 puffs of 75 mcg 3-4 times daily Safety and efficacy for children under age 6 years have not been established.
Mast Cell Stabilizers	

cromolyn sodium (Intal
   Inhaler)
	Adults and Children over 5 years: 20 mg (one capsule) by DPI 4 times daily or 2 puffs of
	   800 mcg by MDI 4 times daily
	Safety and efficacy for children under age 5 years have not been established.

nedocromil sodium (Tilade)	*Adults and Children 6 years and older:* 2 puffs of 1.75 mg 4 times daily Safety and efficacy for children under age 6 years have not been established.

MDI, Metered-dose inhaler.

Common Side Effects
Inhaled Anti-Inflammatory Drugs

Dry mouth, Bad taste   Tearing

Intended Responses
- Swelling of pulmonary mucous membranes is reduced.
- Pulmonary secretions are reduced.
- Airway lumens open, allowing air to move more freely into and out of the alveoli.
- Wheezing decreases or disappears.
- PERF remains within the patient's "personal best" range.

Side Effects. Side effects of inhaled anti-inflammatories and inhaled mast cell stabilizers are local and include cough, bad taste, mouth dryness, and an increased risk for oral infection, specifically a candida fungal infection known as "thrush." Mast cell stabilizers also may cause nausea and vomiting.

Adverse Effects. The propellant and preservatives in inhaled drug mixtures can irritate tissues, causing the patient to cough severely or have bronchospasms.

When inhaled corticosteroids are used as prescribed, they have a low risk for any adverse effect. However, when heavily used, they can be absorbed into the bloodstream and cause adrenal gland suppression just as systemic corticosteroids do (see Chapter 6).

What To Do *Before* Giving Inhaled Anti-Inflammatory Drugs for Respiratory Problems
Inspect the patient's mouth and throat to determine whether an infection or thrush is present. Thrush appears as white or cream-colored patches of a cheesy coating on the mucous membranes, roof of the mouth, and tongue.

Many patients have never used an oral inhaler or a spacer (see Figure 21-5) and may not know the correct technique. If the patient has not used an inhaler or a spacer, teach the correct technique (see Boxes 21-1 and 21-2).

If the patient also is receiving an inhaled bronchodilator, give the bronchodilator first and wait at least 5 minutes before giving the inhaled anti-inflammatory. Giving the bronchodilator first allows the greatest widening effect on the airways so the anti-inflammatory can be inhaled more deeply into the respiratory tract and be more effective.

What To Do *After* Giving Inhaled Anti-Inflammatory Drugs for Respiratory Problems
Assist the patient to rinse with water or mouthwash to remove the drug from the mouth. This practice helps reduce the bad taste and mouth dryness.

What To *Teach* Patients About Anti-Inflammatory Drugs for Respiratory Problems

Anti-inflammatory drugs can be very effective in controlling or preventing an asthma attack and reducing the inflammation of chronic bronchitis in COPD if used correctly. They carry a warning that the risk for death from asthma is increased when using these drugs. This is because the anti-inflammatory drugs for respiratory problems may help prevent inflammation but do not cause bronchodilation.

Remind patients to use anti-inflammatory inhalers at least 5 minutes after using an inhaled bronchodilator.

Teach patients to take the drug as prescribed even when symptoms of asthma are not present because these controller drugs are used to *prevent* an attack, not stop an attack that has already started. However, when acute asthma is present, patients should continue to take these prevention drugs as prescribed in addition to the rescue drugs. Teach patients with COPD the importance of taking the drug daily to prevent worsening of chronic bronchitis. Tell patients to be careful about how the inhaler is used because the risk for oral and respiratory infection increases with increased use. In addition, more systemic side effects are likely to occur.

Tell patients using an inhaled drug that rinsing the mouth after using the drug can reduce the bad taste and mouth dryness.

Teach patients to check the gums, mouth, and throat daily in the mirror for increased redness or the presence of white/cream-colored patches that may indicate an infection. Also tell patients to use good oral hygiene at least three times a day to prevent oral infections.

COMBINATION BRONCHODILATOR AND ANTI-INFLAMMATORY DRUGS

An option for people with asthma and COPD is the use of inhalers that contain both a bronchodilator and a corticosteroid for prevention therapy. These drugs include Advair, Symbicort, BREO, Dulera, and Anoro Ellipta. Advair is a combination of the corticosteroid fluticasone and the long-acting bronchodilator salmeterol. Symbicort is a combination of the corticosteroid budesonide and the long-acting bronchodilator formoterol. BREO is a combination of fluticasone and vilanterol. Dulera is a combination of the corticosteroid mometasone and the long-acting bronchodilator formoterol. Anoro Ellipta is a combination of the anticholinergic drug umeclidinium and the long-acting bronchodilator vilanterol. Symbicort, Anoro Ellipta, and BREO are used more for COPD than for asthma. Dulera is approved only for the treatment of asthma. The therapeutic effects, side effects, adverse effects, precautions, and patient education are the same as for each drug individually.

MUCOLYTICS

Most people with COPD take a **mucolytic** drug daily to reduce the thickness of mucus, allowing the mucus to more easily move out of the airways. Patients with asthma may use mucolytics when increased secretions are a problem.

Guaifenesin (Mucinex, Naldecon Senior EX, Organidin) is a systemic mucolytic that is taken orally. Another mucolytic drug prescribed for a person with COPD is acetylcysteine (Mucomyst). Mucus contains protein molecules and mucus molecules held tightly together. This drug works by breaking the connections that hold the protein and mucus molecules. This results in thinner, less sticky mucus that is easier to cough up and spit out.

Acetylcysteine is most commonly delivered with a nebulizer face mask and is also available as an oral drug. Typically 1 to 10 mL of a 20% solution is placed in a medication nebulizer, and the patient uses a mask to breathe in the mist containing the drug every 6 hours. The drug has few side effects but does have a very unpleasant odor. Some patients experience nausea and even vomiting from the smell.

OTHER SERIOUS RESPIRATORY DISORDERS

Two additional serious respiratory problems that are managed by drug therapy are pulmonary artery hypertension and pulmonary fibrosis. Although drug therapy

Drug Alert!

Teaching Alert

Teach patients not to rely on anti-inflammatory drugs alone to stop or reduce bronchoconstriction.

QSEN: Safety

Memory Jogger

Mucolytics improve airflow by reducing the thickness of mucus in the airways.

does not currently result in a cure for either problem, it can reduce symptoms and prolong life.

PULMONARY ARTERIAL HYPERTENSION

Pulmonary artery hypertension (PAH) is a problem in which the blood vessels of the lungs severely constrict, resulting in reduced blood flow and higher pressures throughout the lungs. Over time, the increased pressures damage lung tissue, greatly reduce gas exchange, and cause heart failure. Some people develop PAH after exposure to drugs such as fenfluramine/phentermine (Pondimin or "Fen-Phen") or dasatinib (Sprycel). For other people, there is no known cause, but there may be a genetic basis. The disorder is rare and occurs mostly in women between the ages of 20 and 40 years. Without treatment, death usually occurs within 2 years after diagnosis.

TYPES OF DRUG THERAPY FOR PULMONARY ARTERY HYPERTENSION

Drug therapy with vitamin K antagonists (warfarin), endothelin-receptor antagonists, prostacyclin agents, phosphodiesterase inhibitors, and guanylate cyclase stimulators can reduce pulmonary pressures and slow the development of heart failure by dilating pulmonary vessels and preventing clot formation. Warfarin (Coumadin) therapy is used to reduce blood clots. See Chapter 20 for a complete discussion of all issues related to warfarin therapy. Phosphodiesterase inhibitors are most commonly used to reduce erectile dysfunction in men. See Chapter 31 for a complete discussion of all issues related to phosphodiesterase inhibitor drug therapy.

How Drugs for Pulmonary Artery Hypertension Work

Prostacyclin agents, either naturally occurring or synthetic, inhibit thromboxane A2 and increase the amount of cyclic adenosine monophosphate (cAMP) in blood vessel smooth muscle. The overall result of this action is dilation of lung blood vessels, decreased resistance in lung blood vessels, increased blood return from the lungs to the heart, and increased cardiac output. Drugs in this class include epoprostenol, iloprost, and treprostinil. **Endothelin-receptor antagonists** block the endothelin-1 receptor on blood vessel cells. Normally endothelin-1 causes vasoconstriction. By blocking these receptors, endothelin-receptor antagonists increase blood vessel dilation and prevent overgrowth of blood vessel cells. Drugs in this class include bosentan and macitentan.

Guanylate cyclase stimulators increase the amount of cyclic guanosine monophosphate (cGMP) in the smooth muscles of pulmonary blood vessels. The increased cGMP works in a similar way to increased cAMP but appears to be more specific to pulmonary blood vessels.

<aside>
Memory Jogger

Types of drugs for treatment of pulmonary artery hypertension include:
- Vitamin K antagonists
- Prostacyclin agents
- Endothelin-receptor antagonists
- Phosphodiesterase inhibitors
- Guanylate cyclase stimulators
</aside>

Dosages for Drugs for Pulmonary Artery Hypertension

Drug	Dosage
Prostacyclin Agents	
epoprostenol (Flolan, VELETRI)	*Adults:* Continuous IV infusion started at 2 ng/kg/min and increased until dose-limiting side effects occur Safety and efficacy for children and adolescents have not been established.
iloprost (Ilomedin, Ventavis)	*Adults:* aerosolized oral inhalation dose by approved pulmonary drug delivery device 2.5-5 mcg every 3-4 hr Safety and efficacy for children and adolescents have not been established.
treprostinil (Orenitram, Remodulin, Tyvaso)	*Adults and children 16 years or older:* 0.625-2.5 ng/kg/min by continuous IV infusion or subcutaneous injection OR 0.25-20 mg orally every 12 hr OR 3 puffs of 6 mcg by oral inhalation every 4 hr while awake. Dosage is gradually increased to 54 mcg (9 puffs) Safety and efficacy for children under age 16 years have not been established.

Dosages for Drugs for Pulmonary Artery Hypertension—cont'd

Drug	Dosage
Endothelin-Receptor Antagonists	
bosentan (Tracleer)	*Adults:* 62.5-125 mg orally twice daily Safety and efficacy for children weighing less than 40 kg have not been established.
macitentan (Opsumit)	*Adults:* 10 mg orally once daily Safety and efficacy for children and adolescents have not been established.
Guanylate Cyclase Stimulators	
riociguat (Adempas)	*Adults:* 0.5-1 mg orally three times daily initially. Gradually increased to 2.5 mg orally three times daily Safety and efficacy for children and adolescents have not been established.

Intended Responses
- Improved blood flow through the lungs
- Reduced pulmonary pressures
- Reduced breathlessness
- Improved cardiac output

Side Effects. The most common side effects of both the prostacyclin agents and the endothelin-receptor antagonists are headache, hypotension, and flushing. Less common side effects include nausea and vomiting.

Adverse Effects. A major adverse effect of prostacyclin agents is severe bleeding. The major adverse effect of the endothelin-receptor antagonists is elevated liver enzymes. Both the prostacyclin agents and the endothelin-receptor antagonists can cause bone marrow suppression with anemia and low white blood cell counts.

What To Do *Before* Giving Drugs to Treat Pulmonary Arterial Hypertension
Before giving any drug for pulmonary arterial hypertension (PAH), check the patient's blood pressure because all of these drugs can cause severe systemic hypotension. Also assess the patient's respiratory and cardiac status to use as a baseline for determining when an increased dose may be needed.

With parenteral prostacyclin agents (epoprostenol and treprostinil), inspect the vial for discoloration or the presence of particles. If either is present, discard the vial and open a new one. Always administer the IV preparation of the product using an appropriate pump infusing into a central line. Use strict aseptic technique to avoid introducing organisms into the patient's bloodstream.

With oral forms of drugs to treat PAH, do not split or crush the tablets.

The endothelin-receptor antagonists (bosentan and macitentan) are not available in regular pharmacies. Patients must be registered into special distribution programs. Assist the prescriber and pharmacy with this process.

Because the endothelin-receptor antagonists and the guanylate cyclase stimulators can cause birth defects, ensure that female patients within childbearing ages have a negative pregnancy test before starting these drugs and use reliable forms of contraception.

What To Do *After* Giving a Drug to Treat Pulmonary Artery Hypertension
With the parenteral forms of these drugs, do not use the line to give any other parenteral drugs. Ensure that there are no interruptions of continuous parenteral therapy. Ensure that all drugs to treat PAH are given on time.

The most appropriate monitoring for the effectiveness of all of these drugs is by assessing arterial blood gas (ABG) levels. Ensure that these are ordered on a regular basis, and monitor the results as soon as they are known. Report changes to the

 Drug Alert!

Administration Alert

It is critical that drugs for pulmonary artery hypertension that are given by continuous infusion are never interrupted. Even an interruption of minutes increases the risk for death. In addition, no other drugs are to be administered through the same line as these drugs.

QSEN: Safety

Common Side Effects

Prostacyclin Agents and Endothelin-Receptor Anatagonists

Headache   Hypotension   Nausea, vomiting

 Drug Alert!

Administration Alert

A major complication of continuous IV infusion is the development of sepsis and septic shock because the IV line is a direct link to the bloodstream. Use sterile technique whenever working with the IV line and always monitor the patient for signs and symptoms of infection.

QSEN: Safety

prescriber as soon as possible. Continue to monitor the respiratory and cardiac status at least every 4 hours.

With the prostacyclin agents, which can cause bleeding, ensure that bleeding times are assessed using the international normalized ratio (INR). Report results higher than 3 to the prescriber immediately. For all drugs to treat PAH, examine the complete blood count for reduced red blood cell (RBC) and white blood cell (WBC) counts.

With parenteral agents given through a central line, assess the patient every shift for signs and symptoms of infection and sepsis. If present, report these to the prescriber immediately.

Ensure that the liver enzyme levels of patients taking an endothelin-receptor antagonist are drawn on a regular basis. Assess the patient for any signs of jaundice and pain in the right upper abdominal quadrant.

What To *Teach* the Patient About Drugs for Pulmonary Artery Hypertension

The most important point to teach patients taking continuous parenteral therapy for PAH is to not stop the therapy and to avoid any interruptions in therapy. Such interruptions greatly increase the risk for death. For all forms of drugs to treat PAH, stress to patients the importance of taking the drug on time, exactly as prescribed, and not to skip or delay doses. Remind patients to always have an adequate supply of the drug or drugs on hand.

Teach patients using parenteral therapy how to self-administer the drugs and work the pump using strict aseptic technique. Teach them how to monitor for infection and sepsis and instruct them to notify the prescriber or go the emergency department at the first sign of infection.

Instruct all patients to notify the prescriber or go to the emergency department immediately if any of these problems occur:

- Increased and persistent shortness of breath
- Chest pain
- Swelling of the feet and legs
- Sudden weight gain

Instruct patients taking oral drugs to not split, crush, or chew the tablets.

Remind female patients of childbearing age who are taking endothelin-receptor antagonists to use reliable forms of contraception.

Teach patients taking endothelin-receptor antagonists how to assess themselves daily for signs or symptoms of liver impairment. Instruct them to report any signs or symptoms to the prescriber,

Teach patients to keep all follow-up appointments for blood tests to monitor effectiveness and identify complications early.

Life Span Considerations for Drugs to Treat Pulmonary Artery Hypertension

Pediatric Considerations. Neither the prostacyclin agents nor the endothelin-receptor antagonists are approved for use in children.

Considerations for Pregnancy and Lactation. The prostacyclin agents have a moderate likelihood of increasing the risk for birth defects or fetal damage. Although drugs with this pregnancy designation are usually not recommended for use during pregnancy, PAH is life threatening when not treated, and drug therapy must continue. Breastfeeding is not recommended while taking prostacyclin agents.

The endothelin-receptor antagonists and guanylate cyclase stimulators are known to cause birth defects and are not to be used during pregnancy or while breastfeeding.

PULMONARY FIBROSIS

Pulmonary fibrosis is a relatively common restrictive lung disease in which a previous lung injury causes inflammation in the lungs, leading to excessive cell division and replacement of normal lung cells with fibrotic scar tissue. These changes thicken the alveoli and make gas exchange difficult. Most often, the patient is an older adult with a history of cigarette smoking, chronic exposure to inhalation irritants, or exposure to the drugs *amiodarone* (Cordarone) or *ambrisentan* (Letairis, Volibris). Most patients have progressive disease with few remission periods. Even with proper treatment, most patients usually survive less than 5 years after diagnosis.

Drug therapy focuses on slowing the fibrotic process. Corticosteroids and other immunosuppressants are the mainstays of therapy. Immunosuppressant drugs include cytotoxic drugs such as cyclophosphamide (Cytoxan, Neosar, Procytox ✦), azathioprine (Imuran), chlorambucil (Leukeran), or methotrexate (Folex). See Chapter 6 for a complete discussion of corticosteroid drug therapy. See Chapter 11 for a discussion of drugs to modulate the immune system.

Get Ready for Practice!

Key Points

- Teach patients with asthma to take drugs exactly as prescribed, even when asthma symptoms have not been present for days.
- Teach patients with asthma to carry a short-acting adrenergic *rescue* inhaler at all times.
- When giving two or more inhalation drugs for asthma at the same time, administer the bronchodilator first and wait at least 5 minutes before giving the second and third drugs.
- Teach patients using dry-powder inhalers not to wash the inhaler or exhale into it.
- Remind the patient who is taking more than one inhaled drug for asthma to take the bronchodilator first and wait at least 5 minutes before taking any other inhaled drug.
- Anti-inflammatory drugs are not used for rescue because they do not cause bronchodilation.
- Inhaled corticosteroids reduce local immune responses and can lead to the development of oral thrush.
- Mucolytic drugs only help reduce thick secretions and do not cause bronchodilation or reduced inflammation.
- Drug therapy for pulmonary artery hypertension (PAH) should not be stopped, delayed, or interrupted.
- To reduce the risk for bloodstream infection and sepsis, use strict aseptic technique when working with continuous parenteral prostacyclin drug therapy.
- Never give any other drugs through the line in use for continuous prostacyclin therapy.
- Endothelin-receptor antagonists can cause birth defects and are not to be used during pregnancy or lactation.
- Do not split or crush endothelin-receptor antagonist tablets.
- Prostacyclin agents can cause severe bleeding.

Additional Learning Resources

evolve Be sure to visit your Evolve website (http://evolve.elsevier.com/Workman/pharmacology/) for additional online resources.

SG Go to your Study Guide for additional learning activities to help you master this chapter content.

Review Questions

See the Answer Keys—In-text Review Questions for answers to these questions.

Test Yourself on the Basics

1. What is the goal of drug therapy for asthma and/or COPD?
   A. To cure asthma or COPD
   B. To improve airflow and reduce symptoms
   C. To thicken bronchiolar cartilage and increase alveolar size
   D. To decrease alveolar recoil and improve contraction of bronchiolar smooth muscle
2. Which drugs are long-acting beta agonists? (Select all that apply.)
   A. budesonide (Pulmicort)
   B. formoterol (Foradil)
   C. ipratropium (Atrovent)
   D. levalbuterol (Xopenex)
   E. nedocromil (Tilade)
   F. salmeterol (Serevent)
   G. tiotropium (Spiriva)
3. Which beta-adrenergic agonist is most effective as a rescue drug?
   A. Arformoterol (Brovana)
   B. Formoterol (Foradil)
   C. Levalbuterol (Xopenex)
   D. Salmeterol (Serevent)
4. A patient who received a bronchodilator 20 minutes ago now has all of the following responses. For which one do you notify the prescriber immediately?
   A. Change in oxygen saturation from 89% to 95%
   B. Bad taste in the mouth
   C. Chest pain on exertion
   D. Dryness of the mouth and throat
5. Which symptoms or conditions are side effects of cholinergic antagonist drugs? Select all that apply.
   A. Anorexia
   B. Blurred vision
   C. Constipation
   D. Diarrhea
   E. Sleepiness
   F. Urinary retention
   G. Watery eyes

6. Which drug classes are used as therapy for pulmonary artery hypertension (PAH)? Select all that apply.
   A. Endothelin-receptor antagonists
   B. Inhaled corticosteroids
   C. Mucolytics
   D. Phosphodiesterase inhibitors
   E. Long-acting beta agonists
   F. Prostacyclin agents
   G. Short-acting beta agonists
   H. Vitamin K antagonists

7. When a patient is prescribed an inhaled bronchodilator and an inhaled corticosteroid at the same time, why must he or she wait 5 minutes after using the bronchodilator before using the inhaled corticosteroid?
   A. When the two drugs are taken one right after the other, the effects of both are reduced.
   B. When the two drugs are taken one right after the other, the side effects are more severe.
   C. Giving the bronchodilator first allows the inhaled corticosteroid to be more effective.
   D. Giving the bronchodilator first reduces the risk for an allergic reaction to the inhaled corticosteroid.

Test Yourself on Advanced Concepts

8. Which sign or symptom in a patient who is using a short-acting beta agonist (SABA) as a rescue drug indicates that he or she is using the inhaler very frequently?
   A. Tremors
   B. Urinary incontinence
   C. Oral candidiasis (thrush)
   D. Widely dilated pupils of the eye

9. A patient who has COPD asks what exactly guaifenesin (Mucinex) does to help him breathe better. What is your best answer?
   A. "It thins the lining of your lung air sacs making it easier for oxygen to enter your body."
   B. "It decreases inflammation and reduces your risk for lung infections."
   C. "It suppressed your cough reflex so that you can breathe better while sleeping."
   D. It thins your lung secretions making it easier for you to cough them out."

10. Which problem indicates that a patient may be excessively using his or her beclomethasone (QVAR) inhaler?
    A. The presence of thick white cheesy material on the tongue and roof of the mouth
    B. The onset of muscle cramps in the legs while at rest
    C. The need to get up to urinate 3 to 4 times every night
    D. The development of a dry, tickling cough

11. What is the most important point to teach a patient using a long-acting beta agonist (LABA)?
    A. Brush your teeth and rinse your mouth 3 times daily to prevent a bad taste.
    B. Take the drug daily as prescribed even when you have no symptoms.
    C. Use a reliable form of contraception while taking this drug.
    D. Keep the inhaler with you at all times.

12. Which precaution should you teach a woman taking bosentan (Tracleer)?
    A. Use strict aseptic technique while handling this drug.
    B. Avoid drinking caffeine while on this drug.
    C. Use a reliable form of contraception
    D. Rinse your mouth 4 times daily

13. A child is prescribed 360 mcg of inhaled budesonide (Pulmicort). You have on hand an inhaler with a concentration of 90 mcg per puff. How many puffs will you give? _____ puff(s)

Critical Thinking Activities

See the Answer Keys—Critical Thinking Activities for answers to these activities.

A 13-year-old girl with asthma is seeing her health care provider for a checkup before going to summer camp for a week. The camp is located in a wooded area of the mountains in Pennsylvania. She takes inhaled mometasone (Asmanex) and salmeterol (Serevent) daily and uses levalbuterol (Xopenex) when symptoms of asthma occur. In the past 4 weeks, she has used the levalbuterol only about 4 times each week. Both she and her mother ask whether she can skip the mometasone and salmeterol for the 7 days she is at camp. They are afraid she will be made fun of for being "different" or may be restricted from activities if the counselors view her as "sick."

1. What type of drug is mometasone, and how does it help asthma?
2. What type of drug is salmeterol, and how does it help asthma?
3. What type of drug is levalbuterol, and how does it help asthma?
4. Is skipping the mometasone and salmeterol a reasonable request for the week this girl is at camp? Why or why not?
5. How will you explain the best plan for this girl's asthma management while she is at camp?

Drug Therapy for Gastrointestinal Problems

Objectives

After studying this chapter you should be able to:

1. List the common names, actions, usual adult dosages, possible side effects, and adverse effects of antinausea drugs and antiemetic drugs.
2. Describe what to do before and after giving antinausea drugs and antiemetic drugs.
3. Explain what to teach patients taking antinausea drugs and antiemetic drugs, including what to do, what not to do, and when to call the prescriber.
4. Describe life span considerations for antinausea drugs and antiemetic drugs.

5. List the common names, actions, usual adult dosages, possible side effects, and adverse effects of drugs for diarrhea and drugs for constipation.
6. Describe what to do before and after giving drugs for diarrhea and drugs for constipation.
7. Explain what to teach patients taking drugs for diarrhea and drugs for constipation, including what to do, what not to do, and when to call the prescriber.
8. Describe life span considerations for drugs for diarrhea and drugs for constipation.

Key Terms

5HT₃-receptor antagonists (rē-SĔP-tŏr ăn-TĂG-ŏ-nĭsts) **(p. 358)** Drugs that work against nausea and vomiting caused by chemotherapy treatments.

adsorbent/absorbent drugs (ăd-SŎRB-ĕnt /ăb-SŎRB-ĕnt DRŬGZ) (p. 368) Drugs that remove substances that cause diarrhea from the body.

anticholinergic drugs (ăn-tĭ-kō-lĭn-ĔRJ-ĭk DRŬGZ) **(p. 358)** Drugs that inhibit pathways of the vomiting reflex; they stop intestinal cramping and inhibit vestibular input (balance and position) into the central nervous system (CNS).

antidiarrheal drugs (ăn-tē-dī-ŭ-RĒ-ŭl DRŬGZ) (p. 368) Drugs that relieve or control diarrhea or some of the symptoms that go along with diarrhea.

antiemetic drugs (ăn-tē-ĕ-MĔT-ĭk DRŬGZ) (p. 357) Drugs that prevent or control nausea and vomiting.

antihistamines (ăn-tĭ-HĬS-tă-mēnz) (p. 357) Drugs that work against nausea and vomiting caused by opiate drugs or motion; they block the action of histamine (a compound released in allergic inflammatory reactions) at the H₁ receptor sites.

antimotility drugs (ăn-tĭ-mō-TĬL-ĭ-tē DRŬGZ) (p. 368) Drugs that slow down peristalsis (movement) in the gastrointestinal (GI) track, used to treat diarrhea.

antisecretory drugs (ăn-tĭ-sĕ-KRĒ-tŏr-ē DRŬGZ) (p. 368) Drugs that inhibit secretory actions in the GI track, used to treat diarrhea

constipation (kŏn-stĭ-PĀ-shŭn) (p. 362) A condition in which bowel movements happen less frequently than is normal for an individual or the stool is small, hard, and difficult or painful to pass.

diarrhea (dī-ŭ-RĒ-ă) (p. 366) Frequent watery bowel movements.

dopamine antagonists (DŌ-pă-mēn ăn-TĂG-ŏ-nĭsts) (p. 358) Drugs that directly block dopamine from binding to receptors in the chemotrigger zone and the intestinal tract, causing food to move more quickly through the GI tract.

laxatives (LĂK-să-tĭvz) (p. 363) Drugs used to produce bowel movements and relieve constipation.

lubricants (LOO-brĭ-kăntz) (p. 364) An oily or slippery substance that can help make bowel movements easier.

nausea (NŎ-zē-ă) (p. 356) The state that precedes vomiting; the urge to vomit brought on by many causes such as influenza, medications, pain, and inner ear disease.

phenothiazines (FĒ-nō-thī-ŭ-zēnz) (p. 357) Drugs that block dopamine receptors in the chemotrigger zone of the brain; this action inhibits one or more of the vomiting reflex pathways

stool softeners (STOOL SŎF-ĕn-ĕrz) (p. 363) A laxative that adds fluid to stool, softening it to make bowel movements easier.

vomiting (VŎM-ĭ-tĭng) (p. 356) The forcing of stomach contents up through the esophagus and out through the mouth.

Memory Jogger

Nausea and vomiting are GI system defenses often used to remove harmful substances from the body.

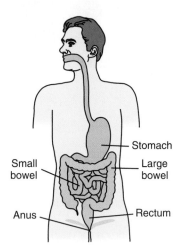

FIGURE 22-1 The gastrointestinal system.

? Did You Know?

Food usually takes 1 to 3 days to be processed by the bowel; about 90% of that time is spent in the colon.

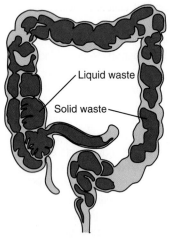

Liquid waste

Solid waste

FIGURE 22-2 Fluid is absorbed from the stool by the large bowel as it moves through the colon.

Memory Jogger

The three phases in the process of vomiting are nausea, retching, and vomiting.

OVERVIEW

Gastrointestinal (GI) system functions include taking in fluids and nutrients (food), breaking down food into forms that the body can use, absorbing useful fluid and nutrients, and eliminating waste products. The GI system begins at the mouth and ends at the anus. It is a hollow tube that is about 25 feet long in an adult (Figure 22-1) and is also called the *digestive system* or the *alimentary canal*.

The bowel is the lower part of the GI system (see Figure 22-1). Its roles include digesting the food we eat, absorbing the nutrients and fluids from digested foods, processing waste products, and expelling the waste products that the body can't use.

The small bowel is where parts of digested food that the body can use are absorbed. It sends waste products to the large bowel *(colon)*. The colon is the waste-processing and fluid-absorbing part of the bowel. Waste products have a consistency similar to that of pea soup when entering the colon. The large bowel absorbs fluids from waste products as they move through the colon and form stool *(feces)* (Figure 22-2). Depending on how long stool remains in the colon and how much water is absorbed, the consistency of stool may vary from soft and loose (watery diarrhea) to very hard lumps (constipation).

The rectum and left side of the colon are where stool is stored before a bowel movement occurs. Mass movements *(peristalsis)* cause stool to enter the rectum (Figure 22-3). These movements can be triggered by food arriving in the stomach or by physical activity such as getting out of bed in the morning, resulting in the sensation that the bowel needs to be emptied. When a person sits on the toilet to move the bowels, first the internal anal sphincter relaxes; then the external sphincter relaxes, and the bowel empties. Bowel movements are complex processes involving several different muscles and nerves located in the pelvic floor. Normal bowel function is different for every person. Bowel movements may occur anywhere between several times per day to several times a week. Consistency of bowel movements is more important than frequency. A person's stool should be soft enough to pass easily out of the bowel but should not be liquid.

NAUSEA AND VOMITING

REVIEW OF RELATED PHYSIOLOGY AND PATHOPHYSIOLOGY

Nausea and vomiting are defenses of the GI system and are signs of altered body function. **Nausea** is the unpleasant sensation of the need to vomit. **Vomiting** *(emesis)* is the forcing of stomach contents up through the esophagus and out the mouth. The process of vomiting consists of three phases: nausea, retching, and vomiting.

Nausea usually occurs before vomiting. It can be accompanied by cold sweats, pallor, salivation, loss of gastric tone, duodenal contractions, and reflux of intestinal contents into the stomach. It is often followed by retching. *Retching* involves labored respiratory movements against a closed throat, with contractions of the abdominal muscles, chest wall muscles, and diaphragm without vomiting. Vomiting does not always follow retching, but retching usually causes enough pressure buildup to lead to vomiting.

Vomiting results from powerful contractions of the abdominal and chest wall muscles, accompanied by lowering of the diaphragm and opening of the sphincter between the stomach and esophagus *(cardiac sphincter)*. It is a reflex, not a voluntary action that involves interactions among the nervous system, vestibular system, vomiting center of the brain, and receptors within the GI tract. The *vestibular apparatus* is the inner ear structures associated with balance and position sense. When balance or sense of position is upset, vomiting can occur. Tension receptors *(mechanoreceptors)* initiate vomiting because of distention and contraction such as with a bowel obstruction. Chemoreceptors are sensory nerve cells that respond to chemical stimuli such as poisonous substances *(toxins)* in the intestines. The mechanoreceptor and chemoreceptor stimuli are sent to the vomiting center in the brain, which controls the act of vomiting (Figure 22-4).

The vomiting center located in the medulla is responsible for initiating the vomiting reflex. It combines the input from the GI tract, vestibular apparatus, and higher brain pressure centers for activation. Once activated, the vomiting center causes vomiting by stimulating the salivary and respiratory centers and the throat (pharyngeal), GI, and abdominal muscles.

There are many causes of nausea and vomiting (Table 22-1). When a person vomits, the body is often trying to remove harmful substances that were ingested. Other possible triggers include disgusting sights, smells, or memories. People often learn to avoid the stimuli that lead to nausea and vomiting because these responses are so unpleasant. Nausea and vomiting are common, severe side effects of chemotherapy.

Nausea and vomiting are not only stressful to a person having these experiences; they can also create complications such as bleeding, aspiration pneumonia, dehydration, and reopening of surgical wounds, which can lead to longer hospital stays.

TYPES OF DRUGS FOR NAUSEA AND VOMITING

ANTIEMETIC DRUGS

How Antiemetic Drugs Work

Antiemetic drugs control nausea and prevent vomiting. Nausea and vomiting often occur together, and the same drugs are used for both problems. In addition to drugs, management of a patient with nausea and vomiting includes identifying and treating or eliminating the cause, controlling the symptoms, and correcting imbalances (electrolyte, fluid, and nutritional).

Antiemetic drugs include the phenothiazines, anticholinergics, antihistamines, $5HT_3$-receptor antagonists, and dopamine receptor antagonists. Each drug affects different receptors, and some drugs affect several sites. For example, $5HT_3$-receptor antagonists work against nausea and vomiting caused by chemotherapy treatments, whereas antihistamines work against nausea and vomiting caused by opiate drugs or motion. Multiple drugs may be used for nausea and vomiting because different drugs affect different parts of the vomiting reflex pathways.

The phenothiazines block dopamine receptors in the chemotrigger zone of the brain. This action inhibits one or more of the vomiting reflex pathways. The sedating effects help control the sensation of nausea.

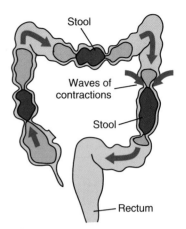

FIGURE 22-3 Peristalsis: mass movements in the colon.

 Did You Know?

As many as 25% of patients who could benefit from chemotherapy refuse treatment because the side effects of nausea and vomiting are so unpleasant.

 Drug Alert!

Action/Intervention Alert

When a patient has nausea and vomiting, be alert for electrolyte, fluid, and nutritional imbalances that must be corrected.

QSEN: Safety

Table 22-1	Causes of Nausea and Vomiting
CAUSE	**AGENTS**
Drug- or treatment-induced	Antibiotics Cancer chemotherapy Opiate drugs Radiation therapy
Labyrinth disorders	Ménière's disease Motion
Endocrine system	Pregnancy
Infection	Gastroenteritis Viral labyrinthitis
Increased intracranial pressure	Hemorrhage Meningitis
Postoperative	Analgesics Anesthetics Procedural
Central nervous system	Anticipatory Bulimia nervosa Migraine

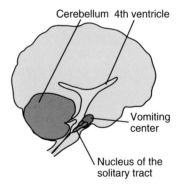

FIGURE 22-4 The vomiting center.

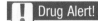

Drug Alert!

Administration Alert

To prevent nausea and vomiting associated with a specific trigger such as cancer chemotherapy or motion, give antiemetics before the triggering events and during the time the person usually has these responses.

QSEN: Safety

Clinical Pitfall

Ask patients about a history of depression. Metoclopramide (Reglan) can cause mild-to-severe depression and should not be prescribed for patients with a history of depression.

QSEN: Safety

Anticholinergic drugs inhibit other pathways of the vomiting reflex. They stop intestinal cramping and inhibit vestibular input (balance and position) into the central nervous system (CNS).

Antihistamines block the action of histamine (a compound released in allergic inflammatory reactions) at the H_1 receptor sites. They inhibit the same pathways as anticholinergic drugs and depress inner ear excitability, reducing vestibular stimulation. These different actions work together to control nausea and prevent vomiting.

The **5HT$_3$-receptor antagonists** bind to and block serotonin receptors in the intestinal tract and the chemotrigger zone of the brain. By blocking the receptors in both of these sites, at least two pathways of the vomiting reflex are interrupted. These drugs are commonly used to manage the nausea and vomiting resulting from cancer chemotherapy.

Dopamine antagonists directly block dopamine from binding to receptors in the chemotrigger zone and the intestinal tract. Food in the intestinal tract moves along more quickly and is less likely to stimulate responses that trigger the vomiting reflex.

Common names and doses of antiemetic drugs are listed in the following table. Be sure to consult a drug reference for information on specific antiemetic drugs.

Dosages for Common Antiemetic Drugs

Drug Class and Name	Dosage
Phenothiazines	
promethazine (Histantil ♣, Phenergan)	*Adults:* Oral—25 mg at bedtime, or 10-12.5 mg 4 times daily; IM, IV, rectal—25 g, may repeat in 2 hr *Children:* Oral—5-12.5 mg 3 times daily or 25 mg at bedtime; Rectal (children over 2 years)—0.125 mg/kg every 4-6 hr or 0.5 mg/kg at bedtime
prochlorperazine (Compazine, Provazin ♣, Stemetil ♣)	*Adults/Children over 12 years:* Oral—5-10 mg 3-4 times daily; IM—5-10 mg every 3-4 hr as needed; IV—2.5-10 mg (do not exceed 40 mg/day); Rectal—25 mg twice daily; Elixir—5-10 mg 3-4 times daily *Children less than 12 years* (weight-based): Oral—2.5 mg 1-3 times daily; IM—132 mcg/kg; Rectal (weight-based)—2.5 mg 1-3 times daily
Anticholinergics	
scopolamine (L-hyoscine)	*Adults:* IM, IV, subcutaneous—0.3-0.6 mg; transdermal—1.5 mg *Children:* IM, IV, subcutaneous—6 mcg/kg
Antihistamines	
cyclizine (Marezine)	*Adults:* Oral—50 mg 30 min before travel; IM—50 mg every 4-6 hr as needed *Children:* Oral—25 mg every 4-6 hr as needed; IM—1 mg/kg 3 times daily as needed
meclizine (Antivert, Bonamine ♣, Dramamine)	*Adults:* Oral—25-50 mg 1 hr before travel for motion sickness, 25-100 mg day for vertigo
5HT$_3$-Receptor Antagonists	
granisetron (Kytril)	*Adults:* Oral—1 mg twice daily, begin 1 hr before chemotherapy; IV—10 mcg/kg over 30 min, begin 30 min before chemotherapy *Children 2-16 years:* Same as adults

Dosages for Common Antiemetic Drugs—cont'd

Drug Class and Name	Dosage
ondansetron (Zofran)	*Adults:* Oral—8 mg 30 min before chemotherapy, then every 8 hr and 16 hr after the initial dose; IV—150 mcg/kg infused over 15 min, begin 30 min before chemotherapy *Children over 4 years:* Oral—4 mg 30 min before chemotherapy, then every 8 hr and 16 hr after the initial dose; IV—same dose as adults
Dopamine Antagonists	
metoclopramide (Emex ♣, Maxeran ♣, Reglan)	*Adults/Children over 14 years:* Oral—10 mg 30 min before symptoms are likely to occur (for example, meals and at bedtime); IV—10 mg *Children 5-14 years:* Dose determined by prescriber
trimethobenzamide (Tigan)	*Adults:* Oral—300 mg 3-4 times daily as needed; IM/rectal—200 mg 3-4 times daily as needed

Intended Responses

- Vomiting reflex is inhibited.
- Vomiting reflex pathways are interrupted or disrupted.
- Patient is sedated.
- Nausea is relieved.
- Vomiting is prevented.

Side Effects. Common side effects of antiemetic drugs vary with the prescribed drug. The most common side effects are listed in the following table. Be sure to consult a drug reference for additional information on any specific antiemetic drug.

Common Side Effects of Antiemetic Drugs

Drug	Common Side Effects
cyclizine (Marezine)	Drowsiness, dry mouth, hypotension
meclizine (Antivert)	Drowsiness
metoclopramide (Reglan)	Drowsiness, fatigue, increased depression, restlessness
prochlorperazine (Compazine)	Blurred vision, constipation, dizziness, dry eyes, dry mouth, involuntary muscle spasms, jitteriness, mouth puckering
promethazine (Phenergan)	Confusion, disorientation, dizziness, dry mouth, nausea, vomiting, rash, sedation
ondansetron (Zofran)	Abdominal pain, constipation, fatigue, headache
granisetron (Kytril)	Headache, constipation, loss of energy
scopolamine (L-hyoscine)	Blurred vision, constipation, dilated pupils, dizziness, drowsiness, dry mouth, lightheadedness, rash, urinary retention
trimethobenzamide (Tigan)	Blurred vision, diarrhea, drowsiness, cramps, headache, hypotension, rectal irritation with suppositories

Additional side effects include insomnia; diplopia (double vision); tinnitus (ringing in the ears); hypertension; photosensitivity; electrocardiogram (ECG) changes such as tachycardia, bradycardia, and supraventricular tachycardia; pink or reddish-brown urine; urinary retention; anxiety; and depression.

⇄ Do Not Confuse

Antivert *with* Axert

An order for Antivert may be confused with Axert. Antivert is an antihistamine used for nausea, vomiting, and dizziness from motion sickness and for vertigo associated with diseases affecting the inner ear vestibular apparatus. Axert is a vascular headache suppressant used to treat migraine headaches.

QSEN: Safety

Common Side Effects

Antiemetic Drugs

Dizziness   Fatigue, Drowsiness   Headache

Blurred vision   Constipation

⚠ Drug Alert!

Action/Intervention Alert

Prochlorperazine (Compazine) can cause a decrease in sweating, increasing the risk of overheating of the patient's body. Check body temperature every 4 to 8 hours while a patient is taking this drug.

QSEN: Safety

Drug Alert!

Action/Intervention Alert

Neuroleptic malignant syndrome is a rare, life-threatening side effect of antiemetic drugs in which dangerously high body temperatures can occur. Be sure to monitor a patient's body temperature every 4 to 8 hours.

QSEN: Safety

Clinical Pitfall

Tardive dyskinesia is an adverse effect of the antiemetic drugs promethazine (Phenergan) and metoclopramide (Reglan). It occurs after a year or more of continuous use of these drugs. If it is not diagnosed early, it is not reversible.

QSEN: Safety

Drug Alert!

Monitoring Alert

Before giving an antiemetic drug, always observe the abdomen for distention and listen for active bowel sounds.

QSEN: Safety

Drug Alert!

Action/Intervention Alert

Carefully monitor respiratory status and rate while patients are taking the antiemetic drugs cyclizine (Marezine), promethazine (Phenergan), and scopolamine (L-hyoscine).

QSEN: Safety

Adverse Effects. Adverse effects of antiemetic drugs also vary with the prescribed drug. Promethazine (Phenergan), prochlorperazine (Compazine), and metoclopramide (Reglan) can cause neuroleptic malignant syndrome, a rare and life-threatening side effect in which dangerously high body temperatures can occur. Without prompt and expert treatment, this condition can be fatal in as many as 20% of those who develop it. Signs and symptoms include fever, respiratory distress, tachycardia, seizures, diaphoresis, blood pressure changes, pallor, fatigue, severe muscle stiffness, and loss of bladder control.

Trimethobenzamide (Tigan) may cause coma and seizures. Promethazine (Phenergan) and metoclopramide (Reglan) can cause *tardive dyskinesia*, a chronic disorder of the nervous system. Signs and symptoms include uncontrolled rhythmic movement of the mouth, face, or extremities; lip smacking or puckering; puffing of cheeks; uncontrolled chewing; and rapid or wormlike movements of the tongue. This adverse effect usually occurs after a year or more of continued use of these drugs and is often irreversible. If diagnosed early, tardive dyskinesia may be reversed by stopping the drug.

Promethazine (Phenergan) and prochlorperazine (Compazine) may cause *neutropenia*, a decrease in the number of neutrophils (white blood cells), putting the patient at higher risk for infections. When given by IV push, undiluted promethazine has been associated with severe tissue necrosis.

Respiratory depression (decreased drive for breathing) is a life-threatening effect that can occur with cyclizine (Marezine), promethazine (Phenergan), and scopolamine (L-hyoscine).

What To Do *Before* Giving Antiemetic Drugs

Check the patient's body temperature, blood pressure, and heart rate and rhythm. Also check his or her baseline respiratory rate and level of consciousness. Obtain a baseline weight and check electrolyte laboratory values. Ask the patient about nausea and vomiting. Ask about any possible causes, allergies, or reactions such as motion sickness.

Use your stethoscope to listen for active bowel sounds in the patient's abdomen. Look for abdominal distention. Ask about the patient's usual diet and fluid intake, bowel movements, constipation, or difficulty swallowing.

Obtain a complete list of drugs the patient is currently taking, including over-the-counter and herbal drugs. Ask whether the patient who is prescribed metoclopramide (Reglan) has experienced depression in the past. If so, notify the prescriber before giving the drug.

If a drug is to be given intravenously, be sure to dilute it first to decrease the risk of tissue necrosis.

What To Do *After* Giving Antiemetic Drugs

Keep track of any episodes of nausea or vomiting to determine the effectiveness of these drugs.

Because ECG changes and dysrhythmias may occur, recheck the patient's blood pressure, heart rate and rhythm, and respiratory rate. Obtain daily weights using the same scale and the same amount of clothing at the same time each day. Ask the patient about nausea and vomiting at least every shift. Continue to listen for active bowel sounds and assess for abdominal distention.

Immediately report any signs of respiratory depression to the prescriber. Instruct the patient to call for help getting out of bed and ensure that the call light is within easy reach. Watch for signs of side effects or adverse effects, especially malignant neuroleptic syndrome and tardive dyskinesia. Report any signs immediately to the prescriber.

Check the patient's level of consciousness and watch for sedation effects, especially with older adults.

Some antiemetic drugs (e.g., cyclizine [Marezine], prochlorperazine [Compazine], promethazine [Phenergan], and scopolamine [L-hyoscine]) may cause hypotension or dizziness. Instruct the patient to change positions slowly and call for help when getting out of bed. Be sure that the call light is within easy reach.

Keep track of intake and output (both food and fluid). Ask about GI upset. If these drugs cause GI symptoms, give them with food, milk, or a full glass of water.

Watch for signs of depression in patients taking metoclopramide (Reglan) because this drug may cause mild-to-severe depression. Notify the prescriber immediately because a different drug may be needed to treat the nausea and vomiting.

What To *Teach* Patients About Antiemetic Drugs

Because these drugs may cause drowsiness, caution patients about driving or operating heavy equipment. Instruct patients to get up slowly because or hypotension and dizziness. Because of sun sensitivity, instruct patients to use sunscreen, wear protective clothing, and avoid tanning beds.

Teach patients about the signs and symptoms of malignant neuroleptic syndrome and tardive dyskinesia. Instruct them to check their body temperature every day and report abnormal signs and symptoms to their prescriber.

Warn patients that prochlorperazine (Compazine) may cause urine to change color to pink or reddish-brown. This condition is temporary and disappears within days after the drug is discontinued.

Tell patients about eating foods with increased bulk and about the importance of drinking enough fluids to prevent constipation. Explain that moderate exercise may also help prevent the side effect of constipation.

Remind patients that for best control of nausea or vomiting, antiemetic drugs should be taken before events that usually cause nausea.

Remind patients to get approval from their prescriber before taking over-the-counter drugs. Advise against using CNS depressants such as alcohol, antihistamines, sedatives, tranquilizers, or sleeping drugs while taking antiemetic drugs.

Suggest the use of a mild analgesic such as acetaminophen for relief from headaches. Teach patients to use frequent mouth rinses and oral care to manage dry mouth. If long-term use of these drugs is planned, remind them to see a dentist regularly to prevent dental disorders.

Remind patients to take a missed dose of the drug as soon as possible but not to take double doses.

Life Span Considerations for Antiemetic Drugs

Pediatric Considerations. Unintentional overdoses of metoclopramide (Reglan) have occurred with infants and children. Teach parents how to read the drug label and correctly give this drug to a child.

Children may have muscle spasms of the jaw, neck, and back, along with jerky movements of the head and face while taking metoclopramide. Balance disturbance is more likely to occur in children with high doses of antiemetic drugs used for cancer chemotherapy.

Considerations for Pregnancy and Lactation. Most of these drugs have a low to moderate likelihood of increasing the risk for birth defects or fetal harm. A woman should check with her prescriber before taking these drugs if she is pregnant or breastfeeding. Some of these drugs, such as metoclopramide, pass into breast milk and should be avoided while breastfeeding.

Considerations for Older Adults. Older adults are more likely to experience side effects such as acute confusion and dizziness. They may develop a shuffling walk, trembling, and shaking of the hands after taking metoclopramide over a long period of time. They are more likely to develop CNS effects of scopolamine (L-hyoscine) such as confusion, memory loss, unusual excitement, and heat-related disorders. Older adults are also more likely to experience symptoms of balance disturbance with high doses of antiemetic drugs used for cancer chemotherapy and may need lower doses of these drugs.

Memory Jogger

Prochlorperazine (Compazine) may cause urine to change color to pink or reddish-brown. This is temporary and disappears within days after the drug is discontinued.

Drug Alert!

Teaching Alert

To prevent nausea and vomiting from cancer chemotherapy, instruct patients to take antiemetic drugs 30 minutes before meals.

QSEN: Safety

Drug Alert!

Teaching Alert

To prevent nausea from motion sickness, teach patients to take antiemetic drugs at least 30 minutes, but preferably 1 to 2 hours, before activities that cause nausea.

QSEN: Safety

Clinical Pitfall

A patient should not take CNS depressants while taking antiemetic drugs because they add to CNS-depressant effects, causing drowsiness and a decreased level of alertness.

QSEN: Safety

REVIEW OF RELATED PHYSIOLOGY AND PATHOPHYSIOLOGY

Memory Jogger

Signs and symptoms of constipation are:
- Fewer than three bowel movements a week
- Sudden decrease in frequency of bowel movements
- Stools that are harder than normal
- Bowels still feeling full after a bowel movement
- Bloated sensation

Constipation occurs when a person has fewer than three bowel movements a week. Stools become very hard, dry, and difficult to eliminate. Having a bowel movement can be uncomfortable, even painful because of straining, bloating, and having a full bowel. Constipation may also include straining or pushing for longer than 10 minutes when trying to have a bowel movement. Figure 22-5 summarizes how constipation occurs.

Constipation is a symptom, not a disease, usually indicating some other health problem. Just about everyone experiences constipation at some time in his or her life, often because of poor diet. Most episodes of constipation are temporary and are not serious.

The most common causes of constipation are low-fiber diet, lack of physical activity, not taking in enough fluid, and delaying going to the bathroom when the urge to have a bowel movement is felt (Box 22-1). Stress, travel, and other changes in bowel habits can lead to constipation. Misuse of laxatives can cause constipation because the body becomes dependent on these drugs, needing higher and higher

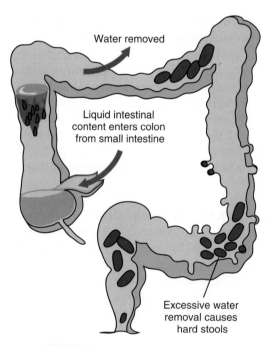

Water removed

Liquid intestinal content enters colon from small intestine

Excessive water removal causes hard stools

FIGURE 22-5 How constipation occurs.

Box 22-1	Common Causes of Constipation

- Abuse of laxatives
- Bowel diseases (e.g., irritable bowel syndrome, cancer)
- Changes in life (e.g., pregnancy, aging, travel)
- Dehydration
- Drugs
- Ignoring the urge to have a bowel movement
- Lack of physical activity
- Medical problems (e.g., hypothyroidism, cystic fibrosis, stroke)
- Mental problems such as depression
- Milk
- Not enough fiber in the diet
- Problems with the colon or rectum
- Problems with intestinal function

Table 22-2	Drug Categories That Cause Constipation
CATEGORY	**EXAMPLES**
Antacids	Drugs containing magnesium
Anticholinergics	amitriptyline, carbidopa-levodopa, dicyclomine, levodopa, nortriptyline, propantheline
Anticonvulsants	phenytoin, valproic acid
Antidepressants	amitriptyline, imipramine, phenelzine
Antihypertensives	clonidine, methyldopa
Antipsychotics	haloperidol, risperidone
Bile acid sequestrants	cholestyramine, colestipol
Calcium channel blockers	diltiazem, nifedipine, verapamil
Calcium supplements	calcium carbonate, PhosCal
Iron supplements	Iron aid (vitamin C, vitamin B_{12}, folic acid), chelated iron
Opiates	oxycodone/acetaminophen, propoxyphene napsylate and acetaminophen, drugs containing morphine or codeine

doses until the bowel no longer works. Bowel diseases, pregnancy, medical illnesses, mental health problems, neurologic problems, and many drugs may also cause constipation (Table 22-2). Drugs may cause constipation by affecting nerve and muscle activity of the colon or binding intestinal fluids. Children often develop constipation when holding back having a bowel movement if they are not yet ready or are afraid of toilet training.

Mild constipation is usually not serious. However, if symptoms are severe, last more than 3 weeks, or complications such as bleeding occur, a health care provider should be informed. Constipation that does not respond to self-treatment, constipation that occurs with rectal bleeding, abnormal pain and cramps, nausea and vomiting, and weight loss should be reported. Patients with severe constipation should be referred to their health care provider to rule out colon cancer. A health care provider should be consulted whenever constipation occurs during pregnancy or breastfeeding.

TYPES OF DRUGS FOR CONSTIPATION

LAXATIVES, LUBRICANTS, AND STOOL SOFTENERS

How Drugs for Constipation Work

Many people buy over-the-counter drugs to self-treat constipation. The purpose of drugs for constipation is to help the body eliminate hard stools. Products that are available include bulk-forming laxatives, stool softeners, lubricants, saline laxatives, and stimulant laxatives. It is important to remember that **laxatives** (drugs used to produce bowel movements and relieve constipation) are not meant for long-term use and should not be used for longer than 1 week unless prescribed for longer. Long-term use of laxatives can cause other health problems. The exception is bulk-forming laxatives such as psyllium (Metamucil) that may be taken once a day to help avoid constipation. This drug is not absorbed from the intestines into the body and is safe for long-term use.

Bulk-forming drugs for constipation add bulk to the stool, which increases stool mass that stimulates peristalsis. This helps stool move through the bowel. These drugs may work in as little as 12 hours but can take as long as 3 days to be effective.

Emollient or **stool softener** drugs soften stool, allowing the stool to mix with fatty substances, making it easier to eliminate. Some drugs combine the softening effect with a stimulant to both soften the stool and increase peristalsis to eliminate stool.

 Memory Jogger

Patients with severe constipation should be referred to a health care provider to rule out colon cancer.

 Clinical Pitfall

Most laxatives should not be used for longer than 1 week, unless a patient is instructed to do so by the prescriber.

QSEN: Safety

Osmotic laxatives cause retention of fluid in the bowel, increasing the water content in stool. Drugs such as **lubricants** coat the surface of stool and help it hold water so the body can more easily expel it.

Common names and doses of drugs for constipation are listed in the following table. Be sure to consult a drug reference for information on any specific constipation drugs.

Dosages for Common Drugs for Constipation

Drug	Dosage
Bulk-Forming Drugs	
methylcellulose (Citrucel)	*Adults:* 1 tsp orally 1-3 times daily with 8 oz of fluid
psyllium (Fiberall, Karacil ♣, Metamucil)	*Children:* Give half the adult oral dose with 8 oz of fluid
Emollients/Stool Softeners	
docusate (Colace, Regulex ♣, Surfak)	*Adults:* 100 mg orally 1-2 times daily
	Children: 10-150 mg orally daily in divided doses; age-based
Emollients Combined with Stimulants	
docusate sodium and casanthranol (Peri-Colace, Diocto C, Silace-C)	*Adults:* 1-4 capsules orally per day
	Children: Not recommended for children <6 years
Stimulants	
bisacodyl (Bisacolax ♣, Dulcolax)	*Adults/Children (>12 years):* 5-15 mg single oral dose; 10 mg rectally
	Children (<12 years): 5-10 mg single oral dose; 5-10 mg rectally
Osmotic Laxatives	
lactulose (Cephulac, Cholac, Constilac, Lactulax ♣)	*Adults:* 15-30 mL orally 1-2 times daily
	Children: 2.5-10 mL orally twice daily; age-based
lubiprostone (Amitiza)	*Adults:* 24 mcg orally twice daily with food
magnesium hydroxide (Phillips' Milk of Magnesia)	*Adults:* 5-15 mL orally every 6 hr as needed
	Children: 2.5-5 mL orally 4 times daily as needed
polyethylene glycol (GoLYTELY, Klean-Prep ♣, MiraLax, Peglyte ♣)	*Adults:* Dissolve 17 g in 8 oz and take orally once daily for up to 2 weeks
sodium phosphate (Fleet Enema)	*Adults:* One 4.5-oz enema given rectally
	Children: One 2.25-oz enema given rectally
Lubricants	
castor oil (Purge, Emulsoil)	*Adults:* 5-30 mL orally at bedtime
	Children: 5-15 mL orally; 4-oz enema given rectally
glycerin suppository (Sani-Supp)	*Adults/Children:* 1 suppository given rectally; hold in rectum 15 min

⇄ **Do Not Confuse**

Colace *with* **Cozaar**

An order for Colace may be confused with Cozaar. Colace is a stool softener, whereas Cozaar is an angiotensin II receptor antagonist used to manage high blood pressure.

QSEN: Safety

Intended Responses

- Stool is softened.
- Stool is passed.
- Constipation is relieved and prevented.

Side Effects. Common side effects of drugs for constipation vary with the prescribed drug. The most common side effects are listed in the following table. Be sure to consult a drug handbook for additional information on any specific constipation drug.

Common Side Effects of Drugs for Constipation

Drug	Common Side Effects
Bulk-Forming Drugs	
psyllium (Metamucil)	Bronchospasm, GI cramps, intestinal or esophageal obstruction, nausea, vomiting
Emollients/Stool Softeners	
docusate (Colace, Surfak)	Mild GI cramps, throat irritation, rashes
Emollients Combined with Stimulants	
docusate sodium and casanthranol (Peri-Colace)	Diarrhea, skin rash, stomach cramps, throat irritation
Stimulants	
bisacodyl (Dulcolax)	Abdominal cramps, diarrhea, hypokalemia (low potassium), muscle weakness, nausea, rectal burning
Osmotic Laxatives	
lactulose (Cephulac, Cholac, Constilac)	Abdominal distention, belching, diarrhea, flatulence, GI cramps, hypoglycemia in patient with diabetes
lubiprostone (Amitiza)	Abdominal pain and distention, diarrhea, dizziness, dry mouth, gas, headache, nausea, peripheral swelling, reflux
magnesium hydroxide (Phillips' Milk of Magnesia)	Diarrhea, flushing, sweating
polyethylene glycol (MiraLax)	Abdominal bloating, cramping, flatulence (gas), nausea
sodium phosphate (Fleet Enema)	Abdominal bloating, abdominal pain, dizziness, electrolyte imbalances (hyperphosphatemia, hypocalcemia, hypokalemia, sodium retention), GI cramping, headache, nausea, vomiting
Lubricants	
castor oil (Purge, Emulsoil)	Belching, cramping, diarrhea, nausea
glycerin suppository (Sani-Supp)	Abdominal cramps, hyperemia (increased blood flow) of rectal mucosa, rectal discomfort

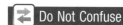

Do Not Confuse

MiraLax *with* Mirapex

An order for MiraLax may be confused with Mirapex. MiraLax is an osmotic diuretic used to treat constipation, whereas Mirapex is a drug used to manage Parkinson's disease.

QSEN: Safety

Common Side Effects

Drugs for Constipation

Diarrhea, Abdominal cramps, Abdominal distention, Nausea

Adverse Effects. Severe life-threatening adverse effects are rare with drugs for constipation. Psyllium (Metamucil) and docusate (Colace) may cause allergic reactions that include difficulty breathing, swelling and closing of the throat, swelling of lips and tongue, or hives.

Side effects of castor oil (Purge) that require medical attention include confusion, irregular heartbeat, muscle cramps, skin rash, and unusual tiredness or weakness.

Lactulose (Cephulac) and bulk-forming drugs containing sugar may cause hyperglycemia (high blood sugar) in patients with diabetes.

Bisacodyl (Dulcolax) may cause hypokalemia, which can lead to life-threatening dysrhythmias.

Fleet Enemas are meant to be used occasionally and can cause electrolyte imbalances when used often.

What To Do *Before* Giving Drugs for Constipation

Obtain a complete list of drugs that the patient is currently using, including over-the-counter and herbal drugs. Ask the patient about current bowel habits and the nature of his or her normal stools. Check the abdomen for distention and bowel

Drug Alert!

Administration Alert

Do not give constipation drugs if a patient has undiagnosed abdominal pain or acute abdomen because of the increased risk for bowel perforation.

QSEN: Safety

Drug Alert!

Administration Alert

Give oral drugs for constipation with 8 ounces of fluid at least 1 hour before or after antacids.

QSEN: Safety

? **Did You Know?**

Normal bowel patterns vary widely from several times a day to several times a week. Patients may need your help to determine their normal pattern.

Drug Alert!

Teaching Alert

Teach older adults that increasing fluid intake often relieves constipation without the need for laxatives.

QSEN: Safety

sounds. Obtain baseline vital signs and the patient's weight. If the patient has diabetes, obtain a baseline blood sugar using a fingerstick test.

Ask the patient about abdominal pain. Drugs for constipation should not be given to a patient experiencing undiagnosed abdominal pain or acute abdomen because these drugs increase peristalsis and the risk of bowel perforation.

Prepare a full glass (8 ounces) of fluid to give with oral drugs. If the patient is also taking antacids, give these drugs at least 1 hour before or after taking them. Be sure to lubricate suppositories before placing them in the rectum.

What To Do *After* Giving Drugs for Constipation

Recheck the patient's abdomen for distention and bowel sounds. Monitor for bowel movements and assess his or her quality of stools.

Instruct the patient to report bowel movements and any drug side effects. Be sure to remind patients to drink at least 1500 to 2000 mL of fluid every day to prevent constipation recurrence.

What To *Teach* Patients About Drugs for Constipation

Instruct patients to take oral drugs for constipation with 8 ounces of fluid to be sure the drugs are safe and effective. Advise them to keep a daily record of bowel movements, including the nature of their stools. Tell them that normal bowel patterns vary from person to person and help them determine their normal pattern. Teach patients to drink at least 1500 to 2000 mL of fluid every day to help prevent constipation from returning.

Remind patients that most laxatives should be used only short term (except for bulk-forming drugs such as psyllium, which are safe to take every day). Instruct them to call the prescriber if constipation is not relieved or if rectal bleeding or signs of electrolyte imbalance such as muscle cramps or pain, weakness, or dizziness occur.

Teach patients not to take oral forms of these drugs within 1 hour of taking an antacid drug because antacids decrease absorption.

Life Span Considerations for Drugs for Constipation

Pediatric Considerations.   Doses of drugs for constipation given to children 6 to 12 years of age are generally half of the adult dose but should still be given with 8 ounces of fluid. Laxatives or enemas should not be given to children without specific instructions from the prescriber.

Considerations for Pregnancy and Lactation. Most drugs for constipation are considered safe for use during pregnancy and have a low likelihood of increasing the risk for birth defects or fetal harm. However, the prescriber must assess the benefits before ordering these drugs. Sodium phosphate (Fleet enema) and lubiprostone (Amitiza) have a moderate likelihood of increasing the risk for birth defects or fetal harm and should not be used.

Considerations for Older Adults. Constipation is common in older adults, and most constipation drugs are safe for them to use. Psyllium is safe for older adults to use on a daily basis to prevent constipation. Older patients often use laxatives for a longer period and at higher dosages than recommended, which places them at risk for diarrhea and fluid imbalance. Remind older adults to follow package directions for laxative use. Reinforce that increasing fluid intake often relieves constipation without the need for laxatives.

DIARRHEA

REVIEW OF RELATED PHYSIOLOGY AND PATHOPHYSIOLOGY

Diarrhea is an increase in the amount of water in bowel movements and in their volume and frequency. It is not a disease but is a symptom of another health problem. Diarrhea may occur suddenly and usually disappears in a few days even without treatment. It is a fairly common occurrence for all age groups, and most cases of diarrhea are not serious. However, in children and infants, diarrhea can cause dehydration fairly rapidly. It may be an acute, self-limiting occurrence, or it may be a severe, life-threatening illness because of fluid and electrolyte imbalances.

An imbalance between the absorption and secretion functions of the intestines can lead to diarrhea. Absorption is decreased, and secretion is increased (Figure 22-6). Acute diarrhea is three or more loose stools within a 24-hour period, continuing for less than 2 weeks. Most often acute diarrhea goes away within 72 hours. Diarrhea that lasts longer than 2 weeks is considered chronic; however, it may not always include frequent daily passing of loose, watery stools.

There are many causes of diarrhea (Box 22-2), but the most common cause is inflammation of the small bowel *(enteritis)*. Most cases of infectious diarrhea are caused by viruses or bacteria taken in with contaminated food or water or with undercooked meat, poultry, fish, or eggs. Many drugs, including antibiotics, cardiac drugs, GI drugs, and neuropsychiatric drugs can cause diarrhea. Examples of these drugs are listed in Box 22-3. Other causes of diarrhea are radiation therapy, medical

Memory Jogger

Signs and symptoms of diarrhea are:
- Frequent need to have a bowel movement
- Abdominal pain and cramping
- Fever, chills, and generally feeling ill
- Weight loss

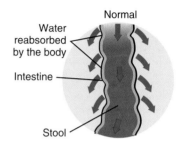
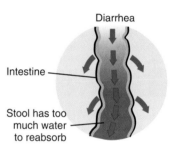

FIGURE 22-6 Pathophysiology of diarrhea.

Box 22-2	Common Causes of Diarrhea

- Drugs (e.g., antibiotics, laxatives, chemotherapy)
- Food poisoning/traveler's diarrhea
- Gastrectomy (partial removal of the stomach)
- High-dose radiation therapy
- Medical conditions (e.g., malabsorption, inflammatory bowel diseases such as Crohn's disease or ulcerative colitis, irritable bowel syndrome, celiac disease)
- Nerve disorders (autonomic neuropathy, diabetic neuropathy)
- Other infections (bacterial, parasites)
- Viral gastroenteritis (most common cause)
- Zollinger-Ellison syndrome

Box 22-3	Examples of Drugs That Can Cause Diarrhea

ANTIBIOTICS
- Ampicillin
- Broad-spectrum antibiotics
- Cephalosporins
- Clindamycin
- Erythromycin
- Sulfonamides
- Tetracycline

ANTIHYPERTENSIVE DRUGS
- Guanabenz
- Guanadrel
- Guanethidine
- Methyldopa
- Reserpine

CARDIAC DRUGS
- Angiotensin-converting enzyme inhibitors
- Beta blockers
- Digitalis/digoxin
- Diuretics
- Hydralazine
- Procainamide
- Quinidine

CHOLINERGICS
- Bethanechol
- Metoclopramide
- Neostigmine

GASTROINTESTINAL DRUGS
- Antacids
- Laxatives
- Misoprostol
- Olsalazine

HYPOLIPIDEMIC DRUGS
- Clofibrate
- Gemfibrozil
- Statin drugs

NEUROPSYCHIATRIC DRUGS
- Alprazolam
- Ethosuximide
- Fluoxetine
- L-dopa
- Lithium
- Valproic acid

MISCELLANEOUS
- Chemotherapy drugs
- Colchicine
- Nonsteroidal anti-inflammatory drugs
- Theophylline
- Thyroid hormones

Table 22-3	Classifications of Diarrhea	
CLASSIFICATION	**MECHANISM**	**CAUSES**
Osmotic	Unabsorbed solutes	Lactose deficiency, magnesium antacid excess
Secretory	Increased secretion of electrolytes	*Escherichia coli* infections, ileal resection, thyroid cancer
Exudative	Defective colonic absorption, outpouring of mucus and/or blood	Ulcerative colitis, Crohn disease, shigellosis, leukemia
Motility disorder	Decreased contact time	Irritable bowel syndrome, diabetic neuropathy

problems, gastrectomy, and nerve disorders. The four major types of diarrhea are osmotic, secretory, exudative, and motility disorder (Table 22-3).

TYPES OF DRUGS FOR DIARRHEA

ANTIMOTILITY, ADSORBENT/ABSORBENT, AND ANTISECRETORY DRUGS

How Antidiarrheal Drugs Work

Drugs for diarrhea (antidiarrheal drugs) are given to control diarrhea and some of the symptoms that occur with this condition. The three types of antidiarrheal drugs are antimotility drugs, adsorbent/absorbent drugs, and antisecretory drugs. The purpose of drugs prescribed for diarrhea is to correct the underlying problem and help the body control diarrhea and its uncomfortable symptoms. Goals of treatment include keeping the patient hydrated, treating the underlying cause, and relieving diarrhea. Be sure to watch for signs and symptoms of electrolyte imbalances that may be caused by diarrhea such as low potassium level (*hypokalemia*).

When diarrhea is caused by an infection from bacteria or parasites antidiarrheal drugs can make the condition worse. This is because the drugs prevent the body from eliminating the organisms causing the diarrhea. These drugs are usually not given for this type of diarrhea. Treatment focuses on preventing dehydration and rehydration.

Drugs for diarrhea act in several ways. **Antimotility drugs** slow the movement of stool through the bowel, allowing more time for water and essential salts to be absorbed by the body. **Adsorbent/absorbent drugs** remove substances that cause diarrhea from the body. **Antisecretory drugs** decrease secretion of intestinal fluids and slow bacterial activity.

Common names and doses of drugs for diarrhea are listed in the following table. Be sure to consult a drug reference for information on specific antidiarrheal drugs.

Memory Jogger

The three types of antidiarrheal drugs are:
- Antimotility drugs
- Adsorbent/absorbent drugs
- Antisecretory drugs

Memory Jogger

Signs and symptoms of hypokalemia include cardiac dysrhythmias, muscle pain, general discomfort or irritability, weakness, and paralysis.

Dosages for Common Antidiarrheal Drugs

Drug	Dosage
Antimotility Drugs	
difenoxin with atropine (Motofen)	*Adults:* 2 tablets orally followed by 1 tablet after each unformed stool; do not exceed 8 tablets per day
diphenoxylate with atropine (Lomotil)	*Adults:* 5 mg orally 4 times daily *Children:* 0.3-0.4 mg/kg orally daily in 4 divided doses (oral solution only; do not use tablets)
loperamide (Imodium)	*Adults:* 4 mg orally followed by 2 mg after each unformed stool; do not exceed 16 mg/day *Children:* 1-2 mg orally 3 times daily

Dosages for Common Antidiarrheal Drugs—cont'd

Drug	Dosage
paregoric (Camphorated Opium Tincture)	*Adults:* 5-10 mL orally after unformed stool; may be given every 2 hr up to 4 times daily *Children:* 0.25-0.5 mL/kg orally 1-4 times daily
Adsorbent/Absorbent Drugs	
attapulgite (Kaopectate ♦) bismuth subsalicylate (Kaopectate)	*Adults:* 1200 mg orally after each unformed stool; up to 7 doses per day *Children:* 300-600 mg orally after each unformed stool; up to 7 doses per day
calcium polycarbophil (FiberCon)	*Adults:* 1 g orally 1-4 times daily as needed; do not exceed 6 g day *Children:* 500 mg orally 1-3 times daily as needed; do not exceed 1.5-3 g day
Antisecretory Drugs	
bismuth subsalicylate (Pepto-Bismol)	*Adults:* 2 tablets or 30 mL orally every 30 min to 1 hr as needed; up to 8 doses per day *Children:* Not recommended for children because it contains subsalicylate, which is similar to aspirin

Intended Responses

- GI motility is decreased.
- Diarrhea is decreased.
- Fluid from bowel is reabsorbed.
- Secretion of fluids into the bowel is decreased.
- Activity of bacteria is decreased.

Side Effects. Side effects of antidiarrheal drugs are uncommon in healthy adults and vary with the prescribed drug. The most common side effect is constipation. Additional side effects are listed in the following table. Be sure to consult a drug reference for additional information on any specific antidiarrheal drug.

 Memory Jogger

The most common side effect of antidiarrheal drugs is constipation.

Common Side Effects of Antidiarrheal Drugs

Drug	Common Side Effects
attapulgite (Kaopectate)	Constipation, bloating, feeling of fullness
bismuth subsalicylate (Pepto-Bismol)	Constipation, gray-black stools, impaction in infants and debilitated patients, tinnitus (ringing in the ears)
calcium polycarbophil (FiberCon)	Abdominal fullness, flatulence (gas), laxative dependence with long-term use
difenoxin with atropine (Motofen)	Blurred vision, constipation, confusion, dizziness, drowsiness, dry eyes, dry mouth, flushing, GI distress, headache, insomnia, nausea, nervousness, tachycardia, urinary retention, vomiting
diphenoxylate with atropine (Lomotil)	Blurred vision, constipation, confusion, dizziness, drowsiness, dry eyes, dry mouth, flushing, GI distress, headache, insomnia, nervousness, tachycardia, nausea, urinary retention, vomiting
loperamide (Imodium)	Abdominal pain/discomfort, allergic reactions, constipation, distention, dizziness, drowsiness, dry mouth, nausea, vomiting
paregoric (Camphorated Opium Tincture)	Abdominal pain, constipation, loss of appetite, nausea, vomiting

Common Side Effects

Antidiarrheal Drugs

Constipation, Abdominal discomfort   Dizziness   Dry mouth

⚠ Drug Alert!

Action/Intervention Alert

After giving an antimotility drug, be sure to check the patient for abdominal distention, a sign of toxic megacolon.

QSEN: Safety

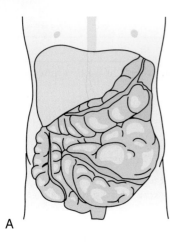

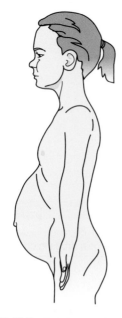

FIGURE 22-7 Toxic megacolon. *A,* Note the enlarged intestines. *B,* Side view.

Clinical Pitfall

Antidiarrheal drugs are not usually given when diarrhea is caused by bacteria or parasites because the drugs prevent the body from eliminating the organisms, which can cause the condition to worsen.

QSEN: Safety

Drug Alert!

Action/Intervention Alert

Bismuth subsalicylate (Pepto-Bismol) contains an aspirin-like drug. Watch for bleeding because this drug can also increase the effects of the anticoagulant warfarin (Coumadin).

QSEN: Safety

Adverse Effects. Adverse effects are rare with antidiarrheal drugs. Calcium polycarbophil (FiberCon) may cause intestinal obstruction.

A potential life-threatening adverse effect of antimotility drugs is *toxic megacolon,* which is a very inflated colon with abdominal distention (Figure 22-7). Other signs and symptoms of this condition include fever, abdominal pain, rapid heart rate, and dehydration. A patient with toxic megacolon may go into shock. When this condition is not recognized and treated early, there is a risk for death.

What To Do *Before* Giving Antidiarrheal Drugs

Obtain a complete list of drugs that the patient is currently using, including over-the-counter and herbal drugs. Check the patient's baseline weight and set of vital signs. Listen to the abdomen with your stethoscope for active bowel sounds and check for abdominal distention. Observe the patient's skin turgor for signs of dehydration. When a patient is dehydrated, gently pinching and lifting the skin over the sternum, back of the hand, or arm will form a "tent." Use the sternum or forehead to test for tenting in the older adult because the skin on the back of hand may tent due to aging. The worse the dehydration, the longer the skin will take to return to its normal position. Ask patients about allergies or unusual reactions to aspirin or other drugs containing aspirin because bismuth subsalicylate (Pepto-Bismol) contains an aspirin-like drug. This drug may interact with and increase the effects of anticoagulant drugs such as warfarin (Coumadin). Determine whether the patient's diarrhea is caused by bacteria or parasites.

What To Do *After* Giving Antidiarrheal Drugs

Reassess the abdomen for bowel sounds and distention. Watch for signs of toxic megacolon if the patient is taking an antimotility drug. If symptoms occur, notify the prescriber immediately.

Recheck and continue to monitor vital signs every 4 to 8 hours. Keep a record of how often the patient has diarrhea stools. Be sure to document the consistency, odor, and appearance of stools. Continue to monitor the skin turgor and encourage the patient to drink plenty of fluids to avoid dehydration.

What To *Teach* Patients About Antidiarrheal Drugs

Instruct patients to take the drug exactly as ordered by their prescriber. Remind them not to take double doses of these drugs because constipation may result.

Because some of these drugs may cause dizziness or drowsiness, advise patients to avoid driving or performing any activities that require alertness until they know how the drugs will affect them. Tell them that frequent mouth rinses, mouth care, and sugarless gum or candy may be useful to relieve dry mouth. If the drug is a liquid, remind patients to shake well before measuring and taking it.

Remind patients to notify their prescriber if the diarrhea is not relieved in 2 days while taking antidiarrheal drugs or if they develop a fever, abdominal pain, or abdominal distention. Patients should also notify their prescriber if any blood or mucus appears in stools.

Advise patients to avoid the use of alcohol and other CNS depressants while taking these drugs.

Remind patients taking bismuth subsalicylate (Pepto-Bismol) that this drug contains an aspirin-like drug and that additional aspirin should not be taken because it may cause ringing in the ears (tinnitus). Also tell them that this drug may turn stool and the tongue gray-black.

Life Span Considerations for Antidiarrheal Drugs

Pediatric Considerations. Children should not be given bismuth subsalicylate because it contains an aspirin-like drug and may cause Reye's syndrome. This is a life-threatening condition that affects the liver and CNS, and it causes vomiting and confusion. It occurs soon after the onset of a viral illness in which a child was treated with aspirin. Children are more sensitive to the drowsiness and dizziness caused by loperamide (Imodium). Bismuth subsalicylate (Kaopectate) and calcium polycarbophil (Fibercon) are not recommended for preschool children. Infants and children are at increased risk for dehydration with diarrhea.

Considerations for Pregnancy and Lactation. Women who are pregnant or breastfeeding should check with their prescriber before using any antidiarrheal drugs. They should also ask about replacing lost fluids because dehydration can cause a woman to go into early labor.

Considerations for Older Adults. Older adults are at higher risk for dehydration from diarrhea. Be sure that they receive adequate fluid replacement to prevent dehydration. Older adults (over 60 years) should not use bismuth subsalicylate (Kaopectate) because they are more likely to experience side effects such as constipation.

 Clinical Pitfall

Antidiarrheal drugs should not be taken for more than 2 days unless instructed to do so by the prescriber.

QSEN: Safety

 Clinical Pitfall

To be safe and prevent Reye's syndrome, children younger than 16 years should never be given bismuth subsalicylate (Pepto-Bismol).

QSEN: Safety

Get Ready for Practice!

Key Points

- Nausea and vomiting are distressing for patients and can cause significant clinical complications and extended hospital stays.
- There are many causes of nausea and vomiting involving several central and peripheral neurotransmitter pathways.
- Nausea and vomiting are GI defense mechanisms.
- Drugs for nausea and vomiting are prescribed to manage these symptoms, eliminate the causes, and correct electrolyte and nutritional imbalances.
- Always check a patient's respiratory status before and after giving drugs for nausea and vomiting because respiratory depression can be an adverse effect of some of these drugs.
- Teach patients taking antinausea drugs for motion sickness to take the drug 30 to 60 minutes before expected travel.
- Normal bowel patterns vary widely from several times a day to several times a week.
- Constipation and diarrhea are symptoms, not diseases.
- The most common causes of constipation are poor diet and lack of exercise.
- Always give drugs for constipation with 8 ounces of fluid.
- A person with diarrhea is at high risk for dehydration because of fluid lost in the stool.
- After giving an antimotility drug for diarrhea such as loperamide (Imodium), be sure to check for signs of the life-threatening adverse effect toxic megacolon.
- Teach patients that antidiarrheal drugs should not be taken for more than 2 days unless instructed to do so by their prescriber.

Additional Learning Resources

evolve Be sure to visit your Evolve website (http://evolve.elsevier.com/Workman/pharmacology/) for additional online resources.

SG Go to your Study Guide for additional learning activities to help you master this chapter content.

Review Questions

See the Answer Keys—In-text Review Questions for answers to these questions.

Test Yourself on the Basics

1. Which type of drug used for nausea and/or vomiting causes food to move more quickly through the GI tract?
   A. Phenothiazines
   B. Anticholinergics
   C. 5HT$_3$-receptor antagonists
   D. Dopamine antagonists

2. Which antiemetic drugs can cause patients to experience decreased sweating, increasing the risk of body overheating?
   A. Cyclizine (Marezine)
   B. Prochlorperazine (Compazine)
   C. Meclizine (Antivert)
   D. Ondansetron (Zofran)

3. For which side effect must you notify the prescriber when a patient is taking metoclopramide (Reglan)?
   A. Depression
   B. Heartburn
   C. Anxiety
   D. Constipation

4. Which drug prescribed to relieve constipation is a lubricant?
   A. Magnesium hydroxide
   B. Milk of Magnesia
   C. Glycerin suppository
   D. Bisacodyl

5. Which electrolyte abnormality must you monitor for when a patient is prescribed bisacodyl (Dulcolax)?
   A. Hypernatremia
   B. Hypercalcemia
   C. Hypophosphatemia
   D. Hypokalemia

6. Which drug when prescribed for diarrhea slows the movement of stool through the bowel?
   A. Loperamide (Imodium)
   B. Bismuth subsalicylate (Pepto-Bismol)

C. Calcium polycarbophil (FiberCon)
D. Attapulgite (Kaopectate)

7. Which drug should not be prescribed to small children because of increased risk for development of Reye's syndrome?
   A. Bismuth subsalicylate (Pepto-Bismol)
   B. Calcium polycarbophil (FiberCon)
   C. Attapulgite (Kaopectate)
   D. Loperamide (Imodium)

Test Yourself on Advanced Concepts

8. Which action of promethazine (Phenergan) helps prevent nausea and vomiting?
   A. Inhibiting the vomiting reflex pathways
   B. Helping food move more rapidly through the GI system
   C. Preventing cancer chemotherapy–induced vomiting
   D. Providing a protective coating to the stomach and esophagus

9. Which actions should you take before giving an antinausea drug? (Select all that apply.)
   A. Listen for active bowel sounds.
   B. Look for abdominal distention.
   C. Check the patient's electrolyte values.
   D. Check the patient's deep tendon reflexes.
   E. Ask about patient coagulation tests.
   F. Ask the patient about usual diet intake.

10. What do you teach a patient who is prescribed prochlorperazine (Compazine)?
    A. Take this drug with food to prevent GI discomfort.
    B. A side effect of this drug is headaches, which can be relieved with acetaminophen (Tylenol).
    C. This drug can cause your urine to change color to pink or reddish-brown.
    D. The action of this drug is to cause food to move rapidly through the GI tract.

11. A child taking chemotherapy drugs for cancer is prescribed metoclopramide for nausea and vomiting. For which side effects do you monitor?
    A. Muscle spasms of the jaw
    B. Confusion
    C. Hypotension
    D. Depression

12. Which electrolyte do you monitor carefully when a patient who has persistent diarrhea?
    A. Sodium
    B. Magnesium
    C. Potassium
    D. Chloride

13. What actions must you be sure to take before giving any drug for constipation? (Select all that apply.)
    A. Listen for active bowel sounds.
    B. Check for abdominal distention.
    C. Ask the patient about previous bacterial infections.
    D. Prepare a full glass of fluid to give with oral drugs.
    E. Ask about the patient's normal bowel habits.

14. After giving a drug for constipation, how many milliliters of fluid do you instruct the patient to drink every day?
    A. 1200-1500
    B. 1500-2000
    C. 2000-2400
    D. 2400-3000

15. What is the dosage of a drug for constipation for a child between 6 and 12 years of age?
    A. One quarter of the adult dose
    B. One half of the adult dose
    C. Three quarters of the adult dose
    D. The same as the adult dose

16. A preoperative patient has been ordered scopolamine (L-hyoscine) 0.3 mg intramuscularly. Scopolamine is available in vials with a concentration of 0.3 mg/mL. How many milliliters will you give? _____ mL

17. A patient on chemotherapy is to receive oral metoclopramide (Reglan) 3 mg/kg 30 minutes before each meal. The patient weighs 48 kg. How many milligrams will you give for each dose? _____ mg

18. A patient with dehydration from diarrhea is prescribed IV fluids 1000 mL over 6 hours. How many milliliters per hour will the patient receive? _____ mL/hr

Critical Thinking Activities

See the Answer Keys—Critical Thinking Activities for answers to these activities.

Mr. Black, who is 93 years old, is admitted to the emergency department with severe dizziness and confusion. Until 2 days ago, he was alert, oriented, and able to ambulate to the dining hall for meals. He was prescribed promethazine (Phenergan) 12.5 mg for frequent episodes of nausea and vomiting 5 days ago. Mr. Black's daughter informs you that her father's urine is now red to pink in color. The patient continues to experience nausea with vomiting.

1. What additional priority assessments are needed at this time?
2. Which side effects of this drugs must you monitor for?
3. What priority teaching will you do with Mr. Black's daughter?
4. What actions are key to providing care for Mr. Black?

Drug Therapy for Gastric Ulcers and Reflux

Objectives

After studying this chapter you should be able to:

1. Explain how different classes of drugs are used to treat peptic ulcer disease (PUD) and gastroesophageal reflux disease (GERD).
2. List the common names, actions, usual adult dosages, possible side effects, and adverse effects of drugs for PUD and GERD.
3. Describe what to do before and after giving drugs for PUD and GERD.
4. Explain what to teach patients taking drugs for PUD and GERD, including what to do, what not to do, and when to call the prescriber.
5. Describe life span considerations for drugs for PUD and GERD.

Key Terms

antacids (ănt-ĂS-ĭdz) (p. 383) Drugs that neutralize the acids produced by the stomach.

cytoprotective drugs (sī-tō-prō-TĔK-tĭv DRŬGZ) (p. 379) Drugs that decrease the acid content of the stomach by coating the stomach mucosa and reducing the risk for developing ulcers.

duodenal ulcer (dŭ-ō-DĒ-nŭl ŬL-sŭr) (p. 374) An open sore (ulcer) in the lining of the first part of the small intestine (duodenum).

esophageal ulcer (ē-sŏf-ŭ-JĔ-ŭl ŬL-sŭr) (p. 374) An open sore (ulcer) in the lining of the esophagus corroded by the acidic digestive juices secreted by the stomach.

gastric ulcer (GĂS-trĭk ŬL-sŭr) (p. 374) An open sore (ulcer) in the stomach lining.

gastroesophageal reflux disease (GERD) (GĂS-trō-ē-sŏf-ŭ-JĔ-ŭl RĒ-flŭks dĭz-ĒZ) (p. 373) Esophageal irritation or inflammation often caused by stomach acid that backs up into the esophagus.

histamine H$_2$ blockers (HĬS-tă-mēn BLŎ-kŭrz) (p. 379) Drugs that treat the gastric effects of histamine in cases of peptic ulcers, gastritis, and GERD by blocking the effects of histamine on the receptor site known as H$_2$.

peptic ulcer disease (PUD) (PĔP-tĭk ŬL-sŭr dĭz-ĒZ) (p. 373) An open sore in the lining of the stomach or duodenum.

proton pump inhibitor (PPI) (PRŌ-tŏn PŬMP ĭn-HĬB-ĭ-tŭr) (p. 379) A drug that blocks acid secretion in the stomach.

OVERVIEW

Gastroesophageal reflux disease (GERD) and **peptic ulcer disease (PUD)** affect the upper gastrointestinal (GI) system, which consists of the mouth, esophagus, stomach, and upper part of the small intestine (duodenum). GERD occurs when stomach contents leak backward into the esophagus. PUD may occur in the esophagus, stomach, or upper part of the duodenum.

REVIEW OF RELATED PHYSIOLOGY AND PATHOPHYSIOLOGY

Food is digested and converted into a form that the body can use. The upper GI system is responsible for taking in and moving food to the stomach. Digestion begins in the mouth, where chewing changes the food to a fine texture; saliva moistens it and begins the conversion of starch into simple sugars. The food is then swallowed, passing through the pharynx and down the esophagus to the stomach. Specialized cells in the stomach *(gastric glands)* secrete digestive enzymes and gastric juices, which act on the partially digested food. The stomach also physically churns and mixes the food. Stomach secretions include the enzyme pepsin, which acts on proteins; hydrochloric acid, needed for the action of pepsin; and an enzyme, gastric

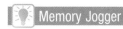 **Did You Know?**

Digestion of food begins in the mouth.

lipase, which begins the breakdown of fats. These acid substances that digest food also have the potential to damage or break down normal GI tissues.

The stomach secretes thick gel-like mucus to coat and protect it from contact with stomach acids. In most people, acid production is balanced by mucus secretion, and ulcers do not form. Whenever acid production exceeds mucus production, the risk for ulcers and tissue damage increases. Health problems, genetic influences, lifestyle influences, and certain drugs can decrease mucus production or increase acid secretion and upset the protective balance. The intestinal tract, unlike the stomach, does not secrete large amounts of the protective mucus. Instead it relies on buffers such as bicarbonate from the pancreas to neutralize stomach acids before they reach the intestines.

GASTROINTESTINAL ULCERS

GI ulcers are fairly common. About 10% of people in the United States develop an ulcer during their lifetime. A GI ulcer is an open sore found in the mucosal lining of the stomach or duodenum where hydrochloric acid and pepsin are located. These ulcers are also commonly referred to as *peptic ulcer disease (PUD)*. When a peptic ulcer occurs in the stomach, it is called a **gastric ulcer**, and when an ulcer is formed in the duodenum, it is called a **duodenal ulcer** (Figure 23-1).

Esophageal ulcers usually occur in the lower part of the esophagus near the stomach. An **esophageal ulcer** is a hole in the lining of the esophagus that has been damaged by the acidic digestive juices secreted by the stomach cells. This type of ulcer is often associated with chronic GERD when acidic stomach contents back up (reflux) into the esophagus.

In the past the causes of peptic ulcers were believed to be excess acids and lifestyle factors such as stress and too many spicy foods. However, research has shown that 80% to 90% of gastric ulcers are caused by infection with the *Helicobacter pylori (H. pylori)* bacteria. *H. pylori* infection is present in 20% to 30% of people in the United States. Some people experience no signs or symptoms, whereas others develop ulcers. Today it is believed that lifestyle (for example, stress and diet), along with excess acids and *H. pylori* infection, have roles in the development of ulcers; but *H. pylori* is the primary cause. Box 23-1 summarizes the factors that are suspected to have a role in the development of peptic ulcers.

Gastric mucosa resists damage, but when there is an increase in gastric acidity or a decrease in prostaglandins, which increase the production of bicarbonate and also produce the protective mucus, there is danger of developing an ulcer (Figure 23-2).

Memory Jogger

The primary cause of 80% to 90% of GI ulcers is infection with the *H. pylori* bacteria.

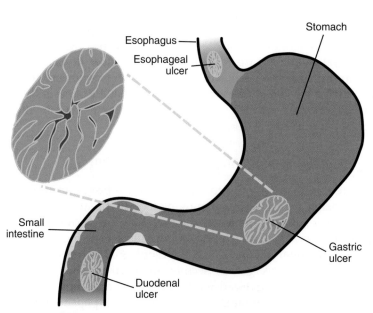

FIGURE 23-1 Locations of gastric, duodenal, and esophageal ulcers.

Box 23-1	Factors in the Development of Peptic Ulcers

- Acid and pepsin
- Alcohol
- Caffeine
- *Helicobacter pylori* bacteria infection
- Nonsteroidal anti-inflammatory drugs
- Smoking
- Stress

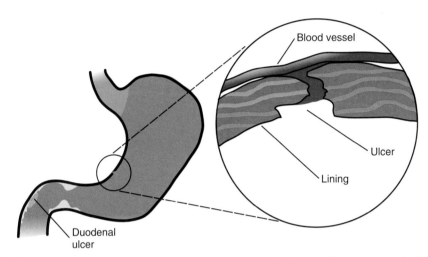

FIGURE 23-2 Gastric ulcer pathophysiology: The mucosa breaks down and an open sore develops.

The mucosa breaks down, and an open sore or raw area develops in the stomach or upper part of the intestine (duodenum).

The most common symptom of a peptic ulcer is burning, gnawing pain caused by stomach acid coming into contact with the open wound (ulcer). The pain usually occurs somewhere between the navel *(umbilicus)* and the breastbone *(sternum)* and may last from a few minutes to many hours. It often occurs when the stomach is empty and can be relieved by eating foods that buffer stomach acids or taking a drug that reduces stomach acid such as an antacid. The pain may flare up at night or come and go for a few days to several weeks. Other symptoms of a gastric ulcer include vomiting blood (bright red or black), dark blood in the stool, nausea or vomiting, belching, unexplained weight loss, and chest pain.

Antibiotics are a very important part of the treatment plan for PUD. They are used to treat *H. pylori* in the GI tract, a major cause of GI ulcers. Commonly prescribed antibiotics include drugs such as clarithromycin (Biaxin), metronidazole (Flagyl), tetracycline (Sumycin), and amoxicillin (Amoxil). Treatment of ulcers involves not only drugs but also lifestyle changes. Recommended lifestyle changes include avoiding irritating foods, caffeine, and excessive alcohol. Smoking cessation is highly recommended because smoking slows ulcer healing and is related to the return of ulcers. Smoking increases acid secretion; reduces prostaglandin, mucus, and bicarbonate production; and decreases mucosal blood flow. Patients with a gastric ulcer are instructed to avoid excess stress and nonsteroidal anti-inflammatory drugs (NSAIDs). NSAIDs are associated with the development of gastric upset and ulcers because they inhibit prostaglandins. As many as 15% of patients on long-term NSAID treatment may develop ulcers of the stomach or duodenum.

Although most ulcers heal within a few weeks with drug treatment, some serious complications may occur. When an ulcer damages GI tissues, blood vessels may also be damaged, resulting in a bleeding ulcer (Figure 23-3). Sometimes an ulcer causes a hole in the wall of the stomach or duodenum, allowing partly digested food and bacteria to enter the sterile abdominal cavity *(peritoneum)* and causing an inflammation and infection of the abdominal cavity *(peritonitis)*. Signs that tell you an ulcer is getting worse are listed in Box 23-2.

 Memory Jogger

The most common symptom of a peptic ulcer is burning, gnawing pain that occurs between the umbilicus and sternum.

 Did You Know?

No special diet is recommended for the prevention or treatment of ulcers. A bland diet has not been shown to be effective.

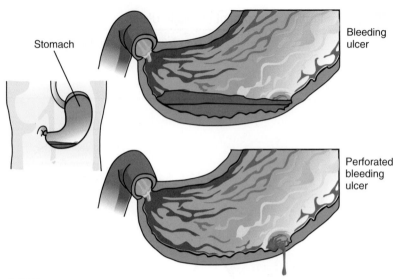

Stomach

Bleeding ulcer

Perforated bleeding ulcer

FIGURE 23-3 A peptic ulcer may lead to bleeding, perforation, or other emergencies.

Box 23-2	Signs That Indicate an Ulcer Is Getting Worse

- Blood in stools
- Continuing nausea or repeated vomiting
- Feeling cold or clammy
- Feeling weak or dizzy
- Losing weight
- Pain that doesn't go away after taking drugs
- Pain that radiates to the back
- Sudden severe pain
- Vomiting blood
- Vomiting food eaten hours or days ago

GASTROESOPHAGEAL REFLUX DISEASE

Most people suffer from occasional heartburn, but when heartburn occurs daily, exposure of the mucosa of the esophagus to stomach acids can cause irritation and inflammation. *Gastroesophageal reflux disease (GERD)* is a condition in which the liquid contents of the stomach back up (*regurgitate* or *reflux*) into the esophagus. At the end of the esophagus where it connects to the stomach is a strong muscle ring called the *lower esophageal sphincter (LES)*. The LES stays tightly shut except when food or liquids pass into the stomach. When closed it prevents stomach contents from backing up into the esophagus. Reflux or *regurgitation* happens when the LES is not working correctly (Figure 23-4). The LES may relax during periods of the day or night, or it may become too weak and constantly allow stomach contents to flow upward into the esophagus. When the LES is very weak and GERD is severe, a patient may need surgery to strengthen the LES.

Most people experience reflux occasionally; a person with GERD has reflux more often, and the stomach contents stay in the esophagus for longer periods of time. The regurgitated stomach contents contain stomach acids and pepsin and may also contain bile. These substances can injure the esophagus, causing inflammation and tissue damage, including ulcers. Risk factors for developing GERD are listed in Box 23-3.

The most common symptom of GERD is *dyspepsia* (heartburn). Other common symptoms include sour or bitter taste; bitter stomach fluid going into the mouth, especially during sleep; hoarseness; *water brash* (regurgitation of watery acid from the stomach); a repeated need to clear the throat; difficulty swallowing food or liquid; wheezing or coughing at night; and worsening of symptoms after eating or when bending over or lying down.

Memory Jogger

The cause of GERD is an LES that is not working correctly and allows stomach contents to back up (reflux) and damage the esophagus.

Memory Jogger

The most common symptom of GERD is dyspepsia (heartburn).

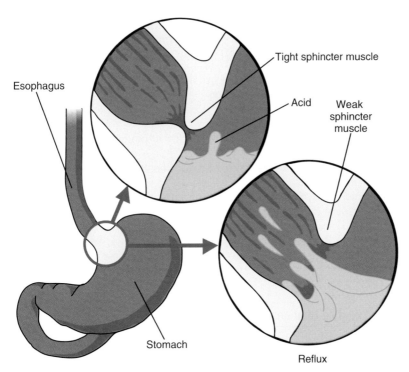

Esophagus

Tight sphincter muscle

Acid

Weak sphincter muscle

Stomach

Reflux

FIGURE 23-4 Acid reflux in the lower esophageal sphincter.

Box 23-3   **Risk Factors for GERD**

- Being overweight
- Being pregnant
- Certain diseases (e.g., diabetes, asthma, peptic ulcers)
- Certain drugs (e.g., nonsteroidal anti-inflammatory drugs)
- Drinking alcohol and caffeinated beverages
- Eating foods with high acid content (e.g., tomatoes, orange juice)
- Eating fatty and spicy foods
- Lying down too soon after meals
- Smoking

GERD is a chronic condition; treatment is lifelong. Treatment of GERD is divided into five stages (Box 23-4) and involves not only drugs but also lifestyle changes (Table 23-1) such as smoking cessation (because nicotine weakens the LES), decreased dietary fat intake, weight reduction, and avoidance of large meals and foods that cause regurgitation. A patient with GERD is instructed to elevate the head of the bed at least 6 to 10 inches using blocks under the top bed legs or a pillow wedge (Figure 23-5). After meals the patient with GERD should remain upright for 3 hours. Patients should also avoid foods that cause increased reflux such as chocolate, peppermint, alcohol, and caffeinated drinks.

Chewing gum after meals may be a useful treatment for GERD because it increases the production of saliva, which contains bicarbonate, and increases the rate of swallowing. The bicarbonate in saliva neutralizes acid in the esophagus and decreases the irritation of refluxed stomach contents.

Complications of GERD occur when the disease is severe or long lasting. The constant irritation of the esophagus by stomach contents can lead to inflammation, ulcers, and bleeding. Bleeding can cause anemia. Over time scarring of the esophagus can cause it to narrow, making swallowing difficult. Narrowing of the esophagus is called an *esophageal stricture*. Chronic GERD can cause changes in the cells of the esophagus, leading to precancerous cells and cancer. This condition is called *Barrett's esophagus* and occurs in about 10% of patients with GERD. Barrett's esophagus increases the risk for developing esophageal cancer.

Clinical Pitfall

Patients with GERD should avoid chocolate, peppermint, alcohol, nicotine, and caffeinated drinks because they lower the pressure of the LES and promote reflux.

QSEN: Safety

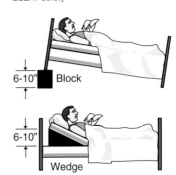

6-10"   Block

6-10"   Wedge

FIGURE 23-5 How to elevate the head of the bed.

? **Did You Know?**

Chewing gum after meals may prevent irritation of the esophagus associated with GERD.

Box **23-4**	**Stages of Treatment for GERD**

Stage I: Lifestyle modifications
Stage II: As-needed drug therapy
- Antacid and/or antacid-containing alginic acid
- Over-the-counter histamine H$_2$ blocker

Stage III: Scheduled pharmacologic therapy
- Histamine H$_2$ blocker for 8 to 12 weeks
- For persistent symptoms: high-dose H$_2$ blocker or proton pump inhibitor for additional 8 to 12 weeks
- Proton pump inhibitors as first choice for documented erosive esophagitis

Stage IV: Maintenance therapy
- For patients with symptoms of relapse or complicated disease
- Lowest effective dosage of histamine H$_2$ blocker or proton pump inhibitor

Stage V: Surgery
- For patients with severe symptoms, erosive esophagitis, or disease complications
- Fundoplication procedure to strengthen lower esophageal sphincter

Table **23-1**	**Lifestyle Changes for Treatment of GERD**

LIFESTYLE CHANGE	RATIONALE
Avoid eating within 3 hours of bedtime	Decreases risk of nighttime reflux
Stop smoking	Nicotine weakens the LES
Avoid alcohol (especially red wine), caffeine, chocolate, citrus fruits and juices, fatty foods, milk, peppermint, pepper seasoning, spearmint, and tomato products	These foods cause increased reflux
Decrease portions at mealtimes	Decreases reflux
Avoid tight-fitting clothes and bending after meals	Decreases reflux
Elevate the head of the bed or mattress 6 to 10 inches	Helps keep acid in stomach by gravity while sleeping
Lose weight if overweight	Relieves pressure on the stomach and LES

LES, Lower esophageal sphincter.

GENERAL ISSUES FOR DRUGS FOR PUD AND GERD

There are several classes of drugs used to treat PUD and GERD that have both different and common actions and effects. Responsibilities for these common actions and effects are listed in the following paragraphs. Specific responsibilities are listed with each individual class of drugs.

Before giving drugs for PUD or GERD, be sure to obtain a complete list of drugs currently being used by the patient, including over-the-counter and herbal drugs. Not only can some drugs increase the risk for PUD or GERD, but the drugs used to treat these problems may interfere with the absorption of other drugs.

Obtain a baseline set of vital signs, including body temperature, and obtain a baseline weight. Ask patients about normal bowel habits, appearance of stools, bleeding, vomiting, and reflux (location, duration, character, and factors that cause it to occur).

Listen to the abdomen with your stethoscope for bowel sounds, check for distention, and ask about abdominal pain. Instruct the patient to report any episodes of heartburn or reflux.

After giving drugs for PUD or GERD, be sure to recheck vital signs every shift and weigh patients every morning. Also watch for abnormal heart rhythms (too fast, too slow, or irregular). Keep track of bowel movement frequency and consistency. Check the abdomen for active bowel sounds and distention every shift. Remind the patient about the potential for altered bowel functions, including constipation and diarrhea. Ask patients about bowel movements every day. Record any episodes of reflux, heartburn, or indigestion.

Teach patients taking a drug for PUD or GERD to take the drug exactly as prescribed for the period of time prescribed, even when they are feeling better. Remind them to take a missed dose as soon as possible but not to take a double dose.

Tell patients to notify their prescriber for difficulty swallowing; persistent abdominal pain; vomiting blood (bright red or coffee grounds–appearing emesis); or black, tarry stools. Remind them that increased fluid intake, fiber-containing foods, and exercise can help prevent constipation.

Advise patients to avoid alcohol, aspirin-containing products, NSAIDs, and foods that cause increased GI irritation. All of these substances increase the risk for ulcer development.

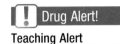

Drug Alert!

Teaching Alert

Teach patients with PUD or GERD to avoid substances that cause increased GI irritation, such as alcohol, NSAIDs, and aspirin.

QSEN: Safety

TYPES OF DRUGS FOR PUD AND GERD

Antiulcer drugs are used to treat ulcers of the stomach and duodenum. **Histamine H₂ blockers** decrease the secretion of gastric acid, and **proton pump inhibitors (PPIs)** block the secretion of gastric acid. **Cytoprotective drugs** such as sucralfate (Carafate) are used to form a thick coating that covers an ulcer to protect the open sore from further damage and allows healing to occur. Antibiotics are used to treat *H. pylori* infections that are the major cause of ulcers.

Several groups of drugs are used to treat GERD. Drugs used to treat PUD such as histamine H₂ blockers and PPIs are also used to treat GERD. Antacids can neutralize stomach acid and decrease the ability of acid to irritate and inflame the esophagus. Metoclopramide (Reglan), a promotility drug, increases LES tone and helps to empty the stomach.

HISTAMINE H₂ BLOCKERS

How Histamine H₂ Blockers Work

Histamine H₂ blockers *(antagonists)* cause decreased stimulation of H₂ receptors in gastric cells that secrete hydrochloric acid *(parietal cells)*, leading to a decrease in gastric acid secretion. When histamine binds to receptors in the stomach lining, acid pumps are activated, releasing acid into the stomach. H₂ blockers prevent histamine from stimulating the pumps in the stomach that produce hydrochloric acid.

Histamine H₂ blockers are used to heal ulcers or relieve the symptoms and pain that occur with GERD. These drugs are available over the counter and by prescription. Over-the-counter H₂ blockers are lower dose and are useful for prevention and relief of mild heartburn, indigestion, or sour stomach. Prescription-strength H₂ blockers come in higher doses and are used for moderate-to-severe forms of GERD.

Common names and doses of drugs for histamine H₂ blockers are listed in the following table. Be sure to consult a drug handbook for information on specific histamine H₂ blockers.

Do Not Confuse

Zantac *with* **Zyrtec**

An order for Zantac may be confused with Zyrtec. Zantac is a histamine H₂ blocker used to decrease secretion of stomach acids, whereas Zyrtec is an antihistamine drug used for allergies.

QSEN: Safety

Dosages for Common Histamine H₂ Blockers

Drug	Dosage
nizatidine (Axid)	*Adults:* 75-150 mg orally twice daily 30-60 min before meals or 300 mg once daily at bedtime
famotidine (Pepcid, Pepcid RPD ✚)	*Adults:* 10-20 mg orally twice daily or 40 mg once daily at bedtime (do not exceed 40 mg/day)
ranitidine (Gen-Ranitidine ✚, Zantac, Zantac-C ✚)	*Adults:* Oral—150 mg twice daily or 300 mg once daily at bedtime (do not exceed 300 mg/day); IV, IM—50 mg every 6 to 8 hr *Children over 12 years:* Oral—75-150 mg every 12 hr or once daily (do not exceed 300 mg/day); IV, IM—3-6 mg/kg/day divided in doses every 6 hr (do not exceed 200 mg/day)

Continued

Dosages for Common Histamine H₂ Blockers—cont'd

Drug	Dosage
cimetidine (Novo-Cimetine ✦, Peptol ✦, Tagamet)	*Adults:* Oral—300 mg 4 times daily or 400 mg twice daily; IM, IV—300 mg every 6 to 8 hr *Children:* Oral, IM, IV—20-40 mg/kg/day in 4 divided doses

Intended Responses
- Secretion of gastric acid is decreased.
- Symptoms of GERD are decreased.
- Ulcers are healed and prevented.

Side Effects. Side effects of these drugs are uncommon. However, the most common side effect of histamine H₂ blockers is confusion. Other common side effects include dizziness, drowsiness, headaches, altered sense of taste, constipation, diarrhea, nausea, impotence and decreased sperm count, anemia, neutropenia (decreased number of neutrophil white blood cells), and thrombocytopenia (low platelet count).

Ranitidine (Zantac) may also cause a blackened tongue and dark stools. Nizatidine (Axid) and cimetidine (Tagamet) may cause drug-induced hepatitis.

Adverse Effects. Adverse life-threatening effects of H₂ blockers include abnormal heart rhythms (dysrhythmias), decreased white blood cell count (*agranulocytosis*), and anemia caused by deficient red blood cell production by the bone marrow (*aplastic anemia*).

What To Do *Before* Giving Histamine H₂ Blockers
In addition to the general responsibilities related to drugs for PUD and GERD (p. 378), check the patient's baseline level of consciousness because drowsiness is a common side effect of these drugs. Use this information to determine patient responses to the drug.

Give the drug with meals to prolong its therapeutic effects. If the patient is prescribed to take a histamine H₂ blocker once a day, give it at bedtime to prolong its effects when there is no food in the stomach and reflux may be worse.

If the patient is to receive an intravenous (IV) drug, be sure to check the IV site at least every 2 to 4 hours for patency and signs of infection.

What To Do *After* Giving Histamine H₂ Blockers
In addition to the general responsibilities related to drugs for PUD and GERD (pp. 378-379), for inpatients, ensure that the call light is within easy reach and remind patients to call for help when getting out of bed because these drugs may cause dizziness or drowsiness.

Watch for other side effects, including nausea or vomiting. Notify the prescriber for any signs of allergic reaction (for example, fever, sore throat, rashes); confusion; black, tarry stools; dizziness; or hallucinations.

What To *Teach* Patients About Histamine H₂ Blockers
In addition to the general precautions related to drugs for PUD and GERD (p. 379), advise patients who have been taking over-the-counter histamine H₂ blockers for more than 2 weeks to see their prescriber if symptoms have not improved, because these drugs are used for short-term treatment of GERD and ulcers. Signs and symptoms of GERD and PUD are similar to those for stomach cancer, which should be ruled out.

Remind patients that smoking interferes with the action of histamine H₂ blockers and encourage them to quit smoking. Because these drugs may cause dizziness or drowsiness, caution patients to avoid driving, operating machines, or engaging in any other activities that require alertness until they know how the drug affects them.

Drug Alert!

Action/Intervention Alert

Watch for confusion, the most common side effect, when giving histamine H₂ blockers.

QSEN: Safety

Common Side Effects

Histamine H₂ Blockers

Confusion   Dizziness   Drowsiness

Headache   Nausea/Vomiting

Drug Alert!

Teaching Alert

Teach patients to notify their prescriber if they have been taking over-the-counter H₂ blockers for more than 2 weeks and are still experiencing reflux.

QSEN: Safety

Clinical Pitfall

Patients taking histamine H₂ blockers should not smoke because smoking interferes with the action of these drugs.

QSEN: Safety

Life Span Considerations for Histamine H$_2$ Blockers

Considerations for Pregnancy and Lactation. Histamine H$_2$ blockers have a low likelihood of increasing the risk for birth defects or fetal harm. However, they have not been studied in pregnant women. A woman should always tell her health care provider if she is pregnant or planning to become pregnant. Pregnant women frequently experience heartburn. They should not take any drugs without consulting their health care provider. Instead they should try nonpharmacologic and lifestyle changes. These drugs pass into breast milk and may cause undesired side effects in the breastfeeding infant. They should be avoided while breastfeeding.

Considerations for Older Adults. Older adults are more likely to experience confusion and dizziness because of increased sensitivity to the side effects of histamine H$_2$ blockers compared with younger adults. Teach family members to watch for changes in cognition or increased confusion. Teach older adults to take special precautions to avoid falls. Instruct them to change positions slowly and to use handrails when going up or down stairs. Suggest that older adults avoid driving or using heavy machinery until they know how the drug affects them.

PROTON PUMP INHIBITORS

How Proton Pump Inhibitors Work

Normally the stomach produces acid to help break down food in the process of digestion. When the acid irritates the mucosal lining of the stomach or duodenum, ulceration or bleeding can occur. Proton pump inhibitors (PPIs) work by completely blocking the production of stomach acid. These drugs block the action of "pumps" located in acid-secreting cells, which totally blocks stomach acid secretion.

PPIs are the most prescribed and powerful drugs used for treating PUD or GERD and should be used for limited periods of time. They are used when H$_2$ blockers are not effective. Often PPIs are used in combination with antibiotics to treat *H. pylori* infections in the stomach.

Some are available over the counter; others require a prescription. Common names and doses of drugs for PPIs are listed in the following table. Be sure to consult a drug reference handbook for information on specific PPIs.

Dosages for Common Proton Pump Inhibitors

Drug	Dosage
omeprazole (Losec , Prilosec, Zegerid)	*Adults:* 20-40 mg orally once daily for 4-8 wk
lansoprazole (Prevacid)	*Adults:* 15-30 mg orally once daily for 4-8 wk
dexlansoprazole (Dexilant)	*Adults:* 30-60 mg orally once daily for up to 8 weeks.
rabeprazole (Aciphex, Pariet)	*Adults:* 20 mg delayed-release tablets orally once daily for 4-8 wk
pantoprazole (Protonix)	*Adults:* 40-80 mg orally once daily
esomeprazole magnesium (Nexium)	*Adults:* 20-40 mg orally once daily for 4 weeks

Intended Responses

- Gastric acid secretion is decreased.
- Acid reflux is decreased.
- Ulcers are healed.

Side Effects. Side effects rarely occur with PPIs. The most common side effects are diarrhea, constipation, belching and gas, abdominal pain, and headaches. Some patients report generally feeling ill while taking these drugs.

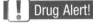

Drug Alert!

Action/Intervention Alert

Monitor older adults closely because they are more likely to experience confusion and dizziness as side effects of histamine H$_2$ blockers.

QSEN: Safety

Do Not Confuse

rabeprazole *with* aripiprazole

An order for rabeprazole may be confused with aripiprazole. Rabeprazole is a PPI used to block gastric secretions, whereas aripiprazole is an antipsychotic drug used for schizophrenia and acute bipolar episodes.

QSEN: Safety

Do Not Confuse

Prilosec *with* Prinivil

An order for Prilosec may be confused with Prinivil. Prilosec is a PPI used to block stomach acid secretion, whereas Prinivil is an angiotensin-converting enzyme inhibitor used to treat high blood pressure.

QSEN: Safety

Common Side Effects

Proton Pump Inhibitors

Diarrhea, Constipation, Gas, Abdominal pain   Headache

Lansoprazole (Prevacid), omeprazole (Prilosec), and rabeprazole (Aciphex) also may cause dizziness. In addition, rabeprazole may cause increased sun sensitivity (photosensitivity).

Long-term use of PPIs may lead to stomach infections because these drugs inhibit production of stomach acids that help to kill bacteria. This may also lead to anemia because the loss of stomach acid reduces digestion of protein essential for making new cells.

Adverse Effects. Allergic reactions are rare and include itching, dizziness, swollen ankles, muscle and joint pain, blurred vision, depression, and dry mouth.

What To Do *Before* Giving Proton Pump Inhibitors

In addition to the general responsibilities related to drugs for PUD and GERD (p. 378), give these drugs before meals, preferably in the morning. PPIs can be given with antacids and with or without food.

If the patient is to be given an IV drug, be sure to check the IV site for patency and signs of infection.

What To Do *After* Giving Proton Pump Inhibitors

In addition to the general responsibilities related to drugs for PUD and GERD (pp. 378-379), report any black, tarry stools to the prescriber immediately. These are indicators of upper GI bleeding, which can lead to severe hemorrhage.

If lansoprazole, rabeprazole, or omeprazole is prescribed, teach the patient to call for help when getting out of bed because these drugs may cause dizziness. Be sure that the call light is within easy reach.

What To *Teach* Patients About Proton Pump Inhibitors

In addition to the general precautions related to drugs for PUD and GERD (p. 379), instruct patients to take the drug exactly as prescribed and to take it for the full time period, even when they are feeling better. These drugs do not cure the ulcer; they just change the GI environment so that healing is more likely to occur. Stopping the drug too soon can allow a partially healed ulcer to reopen.

Instruct patients to report any black, tarry stools; diarrhea; abdominal pain; or persistent headaches to their prescriber immediately because these are signs of bleeding and possible low blood volume (hypovolemia).

Caution patients prescribed lansoprazole, omeprazole, or rabeprazole to avoid driving or engaging in other activities that require increased alertness. These drugs may cause dizziness.

Teach patients taking rabeprazole about the importance of wearing sunscreen and protective clothing when going outdoors because this drug causes photosensitivity (increased sensitivity of the skin to light and other sources of ultraviolet rays).

Life Span Considerations for Proton Pump Inhibitors

Considerations for Pregnancy and Lactation. Omeprazole, pantoprazole, and rabeprazole have a moderate likelihood of increasing the risk for birth defects or fetal harm. They are not safe for use during pregnancy because they may cause harm to the unborn child. The other PPI drugs have a low likelihood of increasing the risk for birth defects or fetal harm. They are considered safe for use during pregnancy, but the benefits must outweigh the risks. PPIs are not recommended for use during breastfeeding. A woman taking a PPI should tell her health care provider if she is pregnant or planning to become pregnant.

Considerations for Older Adults. There is an increased risk for side effects in older adults. PPIs have been associated with an increased risk for hip fractures because of decreased calcium absorption. Some studies have shown that short-term use of PPIs decreases the absorption of vitamin B_{12}. Older adults should have more frequent checkups to determine the effectiveness of the drug. In addition, the drug should be stopped in older adults when ulcers or inflammation have healed completely.

Drug Alert!

Administration Alert

For best effects PPIs should be given before meals, preferably in the morning.

QSEN: Safety

Clinical Pitfall

Black, tarry stools are never normal; they indicate bleeding and should be reported to the prescriber immediately.

QSEN: Safety

Drug Alert!

Teaching Alert

Teach patients to take any PPI for the full period of time prescribed to ensure healing of ulcers.

QSEN: Safety

Drug Alert!

Teaching Alert

Teach older adults who have been prescribed PPIs to take a daily multivitamin because PPIs decrease the absorption of vitamin B_{12} and calcium.

QSEN: Safety

ANTACIDS

How Antacids Work

Antacids, drugs that neutralize acids in the stomach, are given by mouth to relieve heartburn and indigestion. Many antacids are available over the counter without a prescription.

Common names and doses of a few antacids are listed in the following table. Be sure to consult a drug handbook for information on any specific antacid.

Dosages for Common Antacids

Drug	Dosage
magnesium hydroxide/ aluminum hydroxide/ simethicone (Maalox, Milk of Magnesia, Mylanta)	*Adults/Children over 12:* 10-20 mL orally 1 and 3 hr after meals and at bedtime *Children:* Consult the prescriber *Infants:* Consult the prescriber
aluminum hydroxide (AlternaGEL, Alugel ✦, Amphojel)	*Adults:* 80-140 mEq (40-60 mL) liquid orally every 3-6 hr, or 1 and 3 hr after meals and at bedtime.
calcium carbonate (Calcite ✦, Calsan ✦, Rolaids, TUMS)	*Adults:* 1-4 chewable tablets orally every hr as needed, but no more than 16 tablets per day

Antacids are given by mouth to neutralize stomach acids and relieve heartburn and indigestion. Neutralizing stomach acids decreases the irritation and inflammation of the GI mucosa, especially the esophagus. Most antacids use salts of calcium, aluminum, or magnesium to neutralize acid.

Intended Responses
- Gastric acids are neutralized.
- There is relief from heartburn and indigestion.
- Symptoms of GERD are decreased.
- Ulcers are healing, and pain from ulcers is decreased.

Side Effects. Side effects of antacids are very rare when they are taken as directed. They are more likely to occur if the drug is taken in large doses or over a long period of time or if the patient has kidney disease. The most common side effect of antacids containing calcium or aluminum salts is constipation. The most common side effect of antacids containing magnesium salts is diarrhea. Table 23-2 summarizes the side effects of antacids on the basis of their primary ingredients.

Common Side Effects

Antacids

Constipation, Diarrhea, Decreased appetite

Weakness, Fatigue

Table **23-2**	Common Side Effects of Antacids
TYPE OF ANTACID	**SIDE EFFECTS**
Aluminum containing	Bone pain, constipation, discomfort, loss of appetite, mood changes, muscle weakness, swelling of wrists or ankles, weight loss
Calcium containing	Constipation, decreased respiratory rate, difficult and frequent urination, fatigue, loss of appetite, mood changes, muscle pain, nausea and vomiting, nervousness, restlessness, twitching, unpleasant taste
Magnesium containing	Difficult or painful urination, dizziness, fatigue, irregular heart rhythm, light-headedness, loss of appetite, mood changes, muscle weakness, weight loss
Sodium bicarbonate containing	Decreased respiratory rate, fatigue, frequent urination, headache, loss of appetite, mood changes, muscle pain, nausea or vomiting, nervousness, restlessness, swelling of feet and lower legs, twitching

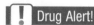 **Drug Alert!**

Action/Interaction Alert

Be sure to ask patients about antacid use because these drugs are readily available over the counter.

QSEN: Safety

 Drug Alert!

Teaching Alert

Teach patients to contact their prescriber if they have been taking an antacid for more than 2 weeks and continue to experience signs of reflux or an ulcer.

QSEN: Safety

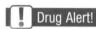 **Clinical Pitfall**

Patients should not take an aluminum hydroxide or a calcium carbonate antacid within 1 to 2 hours of taking other drugs.

QSEN: Safety

 Clinical Pitfall

Patients with heart failure should not take sodium-containing antacids.

QSEN: Safety

 Clinical Pitfall

Older adults with bone problems or Alzheimer's disease should not take aluminum-containing antacids.

QSEN: Safety

Adverse Effects. Adverse effects have not been reported when these drugs are taken appropriately.

What To Do *Before* Giving Antacids

In addition to the general responsibilities related to drugs for PUD and GERD (p. 378), ensure that antacids are given 1 hour after or 2 hours before any other drug therapy. Antacids interfere with absorption of other drugs and should not be taken at the same time.

What To Do *After* Giving Antacids

Be sure to review the general responsibilities related to drugs for PUD and GERD (pp. 378-379). Ask patients about symptom relief. Check patients daily for bowel movements.

What To *Teach* Patients About Antacids

In addition to the general precautions related to drugs for PUD and GERD (p. 378), tell patients to contact their prescriber if they have been taking an antacid for more than 2 weeks and have not obtained relief. The excessive use of antacids may cause or worsen kidney problems. Using calcium-based antacids too much may lead to the formation of kidney stones.

Tell patients not to take an aluminum hydroxide or calcium antacid within 1 to 2 hours of other drugs without consulting their prescriber because these drugs affect absorption of other drugs.

Remind patients with heart failure not to take sodium-containing antacids (for example, Alka-Seltzer, Bromo-Seltzer) because they increase sodium and water retention. This problem causes an increase in the workload of the heart and can worsen heart failure.

Be sure to tell patients taking an aluminum hydroxide or a calcium carbonate antacid about the side effect of constipation; patients taking a magnesium-containing antacid should be told about the side effect of diarrhea.

Teach patients that antacids should be avoided if any signs of appendicitis or inflamed bowel are present. Signs include cramping, pain, and soreness in the lower abdomen; bloating; and nausea and vomiting.

Life Span Considerations for Antacids
Pediatric Considerations. Antacids should not be given to young children unless directed by the prescriber. Excessive amounts of antacids can change the pH of the blood and cause alkalosis.

Considerations for Pregnancy and Lactation. The effects of antacids have not been studied in pregnant women. Magnesium hydroxide antacids have a low likelihood of increasing the risk for birth defects or fetal harm and are generally considered safe for use during pregnancy. Calcium carbonate and aluminum hydroxide antacids have a moderate likelihood of increasing the risk for birth defects or fetal harm. Long-term use of antacids may have negative effects on the fetus, and sodium-containing antacids should not be taken by women who tend to retain body water. Many antacids pass into breast milk, but they have not been reported to cause problems with breastfeeding babies.

Considerations for Older Adults. Older adults should not take aluminum-containing antacids if they have bone problems or Alzheimer's disease because these drugs may cause these conditions to worsen.

CYTOPROTECTIVE DRUGS

How Cytoprotective Drugs Work
Cytoprotective (GI coating) drugs decrease acid damage to the stomach by coating the mucosal lining of the stomach and reducing the risk of developing an ulcer. Some

cytoprotective drugs such as bismuth subsalicylate (Pepto-Bismol) are available over the counter.

Most of these drugs work by coating some part of the GI mucosa and reducing its exposure to stomach acids. Sucralfate (Carafate) is prescribed to protect open-sore areas in the GI tract and allow ulcers to heal. Sucralfate reacts with stomach acids to form a thick coating that covers the surface of an ulcer. This protects the open area from further damage. It also stops the effects of pepsin (a digestive enzyme that breaks down protein). Interestingly, this drug does not coat the normal stomach mucosa. Bismuth subsalicylate also coats the stomach and intestine protecting the mucosa. In addition, this drug inhibits the activity of *H. pylori* bacteria, helping to decrease GI infections. For additional information on bismuth subsalicylate, see Chapter 22.

The common doses of cytoprotective drugs are listed in the following table. Be sure to consult a drug handbook for more information about any specific cytoprotective drug.

Did You Know?

Sucralfate (Carafate) forms a protective coating over an ulcer but does not coat normal stomach mucosa.

Dosages for Common Cytoprotective Drugs

Drug	Dosage
bismuth subsalicylate (Pepto-Bismol)	*Adults:* 524 mg orally 4 times daily (30 mL)
sucralfate (Carafate, Sulcrate ✦)	*Adults:* Treatment of ulcers—1 g orally 4 times daily 1 hr before meals and at bedtime; prevention of ulcers—1 g orally twice daily 1 hr before a meal

Intended Responses
- Ulcers are protected to prevent further tissue damage.
- Ulcers are healed.

Side Effects. Side effects are rare with cytoprotective drugs. The most common side effect of sucralfate is constipation. Other side effects include dizziness; drowsiness; diarrhea; dry mouth; rashes; and gastric discomfort such as flatulence (gas), indigestion, and nausea.

Adverse Effects. No life-threatening adverse effects have been documented with sucralfate.

What To Do *Before* Giving Cytoprotective Drugs
Be sure to review the general responsibilities related to drugs for PUD and GERD (p. 378) before giving these drugs.

What To Do *After* Giving Cytoprotective Drugs
Be sure to review the general nursing responsibilities related to drugs for PUD and GERD (pp. 378-379) after giving cytoprotective drugs.

What To *Teach* Patients About Cytoprotective Drugs
In addition to the general precautions related to drugs for PUD and GERD (p. 379), instruct patients to take the drug exactly as directed by their prescriber for the full period of time (usually 4 to 8 weeks), even when feeling better.

Teach patients that increased fluid intake, dietary fiber (such as extra fruits, vegetables, and bran), and exercise help to prevent constipation, abdominal pain, and gas.

Life Span Considerations for Cytoprotective Drugs
Considerations for Pregnancy and Lactation. Sucralfate has a low likelihood of increasing the risk for birth defects or fetal harm, and appears to be safe to use during

Common Side Effects

Cytoprotective Drugs

Constipation, Abdominal discomfort

Drug Alert!

Teaching Alert

Teach patients taking cytoprotective drugs to prevent constipation by increasing intake of fluids and fiber-containing foods and exercising.

QSEN: Safety

pregnancy. However, extensive studies in pregnant women have not been conducted. A woman of childbearing years should be sure to tell her prescriber if she is breast-feeding an infant because it is not known whether sucralfate passes into breast milk.

Teach patients who continue to breastfeed while taking these drugs to follow the tips in Box 1-1 (in Chapter 1) to reduce infant exposure to the drugs.

PROMOTILITY DRUGS

How Promotility Drugs Work

When used to treat GERD, promotility drugs increase LES tone and the speed of emptying food out of the stomach. Metoclopramide (Reglan) increases stomach and small intestine contractions (peristalsis), helping to move food through the GI system. When food moves more quickly into the intestinal system, it is less likely to back up into the esophagus. Promotility drugs are not used to manage gastric or duodenal ulcers.

Metoclopramide is the promotility drug prescribed for treatment of GERD. It is usually given 30 minutes before meals and may be prescribed for 4 to 12 weeks. The common dosages for this drug are listed in the following table. For additional information on metoclopramide, see Chapter 22.

Dosages for Common Promotility Drugs

Drug	Dosage
metoclopramide (Emex ♣, Maxeran ♣, Octamide, Reglan)	*Adults/Children over 14 years:* Oral—5-10 mg orally 30 min before symptoms are likely to occur (for example, meals and bedtime); IV—10 mg *Children 5-14 years:* Dosage determined by prescriber

⇄ **Do Not Confuse**

metronidazole *with* metformin

An order for metronidazole may be confused with metformin. Metronidazole is an antibiotic, whereas metformin is an antidiabetic drug used for management of type 2 diabetes.

QSEN: Safety

OTHER DRUGS USED TO TREAT ULCERS

ANTIBIOTICS FOR *H. PYLORI* INFECTION

Antibiotics are essential to the treatment plan for PUD and are used to treat *H. pylori* infections of the GI tract. Common drugs and doses used to treat *H. pylori* infections are listed in the following table. Be sure to consult a drug reference handbook for information about specific antibiotics. See Chapter 8 for additional information on antibiotic drugs.

Dosages for Common Antibiotics for *H. pylori* Infections

Drug	Dosage
clarithromycin (Biaxin)	*Adult:* 500 mg orally every 12 hr for 7-14 days *Children:* 15 mg/kg orally in 2 divided doses
metronidazole (Flagyl, Novonidazole ♣, Trikacide ♣)	*Adults:* 250 mg orally 4 times daily when co-administered with bismuth and tetracycline; 500 mg orally twice daily when co-administered with clarithromycin *Children:* Pediatric dosage not established
tetracycline (Novotetra ♣, Sumycin, Tetracap)	*Adults:* 250-500 mg orally 4 times daily for 14 days *Children over 8 years:* 25-50 mg/kg/day orally in 4 divided doses (*not* recommended for children under 8 years)
amoxicillin (Amoxil, Novamoxin ♣, Trimox)	*Adults:* 250-500 mg orally 4 times daily or 1000 mg twice daily for 14 days *Children:* 20-40 mg/kg/day orally in 3 divided doses or 25-45 mg/kg/day in 2 divided doses

Get Ready for Practice!

Key Points

- The most common cause of PUD is infection with the *H. pylori* bacteria.
- Antibiotics are essential to the treatment plan for PUD because of *H. pylori* infections.
- Complications of ulcers include bleeding, perforation, and gastric obstruction.
- GERD may damage the lining of the esophagus, causing inflammation.
- The cause of GERD is a lower esophageal sphincter that is not working correctly and allows stomach contents to back up (reflux) into the esophagus.
- Complications of GERD include ulcers; bleeding; strictures; and Barrett's esophagus, a precancerous condition that may lead to development of esophageal cancer.
- Histamine H_2 blockers are available in lower doses over the counter for mild heartburn and indigestion. They are also available in higher doses by prescription for moderate-to-severe forms of GERD.
- Watch for confusion, the most common side effect, when giving histamine H_2 blockers.
- Smoking interferes with the action of histamine H_2 blockers.
- Black, tarry stools indicate bleeding and should always be reported to the prescriber.
- Teach patients to take proton pump inhibitors for the full period of time recommended by the prescriber, even if they are feeling better.
- Aluminum hydroxide antacids decrease the absorption of other drugs when taken within 1 to 2 hours.
- Patients with heart failure should not take sodium-containing antacids because they can cause salt and water retention and increase the workload of the heart.
- Teach patients taking any drug that causes constipation to increase fluid intake, eat fiber-containing foods, and exercise to help prevent constipation.
- Children should not be given bismuth subsalicylate (Pepto-Bismol) because it contains aspirin and may cause Reye's syndrome.

Additional Learning Resources

evolve Be sure to visit your Evolve website (http://evolve.elsevier.com/Workman/pharmacology/) for additional online resources.

SG Go to your Study Guide for additional learning activities to help you master this chapter content.

Review Questions

See the Answer Keys—In-text Review Questions for answers to these questions.

Test Yourself on the Basics
1. Which drug is a cytoprotective drug?
   A. Ranitidine
   B. Omeprazole
   C. Calcium carbonate
   D. Sucralfate

2. A patient prescribed a proton pump inhibitor tells you that he or she is experiencing black tarry stools. What side effect does this indicate?
   A. Water brash
   B. Reflux
   C. Bleeding
   D. Diarrhea

3. A patient prescribed omeprazole tells you that he had persistent abdominal pain. What should you do?
   A. Administer an antacid
   B. Notify the prescriber
   C. Order a bland diet for the patient
   D. Instruct the patient to drink milk

4. When should you teach a patient prescribed lanzoprazole to take the drug?
   A. Immediately on waking in the morning
   B. One hour after each meal
   C. Before meals in the morning
   D. Only at bedtime

5. An older adult patient is prescribed famotidine for reflux. Which information and precautions would you teach his family? (Select all that apply.)
   A. The patient may experience dizziness.
   B. Be sure to report every episodes of dyspepsia to the prescriber.
   C. Tell the prescriber if you notice LOC changes such as confusion.
   D. Take this drug with an antacid to increase its absorption.
   E. Be aware that the patient is at increased risk for falls.
   F. This drug will form a protective coating in his stomach.

Test Yourself on Advanced Concepts
6. A patient asks you how cytoprotective drugs will help prevent gastric ulcers. What is your best response?
   A. "It will increase movement of digested food through your bowel."
   B. "It will decrease secretion of acids in your stomach."
   C. "It will coat and protect the stomach lining."
   D. "It will neutralize stomach acids."

7. For which common side effect of proton pump inhibitors must you monitor a patient?
   A. Constipation
   B. Confusion
   C. Reflux
   D. Bleeding

8. What must you be sure to do before administering a histamine H_2 blocker? (Select all that apply.)
   A. Check patient's level of consciousness.
   B. Ask the patient about usual bowel habits.
   C. Give a drug to prevent diarrhea.
   D. Give once a day histamine H_2 blockers with a meal.
   E. Ask about bleeding and reflux.

9. A patient has been taking over-the-counter histamine H$_2$ blockers for more than 2 weeks and his GERD symptoms have not improved. What must you instruct the patient to do?
   A. Continue taking the histamine H$_2$ blockers.
   B. Take the histamine H$_2$ blockers more often.
   C. Try taking a different histamine H$_2$ blocker.
   D. Inform his or her health care provider.

10. Which of the following drugs may pass into breast milk and are not recommended when a woman is breastfeeding? (Select all that apply.)
   A. ranitidine (Zantac)
   B. pantoprazole (Protonix)
   C. magnesium hydroxide (Maalox)
   D. aluminum hydroxide (Amphojel)
   E. omeprazole (Prilosec)

11. A 14-year-old child with GERD has been prescribed ranitidine (Zantac) 1.25 mg/kg/day in two divided doses. The child weighs 40 kg. How many milligrams will you give per dose? _____ mg per dose

12. An older adult with a duodenal ulcer is to receive esomeprazole (Nexium) 40 mg once a day. The pharmacy sends esomeprazole 20 mg/tablet. How many tablets will you give? _____ tablet(s) per dose

13. A patient has been prescribed bismuth subsalicylate (Pepto-Bismol) 524 mg 4 times a day. Bismuth subsalicylate comes as an oral suspension of 17.5 mg/mL. How many milliliters will you give with each dose? _____ mL per dose

Critical Thinking Activities

See the Answer Keys – Critical Thinking Activities for answers to these activities.

Ms. Welsh is a 25-year-old graduate student with a new diagnosis or gastroesophageal reflux disease (GERD). The health care provider prescribes ranitidine (Zantac) 150 mg twice daily.

1. What is the purpose of this drug?
2. What side effects will you monitor for while the patient is taking this drug?
3. What lifestyle changes will you recommend for this patient?
4. Ms. Welsh tells you that she plans to marry later in the year and would like to have a child. What teaching must you provide about this drug?

Drug Therapy with Nutritional Supplements

Objectives

After studying this chapter you should be able to:

1. Explain the importance of nutritional supplements including vitamins, minerals, and enteral nutritional supplements.
2. List the common names, actions, usual adult dosages, possible side effects, and adverse effects of vitamins, minerals, and enteral nutritional supplements.
3. Describe what to do before and after giving vitamins, minerals, and enteral nutritional supplements.
4. Explain what to teach patients taking vitamins, minerals, and enteral nutritional supplements.
5. Describe life span considerations for vitamins, minerals, and enteral nutritional supplements.

Key Terms

enteral nutritional supplement (ĔN-tĕr-ăl nū-TRĬSH-ŭn-ăl SŬP-lĕ-mĕnt) (p. 396) A nutritional replacement product that provides nourishment to the body; often given through a tube (e.g., nasogastric, gastrostomy, jejunostomy) that is placed directly into the gastrointestinal tract (stomach or small intestine).

fat-soluble vitamins (FĂT SŎL-ū-bŭl VĬ-tă-mĭnz) (p. 390) Vitamins A, D, E, and K are fat-soluble vitamins. Fat-soluble vitamins are stored in the liver and fatty tissues and are eliminated more slowly than water-soluble vitamins. Fat-soluble vitamins are not lost when the foods that contain them are cooked.

macrominerals (MĂ-krō-MĬN-ĕr-ălz) (p. 392) Minerals the body needs in larger amounts. They include calcium, phosphorus, magnesium, sodium, potassium, chloride, and sulfur.

mineral (MĬN-ĕr-ăl) (p. 389) An inorganic element, such as calcium, iron, potassium, sodium, or zinc, that is essential to the nutrition of humans, animals, and plants.

multivitamin (MŬL-tē-VĬ-tă-min) (p. 389) A pill or other preparation (e.g., liquid, chew) that contains several vitamins essential for health; usually intended as a dietary supplement and often includes essential dietary minerals.

trace minerals (TRĀS MĬN-ĕr-ălz) (p. 392) Minerals the body needs in very small amounts. These include iron, manganese, copper, iodine, zinc, cobalt, fluoride, and selenium

vitamin (VĬ-tă-min) (p. 389) Essential micronutrients the body needs in small amounts for various roles throughout the human body. Vitamins are divided into two groups: water-soluble (B-complex vitamins and C vitamins) and fat-soluble vitamins (A, D, E, and K).

water-soluble vitamins (WĂ-tĕr SŎL-ū-bŭl VĬ-tă-mĭnz) (p. 390) Vitamins that can dissolve in water. Water-soluble vitamins are carried to the body's tissues but are not stored in the body. They are found in plant and animal foods or dietary supplements and must be taken in daily. Vitamin C and members of the vitamin B complex are water soluble.

OVERVIEW

Vitamins and minerals are substances that are essential to the body for normal growth and development. **Vitamins** are essential organic micronutrients the body needs in small amounts for various roles throughout the human body. **Minerals** are also essential micronutrients and are inorganic elements, such as calcium, iron, potassium, sodium, or zinc; they are essential to the nutrition of the human body. The best way to take in vitamins and minerals is through a healthy diet. Although daily consumption of vitamins and minerals is important, it should also be stressed that too much of these substances can cause toxicities. There are also certain conditions in which people may need extra vitamins or minerals (e.g., pregnancy, illness, specific nutritional deficiency). When extra vitamins or minerals are needed, a **multivitamin** (pill or other preparation) containing vitamins and/or minerals may be prescribed. If a specific substance is required, the prescriber may order only that substance or that substance in addition to a multivitamin (e.g., extra calcium for osteoporosis, along with a multivitamin).

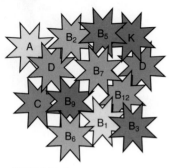

FIGURE 24-1   Essential vitamins.

Memory Jogger

The 13 vitamins needed by the human body are:
- Vitamin A
- B vitamins (thiamine, riboflavin, niacin, pantothenic acid, biotin, vitamin B$_6$, vitamin B$_{12}$, and folate)
- Vitamin C
- Vitamin D
- Vitamin E
- Vitamin K

Memory Jogger

The two major groups of vitamins are water-soluble and fat-soluble vitamins.

Did You Know?

Research has demonstrated that administration of vitamin D supplements is effective in decreasing falls in nursing care facilities.

Common Side Effects

Vitamins

Constipation, Nausea, Upset stomach

REVIEW OF RELATED PHYSIOLOGY AND PATHOPHYSIOLOGY

Vitamins and minerals perform essential functions in the body every day. They strengthen bones, heal wounds, and support the immune system, as well as convert food to energy and repair damage to cells. Sometimes they work together to complete functions. For example, calcium, vitamin D, vitamin K, magnesium, and phosphorus strengthen bones and protect against fractures. Folic acid taken early in pregnancy helps prevent brain and spinal cord birth defects. Fluoride also helps strengthen bone but plays a major role in creating strong teeth and prevention of dental cavities. Adequate intake of vitamin A prevents some types of blindness, vitamin C prevents scurvy, and vitamin D prevents rickets.

VITAMINS

Human bodies need 13 vitamins (Figure 24-1). The two major groups of vitamins are water-soluble (i.e., B-complex vitamins and C vitamins) and fat-soluble vitamins (i.e., A, D, E, and K).

Water-soluble vitamins dissolve in water. They are carried to the body's tissues but are not stored in the body. These vitamins are found in plant and animal foods or dietary supplements and must be taken in each day. Water-soluble vitamins are easily lost during cooking or when improperly stored.

Fat-soluble vitamins are stored in the liver and fatty tissues and are eliminated much more slowly than water-soluble vitamins. Fat-soluble vitamins are not lost when the foods that contain them are cooked and may not need to be taken every day.

How Vitamins Work

Each vitamin has specific functions. Table 24-1 lists the water-soluble vitamins and Table 24-2 lists the fat-soluble vitamins. Each table includes recommended doses, actions, symptoms of deficiencies, and food sources of the vitamins.

Commonly Prescribed Vitamin Supplements

There are numerous brands of multivitamins and individual vitamins available over the counter or by prescription. Most are taken once a day. Although the best way to get necessary vitamins is through a healthy diet, the purpose of these preparations is to ensure that patients receive adequate amounts of essential vitamins. A prescriber may order vitamins to correct specific deficiencies (see Tables 24-1 and 24-2), to correct general dietary deficiencies, for certain illness (e.g., cancer, heart disease), during pregnancy (e.g., specially formulated prenatal vitamins), or to ensure adequate vitamin intake when a patient is unable or unwilling to take in adequate amounts through a healthy diet.

Intended Responses
- Adequate essential vitamin intake
- Avoidance of side effects of deficient vitamin intake

Side Effects. Multivitamins may cause constipation, nausea, or upset stomach. These side effects are usually not permanent and improve as a patient's body gets used to the drug.

Adverse Effects. A rare adverse reaction to multivitamins is an allergic reaction with a rash, itching, swelling (especially of the face/tongue/throat), severe dizziness, or trouble breathing.

What To Do *Before* Giving a Vitamin Supplement

Ask patients about any previous side effects or allergic reactions to multivitamins or specific vitamins. Check the patient's medical history for alcohol abuse, liver problems, or gastrointestinal problems (e.g., colitis, ulcers). Always get a complete list of medications the patient is taking, including over-the-counter drugs.

| Table 24-1 | Water-Soluble Vitamins |

VITAMIN	RECOMMENDED DOSE	ACTION	DEFICIENCY	SOURCES
Vitamin C (ascorbic acid)	Adult male 90 mg/day Adult female 75 mg/day	Holds cells together through collagen synthesis	Scurvy	Citrus fruits and juices, broccoli, cabbage
Niacin (nicotinic acid, vitamin B₃)	Adult male 16 mg/day Adult female 14 mg/day	Involved in energy production, normal enzyme function, digestion, promoting normal appetite, healthy skin, and nerves	Pellagra	Liver, organ meats, fish, poultry, whole and enriched grains, peanuts
Riboflavin (vitamin B₂)	Adult male 1.3 mg/day Adult female 1.1 mg/day	Affects fetal growth, helps to release energy from foods, promotes good vision and healthy skin	Ariboflavinosis (characterized by sores in the mouth), weakness, throat and tongue swelling, skin cracking, dermatitis, anemia	Green leafy vegetables, eggs, milk, enriched cereal, organ meats, peanuts
Thiamine (vitamin B₁)	Adult male 1.2 mg/day Adult female 1.1 mg/day	Carbohydrate metabolism, nerve conduction, energy production	Beriberi	Pork, whole grains, peas, cereal, dry beans, peanuts
Pyridoxine (vitamin B₆)	Adult male/female 1.3 mg/day	Amino acid and protein metabolism; red blood cell formation	Anemia, hair loss, paresthesias	Pork, meats, whole grains, cereals, fish, legumes, green leafy vegetables
Cyanocobalamin (vitamin B₁₂)	Adult male/female 2.4 mcg/day	Helps with building of genetic material, production of normal red blood cells, and maintenance of the nervous system	Megaloblastic anemia	Seafood, egg yolks, organ meats, milk, cheese
Folic acid (folacin)	Adult male/female 400 mcg/day Pregnant female 600 mcg/day	Aids in protein metabolism, promoting red blood cell formation, and lowering the risk for neural tube birth defects	Impaired central nervous system development, anencephaly, spina bifida in pregnancy; anemia, diarrhea, impaired growth	Liver, beans, green leafy vegetables, nuts, fruits
Biotin	Adult male/female 30 mcg/day	Helps release energy from carbohydrates and aids in the metabolism of fats, proteins, and carbohydrates from food	Fatigue, anorexia, nausea, vomiting, muscle pains, depression, anemia	Liver, kidney, egg yolks, milk, fresh vegetables, yeast breads, cereals
Pantothenic acid (vitamin B₅)	Adult male/female 5 mg/day	Involved in energy production, and aids in the formation of hormones and the metabolism of fats, proteins, and carbohydrates from food	Rarely occurs, seen in severe malnutrition	Organ meats, beef, egg yolk, whole grains, legumes

What To Do *After* Giving a Vitamin Supplement

Monitor patients for side effects or adverse effects and report these to the prescriber. A severe allergic reaction with throat swelling and difficulty breathing is an emergency, as described in Chapter 1.

What To Teach Patients Taking Vitamin Supplements

Teach patients about food sources of essential vitamins (see Tables 24-1 and 24-2). Instruct them about the reason vitamins have been prescribed. Tell them about side effects and adverse effects, and explain when to notify the prescriber. Teach patients that too much of any vitamin can lead to toxicity.

Table 24-2 Fat-Soluble Vitamins

VITAMIN NAME	RECOMMENDED DOSE	ACTION	DEFICIENCY	SOURCES
Vitamin A (Retinol)	Adult male: 900 mcg/ day Adult female: 700 mcg/day	Essential for vision, bone growth, reproduction and maintenance of epithelial cells	Night blindness, conjunctival xerosis (abnormal dryness)	Dairy products, fish, liver, carrots, pumpkin, sweet potatoes, spinach, broccoli
Vitamin D (ergocalciferol, cholecalciferol)	Age 1-50: 15 mcg/day Over 50 years: 20 mcg/day	Regulates calcium and phosphorus metabolism	Rickets	Vitamin D enriched milk, fish, sunlight
Vitamin E (alpha-tocopherol)	Over 14 years: 15 mcg/day	Antioxidant protects cell components from oxidation	Poor conduction of electrical impulses along nerves	Vegetable oils, grains, nuts, sunflower seeds, green leafy vegetables
Vitamin K (phytonadione)	Male over 9 years: 60-120 mcg/day Female over 9 years: 60-90 mcg/day	Synthesis of prothrombin and clotting factors	Bleeding, bruising	Green leafy vegetables, vegetable oils

Drug Alert!

Teaching Alert

Teach patients to avoid taking more than one vitamin supplement at a time unless instructed to do so by the prescriber.

QSEN: Safety

Drug Alert!

Teaching Alert

Instruct parents to keep chewable vitamin supplements out of reach for children to prevent vitamin overdose.

QSEN: Safety

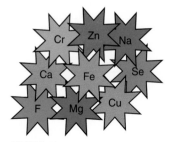

FIGURE 24-2 Essential minerals.

Memory Jogger

The body needs two kinds of minerals: macrominerals and trace minerals.

Tell patients to avoid taking more than one vitamin supplement at the same time unless specifically instructed to do so by the prescriber. Teach patients that vitamin and mineral supplements are not intended to replace a balanced, healthy diet.

Life Span Considerations for Vitamin Supplements

Pediatric Considerations. Children need different vitamin dosages than adults. Be sure to discuss this with the prescriber before giving these drugs to children. Always keep chewable supplements out of reach children because chewable vitamins look like candy, and there is a risk that children may accidentally overdose and have vitamin/mineral toxicities.

Considerations for Pregnancy and Lactation. Vitamin supplements pass into breast milk. Women who plan to breastfeed should discuss this with the prescriber. Vitamin A excess as well as vitamin A deficiency have been associated with birth defects. Excessive doses of vitamin A have been associated with central nervous system malformations.

Considerations for Older Adults. Many older adults do not need vitamin supplements. Most older adults can achieve adequate intake of vitamins through dietary sources but often need extra vitamin D for bone health.

MINERALS

Minerals are inorganic elements (e.g., calcium, iron, potassium, sodium, zinc) that are essential to human nutrition (Figure 24-2). A person's body uses minerals for many purposes, such as building bones, making hormones, and regulating the heartbeat. The two kinds of minerals a person's body needs are macrominerals and trace minerals.

Macrominerals are minerals needed in larger amounts. They include calcium, phosphorus, magnesium, sodium, potassium, chloride, and sulfur. **Trace minerals** are needed in very small amounts. These include iron, manganese, copper, iodine, zinc, cobalt, fluoride, and selenium. The best way to take in adequate minerals is though a healthy diet. However, in some cases a prescriber may order a mineral supplement to correct deficiencies. Often vitamin and mineral supplements are combined in one pill.

How Minerals Work

Minerals are found in soil and water. They easily find their way into a person's body through plants, fish, animals, and fluids that are consumed. Macrominerals travel through the body in a variety of ways. For example, potassium is quickly absorbed into the bloodstream, where it circulates freely and is excreted by the kidneys, similar to a water-soluble vitamin. Calcium is more like a fat-soluble vitamin because it requires a carrier for absorption and transport. Some minerals help to maintain the proper balance of water in the body. Sodium, chloride, and potassium take the lead in doing this. Three macrominerals, calcium, phosphorus, and magnesium, are important for healthy bones. Sulfur helps stabilize protein structures, including those that help make up hair, skin, and nails.

Trace minerals carry out a wide variety of tasks. Some examples include:

- Iron goes into hemoglobin, which carries oxygen throughout the body.
- Fluoride strengthens bones and prevents tooth decay.
- Zinc helps blood clot, is essential for taste and smell, and supports the immune response.
- Copper helps form several enzymes, one of which assists with iron metabolism and the creation of hemoglobin, which carries oxygen in the blood.

Other trace minerals perform equally vital jobs, such as helping to block damage to body cells and forming parts of key enzymes or enhancing their activity.

Commonly Prescribed Mineral Supplements

There are many over-the-counter or prescription mineral supplements available. Most are taken once or twice a day in combination with vitamins. Although the best way to consume adequate minerals is through a healthy diet, a prescriber may order mineral supplements to ensure that a patient has adequate intake or to correct a deficit (e.g., calcium to strengthen bones; iron to correct anemia). Table 24-3 lists minerals needed by the body along with recommended doses, actions, symptoms of deficiencies, and food sources of the minerals.

Intended Responses

- Adequate essential mineral intake
- Avoidance of side effects of deficient mineral intake

Side Effects. When taken as directed minerals are not expected to cause side effects. However, the side effects that may occur include upset stomach, headache, and an unusual or unpleasant taste in the mouth.

Minerals taken in large doses can cause staining of teeth, increased urination, stomach bleeding, irregular heart rate, confusion, and muscle weakness.

Adverse Effects. Adverse effects are rare and may include signs of an allergic reaction such as hives; difficulty breathing; and swelling of the face, lips, tongue, or throat (see Chapter 1).

What To Do *Before* Giving a Mineral Supplement

Ask patients about use of over-the-counter mineral supplements. Question patients about previous side effects or adverse reactions to mineral supplements. Check patients' medical histories for anemia, liver problems, or metabolic problems.

If patients experience upset stomach, supplements can be given with food to avoid this side effect.

What To Do *After* Giving a Mineral Supplement

Monitor patients for side effects or adverse effects from the supplement and notify the prescriber if these occur.

What To Teach Patients Taking Mineral Supplements

Remind patients to avoid salt substitutes if the mineral supplement includes potassium. If the patient is ordered a low-salt diet, instruct them to talk with the prescriber before taking over-the-counter mineral supplements.

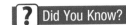

Did You Know?

The minerals iron and copper are essential in the formation of hemoglobin, which carries oxygen in the blood.

Common Side Effects

Mineral Supplements

Upset stomach   Headache   Unpleasant taste

Drug Alert!

Teaching Alert

Teach patients to avoid salt substitutes if they are receiving mineral supplementation with potassium.

QSEN: Safety

Table **24-3**   Minerals

MINERAL	RECOMMENDED DOSE	ACTION	DEFICIENCY	SOURCES
Calcium	1000 mg/day	Important for healthy bones and teeth; helps muscles relax and contract; important in nerve functioning, blood clotting, blood pressure regulation, immune system health	Decreased bone density (osteopenia), osteoporosis	Milk and milk products; canned fish with bones (salmon, sardines); fortified tofu and fortified soy milk; greens (broccoli, mustard greens); legumes
Chloride	3400 mg/day	Needed for proper fluid balance, stomach acid	Decreased chloride: loss of appetite, muscle weakness, lethargy, dehydration, alkalosis	Table salt, soy sauce; large amounts in processed foods; small amounts in milk, meats, breads, and vegetables
Chromium	120 mcg/day	Works closely with insulin to regulate blood sugar (glucose) levels	Decreased chromium level: development of diabetes and metabolic syndrome; anxiety, fatigue	Unrefined foods, especially liver, brewer's yeast, whole grains, nuts, cheeses
Cobalt	No specific RDA Average intake: 5-8 mcg/day	Essential to red blood cell formation and is also helpful to other cells	Low cobalt level: related to vitamin B_{12} deficiency; can cause pernicious anemia	Meat, organ meats, oysters, clams, milk, ocean fish
Copper	2 mg/day	Part of many enzymes; needed for iron metabolism	Copper deficiency may cause neutropenia, impaired bone calcification, myelopathy, neuropathy, and hypochromic anemia not responsive to iron supplements	Legumes, nuts and seeds, whole grains, organ meats, drinking water
Fluoride	3.5 mg/day	Involved in formation of bones and teeth; helps prevent tooth decay	Fluoride deficiency can lead to dental cavities as well as weal bones and teeth	Drinking water (either fluoridated or naturally containing fluoride), fish, and most teas
Iodine	150 mcg/day	Found in thyroid hormone, which helps regulate growth, development, and metabolism	Iodine deficiency: goiter (a swollen thyroid gland) and reduced production of thyroid hormones; severe deficiency early in life may cause a form of mental and physical retardation called cretinism	Seafood, foods grown in iodine-rich soil, iodized salt, bread, dairy products
Iron	15 mg/day	Part of a molecule (hemoglobin) found in red blood cells that carries oxygen in the body; needed for energy metabolism	Iron deficiency anemia	Organ meats, red meats; fish; poultry; shellfish (especially clams); egg yolks; legumes; dried fruits; dark, leafy greens; iron-enriched breads and cereals; and fortified cereals

Table 24-3 | Minerals—cont'd

MINERAL	RECOMMENDED DOSE	ACTION	DEFICIENCY	SOURCES
Magnesium	350 mg/day	Found in bones; needed for making protein, muscle contraction, nerve transmission, immune system health	Early signs: fatigue, weakness, loss of appetite, nausea, and vomiting. Left untreated: numbness, tingling, muscle cramps, seizures, or abnormal rhythms of the heart	Nuts and seeds, legumes, leafy green vegetables, seafood, chocolate, artichokes, "hard" drinking water
Phosphorus	1000 mg/day	Important for healthy bones and teeth; found in every cell; part of the system that maintains acid-base balance	Phosphorus deficiency can lead to weak teeth and bones, joint pain and stiffness, decreased energy, and decreased appetite	Meat, fish, poultry, eggs, milk, processed foods (including sodas)
Potassium	3500 mg/day	Needed for proper fluid balance, nerve transmission, and muscle contraction	Symptoms of potassium deficiency: muscle cramping and weakness, and constipation, bloating, or abdominal pain caused by paralysis of the intestines; severe potassium deficiency: paralysis of the muscles or irregular heart rhythms that may lead to death	Meats, milk, fresh fruits and vegetables, whole grains, legumes
Selenium	35 mcg/day	Antioxidant	Muscle pain; weakness	Meats, seafood, grains
Sodium	2400 mg/day	Needed for proper fluid balance, nerve transmission, and muscle contraction	Low blood serum sodium: headache, nausea, vomiting, muscle cramps, fatigue, disorientation, and fainting	Table salt, soy sauce; large amounts in processed foods; small amounts in milk, breads, vegetables, and unprocessed meats
Sulfur	No specific RDA Average intake: 800-900 mg/day	Found in protein molecules	Sulfur deficiency may contribute to obesity, Alzheimer's disease, heart disease, and chronic fatigue	Occurs in foods as part of protein: meats, poultry, fish, eggs, milk, legumes, nuts
Zinc	15 mg/day	Part of many enzymes; needed for making protein and genetic material; has a function in taste perception, wound healing, normal fetal development, production of sperm, normal growth and sexual maturation, immune system health	Zinc deficiency: loss of appetite, decreased function of the immune system. and slowed growth. Severe deficiency: diarrhea, loss of hair, impotence, and slow healing of wounds	Meats, fish, poultry, leavened whole grains, vegetables

RDA, Recommended dietary allowance.

Drug Alert!

Teaching Alert

Tell patients that side effects from mineral supplements are usually temporary and resolve when the body becomes accustomed to the supplement.

QSEN: Safety

Drug Alert!

Teaching Alert

Teach patients that iron supplements can cause stools to appear black.

QSEN: Safety

Memory Jogger

Older adults often are prescribed calcium supplements for bone health and to prevent osteoporosis.

Memory Jogger

Enteral nutrition is the preferred route for supplementation as long as the GI tract is working.

Teach patients the signs of allergic reaction (e.g., hives, difficulty breathing, or swelling of the face) and to call for help immediately when this occurs.

Instruct patients to avoid taking mineral supplements after taking antacids, which may interfere with absorption. Tell them to take the supplement with food if upset stomach occurs. Teach patients that side effects are usually temporary and resolve as the body becomes accustomed to the supplement. Remind patients that iron supplements can cause stool to appear black, but this is not harmful.

Life Span Considerations for Mineral Supplements

Pediatric Considerations. Mineral and vitamin supplements for children are usually in liquid or chewable form. Chewable supplements should be chewed and swallowed. Keep chewable supplement bottles out of reach of children to avoid overdose.

Considerations for Pregnancy and Lactation. Mineral and vitamin supplements pass into breast milk. Women who plan to breastfeed should discuss this with the prescriber.

Considerations for Older Adults. Older adults experience changes in lifestyle and appetite. Decreased appetite or reduced ability to buy and prepare healthy foods can lead to older people not getting enough essential vitamins or minerals. Supplements are often ordered by prescribers to make up for these deficits. Older adults often need additional calcium for bone health and to prevent osteoporosis.

TYPES OF NUTRITIONAL SUPPLEMENTS

When patients are unable to take in adequate nutrition, they may need nutritional supplements. Supplements may be provided by way of the gastrointestinal (GI) tract if it is functional (enteral nutrition) or parenterally (intravenous formula) with total parenteral nutrition (TPN).

TPN provides all of a patient's daily nutritional needs. A peripheral intravenous (IV) line can be used for a short period with a less concentrated formula. When nutritional support is needed for a long period of time, concentrated solutions are used and require central venous access (e.g., peripherally inserted central catheter [PICC line]; triple lumen catheter [TLC]). TPN formulas are individualized and prepared by pharmacists according to patient needs. This form of nutrition is given in the hospital and at home. In many cases TPN allows people who have lost small intestine function to lead fairly normal lives.

ENTERAL NUTRITIONAL SUPPLEMENTS

Enteral feedings are preferred as long as the GI tract is working. **Enteral nutritional supplements** are often given through a tube directly into the stomach or more commonly into the small intestine. Enteral feedings can be provided in the hospital, long-term care facility, or home. Some reasons for this type of nutrition include cancer, neurological or GI problems, and traumatic injury to the GI tract. Feeding tubes may be passed through the nose (e.g., nasogastric or nasojejunal tubes) (Figure 24-3, *A*) or through the skin on the abdomen (e.g., gastrostomy, jejunostomy, percutaneous endoscopic gastrostomy [PEG] tubes) (Figure 24-3, *B*).

How Enteral Nutritional Supplements Work

When a patient with a working GI tract is unable to take in enough nutrition to meet the body's needs, nutritional supplements given orally or through a feeding tube can be prescribed to make up the deficits. Examples of when enteral nutrition may be needed include prolonged anorexia, inadequate protein intake, coma or decreased sensorium, head or neck trauma, and critical illnesses such as burns. A

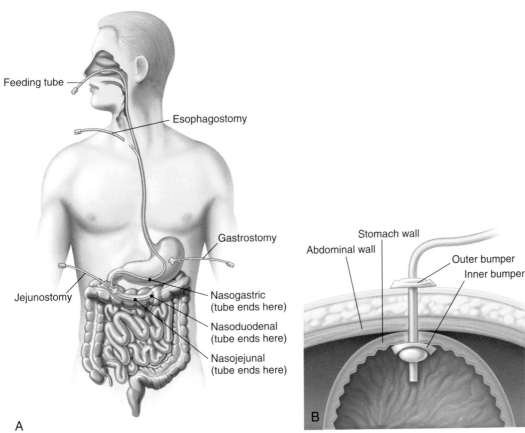

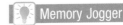

FIGURE 24-3   Feeding tubes and routes of access. **A,** Nasogastric and surgically placed feeding tubes. **B,** Percutaneous endoscopic gastrostomy tube. (From Harkreader, H. (2007). *Fundamentals of nursing: caring and clinical judgment* (3rd ed.). St. Louis: Saunders.)

nutritional formula is prescribed and administered to meet the nutritional needs of the patient.

Commonly Prescribed Enteral Nutritional Supplements

There are more than 100 varieties of enteral feeding formulas available. Enteral formulas include those for renal failure, GI disease, hyperglycemia/diabetes, liver failure, acute and chronic pulmonary disease, and immunocompromised states. There are three classifications of enteral formulas: standard, elemental, and specialized.

Standard enteral formulas are defined as those with intact protein containing balanced amounts of macronutrients that will often meet a patient's nutrient requirements at much lower cost than specialized formulas (e.g., Osmolite, Jevity, Isocal, Nutren). *Elemental* formulas are often predigested formulas for patients with limited GI function (e.g., Optimental, Peptamen, Vivonex). *Specialized* formulas are designed for supplement in a variety of clinical conditions or disease states. Examples of specialized formulas are listed in Table 24-4. Both elemental and specialized formulas are much more expensive compared with standard formulas.

Intended Responses
- Nutritional requirements are met.
- Functional GI tract is maintained.
- Side effects of nutritional deficits are avoided.

Side Effects. Diarrhea is the main side effect of enteral nutritional supplemental feedings. Other GI side effects may include constipation, nausea, and vomiting. Often these side effects disappear once a patient's body adjusts to the nutritional supplement.

> **Memory Jogger**
>
> The three classes of enteral nutritional formulas are standard, elemental, and specialized.

> **Common Side Effects**
> **Enteral Nutritional Supplements**
>
>
>
> Diarrhea, Constipation, Nausea, Vomiting

Table 24-4	Examples of Specialized Formulas
FORMULA	**CLINICAL CONDITION/DISEASE STATE**
Choice DM, Glucerna Select, Glytrol	Diabetes mellitus
Hepatic Aid II, NutriHep	Hepatic (liver) disease
Nutri-renal, Nepro, Magnacal Renal	Renal (kidney) disease
Nutri-vent, Pulmocare, Respalor	Chronic obstructive pulmonary disease (COPD)

Adverse Effects. Prolonged, severe diarrhea can lead to fluid and electrolyte imbalances. An adverse effect of enteral nutritional supplements administered by a feeding tube is the risk for aspiration and aspiration pneumonia.

What To Do *Before* Giving an Enteral Nutritional Supplement

Tell the patient what to expect. If a special tube is necessary, explain why and tell the patient about the insertion procedure. Nasogastric (NG) and nasojejunal (NJ) tubes can be placed at the bedside but cannot be used until correct placement is confirmed by an x-ray. Tubes placed through the skin require that the patient be prepared for a surgical procedure to insert them.

When a patient has a tube for administration of an enteral nutritional supplement, always check the tube for patency and placement before administering. Refer to fundamentals textbooks and facility procedures for guidelines. Always elevate the head of the bed 30 to 45 degrees to prevent aspiration.

Review patient nutrition related laboratory values (e.g., electrolytes, albumin, prealbumin). Continue to record intake and output for each patient.

Make sure that appropriate equipment is at the patient's bedside (e.g., feeding pump, tubing, container, correct nutritional supplement). Most patient care units stress that only 4 hours of the supplement is hung at a time to prevent bacterial overgrowth at room temperature. Check the prescriber's orders for flow rate.

Get and record a baseline weight and height for the patient. Assess for gag reflex.

What To Do *After* Giving an Enteral Nutritional Supplement

Keep track of intake and output. When a supplement is administered intermittently, be sure to flush the tubing after each dose so that the tube does not become clogged. Refer to a fundamentals textbook or facility policies for guidelines. Continue to monitor gag reflex and to follow safety measures to prevent aspiration of supplements (e.g., elevation of head of bed, assessment of adequate gag reflex).

Continue to monitor laboratory values. Assess for side effects, especially diarrhea. Change administration containers and tubing according to facility policies. Most facilities instruct changes every 24 hours. Be sure to check for residual feeding and notify the prescriber.

Check weights for patients on a daily basis. Remember to use the same scale, same time, and same amount of clothing each day. Assess bowel habits and record bowel movements. Report constipation to the prescriber.

Check precautions for the patient's other drugs. Some drugs require that enteral feeding be held for a period before and after administration (e.g., phenytoin). Place feedings on hold when performing procedures or patient care that requires lowering the head of the bed, to protect against aspiration.

What To Teach Patients Taking Enteral Nutritional Supplements

Teach patients and families about the specific nutritional supplement prescribed.

If the patient is to be discharged with a special feeding tube, teach the patient and his or her family how to care for the tube including how to check placement, flush, change tubing, and care for the feeding pump. Instruct patients and families about

---

! Drug Alert!

Intervention Alert

Before giving an enteral nutritional supplement through a feeding tube, always check for placement and residual volume. Also elevate the head of the bed to protect the patient from aspiration of the formula.

QSEN: Safety

! Drug Alert!

Intervention Alert

After giving an intermittent enteral supplement flush the tube to prevent clogging.

QSEN: Safety

! Drug Alert!

Intervention Alert

Change enteral feeding containers and tubing every 24 hours to prevent organism growth and infection.

QSEN: Safety

the importance of flushing the tube after intermittent feedings to prevent clogging of the tube. Tell them how to clean and protect skin around the tube.

Remind patients and families to notify the prescriber if diarrhea occurs, especially if it is severe, because of the risk for fluid and electrolyte imbalances. Show them how to provide skin care to prevent skin breakdown. For continuous administration of a nutritional supplement, remind patients and family members to hang only 4 hours volume of the supplement. Teach them that with supplements hung for longer than 4 hours, there is an increased risk of growth of infectious organisms. Remind patients and family members to keep the patient's head elevated during and after giving the supplement.

Life Span Considerations for Enteral Nutritional Supplements

Pediatric Considerations. Enteral nutritional supplements may be prescribed for children who are unable to or unwilling to take in enough nutrients for normal growth and development. These children are often diagnosed with malnutrition or failure to thrive.

Considerations for Pregnancy and Lactation. Enteral nutrition is considered during pregnancy when a woman experiences persistent nausea and vomiting along with weight loss that does not respond to treatment with diet changes or antiemetic drugs. A small-bore feeding tube may be placed and a supplement prescribed to meet the needs of mother and fetus.

Considerations for Older Adults. Older adults are at increased risk for inadequate nutrition due to aging changes, loss of appetite, decreased sensation, problems with chewing and swallowing, chronic diseases, and multiple prescribed drugs.

Drug Alert!

Teaching Alert

Teach patients (and families) who will be going home on continuous enteral nutritional supplements to hang only 4 hours of formula to prevent organism growth and infection.

QSEN: Safety

Get Ready for Practice!

Key Points

- Vitamins and minerals are essential for normal growth and development.
- Vitamins and minerals perform essential body functions every day.
- Human bodies need two types of vitamins: water soluble and fat soluble.
- Water-soluble vitamins must be taken in daily.
- Fat-soluble vitamins can be stored in the body.
- The best way to take in adequate vitamins and minerals is through a healthy diet.
- Prescribers may order vitamin and mineral supplements to correct deficiencies.
- The body needs two kinds of minerals: macrominerals and trace minerals.
- Taking in excess vitamins or minerals can cause toxicities.
- Enteral nutrition is prescribed when a person cannot or will not take in adequate nutrition.
- Enteral nutrition is preferred as long as the GI tract is functioning.
- There are three types of enteral formulas: standard, elemental, and specialized.
- Enteral formulas are often administered through a feeding tube that is placed in the stomach or small intestine.
- The major side effect of enteral nutritional supplements is diarrhea.

- Monitor patients receiving enteral nutrition for fluid or electrolyte imbalances.
- Protect patients receiving enteral nutrition from aspiration.

Additional Learning Resources

evolve Be sure to visit your Evolve website (http://evolve.elsevier.com/Workman/pharmacology/) for additional online resources.

SG Go to your Study Guide for additional learning activities to help you master this chapter content.

Review Questions

See the Answer Keys—In-text Review Questions for answers to these questions.

Test Yourself on the Basics
1. Which vitamin supplement can prevent some types of blindness?
   A. Vitamin A
   B. Vitamin B
   C. Vitamin D
   D. Vitamin K

2. What is the most common side effect of enteral feeding supplements?
   A. Muscle aches
   B. Constipation
   C. Diarrhea
   D. Nausea
3. What must be done before beginning the first enteral supplementation through a feeding tube?
   A. Check for residual.
   B. Inject air while listening with a stethoscope.
   C. Flush the tube to prevent clogging.
   D. Get an x-ray to check placement.
4. Which teaching point about vitamin and mineral supplements is accurate?
   A. Do not take more than one supplement unless instructed to do so by the prescriber.
   B. Vitamin and mineral supplements are always given in separate pills.
   C. Children often need additional calcium supplements to grow strong bones.
   D. Fat-soluble vitamins must be taken every day.
5. What precaution must be taken for children who are prescribed chewable vitamin and mineral supplements?
   A. Give the supplement in the evening before bedtime.
   B. Keep the supplements out of the reach of children.
   C. Teach parents to administer two supplements when the child is ill.
   D. If the child will not take the supplement, tell him or her that it is candy.

Test Yourself on Advanced Concepts
6. Which vitamins and minerals are essential for bone health? (Select all that apply.)
   A. Calcium
   B. Vitamin K
   C. Phosphorus
   D. Vitamin D
   E. Folic acid
   F. Potassium
7. The patient is receiving an enteral nutritional supplement. For which major side effect should you monitor?
   A. Upset stomach
   B. Constipation
   C. Diarrhea
   D. Unpleasant taste

8. What priority action must be taken after a patient is administered an intermittent enteral nutritional supplement through a feeding tube?
   A. Check the patient's gag reflex.
   B. Assess the feeding tube for correct placement.
   C. Double check the feeding rate with another nurse.
   D. Flush the feeding tube to prevent clogging.
9. Which important teaching point will be included when teaching a patient about iron supplements?
   A. This mineral may cause stools to appear black.
   B. This mineral is essential for strong teeth.
   C. This mineral is found mostly in dairy products.
   D. This mineral should always be taken on an empty stomach.
10. Which vitamin must you caution a woman who plans to become pregnant to avoid taking in excess?
    A. Vitamin E
    B. Vitamin C
    C. Vitamin B
    D. Vitamin A
11. The patient receiving an enteral nutritional supplement has 500 mL hanging to infuse over 4 hours. At how many mL/hr should the feeding pump be set? ____mL/hr

Critical Thinking Activities

See the Answer Keys—Critical Thinking Activities for answers to these activities.

Ms. Day is a 58-year-old who weighs 112 pounds and is 5 feet 6 inches tall. Her health history includes type 1 diabetes since she was a child, advanced MS (multiple sclerosis), and a 6 × 5 cm stage III pressure ulcer on her left hip. She is from a long-term care facility, where she is confined to bed, uses adult diapers, and has a percutaneous endoscopic gastrostomy (PEG) feeding tube in place. The patient's daughter tells you that she is incontinent of both urine and stool.
1. What type of feeding would be of most benefit for Ms. Day and why?
2. What type of tube feeding should you expect the prescriber to order?
3. For which main side effect of liquid nutritional supplements should you monitor? Why?

chapter

25

Drug Therapy for Seizures

http://evolve.elsevier.com/Workman/pharmacology/

Objectives

After studying this chapter you should be able to:

1. Explain how different classes of drugs are used to treat seizures.
2. List the common names, actions, usual adult dosages, possible side effects, and adverse effects of drugs for seizures.
3. Describe what to do before and after giving drugs for seizures.
4. Explain what to teach patients taking drugs for seizures, including what to do, what not to do, and when to call the prescriber.
5. Describe life span considerations for drugs for seizures.

Key Terms

aura (ŌR-ă) (p. 402) Strange sensations such as tingling, smell, or emotional changes that occur before a seizure.

epilepsy (ĔP-ĭl-ĕp-sē) (p. 401) A disorder of the brain that causes recurrent, unprovoked seizures.

first-line drugs for seizures (p. 406) The exact action of first-line drugs for partial or generalized seizures is not known, but these drugs causes a decrease in the voltage, frequency, and spread of electrical impulses within the motor cortex of the brain, which leads to decreased seizure activity.

generalized seizure (JĔN-ŭr-ăl-īzd SĒ-zhŭr) (p. 404) A seizure that involves the entire brain; caused by electrical discharges originating from both sides of the brain.

partial seizure (PĂR-shŭl SĒ-zhŭr) (p. 404) A seizure that starts in one part of the brain. The abnormal electrical activity may remain confined to one area or spread to the entire brain; also called a focal or local seizure.

postictal phase (pōst-ĬK-tŭl FĀZ) (p. 402) "After the seizure" phase often characterized by confusion, headache, sore muscles, and fatigue.

second-line drugs for seizures (p. 410) Alternative drugs used for treatment of seizures.

seizure (SĒ-zhŭr) (p. 401) Uncontrolled electrical activity in the brain that may produce a physical convulsion, minor physical signs, thought disturbances, or a combination of symptoms.

seizure disorder (SĒ-zhŭr dĭs-ŌR-dŭr) (p. 401) A pathologic condition resulting in a sudden episode of uncontrolled electrical activity in the brain.

status epilepticus (STĂT-ŭs ĕp-ĭl-LĔP-tĭ-kŭs) (p. 404) A prolonged seizure (usually defined as lasting longer than 30 minutes) or a series of repeated seizures; a continuous state of seizure activity that may occur in almost any seizure type.

OVERVIEW

A **seizure** results from excessive or disordered electrical activity in the brain. A person with repeated seizures has a **seizure disorder**, sometimes called **epilepsy**. About 2 million people in the United States have this brain disorder, and 10% of Americans will experience a seizure sometime during their lives. Most of them (60%) never experience another seizure. Although seizures may begin at any age, most begin during early childhood or late adulthood. Seizures are frightening and can range from minor to life threatening.

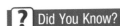
? Did You Know?

Although 10% of Americans experience a seizure at some time during their lives, about 60% of these people never experience another seizure.

REVIEW OF RELATED PHYSIOLOGY AND PATHOPHYSIOLOGY

When the brain is working normally, electrical impulses are orderly and organized. These impulses help the brain communicate with the spinal cord, nerves, muscles, and other parts of the brain. Abnormal electrical impulses can lead to seizures

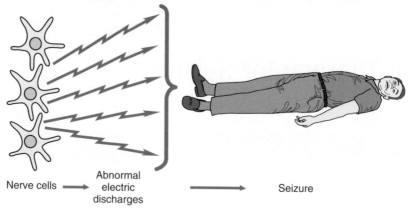

FIGURE 25-1 The cause of seizures.

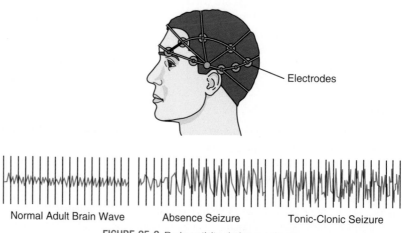

FIGURE 25-2 Brain activity during a seizure.

(Figure 25-1). Often seizures occur when nerve cells fire in a more rapid and less controlled manner (Figure 25-2). Seizures can affect movements, senses, concentration, communication, and level of consciousness. After a seizure, most people experience confusion for a period of time.

CAUSES OF SEIZURES

Although certain factors are known to cause seizures (Table 25-1), for the most part their cause is unknown. Several risk factors increase the possibility of seizures (Box 25-1). For adults the most common causes include head injury, stroke, and tumor. Certain drugs may lead to seizures (Box 25-2). For children, the most common causes include fever, head injury, central nervous system infection, hypoxia, and electrolyte imbalances.

Stimuli that cause irritation to the brain such as injury, drugs, lack of sleep, infections, and low levels of oxygen may cause a seizure in anyone. However, when a person has a seizure disorder, seizures are more likely to occur during periods of increased emotional or physical stress. Risk factors associated with worsening of a well-controlled seizure disorder include pregnancy and lack of sleep (Box 25-3).

TYPES OF SEIZURES

Signs and symptoms of a seizure may vary widely, ranging from staring off into space to loss of consciousness and violent jerky movements. The type of seizure experienced depends on the part of the brain that is affected, the cause of the seizure, and the person's response. Some people experience an **aura**, a strange sensation (for example, smell, visual, sound, or taste) that occurs before each seizure. Commonly a seizure consists of an aura followed by the seizure and then a **postictal phase**

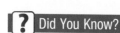

Did You Know?

The cause of most seizures is unknown.

Monitoring Alert

A person who has seizures is more likely to have a seizure during times of increased emotional or physical stress.

QSEN: Safety

Table 25-1 Common Causes of Seizures

CAUSE	CHARACTERISTICS
Brain injury	Any age—mostly young adults Damage to brain membranes Seizures begin within 2 years of injury
Degenerative disorders (for example, dementias)	Mostly affect older adults
Developmental/genetic	Condition present at birth Injury near birth; hypoxia at birth Seizures begin during infancy or early childhood
Disorders affecting blood vessels (stroke, transient ischemic attacks)	Most common cause of seizures after age 60
Idiopathic (no known cause)	Usually begin between ages 5 and 20 Can occur at any age No other neurologic abnormalities present Family history of seizures present
Infections (for example, meningitis, encephalitis, brain abscess, immune disorders)	Affect any age Reversible cause of seizures May be caused by acute severe infection in any part of the body Sometimes related to chronic infections
Metabolic abnormalities	Affect any age Diabetic complications Electrolyte abnormalities Kidney failure Nutritional deficiencies Phenylketonuria—causes seizures during infancy Metabolic diseases Use of cocaine, amphetamines, alcohol, other illicit drugs Alcohol or drug withdrawal
Tumors	Affect any age—most likely after age 30 Partial (focal) seizures more common May progress to generalized seizures

---

Box 25-1 Risk Factors for Seizures

- Brain infections
- Drugs (see Box 25-2)
- Drug withdrawal
- Emotional stress
- Family history
- Fevers
- Head injury
- Hormone changes
- Hyperventilation
- Lack of food
- Metabolic disorders
- Sensory stimuli (for example, flashing lights)
- Sleep deprivation
- Tumors

Box 25-2 Common Seizure-Causing Drugs

- Antidepressants
- Bupropion alcohol
- Cocaine and other street drugs
- Excessive doses of antiseizure drugs
- Oral contraceptives
- Phenothiazines
- Theophylline

Box 25-3 Risk Factors for Worsening of Seizures with a Well-Controlled Seizure Disorder

- Illness
- Lack of sleep
- Pregnancy
- Prescribed drugs (see Box 25-2)
- Skipping doses of antiseizure drugs
- Use of alcohol or street drugs

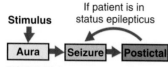

FIGURE 25-3 Typical seizure. During status epilepticus the patient experiences a state of continuous seizure.

 Memory Jogger

Before a seizure, a strange sensation called an aura may occur. After a seizure, a period of confusion, lethargy, and decreased responsiveness (postictal phase) usually occurs.

 Memory Jogger

The two major groups of seizures are generalized and partial seizures.

 Memory Jogger

The six types of generalized seizures are tonic-clonic, tonic, clonic, absence, myoclonic, and atonic.

 Memory Jogger

The two major types of partial seizures are simple and complex.

 Clinical Pitfall

Without rapid recognition and treatment, status epilepticus can result in brain damage, coma, and death.

QSEN: Safety

usually characterized by confusion, lethargy, and decreased responsiveness (Figure 25-3). Most seizures are brief, lasting a few seconds to a few minutes. Status epilepticus is a life-threatening, continuous state of seizure that lasts from 5 to 30 minutes or is a series of repeated seizures without recovery (postictal period). The risk of status epilepticus increases when a seizure is prolonged or when a series of seizures occur.

Seizures are divided into two groups, generalized seizures and partial seizures.

Generalized Seizures
Generalized seizures affect most or all of the brain. There are six types of generalized seizures (Table 25-2).

Tonic-clonic seizures (also known as grand mal seizures) last 2 to 5 minutes, with stiffening or rigidity of the arm and leg muscles and immediate loss of consciousness. Spasm of the respiratory muscles can cause forced exhalation, sounding like a scream, called the *epileptic cry*. *Clonic seizures* are characterized by muscle contraction and relaxation. Patients may bite their tongues or become incontinent. *Tonic seizures* include sudden increase in muscle tone; loss of consciousness; and autonomic signs such as rapid heart rate, sweating, pupil dilation, flushing, and loss of bowel function and bladder control for 30 seconds to several minutes. After the seizure, patients are often tired, confused, or lethargic for an hour or more.

Absence seizures (also known as petit mal seizures) are more common in children and tend to occur in families. They are brief (a few seconds) with loss of consciousness and blank staring (a child may appear to be daydreaming). After the seizure, the child returns to normal immediately.

A *myoclonic seizure* involves brief jerking or stiffening of the extremities that lasts a few seconds. It may involve one or more extremities, and the jerking contractions may be asymmetric (stronger on one side of the body) or symmetric (the same on both sides of the body). With an *atonic seizure* typically there is sudden loss of muscle tone for a few seconds, followed by postictal (after the seizure) confusion.

Partial Seizures
Partial seizures are also called focal or local seizures. The two major types of partial seizures are simple and complex (Table 25-3). With a *simple partial seizure,* the patient remains conscious. Before the seizure a patient may report an aura. During the seizure, the patient remains conscious. One-sided movement of an extremity, unusual sensations, or autonomic changes (e.g., heart rate, flushing, epigastric discomfort) may occur. *Complex partial seizures* cause patients to lose consciousness for 1 to 3 minutes. During a complex partial seizure, patients may have *automatisms* (automatic, unconscious actions) such as lip smacking, patting, or picking at clothes. Often they experience amnesia during the period after a seizure.

Status epilepticus is a prolonged seizure (usually defined as lasting longer than 30 minutes) or a series of repeated seizures that may occur in almost any type of seizure. Rapid recognition and treatment of this disorder are essential to prevent brain damage. Actions for treating this life-threatening condition include protecting the airway, providing oxygen, establishing intravenous (IV) access to give 5 to 10 mg of diazepam (Valium) by slow IV injection, and determining and treating the cause.

Table 25-2 Types of Generalized Seizures

TYPE	SYMPTOMS
Tonic-clonic (grand mal)	Convulsions, muscle rigidity, unconsciousness
Tonic	Muscle stiffness, rigidity
Atonic	Loss of muscle tone
Absence (petit mal)	Brief loss of consciousness
Myoclonic	Sporadic (isolated) jerking movements
Clonic	Repetitive jerking movements

Table 25-3	Types of Partial Seizures
TYPE	**SYMPTOMS**
Simple	
Simple partial motor	Head-turning, jerking, muscle rigidity, spasms,
Simple partial sensory	Unusual sensations affecting either vision, hearing, smell, taste, or touch
Simple partial psychologic	Memory or emotional disturbance
Complex	Automatisms (for example, chewing, fidgeting, lip smacking, walking and other repetitive involuntary but coordinated movements)
Partial with secondary generalization	Symptoms that are initially associated with a preservation of consciousness, which then evolves into a loss of consciousness and convulsions

  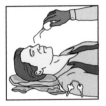 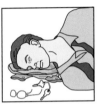

Help the person to the floor and cushion the head | Loosen any clothing around the neck | Remove any sharp objects | Turn the person on one side

FIGURE 25-4 What to do if you witness a generalized or complex partial seizure.

TREATMENT OF SEIZURES

Controlling and preventing seizure activity are important for many reasons. During a seizure, the patient has no control over motor activities, which can lead to accidents when the person is driving a car or handling heavy or dangerous equipment. Falls are common during a seizure. So the patient having a seizure is at risk for trauma and loss of motor control and could endanger other people. In addition, the confusion and incontinence (common during or after a seizure) reduce a person's productivity and are embarrassing.

Although antiseizure drugs are a major part of treating and controlling seizures, other important components include precautions such as keeping the airway open, placing a saline lock to give IV drugs, raising side rails, and keeping the bed in its lowest position.

The actions taken during a seizure should be correct for the type of seizure. For example, for a simple partial seizure, watch the patient and document the time the seizure occurred and how long it lasted. For a generalized or complex partial seizure, remove anything that could cause injury to the patient and turn him or her to one side to prevent aspiration and let secretions drain (Figure 25-4).

TYPES OF ANTISEIZURE DRUGS

Antiseizure drugs are a major part of the management and control of seizures. These drugs are started one at a time. If a prescribed drug does not work, either the dose may be increased, or another drug may be tried. Sometimes it takes more than one drug to control a patient's seizure disorder. Use of these drugs involves a balance between keeping a therapeutic level of the drug in the blood and avoiding important side effects. Drugs include first-line and second-line medications. Drugs must be taken on time to maintain the blood level and control seizures.

The best outcome for seizure drug therapy is the control and elimination of seizures. The choice of drugs prescribed is based on the type of seizure. Certain drugs

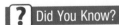 **Did You Know?**

The use of padded side rails is controversial because it is not known whether they help maintain safety, and they may cause the patient and family to feel embarrassed.

Did You Know?

Often more than one drug is needed to control seizures.

are used as first line, or first choice, for each type of seizure, whereas other drugs are considered alternatives, or second line.

GENERAL ISSUES RELATED TO DRUG THERAPY FOR SEIZURES

Antiseizure drugs include first-line and second-line medications. Responsibilities for common actions and effects are listed in the following paragraphs. Specific responsibilities are listed in the discussions of each group of antiseizure drugs.

Before giving any antiseizure drug, always get a complete list of drugs that the patient is taking, including over-the-counter and herbal preparations. Antiseizure drugs, especially phenytoin, interact with many other drugs. For example, the effects of anticoagulants may be increased, putting the patient at greater risk for bleeding.

Check baseline vital signs, level of consciousness, and gait. Ask a patient to describe the nature of his or her seizures. Find out whether an aura occurs before each seizure. If an aura occurs, ask the patient to describe it. Instruct patients to notify the health care providers if they sense that a seizure may occur.

To reduce the risk of injury during a seizure, be sure the patient's bed is in the lowest position and the side rails are raised. Ensure that the call light is within easy reach.

Ask female patients of childbearing age if they are pregnant, planning to become pregnant, or breastfeeding.

After giving any antiseizure drug, recheck the patient's level of consciousness. Check his or her vital signs. Because these drugs can cause dizziness or drowsiness, remind the patient to call for help when getting out of bed and make sure that the call light is within easy reach.

Monitor the patient for seizure activity and be prepared to manage a seizure if one occurs (for example, protect the airway and protect the patient from injury; see Figure 25-4).

Teach patients receiving any antiseizure drug about the importance of keeping follow-up appointments with the prescriber to monitor control of the seizures and having periodic laboratory tests done to monitor blood levels of these drugs

Instruct patients to take the drug exactly as prescribed and explain that suddenly stopping an antiseizure drug may cause seizures to occur. Remind them to take a missed dose as soon as possible but not to take a double dose. Teach about symptoms to report immediately to their prescriber. Tell them to ask their prescriber before taking any over-the-counter drugs.

Because these drugs can cause dizziness or drowsiness, caution patients to avoid driving, operating machinery, or doing anything that requires mental alertness. Instruct them to get out of bed slowly. Tell them to avoid alcohol while taking these drugs because it can cause increased drowsiness or dizziness.

Suggest that patients wear a medical alert bracelet and carry an identification card with them that states their diagnosis, prescribed drugs, and their prescriber's name.

Instruct patients to take these drugs with food if gastrointestinal (GI) symptoms occur and to drink plenty of water. Remind patients taking any antiseizure drug to avoid grapefruit and grapefruit juice because they increase the action of the drug and can lead to more side effects or adverse effects.

If a patient is to have surgery of any kind, including dental surgery, teach him or her that the surgeon or dentist should be notified about the use of these drugs because of the increased risk for bleeding.

FIRST-LINE DRUGS FOR PARTIAL AND GENERALIZED SEIZURES

How Drugs for Partial and Generalized Seizures Work

The exact action of **first-line drugs for seizures** (generalized or partial) is not known, but they act on the brain and nervous system. Use of these drugs causes a decrease in the voltage, frequency, and spread of electrical impulses within the motor cortex of the brain, which leads to decreased seizure activity.

Commonly prescribed first-line drugs for partial or generalized seizures include carbamazepine (Tegretol), valproic acid (Depakote, Depacon), and phenytoin

Drug Alert!

Action/Intervention Alert

Drugs for partial and generalized seizures can increase the effects of anticoagulant drugs. Watch for abnormal bleeding.

QSEN: Safety

Clinical Pitfall

Because drugs for partial and generalized seizures can cause dizziness and drowsiness, a patient should not get out of bed without assistance until the effects of the drug are known.

QSEN: Safety

Clinical Pitfall

Patients taking drugs to prevent generalized or partial seizures should not drink alcohol because it can increase the side effects of dizziness or drowsiness.

QSEN: Safety

Drug Alert!

Teaching Alert

While prescribed and taking any antiseizure drug, patients should be taught to avoid grapefruit and grapefruit juice because they may increase the effects of these drugs.

QSEN: Safety

(Dilantin). The action of valproic acid may be related to increased availability of the neurotransmitter gamma-aminobutyric acid (GABA). Carbamazepine decreases impulse transmission by affecting sodium channels in neurons. Phenytoin (Dilantin) changes ion transport, but the exact action is not known.

Generic names, brand names, and common dosages of these drugs are listed in the following table. Be sure to consult a drug handbook for specific information about each of these drugs.

Dosages for Common First-Line Drugs for Partial and Generalized Seizures

Drug	Dosage
carbamazepine (Carbamax ✦, Tegretol)	*Adults:* 600-1600 mg orally daily in 3-4 divided doses *Children less than 6 years:* 10-35 mg/kg/day orally in 3-4 divided doses *Children over 6 years:* 200-1000 mg/day orally in 3-4 divided doses
phenytoin (Dilantin)	*Adults:* Oral loading dose—400 mg followed by 300 mg after 2 and 4 hours; maintenance dose—300 mg daily (extended release) or 100 mg 3 times daily (immediate release); IV—15-18 mg/kg loading dose followed by 100 mg 3 times daily *Children:* Oral—5 mg/kg/day in 2-3 divided doses, maximum 300 mg/day; IV—15-20 mg/kg loading dose, then 100 mg every 6-8 hr
valproic acid (Depakote; Depacon IV)	*Adults/Children 10 years or older:* Oral and IV—10-15 mg/kg/day in divided doses; can increase by 5-10 mg/kg/day until seizures are controlled; maximum dosage 60 mg/kg/day

Intended Responses
- Seizures are controlled and prevented.
- Abnormal electrical impulses are decreased.

Side Effects. Common side effects of drugs for generalized and partial seizures include *ataxia* (loss of coordination, clumsiness), dizziness, light-headedness, and drowsiness. Valproic acid and phenytoin often cause GI symptoms such as indigestion, nausea, and vomiting. Phenytoin also may cause double vision (*diplopia*), rapid involuntary movement of the eyes (*nystagmus*), hypotension, excessive growth of gum tissue (*gingival hyperplasia*), excessive growth of hair in areas not normally hairy (*hypertrichosis*), and rashes.

Side effects for which the patient should be instructed to call the prescriber immediately include difficulty coordinating movements; skin rashes; easy bruising; tiny, purple-colored skin spots (*petechiae*, an indication of bleeding beneath the skin); bloody nose; or unusual bleeding. These side effects likely indicate allergic and adverse reactions to these drugs.

Adverse Effects
Adverse effects of both carbamazepine and phenytoin include *neutropenia* (a decrease in the number of white blood cells [WBCs] with sore throat, fever, and chills), and *aplastic anemia* (anemia caused by too few red blood cells [RBCs] produced by the bone marrow). A patient who develops neutropenia is at risk for life-threatening infections, whereas a patient with aplastic anemia does not have enough RBCs to carry oxygen to the tissues and cells.

Carbamazepine can also cause *thrombocytopenia* (low platelet count), increasing a patient's risk for severe bleeding. Phenytoin can lead to Stevens-Johnson syndrome (see Chapter 1), a serious and life-threatening body-wide (*systemic*) allergic reaction with a rash involving burnlike sores on the skin and mucous membranes. This syndrome usually indicates a serious allergic reaction to a drug.

🔁 **Do Not Confuse**

Tegretol *with* Tegretol XR or Tequin

An order for Tegretol may be confused with Tequin or Tegretol XR. Tegretol is an antiseizure drug, whereas Tegretol XR is an extended-release form of the drug. Tequin is an antibiotic.

QSEN: Safety

💡 **Memory Jogger**

Most first-line antiseizure drugs used for partial and generalized seizures cause side effects of dizziness, hypotension, and sedation.

Common Side Effects

First-Line Drugs for Generalized and Partial Seizures

Dizziness Loss of coordination   Drowsiness/ Sedation   Nausea/ Vomiting

Hypotension

❗ **Drug Alert!**

Teaching Alert

Teach patients taking drugs for generalized and partial seizures to notify their prescriber immediately for signs of allergic or adverse reactions.

QSEN: Safety

! **Drug Alert!**

Administration Alert

Do *not* use dextrose solutions with IV phenytoin because it causes precipitation as a result of chemical incompatibility.

QSEN: Safety

! **Drug Alert!**

Teaching Alert

Drugs for generalized and partial seizures interfere with the effects of birth control pills. Women may need to use another form of contraception to avoid becoming pregnant.

QSEN: Safety

! **Drug Alert!**

Teaching Alert

Patients taking phenytoin (Dilantin) should see their dentist regularly because of extra growth of the gums that occurs while taking this drug.

QSEN: Safety

! **Drug Alert!**

Action/Intervention Alert

Monitor a patient who is taking valproic acid (Depakote) closely for wound healing and signs of infection.

QSEN: Safety

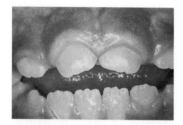

FIGURE 25-5 Developmental gingival enlargement (overgrowth)

Serious adverse effects of valproic acid include damage to the liver *(hepatotoxicity)* and inflammation of the pancreas *(pancreatitis)*.

What To Do *Before* Giving First-Line Drugs for Partial and Generalized Seizures

In addition to the general responsibilities related to antiseizure drugs (p. 406), if the patient is to receive an IV drug such as phenytoin, make sure to check the IV site for patency and solution compatibility. Use normal saline because this drug *precipitates* (forms solid particles) due to chemical incompatibility with dextrose solutions.

What To Do *After* Giving First-Line Drugs for Partial and Generalized Seizures

In addition to the general responsibilities related to antiseizure drugs (p. 406), check his or her gait. Remind him or her about the importance of frequent and careful mouth care.

Be sure to ask the patient about nausea and vomiting. If GI symptoms develop, give these drugs with food. Remind the patient to drink plenty of water because these drugs dry the mouth and increase urine excretion.

Watch for side effects such as abnormal bleeding and report these to the prescriber.

What To *Teach* Patients About First-Line Drugs for Partial and Generalized Seizures

In addition to the general precautions related to antiseizure drugs (p. 406), tell patients that they may need to have occasional laboratory tests done to check blood levels of these drugs or to check for liver damage.

Teach female patients of childbearing age that birth control pills may not work effectively while taking these drugs. To prevent pregnancy they may need to use another form of contraception.

Carbamazepine (Tegretol) can make skin more sensitive to sunlight. Instruct patients to wear protective clothing and sunscreen and to avoid the use of sun lamps or tanning beds.

Phenytoin (Dilantin) can cause extra growth of gum tissues. Tell patients to visit their dentist regularly and to brush and floss teeth carefully.

Teach patients to take phenytoin at least 2 to 3 hours before or after using antacids. Antacids decrease absorption of phenytoin. Valproic acid (Depakote, Depacon) can lead to blood problems that can cause slowed healing and increased risk for infection.

Life Span Considerations for First-Line Drugs for Partial and Generalized Seizures

Pediatric Considerations. Phenytoin must be used carefully for children because of extra growth of gums while taking the drug. Children are more likely to have behavioral changes while taking carbamazepine. Adolescents often require increased dosages of antiseizure drugs because of growth and hormone changes. Adolescents are at risk to stop taking this drug to avoid changes to the skin and gums and to fit in more closely with their peers (Figure 25-5).

Considerations for Pregnancy and Lactation. Carbamazepine, phenytoin, and valproic acid have a high likelihood of increasing the risk for birth defects or fetal damage and may be used during pregnancy only if potential benefits outweigh risks to the fetus. A seizure during pregnancy can result in oxygen loss to the fetus or physical injury to the mother or fetus if a fall occurs. Some infants have been born with low birth weight, small head sizes, skull or facial defects, underdeveloped fingernails, and delayed growth when mothers took large doses of these drugs during pregnancy. Carbamazepine passes into breast milk.

Safe use of phenytoin during pregnancy or breastfeeding has not been established. Taking phenytoin during pregnancy increases the risk of children born with cleft palate. Valproic acid during pregnancy has been associated with developmental defects, low IQ, birth defects, congenital anomalies, and damage to the infant's liver. This drug also passes into breast milk and should not be taken while a mother is breastfeeding. Fetal hydantoin syndrome is a rare disorder that is caused by exposure of a fetus to phenytoin. The symptoms of this disorder may include abnormalities of the skull and facial features, growth deficiencies, underdeveloped nails of the fingers and toes, and/or mild developmental delays.

Considerations for Older Adults. Older adults are more sensitive to the effects of these drugs and may experience confusion, restlessness, nervousness, and abnormal heartbeats. Older adults may also experience chest pain. Monitor heart rate and rhythm more frequently. Teach older adults to check their pulse at least once daily and to report abnormal beats to the prescriber. Stress the importance of calling 911 or getting to the nearest emergency department if chest pain occurs, especially if it is accompanied by shortness of breath.

FIRST-LINE DRUGS FOR ABSENCE SEIZURES

How Drugs for Absence Seizures Work

First-line drugs for absence seizures include ethosuximide (Zarontin) and valproic acid (Depakote). Ethosuximide depresses the motor cortex and increases the central nervous system (CNS) threshold to stimuli. The action of valproic acid may be related to increased availability of the neurotransmitter GABA.

Generic names, brand names, and common dosages of these drugs are listed in the following table. Be sure to consult a drug handbook for specific information about each of these drugs.

Dosages for Common First-Line Drugs for Absence Seizures

Drug	Dosage
ethosuximide (Zarontin)	*Adults/Children 6-12 years:* 250 mg orally twice daily; maximum dosage 1.5 g/day *Children 3-6 years:* 250 mg orally daily; maximum dosage 1.5 g/day
valproic acid (Depakote; Depacon IV)	*Adults/Children 10 years or older:* Oral and IV—10-15 mg/kg/day in divided doses; can increase by 5-10 mg/kg/day until seizures are controlled; maximum dosage 60 mg/kg/day

Intended Responses
- Seizures are controlled and prevented.
- Abnormal electrical impulses are decreased.
- Resistance of CNS to abnormal stimuli is increased.

Side Effects. Common side effects of these drugs include the GI symptoms of nausea, vomiting, and indigestion. They also may cause loss of appetite (anorexia) and weight loss. Valproic acid may cause prolonged bleeding time.

Other side effects of these drugs include mental confusion, drowsiness, dizziness, headaches, constipation, depression, and nervousness.

Patients taking these drugs should notify their prescriber immediately about symptoms of allergic reaction such as rashes, fever, and sore throat. The prescriber should also be notified immediately about signs of bleeding such as easy bruising, petechiae, bloody nose, or any unusual bleeding.

Adverse Effects. Adverse effects of ethosuximide (Zarontin) include a decrease in the number of WBCs *(neutropenia)*; reduction in the number of erythrocytes, all types

 Drug Alert!

Monitoring Alert

Assess older adults who have been prescribed first-line drugs for partial or generalized seizures for abnormal heart rhythms and chest pain. Report these occurrences immediately to the prescriber.

QSEN: Safety

 Memory Jogger

Ethosuximide (Zarontin) causes CNS depression.

Common Side Effects

First-Line Drugs for Absence Seizures

Nausea/Vomiting, Indigestion, Decreased appetite, Weight loss

 Drug Alert!

Action/Intervention Alert

Report signs of allergic reaction or abnormal bleeding immediately to the prescriber.

QSEN: Safety

of WBCs, and blood platelets in the circulating blood *(pancytopenia)*; and anemia caused by deficient RBC production in the bone marrow *(aplastic anemia)*.

Valproic acid can lead to damage or destruction in the liver *(hepatotoxicity)*, inflammation of the pancreas *(pancreatitis)*, and bone marrow depression. Bone marrow depression can result in reduced production of RBCs, which causes anemia; reduced WBCs, which can result in infection; and reduced platelets, which can result in bleeding.

What To Do *Before* Giving First-Line Drugs for Absence Seizures

In addition to the general responsibilities related to antiseizure drugs (p. 406), check the patient's baseline coagulation laboratory test results. Obtain a baseline weight for the patient.

What To Do *After* Giving First-Line Drugs for Absence Seizures

In addition to the general responsibilities related to antiseizure drugs (p. 406), check the patient's weight every day. If the patient develops GI distress, give these drugs with food.

What To Teach Patients Taking First-Line Drugs for Absence Seizures

In addition to the general precautions related to antiseizure drugs (p. 406), instruct patients to take these drugs exactly as prescribed and to take missed doses as soon as possible but not to take double doses. Tell patients not to stop taking these drugs suddenly because seizures may occur.

If a patient is scheduled for surgery, including dental surgery, instruct him or her to notify the surgeon or dentist about the use of these drugs.

Ethosuximide (Zarontin) can make the eyes more sensitive to light. Instruct patients to protect their eyes by wearing dark glasses in bright light.

Life Span Considerations for First-Line Drugs for Absence Seizures

Pediatric Considerations. Children younger than 2 years of age are at increased risk for liver damage that may lead to death with valproic acid. Safe use of ethosuximide in children younger than 3 years has not been studied or established. Growing children who take drugs for seizures often need dose increases as they grow. Adolescence is a physically and emotionally stressful time with an increased risk for seizure occurrences.

Considerations for Pregnancy and Lactation. Safe use of ethosuximide has not been established. Valproic acid has a high likelihood of increasing the risk for birth defects or fetal damage. During pregnancy it has been associated with developmental defects, low IQ, birth defects, congenital anomalies, and damage to the infant's liver. This drug also passes into breast milk and should not be used while a mother is breastfeeding.

Considerations for Older Adults. Valproic acid should be used cautiously in older adults because they may be more sensitive to its side effects such as sleepiness and dizziness. Teach older adults to take special precautions to avoid falls. Instruct them to change positions slowly and to use handrails when going up or down stairs. Suggest that older adults avoid driving or using dangerous machines until they know how the drugs will affect them.

SECOND-LINE (ALTERNATIVE) DRUGS FOR SEIZURES

How Second-Line Drugs for Seizures Work

Second-line drugs for seizures are alternative drugs for the treatment of seizures. Included in this group are phenobarbital (Luminal) and primidone (Mysoline), which increase the body's threshold against seizure activity by blocking or slowing the spread of abnormal impulses. The disadvantage of phenobarbital is that it can lead to physical dependence. Primidone is turned into phenobarbital by the body

Drug Alert!

Action/Intervention Alert

Give drugs for seizures with food if GI symptoms such as nausea, vomiting, and stomach upset develop.

QSEN: Safety

Clinical Pitfall

Patients should *never* suddenly stop taking seizure drugs because this may cause seizures to occur.

QSEN: Safety

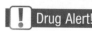

Drug Alert!

Teaching Alert

Teach patients taking ethosuximide (Zarontin) to wear dark glasses when going out into bright light.

QSEN: Safety

and acts in the same way as phenobarbital. Gabapentin (Neurontin) and lamotrigine (Lamictal) stabilize the membranes of neurons to decrease seizure activity. The action of clonazepam (Klonopin) is not well understood but may be related to inhibition (slowing or stopping) of transmission of abnormal impulses. Pregabalin (Lyrica) is used to decrease the frequency of partial seizures.

Commonly prescribed second-line drugs for seizures are listed in the following table. Be sure to consult a drug handbook for specific information on each of these drugs.

Dosages for Common Second-Line Drugs for Seizures

Drug	Dosage
clonazepam (Klonopin, Novo-Clonazepam ♣, Rivotril)	*Adults:* 1.5 mg orally daily in 3 divided doses; maximum dosage 20 mg/day *Children less than 10 years:* 0.01-0.03 mg/kg orally daily in 3 divided doses; maximum dosage 0.2 mg/kg/day
gabapentin (Neurontin)	*Adults/Children over 12 years:* 300-400 mg orally 3 times daily; maximum dosage 1800-2400 mg/day
lamotrigine (Lamictal)	With valproic acid: *Adults:* 25 mg orally every day during weeks 1-2; increase to 100-200 mg/day slowly over several weeks; maximum dosage 200 mg/day *Children 2-12 years:* 0.2-1 mg/kg orally daily; increase slowly over several weeks; maximum dosage 5 mg/kg/day With other seizure drugs: *Adults:* 50-500 mg orally daily in 2 divided doses *Children 2-12 years:* 5-15 mg/kg orally daily in 2 divided doses; maximum dosage 400 mg/day
phenobarbital (Ancakuxur ♣, Barbita, Luminal)	*Adults:* Oral—100-300 mg/day; IV/IM—200-600 mg/day *Children:* Oral, IV—3-8 mg/kg/day *Neonates:* Oral, IV—4 mg/kg/day; maximum dosage 5 mg/kg/day
pregabalin (Lyrica)	*Adults and children >12 years:* 150 mg/day in 2-3 divided doses; may increase to 600 mg/day in 2-3 divided doses *Children <12 years:* Safety/efficacy not established
primidone (Mysoline, Primidone ♣, Sertan ♣)	*Adults/Children 8-12 years:* 250 mg orally daily; maximum dosage 2 g in 2-4 divided doses *Children less than 8 years:* 125 mg orally daily; maximum dosage 1 g in 2-4 divided doses

Intended Responses
- Seizures are controlled and prevented.
- Abnormal electrical impulses are decreased.
- Resistance of CNS to abnormal stimuli is increased.

Side Effects. Common side effects of second-line drugs for seizures vary with the prescribed drug. The most common side effects of these drugs are listed in the following table. Be sure to consult a drug handbook for additional information on a specific drug.

Common Side Effects of Second-Line Drugs for Seizures

Drug	Common Side Effects
clonazepam (Klonopin)	Dizziness, sedation, weakness
gabapentin (Neurontin)	Drowsiness, fatigue, dizziness, swelling in ankles, weight gain

Continued

 Memory Jogger

Gabapentin (Neurontin) is often used to control pain from chronic neuropathy and fibromyalgia.

 Do Not Confuse

Neurontin *with* Noroxin

An order for Neurontin may be confused with Noroxin. Neurontin is an antiseizure drug, whereas Noroxin is an anti-infective drug.

QSEN: Safety

 Do Not Confuse

Lamictal *with* Lamisil

An order for Lamictal may be confused with Lamisil. Lamictal is an antiseizure drug, whereas Lamisil is an antifungal, anti-infective drug.

QSEN: Safety

 Do Not Confuse

lamotrigine *with* lamivudine

An order for lamotrigine may be confused with lamivudine. Lamotrigine is an antiseizure drug, whereas lamivudine is an anti-infective, antiretroviral drug used to treat human immune deficiency virus.

QSEN: Safety

Common Side Effects

Second-Line Drugs for Seizures

Dizziness

Drowsiness

GI upset

Clumsiness, Unsteadiness

Common Side Effects of Second-Line Drugs for Seizures—cont'd

Drug	Common Side Effects
lamotrigine (Lamictal)	Dizziness, upset stomach, headache, unsteadiness, double vision, rash
pregabalin (Lyrica)	Dizziness, drowsiness, ataxia, peripheral edema
phenobarbital (Luminal)	Drowsiness, dizziness
primidone (Mysoline)	Anorexia, ataxia, clumsiness, dizziness, unsteadiness, vertigo

⚠ Drug Alert!

Interaction Alert

When a patient takes morphine at the same time as gabapentin (Neurontin), the blood level of gabapentin is increased and could become toxic.

QSEN: Safety

⚠ Drug Alert!

Administration Alert

Antacids interfere with absorption of gabapentin (Neurontin). Schedule at least 2 hours between giving gabapentin and an antacid.

QSEN: Safety

Clinical Pitfall

If a patient develops a rash, do not give the drug and notify the prescriber immediately.

QSEN: Safety

Second-line drugs for seizures are often prescribed with other seizure medications, causing an increased risk for side effects. When seizure drugs are prescribed together, lower doses may be needed. When gabapentin is prescribed for a patient who is taking morphine, increased blood levels of gabapentin can occur, possibly leading to toxicity. A lower dose of gabapentin, morphine, or both may be required to avoid side effects.

Primidone decreases the effects of anticoagulant drugs, so higher doses of an anticoagulant may be needed to achieve therapeutic effects.

Adverse Effects. Clonazepam is a benzodiazepine CNS drug with the life-threatening adverse reaction of respiratory depression. Lamotrigine can lead to Stevens-Johnson syndrome, a serious and life-threatening body-wide (systemic) allergic reaction with a rash involving the skin and mucous membranes (see Chapter 1). It can also lead to toxic epidermal necrolysis, a life-threatening skin disorder characterized by blistering and peeling of the top layer of skin. Sudden withdrawal of pregabalin can increase the frequency of seizure activity. The drug should be gradually withdrawn over a week.

Several life-threatening adverse effects are associated with phenobarbital, including closure of the larynx, which blocks the passage of air to the lungs (*laryngospasm*); circulatory collapse (*shock*); and decreased number of WBCs (*neutropenia*). Additional adverse effects include respiratory depression when high doses are prescribed, CNS depression, coma, and death. Swelling similar to that seen in urticaria (hives) can occur beneath the skin instead of on the surface. Other adverse effects include deep swelling around the eyes and lips and sometimes of the hands and feet (*angioedema;* see Chapter 1) and hypersensitive reaction to the administration of a foreign serum (*serum sickness*), which is characterized by fever, swelling, skin rash, and enlargement of the lymph nodes.

What To Do *Before* Giving Second-Line Drugs for Seizures

In addition to the general responsibilities related to antiseizure drug therapy (p. 406), be sure to schedule at least 2 hours between gabapentin and antacid drugs.

Ask older adults about the presence of liver or kidney problems.

If the patient is to receive an IV drug form such as phenobarbital, be sure to check that the IV site is patent and the IV solution is compatible with the drug.

What To Do *After* Giving Second-Line Drugs for Seizures

In addition to the general responsibilities related to antiseizure drug therapy (p. 406), be sure to assess for and ask about side effects and watch for adverse effects of these drugs. Notify the prescriber if side effects or adverse effects occur. If the patient develops a rash, hold the drug and notify the prescriber immediately. To minimize the risk of severe rashes, the dose of lamotrigine (Lamictal) can be increased very slowly over 6 to 7 weeks. If the patient is taking lamotrigine, skin rash can be the first sign of Stevens-Johnson syndrome (see Chapter 1) or toxic epidermal necrolysis.

Give these drugs with food if the patient develops nausea, vomiting, or stomach upset. Make sure that any ordered laboratory tests are completed.

What To Teach Patients Taking Second-Line Drugs for Seizures

In addition to the general precautions related to antiseizure drug therapy (p. 406), instruct patients to notify their prescriber immediately about any signs of allergic reactions to these drugs, including skin rashes, fever, flulike symptoms, and swollen glands. They should also notify their prescriber immediately if seizure activity increases.

Remind patients that phenobarbital and clonazepam may become habit forming and should only be taken for the period of time prescribed.

Phenobarbital and primidone (Mysoline) interfere with the actions of birth control pills. Women taking these drugs should be instructed to use another form of contraception to prevent pregnancy. Remind female patients to notify their prescriber immediately if they are pregnant, breastfeeding, or planning to become pregnant.

Patients taking phenobarbital, primidone, or lamotrigine should be taught to avoid alcohol because it adds to the drowsiness that these drugs may cause.

Tell patients with diabetes that gabapentin may affect a dipstick test for protein in the urine (*proteinuria*). Gabapentin (Neurontin) should be taken at least 2 hours after an antacid because antacids can decrease absorption of this drug.

Patients taking lamotrigine should be taught to wear sunscreen and protective clothes to prevent photosensitivity reactions. Remind patients about these precautions even if they have dark skin that does not usually get sunburned.

Remind patients who smoke while taking clonazepam (Klonopin) that cigarette smoking may decrease the effectiveness of this drug. If he or she smokes, a higher dose of the drug may be needed to be effective.

Teach patients prescribed pregabalin (Lyrica) to avoid suddenly stopping the drug because the frequency of seizures may increase.

Life Span Considerations for Second-Line Drugs for Seizures

Pediatric Considerations. Children have a higher incidence of rashes with lamotrigine. Gabapentin may cause fever, hyperactivity, and hostile or aggressive behavior in children. They are much more sensitive to the effects of gabapentin and are at increased risk of side effects.

Considerations for Pregnancy and Lactation. Second-line drugs for seizures have a moderate to high likelihood of increasing the risk for birth defects or fetal damage. These drugs have not been tested in pregnant women. Women are more likely to experience dizziness when taking lamotrigine. Primidone may cause increased birth defects, and there have been reports of newborns with bleeding problems. Lamotrigine limits the body's production of folic acid. Folic acid deficiency during pregnancy is associated with a variety of birth defects. To prevent deficiency during pregnancy, a woman taking lamotrigine should take folic acid supplements throughout the pregnancy. Gabapentin has been associated with bone and kidney problems in pregnant animals but has not been tested in women. With phenobarbital, clonazepam, and primidone, animal studies have shown that newborns have lower weight and have a lower survival rate. These drugs pass into breast milk and should not be taken by a woman who is breastfeeding because they may cause unwanted side effects in infants.

Considerations for Older Adults. Older adults are also more sensitive to these drugs and more likely to develop side effects. They may develop unusual restlessness or excitement with primidone. Lamotrigine and gabapentin are more slowly eliminated from an older adult's body. Because of this, older adults may need to be started on a lower drug dose.

 Drug Alert!
Teaching Alert
Patients should be taught to notify their prescriber immediately if seizure activity increases or changes in any way.
QSEN: Safety

 Clinical Pitfall
Patients should not smoke while taking clonazepam (Klonopin).
QSEN: Safety

 Drug Alert!
Action/Intervention Alert
Children and older adults are more sensitive to the effects of second-line antiseizure drugs and are more likely to develop side effects. Monitor these patients carefully.
QSEN: Safety

Get Ready for Practice!

Key Points

- Abnormal electrical impulses in the brain cause seizures to occur.
- The most common ages for onset of seizures are early childhood and late adulthood.
- A typical seizure consists of an aura, the seizure, and a postictal period.
- The two major groups of seizures are generalized and partial.
- Status epilepticus is a prolonged seizure or a series of repeated seizures without enough time for recovery between seizures.
- The exact action of most antiseizure drugs is not known, but these drugs decrease the voltage, frequency, and spread of abnormal electrical impulses in the brain.
- Many drugs for seizures interfere with the effects of birth control pills, and women should be taught to use an alternative form of contraception to prevent pregnancy.
- Antacids decrease the absorption of antiseizure drugs and should be given at least 2 to 3 hours before or after taking these drugs.
- Patients who suddenly stop taking antiseizure drugs are at high risk for having a seizure.
- Patients should be instructed to notify their prescriber immediately if seizure activity increases or changes in any way.

Additional Learning Resources

evolve Be sure to visit your Evolve website (http://evolve.elsevier.com/Workman/pharmacology/) for additional online resources.

SG Go to your Study Guide for additional learning activities to help you master this chapter content.

Review Questions

See the Answer Keys—In-text Review Questions for answers to these questions.

Test Yourself on the Basics

1. Which phrase best describes second-line drugs for treatment of seizures?
   A. Used when first-line drugs do not work
   B. Used as alternative drugs to treat seizures
   C. Used for only generalized seizures
   D. Used as adjuncts to first-line drugs for partial seizures
2. Which side effects are common with first-line drugs used to treat partial and generalized seizures? (Select all that apply.)
   A. Dizziness
   B. Constipation
   C. Hypotension
   D. Sedation
   E. Rashes
   F. Nausea

3. A patient is prescribed an IV dose of phenytoin (Dilantin). Which solution should be used to dilute this drug?
   A. 5% dextrose
   B. 5% dextrose with 0.45 saline
   C. 0.9% normal saline
   D. Lactated ringer's solution
4. A patient tells you that his seizure activity has increased over the past month. What important teaching point will you stress with this patient?
   A. "You should take an extra dose of your antiseizure medication each day."
   B. "You must go to the lab to have some blood tests done."
   C. "You need to contact your prescriber whenever seizures increase or change."
   D. "You should not worry about this because stress can cause increased seizures."
5. A child is prescribed phenytoin (Dilantin) for a seizure disorder. What precaution should you discuss with the parents?
   A. Be sure to take your child to see a dentist regularly.
   B. Always give this drug on an empty stomach.
   C. Administer the phenytoin within 30 minutes after an antacid.
   D. Report any facial swelling due to the risk for angioedema.

Test Yourself on Advanced Concepts

6. Which drug used to treat seizures decreases impulse transmission by affecting sodium channels in neurons?
   A. phenobarbital (Luminal)
   B. carbamazepine (Tegretol)
   C. valproic acid (Depakote)
   D. phenytoin (Dilantin)
7. For which adverse effects must you watch after giving a patient phenytoin (Dilantin)? (Select all that apply.)
   A. Neutropenia
   B. Stevens-Johnson syndrome
   C. Aplastic anemia
   D. Thrombocytopenia
   E. Pancreatitis
8. What safety intervention must you take when giving the first-line drug for seizures phenytoin (Dilantin) by the intravenous (IV) route?
   A. Make sure that the IV catheter is 18 gauge or larger.
   B. Question the order because this drug is not given IV.
   C. Ensure that the IV solution infusing is normal saline.
   D. Place a padded tongue blade at the patient's bedside.
9. A patient is taking carbamazepine (Tegretol). What must you be sure to teach the patient about this drug?
   A. Visit a dentist regularly.
   B. You may experience delayed healing and increased risk of infection.
   C. Always take the drug on an empty stomach.
   D. Wear protective clothing and a strong sunscreen.

10. Which is an important consideration when administering first-line drugs for absence seizures to growing children?
    A. They may develop high fevers.
    B. They will have a higher incidence of rashes.
    C. They may develop hostile, aggressive behavior.
    D. They may need dose increases.
11. A patient has been prescribed phenobarbital (Luminal) 300 mg per day. The pharmacy sent 100 mg tablets. How many tablets do you give with each dose? _____ tablets
12. A 4-year-old child is to be given phenytoin (Dilantin) 5 mg/kg/day in two divided doses. The child weighs 20 kg. How many milligrams do you give for each dose? _____ mg/dose

Critical Thinking Activities

See the Answer Keys—Critical Thinking Activities for answers to these activities.

Ms. Plant, aged 48 years, is admitted to the hospital with a seizure disorder. She experiences generalized seizures approximately once a month. Her prescribed drugs include carbamazepine (Tegretol) 300 mg three times a day. Carbamazepine comes in 100-mg tablets. The patient states that while taking this drug, she sometimes experiences nausea and vomiting, as well as dizziness.

1. How many tablets will you give Ms. Plant with each dose of medication?
2. What important teaching points will you share with the patient about this drug?
3. What safety measures will you take when admitting Ms. Plant to your hospital unit?

Drug Therapy for Alzheimer's and Parkinson's Diseases

Objectives

After studying this chapter you should be able to:

1. Explain how different classes of drugs are used to treat Alzheimer's disease and Parkinson's disease.
2. List the names, actions, usual adult dosages, possible side effects, and adverse effects of drugs for Alzheimer's disease.
3. Describe what to do before and after giving drugs for Alzheimer's disease.
4. Explain what to teach patients and their families or caregivers about drugs for Alzheimer's disease, including what to do, what not to do, and when to call the prescriber.
5. Describe life span considerations for drugs for Alzheimer's disease.

6. List the names, actions, usual adult dosages, possible side effects, and adverse effects of drugs for Parkinson's disease.
7. Describe what to do before and after giving drugs for Parkinson's disease.
8. Explain what to teach patients and their families or caregivers about drugs for Parkinson's disease, including what to do, what not to do, and when to call the prescriber.
9. Describe life span considerations for drugs for Parkinson's disease.

Key Terms

Alzheimer's disease (ĂLZ-hī-mŭrz dĭz-ÊZ) (p. 417) A progressive, incurable condition that destroys brain cells, gradually causing loss of intellectual abilities such as memory and extreme changes in personality and behavior.

anticholinergic drugs (ăn-tĭ-kō-lĭn-ĔRJ-ĭk DRŬGZ) (p. 423) (See Chapter 23.)

catechol-*O*-methyltransferase (COMT) inhibitors (KĂ-tĕ-kŏl Ō MĔ-thŭl-TRĂNS-fŭr-ās ĭn-HĬB-ĭ-tŏrz) (p. 423) A group of drugs used to treat Parkinson's disease that allow a larger amount of levodopa to reach the brain, which raises dopamine levels in the brain.

cholinesterase/acetylcholinesterase inhibitors (KŌ-lĭn-ĔS-tĕr-ās/ăs-ĕ-tĭl-KŌ-lĭn-ĔS-tĕr-ās ĭn-HĬB-ĭ-tŏrz) (p. 418) A group of drugs used to treat Alzheimer's disease that reduce the activity of the enzyme acetylcholinesterase which breaks down acetylcholine in the synapses of neurons to keep

levels of acetylcholine higher and slow the progress of the disease.

dopaminergic/dopamine agonists (DŌ-pă-mĭ-nĕr-jĭk/DŌ-pă-mēn ĂG-ŏ-nĭsts) (p. 422) A group of drugs used to treat Parkinson's disease that increase the amount of dopamine activity in the brain, reducing tremor and muscle rigidity and improving movement.

monoamine oxidase B (MAO-B) inhibitors (MŎ-nō-ă-mēn ŎK-sĭ-dās ĭn-HĬB-ĭ-tŏrz) (p. 423) A group of drugs used to treat Parkinson's disease that inhibit the enzyme that breaks down dopamine in the brain.

Parkinson's disease (PĂR-kĭn-sŭnz dĭz-ÊZ) (p. 420) A progressive disorder of the nervous system marked by muscle tremors, muscle rigidity, decreased mobility, stooped posture, slowed voluntary movements, and a masklike facial expression.

OVERVIEW

Alzheimer's disease and Parkinson's disease are both progressive neurologic disorders that are more common as people age. Alzheimer's disease is the most common form of dementia. Parkinson's disease is a neurodegenerative disease with slow and progressive degeneration of the nervous system. Both illnesses involve interrupted transmission of nerve impulses. Transmission of these impulses is normally helped by the presence of *neurotransmitters* (for example, dopamine, acetylcholine), which are chemicals that transmit messages from one nerve cell (*neuron*) to another (see Figure 27-3 in Chapter 27).

ALZHEIMER'S DISEASE

Alzheimer's disease is a progressive and incurable condition that destroys brain cells, with gradual loss of intellectual abilities such as memory and extreme changes in personality and behavior. It is the most feared and common form of dementia. *Dementia* is a brain disorder that seriously affects a person's ability to perform activities of daily living (ADLs), including loss of intellectual functions (for example, thinking, remembering, and reasoning). It is estimated in 2014 that 5.2 million people in the United States have Alzheimer's disease, and it affects about 44.4 million people worldwide. About 10% of people over age 65 are affected, and as many as 50% of people over age 85 have Alzheimer's disease. About 200,000 people develop early-onset Alzheimer's disease in their 40s and 50s.

REVIEW OF RELATED PHYSIOLOGY AND PATHOPHYSIOLOGY

There are two main pathologic changes in Alzheimer's disease. First is the presence of large amounts of the protein beta-amyloid (Abeta), which clumps together and forms plaques between cells in the brain. Second, other proteins twist and form tangles within the neurons. As a result, neurons die in the areas of the brain that are important to memory and other essential mental abilities (Figure 26-1). Connections between nerve cells are also disrupted. Levels of chemicals (for example, acetylcholine and acetylcholinesterase) in the brain that carry messages between nerve cells are lower.

No single cause has been established for Alzheimer's disease. Instead, a combination of factors has been proposed. Age is the greatest risk factor. Genetics may play a role in development of this condition. People with Down syndrome, a common disorder involving an extra chromosome number 21 (trisomy 21), have an increased risk for Alzheimer's disease by age 50 to 60 years. A person who has a severe head injury or whiplash injury may also be at increased risk of developing dementia. People who smoke or have high blood pressure or high cholesterol levels also seem to have a higher risk for Alzheimer's disease.

Alzheimer's disease symptoms begin very slowly. In the early stage, the first symptom may be mild forgetfulness, which can be confused with age-related memory changes. Table 26-1 provides a list of symptoms that occur during stages of the disease. As the disease progresses, symptoms are more noticeable, and family

> **? Did You Know?**
>
> Alzheimer's disease is more common in older adults, but it can affect people as young as age 30.

> **💡 Memory Jogger**
>
> With Alzheimer's disease, neurons die in the areas of the brain that are essential for memory and important mental abilities such as language.

> **? Did You Know?**
>
> A person with Down syndrome who lives to the age of 50 to 60 years is at increased risk for developing Alzheimer's disease.

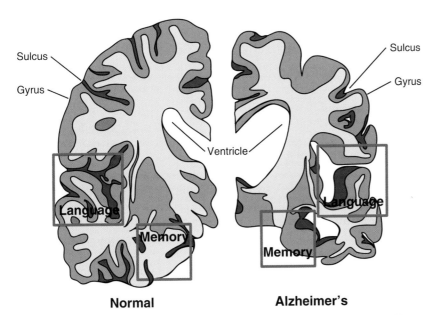

FIGURE 26-1 Cross sections of a normal brain and a brain affected by Alzheimer's disease. Neurons die in areas of the brain important to memory and language.

Table 26-1	Symptoms of Alzheimer's Disease
STAGE	**SYMPTOMS**
Early	Forgetfulness • Difficulty recalling events and activities • Difficulty remembering names of familiar people and things • Inability to solve simple mathematics problems
Middle	Beginning to have difficulty speaking, understanding, reading, and writing Failure to recognize familiar people and places Forgetting how to perform simple tasks such as brushing teeth and combing hair Inability to think clearly
Late	Aggressiveness Anxiety Need for total care Wandering away from home

members seek medical help. In the late stages of the disease, the patient will need total care to prevent complications of immobility, aspiration, urinary tract infections, pneumonia, and pressure ulcers, which commonly lead to death in these patients.

There is no test that diagnoses Alzheimer's disease. The only absolute way to confirm that a patient has this illness is to see the plaques and tangles in the brain tissue, which can be done only by autopsy after the patient dies. Diagnosis is made by excluding other possible causes (for example, thyroid problems, drug reactions, depression, brain tumors, and blood vessel diseases). On the basis of symptom assessment, health history, tests of memory and problem solving, and brain scan, a diagnosis of probable Alzheimer's disease can be made.

There is no cure for Alzheimer's disease. Early diagnosis is important because it helps patients and families plan for the future, makes it possible for the patient with dementia to benefit from drugs that can slow the progress of the disease, and helps the patient and family to identify sources of advice and support. No treatment can stop the progression of Alzheimer's disease. Drug therapy may help prevent symptoms from becoming worse for a limited time and allow the patient to continue performing some daily activities for a longer period. Drugs may also be prescribed to help control behavioral symptoms such as sleeplessness, agitation, wandering, anxiety, and depression.

TYPES OF DRUGS FOR ALZHEIMER'S DISEASE

CHOLINESTERASE/ACETYLCHOLINESTERASE INHIBITORS AND MEMANTINE

How Drugs for Alzheimer's Disease Work

No drug has been developed that protects neurons from the changes that occur with Alzheimer's disease. Drug treatments have been developed that can temporarily slow the progression of symptoms in some patients.

Cholinesterase/acetylcholinesterase inhibitors reduce the activity of the enzyme acetylcholinesterase that breaks down acetylcholine in the synapses of neurons. This action keeps levels of acetylcholine higher. These drugs are used for early to moderate stages of Alzheimer's disease and their effects are temporary. The three drugs in this category, donepezil (Aricept), rivastigmine (Exelon), and galantamine (Reminyl), are the main ones used for Alzheimer treatment.

Memantine (Namenda) blocks the amino acid glutamate at N-methyl-D-aspartate receptors in the brain, preventing overstimulation (overstimulation of these receptors damages neurons and appears to be one cause of Alzheimer's disease). It can be effective in helping modify dementia (temporarily) in some patients with moderate-to-severe Alzheimer's disease.

Did You Know?

The only way to absolutely diagnose Alzheimer's disease is to look for plaques and tangles in brain tissue by autopsy after the patient's death.

Memory Jogger

Drugs prescribed for Alzheimer's disease and Parkinson's disease can help control the symptoms but cannot cure the disease.

Generic names, trade names, and common dosages of these drugs are listed in the following table. Be sure to consult a drug reference for specific information about any drugs used for Alzheimer's disease.

Dosages for Common Drugs for Alzheimer's Disease

Drug	Dosage
donepezil (Aricept)	*Adults:* 5 mg orally at bedtime; increase to 10 mg after 4-6 weeks
galantamine (Reminyl , Razadyne)	*Adults:* 4 mg orally twice daily with food, increase at 4-week intervals to 12 mg twice daily; extended-release—8 mg once daily in the morning, increase at 4-week intervals to 24 mg daily
memantine (Namenda, Ebixa)	*Adults:* 5 mg orally daily; increase to 5 mg twice daily, then 5 mg in AM and 10 mg in PM; maximum dosage 10 mg twice daily
rivastigmine (Exelon)	*Adults:* Oral—1.5 mg twice daily with food, increase at 2-week intervals to 6 mg twice daily; Patch—apply 1 patch (4.6 mg) at a different body site once daily, may increase to a 9.5-mg patch

Intended Responses
- Dementia with Alzheimer's disease decreases temporarily.
- Degradation of acetylcholine is inhibited.
- Progression of Alzheimer's disease symptoms is slowed.
- Cognitive function in patients with Alzheimer's disease is improved.

Side Effects. The most common side effects of cholinesterase/acetylcholinesterase inhibitors are nausea, vomiting, diarrhea, stomach cramps, headaches, dizziness, fatigue, weakness, insomnia, and loss of appetite *(anorexia).* Common side effects of memantine (Namenda) include dizziness, headache, constipation, and confusion. This drug may also cause anemia.

Adverse Effects. Adverse effects of cholinesterase/acetylcholinesterase inhibitors include abnormal heart rhythms such as bradycardia and atrial fibrillation. Although uncommon, all of these drugs may cause gastrointestinal (GI) bleeding. Two additional uncommon but serious adverse effects include difficulty urinating and seizures. Adverse effects of memantine include shortness of breath and hallucinations. Risks associated with these drugs when a patient needs surgery with general anesthesia include awakening more slowly, respiratory depression, and increased likelihood for experiencing confusion and delirium.

Symptoms of overdose with these drugs include upset stomach, vomiting, drooling, sweating, slow heartbeat (bradycardia), difficulty breathing, muscle weakness, and seizures. Report these effects to the prescriber immediately.

What To Do *Before* Giving Drugs for Alzheimer's Disease
Obtain a complete list of drugs currently being used by the patient, including over-the-counter and herbal products. Assess the patient for baseline cognitive function (for example, memory, attention, reasoning, language, and ability to perform simple tasks).

Obtain a baseline weight. Check baseline blood pressure and heart rate and rhythm. Ask about recent nausea, vomiting, loss of appetite, and weight loss. Have the patient or caregiver tell you about usual urinary output pattern. Check the patient's hemoglobin and hematocrit levels.

Assess swallowing because patients may develop difficulty as the disease progresses and be at risk for aspiration. Drugs may need to be crushed or given in liquid form. Do not crush time-released pills or open time-released capsules.

Ask about a history of liver or kidney problems that may affect metabolism of these drugs. Also ask about previous problems with GI bleeding or ulcers.

Do Not Confuse

Aricept *with* **Aciphex**

An order for Aricept may be confused with Aciphex. Aricept is an acetylcholinesterase inhibitor used for Alzheimer's disease, whereas Aciphex is a proton pump inhibitor used to treat gastroesophageal reflux disease (GERD) and gastric ulcers.

QSEN: Safety

Do Not Confuse

Reminyl *with* **Robinul**

An order for Reminyl may be confused with Robinul. Reminyl is an acetylcholinesterase inhibitor used for Alzheimer's disease, whereas Robinul is an anticholinergic agent that inhibits salivation and excessive respiratory secretions.

QSEN: Safety

Common Side Effects

Drugs for Alzheimer's Disease

Nausea/ Vomiting, Diarrhea   Dizziness   Headache

Fatigue, Insomnia

Drug Alert!

Administration Alert

Assess a patient's ability to swallow before giving drugs for Alzheimer's disease because he or she may be at risk for aspiration.

QSEN: Safety

(!) Drug Alert!

Action/Intervention Alert

Because acetylcholinesterase inhibitors may cause GI bleeding, monitor the patient carefully for any signs of bleeding.

QSEN: Safety

(!) Drug Alert!

Administration Alert

Give galantamine (Reminyl, Razadyne) and rivastigmine (Exelon) twice a day with food to minimize the GI upset that is common with these drugs.

QSEN: Safety

(!) Drug Alert!

Teaching Alert

Teach care providers to remind patients to use the bathroom every 2 hours to avoid incontinence episodes while taking drugs for Alzheimer's disease.

QSEN: Safety

What To Do *After* Giving Drugs for Alzheimer's Disease

Reassess the patient's cognitive function often. Watch for changes in memory, attention, reasoning, language, and ability to perform simple tasks. Cognitive assessment is a long-term task because changes may take time to appear.

Recheck and monitor the patient's heart rate and rhythm, and blood pressure. Monitor intake and output and daily weights. Assess for signs of low hemoglobin or hematocrit. Continue to monitor the patient's swallowing ability. Watch him or her for potential seizure activity.

Because these drugs may cause dizziness and fatigue, instruct any in-patient to call for help when getting out of bed and ensure that the call light is within easy reach. Instruct patients at home to also call for help getting up. Suggest the use of a bell or other call device for help.

Ask the patient about nausea, vomiting, and GI discomfort. Check stools or emesis for signs of GI bleeding. Notify the prescriber if side effects occur.

What To Teach Patients Taking Drugs for Alzheimer's Disease

Always include the person providing home care for the patient when teaching about these drugs. Include information about safe dosage and proper storage. Patients with difficulty swallowing may need medications crushed or in liquid form. Remind caregivers not to crush extended-release drugs.

Teach patients and caregivers that these drugs should be taken exactly as instructed by their prescriber. Tell them about the importance of keeping follow-up appointments to monitor the progress of controlling the symptoms of the disease. Instruct them to report side effects and signs of allergic or toxic reactions to their prescriber immediately.

Caution patients and caregivers that these drugs may cause dizziness, weakness, and fatigue. Remind them to get up slowly. Teach about the side effects of these drugs and the importance of notifying their prescriber for any signs of bleeding.

Tell patients and their caregivers to administer donepezil (Aricept) at bedtime and galantamine (Reminyl, Razadyne) and rivastigmine (Exelon) twice a day with food.

Instruct patients and caregivers about the desired outcomes of temporary improved memory, attention, reasoning, language, and ability to perform simple tasks. Remind patients and caregivers to notify their prescriber about any changes in cognitive function.

Life Span Considerations for Drugs for Alzheimer's Disease

Considerations for Older Adults. All of these drugs should be used cautiously in patients with histories of GI bleeding, liver disease, kidney disease, or heart disease. Rivastigmine should also be used cautiously for patients with asthma or chronic obstructive pulmonary disease (COPD). Older, frail women should not take more than 5 mg/day of donepezil because the drug has been associated with significant weight loss. This drug should be used with caution in any older adult with a low body weight.

Because these drugs increase urination, the older adult, especially one who is confused, may have more episodes of incontinence. Remind family members to ensure that the older adult has the opportunity to use the bathroom every 2 hours while awake and at least once during the night.

PARKINSON'S DISEASE

Parkinson's disease is a slow, progressive, degenerative disease of the nervous system. In the United States about 1 million people are affected by this disease. It affects 1 in 20 people older than 80 and commonly begins between the ages of 50 and 79.

The exact cause of Parkinson's disease is not known; many factors may play a part. Age, especially age 50 and older, is a major risk factor. Genetic and environmental factors may cause development of this condition. Two abnormal genes have

Table 26-2	Drugs That Cause Secondary Parkinson's Disease
CATEGORY	**DRUG NAME**
Antiemetics	prochlorperazine (Compazine)
Antihypertensives	reserpine (Serpasil)
Antipsychotics	chlorpromazine (Thorazine) fluphenazine (Prolixin) haloperidol (Haldol) mesoridazine (Serentil) perphenazine (Trilafon) risperidone (Risperdal) thioridazine (Mellaril) trifluoperazine (Stelazine)
Gastrointestinal motility drugs	metoclopramide (Reglan)
Illicit drugs	methcathinone—a psychoactive stimulant N-MPTP (1-methyl-4-phenyl-1,2,3,6-tetrahydropyridine)—a contaminant found in illicit drugs

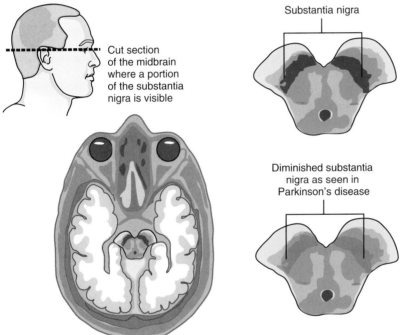

FIGURE 26-2 In Parkinson's disease, nerve cells in the substantia nigra degenerate, and less dopamine is produced. This results in fewer connections between the nerve cells in the basal ganglia and in decreased smooth movements.

been identified in people affected by Parkinson's disease before age 40. Environmental factors such as exposure to weak toxins over a long period of time are thought to lead to Parkinson's disease in genetically predisposed people. Several drugs have caused secondary Parkinson's disease (Table 26-2).

REVIEW OF RELATED PHYSIOLOGY AND PATHOPHYSIOLOGY

Normally, when the brain initiates an impulse to move a muscle, the impulse passes through the basal ganglia. The function of the basal ganglia is to make muscle movements smooth and coordinate changes in posture. Basal ganglia release chemical messengers called *neurotransmitters* (for example, dopamine) that trigger the next nerve cell in the pathway to send an impulse. In Parkinson's disease nerve cells degenerate in a part of the basal ganglia called the *substantia nigra* (Figure 26-2). This

---

Box 26-1 Symptoms of Parkinson's Disease

MOTOR SYMPTOMS	NONMOTOR SYMPTOMS
• Bradykinesia	• Constipation
• Decreased arm swing when walking	• Decreased sense of smell
• Difficulty rising from a chair	• Depression
• Difficulty turning in bed	• Drooling
• Lack of facial expression	• Increased sweating
• Micrographia (small handwriting)	• Low voice volume
• Postural instability	• Male erectile dysfunction
• Rigidity and freezing in place	• Painful foot cramps
• Stooped, shuffling gait	• Sleep disturbance
• Tremor	• Urinary frequency and urgency

Memory Jogger

The four major symptoms of Parkinson's disease are:
• Tremor at rest
• Rigidity
• Bradykinesia (slow movements and difficulty starting to move)
• Abnormal gait

Memory Jogger

The goals of treatment for Parkinson's disease are to minimize disability, reduce possible side effects of drug therapy, and help the patient maintain a high quality of life.

causes a decrease in the production of dopamine and in the number of connections between nerve cells in the basal ganglia. As a result the basal ganglia are less able to produce smooth movements. These changes cause symptoms of increased tremor, lack of coordination, and slowed or reduced movements *(bradykinesia).* Parkinson's disease begins subtly and progresses gradually. Symptoms appear when the amount of dopamine decreases in the brain.

The symptoms appear gradually and increase in severity as the disease progresses. Symptoms may be motor or nonmotor (Box 26-1). For many patients, the initial symptom is a coarse, rhythmic *tremor* of the hand while the hand is at rest, also called *pill-rolling tremor.* As the disease progresses, muscles become rigid, movements become slow and difficult to initiate, and stiffness occurs. When the disease is advanced, the patient may suddenly stop walking, quicken his or her steps, or stumble-run to avoid falling. Posture becomes stooped, and balance becomes difficult to maintain.

There is no specific test or marker for diagnosing Parkinson's disease. Diagnosis is based on symptoms. A diagnosis of Parkinson's disease is probable if drug therapy improves symptoms and other diseases have been ruled out.

There is no cure for Parkinson's disease. Goals of drug therapy include minimizing disability, reducing possible side effects of drug therapy, and helping the patient maintain a high quality of life. Drug therapy may make movement easier and prolong normal function for several years.

TYPES OF DRUGS FOR PARKINSON'S DISEASE

DOPAMINERGIC/DOPAMINE AGONISTS, COMT INHIBITORS, MAO-B INHIBITORS, ANTICHOLINERGICS

How Drugs for Parkinson's Disease Work

No drugs have been developed that will reverse the progression of Parkinson's disease. However, certain drugs can be used effectively to control the symptoms of the disease.

Drugs are prescribed to improve movement and enable patients to function effectively. The period of time that drugs for Parkinson's disease remain effective varies. For some patients they may work for several years, whereas for others they may work for only a short period.

Dopaminergic and dopamine agonists increase the amount of dopamine activity in the brain, thereby reducing tremor and muscle rigidity and improving movement. Carbidopa prevents levodopa from being converted to dopamine before it reaches the brain. When carbidopa is added to levodopa, lower doses of levodopa can be used, leading to reduced side effects such as nausea and vomiting. Dopamine agonist drugs stimulate dopamine receptors to relieve symptoms and delay onset of motor complications. The mechanism of action for the dopamine agonist rotigotine (Neopro) is unknown.

Catechol-*O*-methyltransferase (COMT) inhibitors allow a larger amount of levodopa to reach the brain, which raises dopamine levels in the brain. They help provide a more stable, constant supply of levodopa, which makes its beneficial effects last longer.

Monoamine oxidase B (MAO-B) inhibitors inhibit the enzyme that breaks down dopamine in the brain. As a result, more dopamine is available, and the progression of Parkinson's disease is slowed.

Anticholinergic drugs are effective against tremors and rigidity. These drugs block cholinergic nerve impulses that help control the muscles of the arms, legs, and body. They also restrict the action of acetylcholine, an important chemical messenger in the brain that helps regulate muscle movement, sweat gland function, and intestinal function.

Generic names, trade names, and dosages of the most commonly prescribed drugs are listed in the following table. Be sure to consult a drug reference for specific information about any drug used to treat Parkinson's disease.

Dosages for Common Drugs for Parkinson's Disease

Drug	Dosage (Adults Only)
Dopaminergic/Dopamine Agonists	
apomorphine (Apokyn)	Subcutaneous—0.2 mL; can be increased by 0.1 mL; each dose should not exceed 0.6 mL
bromocriptine (Apo-Bromocriptine ♣, Parlodel)	1.25-2.5 mg orally twice daily with meals; increase at 14- to 28-day intervals by 2.5 mg/day to a maximum dosage 100 mg/day in divided doses; always give with meals
carbidopa/levodopa (Sinemet, Sinemet CR)	25 mg carbidopa / 100 mg levodopa orally 3-4 times daily; extended-release—50 mg carbidopa/200 mg levodopa twice daily
pramipexole (Mirapex)	0.125 mg orally 3 times daily initially; dosage range 1.5-4.5 mg/day in 3 divided doses
ropinirole (Requip)	0.25 mg orally 3 times daily for 1 week, then gradually increase at weekly intervals up to 24 mg/day; extended-release—2 mg once daily, increase at 1- to 2-week intervals by 2 mg/day, maximum dosage 24 mg/day
COMT Inhibitors	
entacapone (Comtan)	200 mg orally given with each dose of carbidopa/levodopa; maximum dosage 1600 mg/day (8 doses)
tolcapone (Tasmar)	100 mg orally 3 times daily given with each dose of carbidopa/levodopa; may increase to 200 mg 3 times daily
MAO-B Inhibitors	
rasagiline (Azilect)	1 mg orally once daily; 0.5-1 mg once daily when combined with levodopa
selegiline (Eldepryl, Novo-Selegiline ♣, Zelapar)	5 mg orally twice daily with breakfast and lunch; oral dissolving tablet—1.25 mg dissolved in mouth once daily (in the morning before breakfast) for 6 weeks, then may increase to 2.5 mg once daily
Anticholinergic Drugs	
benztropine (Apo-Benztropine ♣, Cogentin)	1-2 mg orally per day in 1-2 divided doses

Continued

Memory Jogger

Drug classes for Parkinson's disease are:
- Dopaminergic/dopamine agonists
- COMT inhibitors
- MAO-B inhibitors
- Anticholinergic drugs

Do Not Confuse

Mirapex *with* MiraLax

An order for Mirapex can be confused with MiraLax. Mirapex is a DOPamine agonist used to treat the symptoms of Parkinson's disease, whereas MiraLax is an osmotic laxative used to treat constipation.

QSEN: Safety

Dosages for Common Drugs for Parkinson's Disease—cont'd

Drug	Dosage (Adults Only)
trihexyphenidyl (Apo-Trihex ❧, Artane, Novohexidyl ❧, Trihexane)	1 mg orally day 1, 2 mg day 2, then increase by 2 mg every 3-5 days up to 6-10 mg/day in 3 divided doses; maximum dosage 15 mg/day
Dopamine Agonist	
rotigotine (Neupro)	Early Stage: 2-6 mg/24-hour transdermal patch Advanced Stage: 2-8 mg/24-hour transdermal patch

Common Side Effects

Drugs for Parkinson's Disease

Dizziness

Nausea

Hypotension

Intended Responses
- Signs and symptoms of Parkinson's disease are decreased
- Tremor and rigidity of Parkinson's disease are relieved.

Side Effects. The most common side effects of drugs to treat Parkinson's disease are dizziness, nausea, and hypotension. Common side effects of these drugs are summarized by drug or drug group in the following table.

Common Side Effects of Drugs for Parkinson's Disease

Drugs or Drug Groups	Side Effects
Anticholinergic drugs	Blurred vision, constipation, dizziness, dry eyes, dry mouth, nervousness, sedation
carbidopa-levodopa (Sinemet)	Involuntary movements (dyskinesia), nausea and vomiting
COMT inhibitors	Constipation, diarrhea, dyskinesia, dystonia (slow movement or extended spasm in a group of muscles), headache, sleep disorder
Dopamine agonists	Amnesia, chest pain, constipation, dizziness, dry mouth, dyskinesia, dyspepsia, flushing, hallucinations, hypotension, nausea and vomiting, pallor, rhinorrhea (runny nose), somnolence, sweating, weakness, yawning
MAO-B inhibitors	Confusion, dizziness, dry mouth, nausea, vivid dreams and hallucinations

Adverse Effects. Serious adverse effects of carbidopa-levodopa (Sinemet) include depression with suicidal tendencies; neutropenia (decreased number of white blood cells), and neuroleptic malignant syndrome (dysfunction of the autonomic nervous system, the branch of the nervous system responsible for regulating involuntary actions such as heart rate, blood pressure, digestion, and sweating; muscle tone; body temperature; and consciousness).

Apomorphine (Apokyn) can cause life-threatening central nervous system (CNS) depression, including respiratory depression, coma, and cardiac arrest.

Bromocriptine (Parlodel) may lead to shock, or acute myocardial infarction. Pramipexole (Mirapex) can cause sleep attacks *(narcolepsy).*

COMT inhibitors can cause neuroleptic malignant syndrome or rhabdomyolysis, a serious and potentially fatal effect involving destruction or degeneration of skeletal muscle. Signs and symptoms of this disorder include muscle aches; muscle weakness; and dark, cola-colored urine.

What To Do *Before* Giving Drugs for Parkinson's Disease

Obtain a complete list of drugs currently being used by the patient, including over-the-counter and herbal products. Check blood pressure, heart rate, and respiratory rate for a baseline. Assess baseline neurologic and mental status. Check for baseline dyskinesia, rigidity, tremors, and gait. Assess swallowing ability.

ⓘ Drug Alert!

Administration Alert

Always ask patients taking COMT inhibitor drugs about muscle aches or weakness; these are symptoms of rhabdomyolysis, which is an adverse effect of these drugs.

QSEN: Safety

Ask women of childbearing age if they are pregnant or planning to become pregnant. Ask the patient about kidney or liver disease, which may affect metabolism of these drugs.

Teach patients and their caregivers that extended-release forms of these drugs must be swallowed whole and not chewed or split in half. Be sure to give apomorphine (Apokyn) subcutaneously and not intravenously.

Remove the old patch before applying a new rotigotine (Neupro) patch to an area of clean, dry skin at the same time daily. Press firmly for 20 to 30 seconds, especially around the edges for good adherence. After removing the old patch, be sure to wash the site with soap and water to remove any adhesive or drug.

What To Do *After* Giving Drugs for Parkinson's Disease

Regularly reassess the patient's vital signs, including blood pressure, heart rate, and respiratory rate every 4 to 8 hours. Because of side effects such as dizziness and hypotension, instruct the patient to call for help when getting out of bed and ensure that the call light is within easy reach. Tell the patient to change positions slowly.

Reassess the patient's mental status and watch for confusion or hallucinations. Watch the patient taking ropinirole (Requip) for episodes of falling asleep suddenly (narcolepsy). Report this immediately to the prescriber because the drug may need to be discontinued.

Ask the patient about side effects such as nausea and vomiting. Watch for side effects or adverse effects and report them immediately to the prescriber. Signs and symptoms of such adverse effects as neutropenia, neuroleptic malignant syndrome, and rhabdomyolysis are summarized in Table 26-3. Observe the patient for signs of drug allergic reactions such as rashes, hives, or changes in respiratory status.

After giving these drugs, be sure to monitor the patient's intake and output and assess for bladder distention because some drugs can cause urine retention. Monitor the patient for difficulty swallowing, which could increase the risk for aspiration.

Keep track of bowel movements and check bowel sounds because some drugs for Parkinson's disease can cause constipation or diarrhea.

Reassess dyskinesia, rigidity, tremors, and gait while the patient is taking drugs for Parkinson's disease.

Monitor skin condition for patients receiving the rotigotine (Neupro) patch. Be sure to rotate the site and do not apply to the same site more than once every 14 days. Always wash your hands after handling these patches.

 Drug Alert!

Administration Alert

Always press firmly on the rotigotine (Neupro) patch for good adherence.

QSEN: Safety

 Clinical Pitfall

Be sure to give apomorphine subcutaneously and not intravenously because intravenous drugs are immediately absorbed and act very rapidly.

QSEN: Safety

 Drug Alert!

Action/Intervention Alert

Immediately report episodes of narcolepsy to the prescriber for a patient taking ropinirole (Requip).

QSEN: Safety

 Drug Alert!

Action/Intervention Alert

To determine the effectiveness of drug therapy for Parkinson's disease, regularly reassess the patient for dyskinesia, rigidity, tremors, and gait.

QSEN: Safety

Table 26-3 Signs and Symptoms of Adverse Effects of Drugs Used to Treat Parkinson's Disease

ADVERSE EFFECT	SIGNS AND SYMPTOMS	ADVERSE EFFECT	SIGNS AND SYMPTOMS
Neuroleptic malignant syndrome	Changes in cognition, including agitation, delirium, and coma High fever Muscle rigidity Muscle tremors Pharyngitis Unstable blood pressure	Rhabdomyolysis	Dark red or cola-colored urine Fatigue Generalized weakness Joint pain Muscle stiffness or aching Muscle tenderness Seizures Unintentional weight gain Weakness of the affected muscle(s)
Neutropenia	Anal ulcers Decreased immune response Fever Increased risk of bacterial infections Painful mouth ulcers Sore throat		

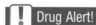 **Drug Alert!**

Teaching Alert

Patients should be taught to notify their prescriber immediately if symptoms of Parkinson's disease (for example, shaking, stiffness, and slow movement) become worse.

QSEN: Safety

What To Teach Patients Taking Drugs for Parkinson's Disease

Always include the person providing home care when teaching about these drugs. Instruct the caregiver to report any changes in swallowing ability to the prescriber because of the increased risk of aspiration.

Instruct patients to take drugs for Parkinson's disease exactly as prescribed and stress the importance of keeping follow-up appointments to monitor the progress of treatment. Remind them to notify the prescriber if symptoms of Parkinson's disease (for example, shaking, stiffness, and slow movement) become worse. Teach them to report any side effects immediately to their prescriber. Tell them to consult their prescriber or pharmacist before taking any over-the-counter or herbal products.

Missed doses of drugs for Parkinson's disease should be taken as soon as possible. However, if it is almost time for the next dose, teach patients to skip the missed dose to avoid taking a double dose of these drugs.

Tell patients that some drugs for Parkinson's disease are started at lower doses and gradually increased by the prescriber to best control the symptoms. Remind them that these drugs can be used to control symptoms but do not cure the disease. Instruct them to avoid stopping these drugs suddenly because symptoms may become much worse.

Teach patients to be careful not to overdo physical activities but to gradually increase activities to avoid falls and injuries.

Remind patients to always notify their surgeons or dentists that they are taking these drugs before having any surgical procedure.

Drugs such as selegiline (Carbex) may cause photosensitivity. Tell patients to wear protective clothing and sunscreen and to avoid excessive sun exposure. Because of side effects such as dizziness and drowsiness, caution patients to avoid driving, operating machines, or doing anything that requires increased alertness. Teach them to avoid alcohol or other CNS depressants because they can add to the drowsiness sometimes caused by these drugs. Instruct them to change positions slowly because of the possible side effect of hypotension.

Tell patients to take drugs that cause GI upset with food or milk. Teach patients prescribed anticholinergic drugs to have regular eye examinations because these drugs can cause blurred vision. Dry mouth can be kept to a minimum by frequent mouth care, ice chips, or sugarless candy.

Tell patients who are prescribed entacapone (Comtan) that this drug may change urine to a brownish-orange color and explain that this side effect is not harmful.

Instruct patients who are prescribed an MAO-B inhibitor such as selegiline (Carbex) or rasagiline (Azilect) to avoid the foods listed in Box 26-2 while taking these drugs and for 2 weeks after stopping them. Teach them also to avoid large amounts of chocolate, coffee, tea, or colas with caffeine. These foods contain tyramine, an amino acid that can cause a hypertensive crisis in patients receiving MAO inhibitor therapy.

Anticholinergic drugs can cause decreased perspiration. Caution patients taking these drugs to be careful about overheating in hot weather.

 Drug Alert!

Teaching Alert

While taking selegiline (Carbex) or rasagiline (Azilect), patients should avoid foods that contain tyramine (see Box 26-2).

QSEN: Safety

 Drug Alert!

Teaching Alert

Teach patients taking anticholinergic drugs to remain indoors in an air-conditioned setting during hot weather.

QSEN: Safety

Box 26-2	Foods to Avoid When Taking MAO Inhibitors
• Aged cheeses	• Pickled herring
• Avocados	• Poultry
• Bananas	• Raisins
• Figs	• Red wine
• Beer	• Salami
• Broad beans	• Sauerkraut
• Dried sausage	• Sour cream
• Fish	• Soy sauce
• Liver	• Yeast extract
• Meats prepared with tenderizer	• Yogurt

Inform patients taking the combination of carbidopa-levodopa (Sinemet) that this drug can cause darkening of urine or perspiration. Caution them to report any changes in skin lesions immediately to the prescriber because carbidopa-levodopa can activate malignant melanoma. This drug may be contraindicated in patients with a history of melanoma.

Patients prescribed apomorphine (Apokyn) at home need special teaching about how to give the subcutaneous injections and how to care for the special dosing pen used to give this drug. Include the caregiver in your teaching because the patient's muscle rigidity and tremors may make it impossible to self-inject.

Teach patients and caregivers how to apply the rotigotine (Neupro) patch system correctly including care of sites, rotation of sites, and washing hands after handling the patches.

Life Span Considerations for Drugs for Parkinson's Disease

Considerations for Pregnancy and Lactation. Although Parkinson's disease is very rare in women of childbearing age, bromocriptine (Parlodel) is usually not recommended during pregnancy or breastfeeding. It stops the production of breast milk. Most drugs for Parkinson's disease have a moderate likelihood of increasing the risk for birth defects or fetal harm. They have not been tested in pregnancy or breastfeeding and should not be used unless the benefits outweigh the risks.

Considerations for Older Adults. Older adults should be aware that they may experience confusion, hallucinations, and uncontrolled body movements because they are more sensitive to the effects of these drugs.

The older adult with Parkinson's disease is already unstable when walking and is at increased risk for falls. The drugs can cause a rapid decrease in blood pressure. Remind older adults to sit on the side of the bed for a few moments before attempting to stand and to change positions slowly. Instruct them to wear shoes, rather than slippers, for better stability and to use handrails when going up or down stairs. Assess the older adult's need for assistive devices, such as a cane or a walker for ambulating.

> **! Drug Alert!**
>
> **Teaching Alert**
>
> Because carbidopa-levodopa may activate malignant melanoma, instruct patients to watch for and report any changes in skin lesions to their prescriber immediately.
>
> QSEN: Safety

Get Ready for Practice!

Key Points

- Alzheimer's disease and Parkinson's disease are both progressive neurologic disorders that occur more often with aging.
- There is no cure for either Alzheimer's disease or Parkinson's disease. Treatment focuses on controlling symptoms.
- Alzheimer's disease is the most common form of dementia and affects a person's ability to perform activities of daily living.
- With Alzheimer's disease, neurons essential to memory and cognitive function die.
- Mild forgetfulness, the first symptom of Alzheimer's disease, can be confused with age-related memory changes.
- With Parkinson's disease, there is a deficit of chemical messengers called *neurotransmitters* that facilitate transmission of brain impulses.
- The major symptoms of Parkinson's disease are tremor at rest, rigidity, bradykinesia, and abnormal gait. (Tremor is often the initial symptom.)

- The goals of treatment for Parkinson's disease are minimizing disability, reducing possible side effects of drug therapy, and helping the patient to maintain a high quality of life.
- Patient safety is a major concern for patients with Parkinson's disease and Alzheimer's disease.
- Teach a patient to report worsening of Parkinson's disease symptoms immediately to his or her prescriber.

Additional Learning Resources

evolve Be sure to visit your Evolve website (http://evolve.elsevier.com/Workman/pharmacology/) for additional online resources.

SG Go to your Study Guide for additional learning activities to help you master this chapter content.

Review Questions

See the Answer Keys—In-text Review Questions for answers to these questions.

Test Yourself on the Basics

1. Which statement about drug therapy for Alzheimer's disease is accurate?
   A. Lifelong drug prescriptions are the cure for Alzheimer's disease.
   B. Drug therapy for Alzheimer's disease must be taken until the symptoms resolve.
   C. Medications prescribed to treat Alzheimer's disease slow progression of the illness.
   D. A combination of drug therapy, diet, and exercise is necessary to cure the illness.

2. A patient is prescribed memantine (Namenda) for Alzheimer's disease. For which common side effects should you monitor? (Select all that apply.)
   A. Diarrhea
   B. Constipation
   C. Dizziness
   D. Confusion
   E. Fatigue
   F. Headache

3. Which lab tests should you check before and after administering memantine to a patient?
   A. Hematocrit and hemoglobin
   B. Clotting studies including activated partial thromboplastin time (aPTT) and international normalized ratio (INR)
   C. Serum electrolytes
   D. White blood cell count

4. When should you teach a patient and his or her caregivers to administer donepezil (Aricept)?
   A. In the morning before breakfast
   B. Thirty minutes before lunch
   C. With the first bite at any meal
   D. In the evening at bedtime

5. A patient with Parkinson's disease is prescribed the rotigotine (Neupro) patch. What must you do to ensure proper adherence of the patch to the patient's skin?
   A. Wash the skin with soap and warm water before applying the patch.
   B. Place a skin protective lotion on the skin around the patch.
   C. Press firmly on the patch especially around the edges for 20 to 30 seconds.
   D. Remove the old patch and apply the new patch to the same area.

Test Yourself on Advanced Concepts

6. How do cholinesterase/acetylcholinesterase inhibitor drugs used for Alzheimer's disease work?
   A. They prolong the availability of dopamine.
   B. They inhibit the breakdown of acetylcholine.
   C. They inhibit transmission of abnormal nerve impulses.
   D. They act in the brain to degrade dopamine more rapidly.

7. The spouse of a patient with Alzheimer's disease asks you how memantine (Namenda) will help his wife. What is your best response?
   A. "Memantine will prevent overstimulation of certain receptors in the brain which seems to be one cause of Alzheimer's disease."
   B. "This drug treatment will cure your wife's Alzheimer's disease."
   C. "The action of memantine will slow the progression of the disease by keeping levels of acetylcholine higher."
   D. "This drug will not cure your wife's disease, but it will prevent it from getting worse."

8. Which assessments are essential before and after giving a drug for Alzheimer's disease? (Select all that apply.)
   A. Language skills
   B. Weight
   C. Bowel function
   D. Swallowing
   E. Ability to perform simple tasks

9. What do you teach the spouse and the patient who has been prescribed rivastigmine (Exelon) about common side effects? (Select all that apply.)
   A. "Give this drug once a day at bedtime."
   B. "Check the patient's blood pressure before giving the drug."
   C. "Rivastigmine can cause you to feel tired and weak."
   D. "The drug works best when given on an empty stomach."
   E. "Remember to get up slowly because this drug can cause dizziness."

10. What precaution must you teach the spouse of an older, frail female patient with Alzheimer's disease who is prescribed donepezil (Aricept)?
    A. Be sure to keep your wife on bedrest after she takes this drug.
    B. Have your wife drink extra water because this drug decreases urination.
    C. Be sure to monitor your wife's weight and report weight loss to the prescriber.
    D. Monitor your wife's breathing because this drug can cause chronic difficulty with breathing.

11. Which patient response indicates to you that benztropine (Cogentin) therapy for Parkinson's disease is effective?
    A. Reduced tremor and muscle rigidity
    B. Improved memory and attention span
    C. Increased ability to perform simple tasks
    D. Prevention of seizures

12. For which dangerous adverse effects must you monitor in a patient who is taking carbidopa-levodopa (Sinemet)? (Select all that apply.)
    A. Decreased white blood cells
    B. Suicidal thoughts
    C. Rhabdomyolysis
    D. Respiratory depression
    E. Neuroleptic malignant syndrome

13. Which foods should you teach the patient prescribed rasagiline (Azilect) to avoid? (Select all that apply.)
    A. Avocadoes
    B. White wines
    C. Yogurt
    D. Raisins
    E. Pasta
    F. Sauerkraut

14. About which safety measures must you instruct the older adult who has been prescribed carbidopa-levodopa for Parkinson's disease? (Select all that apply.)
    A. Apply sunscreens and wear protective clothing whenever outdoors.
    B. Always wear shoes and use handrails for stability when going up or down stairs.
    C. Monitor fluid intake and urine output to prevent dehydration.
    D. Sit on the side of the bed for a few minutes before getting up.
    E. Be sure to have regular eye examinations because this drug can cause blurred vision.

15. A patient with Alzheimer's disease is prescribed rivastigmine (Exelon) 4.5 mg twice a day. The drug comes in 1.5-mg tablets. How many tablets do you give for each dose? _____ tablet(s)

16. A patient with Parkinson's disease is ordered apomorphine (Apokyn) 0.6 mg subcutaneously. The drug comes in 10 mg/1 mL. How many milliliters do you inject for each dose? _____ mL

Critical Thinking Activities

See the Answer Keys—Critical Thinking Activities for answers to these activities.

Mr. Gates is a 71-year-old man who was diagnosed with Alzheimer's disease 5 years ago. His prescribed medications include donepezil (Aricept) 10 mg once a day at bedtime and memantine (Namenda) 5 mg each morning and evening. His wife tells you that he is still able to feed and dress himself as well as help with simple tasks, such as feeding the dog. He is admitted to the hospital for spinal surgery, which will be done under general anesthesia. Mrs. Gates tells you that she is worried about how her husband will react to general anesthesia.

1. What assessment questions will you be sure to ask Mr. Gates's wife?
2. Which teaching points will you be sure to include about Mr. Gates's medications and surgery?
3. What will you discuss with Mrs. Gates about Alzheimer's disease and the risks of general anesthesia?

Drug Therapy for Psychiatric Problems

Objectives

After studying this chapter you should be able to:

1. Explain how different classes of drugs are used to treat depression, anxiety, and psychosis.
2. List the common names, actions, usual adult dosages, possible side effects, and adverse effects of drugs for depression and anxiety.
3. Describe what to do before and after giving drugs for depression and anxiety.
4. Explain what to teach patients taking drugs for depression and anxiety, including what to do, what not to do, and when to call the prescriber or pharmacist.
5. Describe life span considerations for drugs for depression and anxiety.

6. List the common names, actions, usual adult dosages, possible side effects, and adverse effects of drugs for psychosis.
7. Describe what to do before and after giving drugs for psychosis.
8. Explain what to teach patients taking drugs for psychosis, including what to do, what not to do, and when to call the prescriber or pharmacist.
9. Describe life span considerations for drugs for psychosis.

Key Terms

antianxiety drug (ăn-tē-ăng-ZĪ-ĕ-tē DRŬG) (p. 441) A drug that eases anxiety; also known as an anxiolytic.

antidepressant drug (ăn-tē-dē-PRĔS-sĕnt DRŬG) (p. 434) A drug used to treat the symptoms of depression.

antipsychotic drug (ăn-tē-sī-KŎT-ĭk DRŬG) (p. 444) A drug used to treat psychosis; also called major tranquilizers and neuroleptics.

anxiety (ăng-ZĪ-ĕ-tē) (p. 438) A multiple-system response sometimes described as a feeling of dread about a perceived threat or danger thought to be unique to humans.

benzodiazepine (bĕn-zō-dī-ĂZ-ĕ-pēn) (p. 441) A type of drug commonly used to treat anxiety, produce sedation, or relax muscles.

depression (dē-PRĔSH-ŭn) (p. 432) An illness characterized by feelings of sadness, despair, loss of energy, and difficulty dealing with normal daily life.

psychosis (sī-KŌ-sĭs) (p. 443) An illness that prevents a person from being able to distinguish between the real world and the imaginary world; it commonly includes delusions or hallucinations.

selective serotonin reuptake inhibitors (SSRIs) (sĕ-LĔK-tĭv sĕr-ō-TŌ-nĭn rē-ŬP-tāk ĭn-HĬB-ĭ-tŭrz) (p. 435) Antidepressant drugs that act by blocking the reuptake of serotonin, making more serotonin available to act on receptors in the brain.

tricyclic antidepressants (TCAs) (trī-SĪK-lĭk ăn-tē-dē-PRĔS-sĕnts) (p. 435) Antidepressant drugs that act by blocking the reuptake of norepinephrine and serotonin and making more of these substances available to act on receptors in the brain.

OVERVIEW

Psychiatric disorders are a broad group of illnesses that may include affective or emotional instability, behavioral problems, and cognitive dysfunction or impairment. Mental illness may be of biological (for example, anatomic, chemical, or genetic) or psychologic (for example, emotional trauma or conflict) origin and may affect a person's ability to function in society or relationships. Specific illnesses include major depression, generalized anxiety disorder, bipolar disorder, and schizophrenia.

Major mental illnesses are the most common cause of disability in the United States. About 26.2% of U.S. adults experience a clinically diagnosable mental illness each year. Between 13% and 20% of children younger than age 18 experience serious emotional disturbance with functional impairment, whereas 5% to 9% have serious emotional disturbance with extreme functional impairment caused by a mental illness.

Depression, anxiety, and psychosis are major psychiatric illnesses. As many as 30% of patients in the United States report symptoms of depression, but only about 10% experience major depression. Anxiety affects as much as 18% of the population in the United States each year. The incidence of schizophrenia, a major psychotic disorder, is about 1% in the United States. The chronic nature of these illnesses presents many challenges for treatment.

GENERAL ISSUES RELATED TO DRUG THERAPY FOR PSYCHIATRIC PROBLEMS

Drug therapy is extremely important in the management of psychiatric problems. General responsibilities with drugs for depression, anxiety, and psychosis are discussed in the following paragraphs, followed by chapter sections related to specific drugs for each illness. Be sure to use the principles listed in Chapter 2 when administering any drug for a psychiatric problem.

Before giving any drug for a psychiatric problem, always obtain a complete list of the patient's current drugs including over-the-counter and herbal preparations. Check vital signs including blood pressure, heart rate, and respiratory rate to establish a baseline. Assess any patient's risk for falls and apply precautions if needed. If the drug is to be given intravenously, assess the site and ensure that it is patent. Ask women of childbearing age if they are pregnant or breastfeeding, or if they plan to become pregnant.

Assess each patient's mental status and ask about suicidal thoughts. Notify the prescriber immediately if the patient has a suicide plan. Place patients on suicide precautions if needed.

After giving any drug for a psychiatric problem recheck the patient's blood pressure and heart rate and rhythm and monitor for decreased blood pressure and abnormal heart rhythms. Because of the increased risk for dizziness, instruct patients to call for assistance when getting out of bed and ensure that the call light is within easy reach. Continue to monitor patients for dizziness, drowsiness, or light-headedness. Watch for side effects and adverse effects and report changes to the prescriber.

Reassess a patient's mental status and continue to monitor for suicidal ideation or a suicide plan.

Teach patients receiving any psychiatric drug to take these drugs exactly as directed by their prescriber and pharmacist. Tell patients about the importance of keeping follow-up appointments to monitor the progress of treatment. Tell patients to report any side effects to their prescriber or pharmacist immediately.

If a drug dose is missed, tell the patient to take the dose as soon as possible unless it is almost time for the next dose. Remind him or her not to double the doses of these drugs.

Caution patients to avoid driving, operating heavy or complicated equipment, or doing anything requiring alertness because of drowsiness, dizziness, and impaired (blurred) vision until the effects of the drug are known. Remind them to change positions slowly because of hypotension and dizziness.

Remind women of childbearing age to notify their prescriber if they are pregnant, plan to become pregnant, or are breastfeeding.

Tell patients to avoid alcohol while taking these drugs because alcohol may increase drowsiness and central nervous system (CNS) depression.

Remind patients to tell all health care providers about taking these drugs before having any surgical procedures, including dental surgery, because many of these drugs work on the CNS, causing side effects such as hypotension, dizziness, and drowsiness.

Advise patients to wear a medical alert bracelet or carry an identification card stating the name of the drug and the reason for taking it.

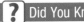 **Did You Know?**

As many as 30% of patients in the United States report symptoms of depression, and about 10% experience major depression.

 Clinical Pitfall

Immediately report any suicidal thoughts or suicide plans to the prescriber.

QSEN: Safety

 Drug Alert!

Interaction Alert

Patients taking an antidepressant that causes drowsiness should avoid alcohol because it can increase the drowsiness.

QSEN: Safety

DEPRESSION

Depression is an illness characterized by persistent feelings of sadness, despair, loss of energy, and difficulty dealing with normal daily life. It involves the body, mood, and thoughts and affects how a person eats and sleeps, how a person feels about himself or herself and relates to others, and how he or she thinks about things. It interferes with the ability to function normally and causes pain and suffering for patients with this disorder and their loved ones. Figure 27-1 gives some examples of depression.

Depression can occur at any age but typically develops in the middle teens, 20s, or 30s. Women are twice as likely as men to experience depression, and men are less likely than women to seek treatment. Because depression is often mistaken for a normal part of aging, many older adults with depression may be undiagnosed or untreated. Children and adolescents with depression often pretend to be sick, refuse to go to school, get into trouble in school, have negative outlooks, and feel misunderstood. Many people with depression do not seek treatment because they do not recognize the condition as a treatable illness.

There are three forms of depressive disorders: major depression, dysthymia, and bipolar disorder. *Major depression* is a disabling mental disorder marked by a persistent low mood, lack of pleasure in life, and increased risk of suicide. Diagnosis is based on the presence of five or more depression symptoms that last 2 weeks or more (Box 27-1). Major depression may occur just once or several times during a lifetime.

Dysthymia is a chronic but less severe form of depression characterized by moods that are persistently low. The symptoms may be daunting but are not disabling. A person with dysthymia may experience episodes of major depression.

? Did You Know?

Women are twice as likely as men to experience depression; men are less likely to seek treatment.

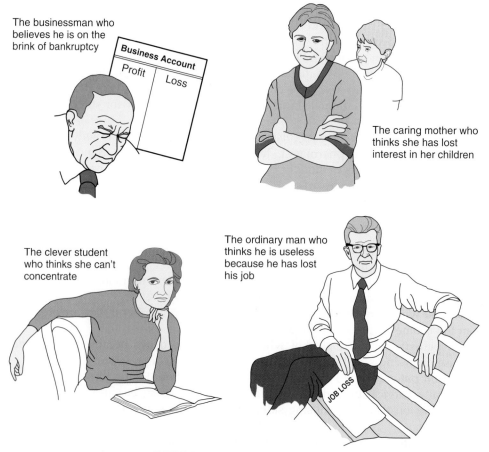

FIGURE 27-1 Examples of depression.

| Box 27-1 | Symptoms of Depression |

- Abrupt changes in eating habits
- Chronic fatigue; being slowed down
- Decreased ability to perform normal daily tasks
- Decreased appetite and/or weight loss or overeating and weight gain
- Difficulty concentrating, remembering, or making decisions
- Feelings of hopelessness or pessimism
- Inability to experience pleasure in hobbies and activities that were once enjoyed
- Insomnia, early morning awakening, or oversleeping
- Irritability
- Numb or empty feeling or absence of any feelings at all
- Persistent feeling of worthlessness, guilt, helplessness, or sadness
- Persistent physical symptoms that do not respond to treatment (for example, headaches, digestive disorders, chronic pain)
- Recurrent thoughts of death or suicide
- Restlessness

| Box 27-2 | Symptoms of Mania |

- Abnormal or excessive elation
- Decreased need for sleep
- Grandiose notions
- Inappropriate social behavior
- Increased sexual desire
- Increased talking
- Markedly increased energy
- Poor judgment
- Racing thoughts
- Unusual irritability

Bipolar disorder, formerly called manic depression, is characterized by cycling moods from severe highs (*mania*) to severe lows (depression). Mood changes may be sudden and dramatic, or they may be gradual. During a low cycle, the person has symptoms of depression (see Box 27-1). During a high cycle, he or she may be overactive, overly talkative, and full of energy. Mania can affect thought processes, judgment, and social behavior. Box 27-2 summarizes symptoms of mania. Untreated mania may progress to psychosis.

Diagnosis of depression is based on identifying symptoms (see Box 27-1). A complete physical examination is important to rule out physical disorders such as thyroid disease, anemia, and viral infections. A detailed history by a qualified health care professional is important to discover specific factors in a patient's life that may contribute to depression.

The most common treatments for depression include counseling or psychotherapy and antidepressant drugs. Depression treatment is individualized, taking into account the severity and cause of the depression episode. Most patients with depression are treated as outpatients; however, when a person has suicidal thoughts (also called *suicidal ideation*), and particularly if the person has a suicide plan, hospitalization may be required. With treatment, symptoms can be well controlled. Figure 27-2 shows the cycle of depression, including how and when to intervene for effective treatment with medications and psychotherapy.

REVIEW OF RELATED PHYSIOLOGY AND PATHOPHYSIOLOGY

The exact cause of depression is not known, but theories include heredity, changes in neurotransmitter levels, altered neuroendocrine function, and psychosocial factors. Table 27-1 summarizes factors often associated with depression.

Research suggests that depression may be caused by an imbalance of brain chemicals called *neurotransmitters* (for example, serotonin, dopamine, and norepinephrine). Communication between neurons in the brain occurs by the movement of these chemicals across a small gap called the *synapse*. Neurotransmitters are released from

 Memory Jogger

Bipolar disorder is characterized by cycling moods—from severe highs to severe lows.

 Clinical Pitfall

When a patient with depression has suicidal thoughts and a suicide plan, hospitalization may be required for the patient's safety.

QSEN: Safety

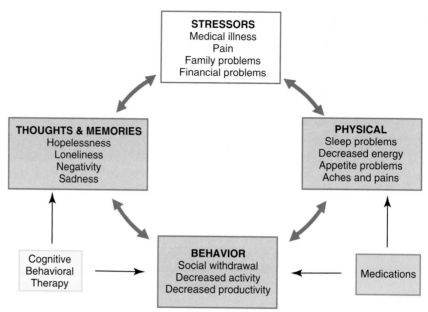

FIGURE 27-2   The cycle of depression.

Table 27-1   Factors Associated with Depression

FACTOR	EXAMPLES	FACTOR	EXAMPLES
Chemicals	Dopamine	Heredity	First-degree relatives
Physical factors	Norepinephrine	Physical illness	(for example,
Drugs	Serotonin	Psychosocial factors	mother, father)
Gender	Environmental	Seasonal	Acquired immune
	conditions		deficiency syndrome
	Extreme stress		Adrenal disorders
	Trauma		Brain tumors
	Abuse of alcohol or		Multiple sclerosis
	amphetamines		Parkinson's disease
	Antipsychotics		Stroke
	Beta blockers		Thyroid disorders
	Corticosteroids		Abuse
	Reserpine		Introversion
	Postmenopause		Separations or losses
	Postpartum		Climates with long,
	Thyroid dysfunction		severe winter
	Women twice as		
	susceptible as men		

one neuron at the presynaptic nerve terminal and then cross the synapse, where they may be accepted by the next neuron at a specialized site called a receptor (Figure 27-3). When neurotransmitter levels decrease or become imbalanced, the neurons may be less able to communicate with each other, which may lead to depression and other mood changes.

TYPES OF DRUGS FOR DEPRESSION

ANTIDEPRESSANTS

How Antidepressants Work

Antidepressant drugs are used to treat people with depression. Prescribing and using these prescription drugs can lead to the improvement of symptoms, particularly when patients also receive some form of psychotherapy or counseling.

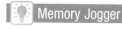

Memory Jogger

The two most common groups of drugs to treat depression are SSRIs and TCAs.

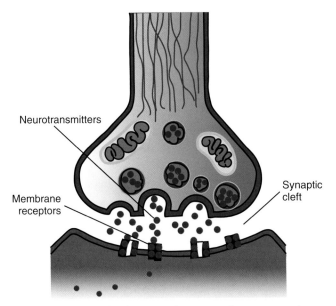

FIGURE 27-3   Neurotransmitters carry signals across the synapse from a neuron to receptors on the next neuron.

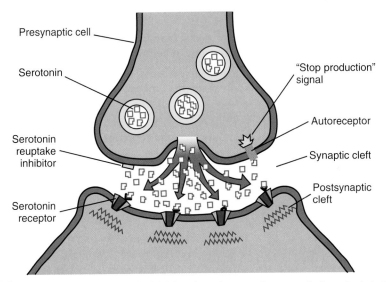

FIGURE 27-4   Selective serotonin reuptake inhibitor drugs increase the amount of serotonin in the brain by blocking reuptake of neurotransmitters by neurons.

The two most common groups of drugs used to treat depression are **selective serotonin reuptake inhibitors (SSRIs),** and **tricyclic antidepressants (TCAs).** SSRIs have fewer side effects and are more commonly prescribed than TCAs. With most of these drugs, it can take as long as 8 weeks for symptoms of depression to improve. Often depression is chronic, and patients must continue to take antidepressants even when they have no symptoms to keep the depression from returning.

SSRIs work by increasing the amount of serotonin in the brain by inhibiting reuptake (Figure 27-4). TCAs inhibit the reuptake of the neurotransmitters norepinephrine, dopamine, and serotonin by nerve cells. The effects of these drugs occur immediately, but the patient's symptoms often do not respond for 2 to 8 weeks. Other drugs such as norepinephrine and dopamine reuptake inhibitors (NDRIs; for example, bupropion [Wellbutrin]) correct the imbalance of the neurotransmitters dopamine and norepinephrine.

 Do Not Confuse

Celexa *with* Zyprexa or Celebrex

An order for Celexa may be confused with Zyprexa or Celebrex. Celexa is an SSRI drug used to treat depression, whereas Zyprexa is an antipsychotic drug used to treat psychotic disorders. Celebrex is a nonsteroidal anti-inflammatory drug (NSAID) used to treat osteoarthritis and rheumatoid arthritis.

QSEN: Safety

 Do Not Confuse

buPROPion *with* busPIRone

An order for bupropion can be confused with buspirone. Bupropion is an antidepressant drug, whereas buspirone is an antianxiety drug.

QSEN: Safety

 Do Not Confuse

Wellbutrin SR *with* Wellbutrin XL

An order for Wellbutrin SR can be confused with Wellbutrin XL. Both drugs are norepinephrine and dopamine reuptake inhibitors used to treat depression. But Wellbutrin SR is a slow-release form of the drug given twice a day, whereas Wellbutrin XL is an extended-release form of the drug given once a day.

QSEN: Safety

 Do Not Confuse

trazodone *with* tramadol

An order for trazodone may be confused with tramadol. Trazodone is a combined reuptake inhibitor and receptor blocker used to treat depression, whereas tramadol is an analgesic used to treat moderate to moderately severe pain.

QSEN: Safety

Generic names, trade names, and dosages of common antidepressants are listed in the following table. Be sure to consult a drug handbook for specific information about any drug used to treat depression.

Dosages for Common Antidepressant Drugs

Drug	Dosage
SSRIs	
citalopram (Celexa)	*Adults:* 20 mg orally once daily; may increase by 20 mg per week up to 60 mg/day; usual dosage is 20-40 mg/day
escitalopram (Lexapro)	*Adults:* 10 mg orally once daily; may increase to 20 mg after 1 week
fluoxetine (Prozac, Prozac Weekly)	*Adults:* 20 mg orally daily in the morning; may increase by 20 mg every 4 weeks up to 80 mg; doses over 20 mg/day should be given in 2 divided doses every 12 hours; 90 mg once a week *Children (8-18 years):* 10-20 mg orally daily; may increase to 20 mg/day after 1 week
paroxetine (Paxil, Paxil CR)	*Adults:* 20 mg orally daily, may increase by 10 mg per week up to 50 mg/day; controlled-release (CR)—12.5 mg/day, may increase by 12.5 mg per week to a maximum dosage of 62.5 mg/day
sertraline (Zoloft)	*Adults:* 50 mg orally daily; may increase by 25 mg/day each week; maximum dosage 200 mg/day *Children (13-17 years):* 50 mg orally once daily *Children (6-12 years):* 25 mg orally once daily
TCAs	
amitriptyline (Apo-Amitriptyline ♣, Elavil)	*Adults:* 75 mg orally daily in divided doses; may increase to 150 mg/day; maintenance dose 50-100 mg once a day at bedtime.
desipramine (Norpramin, Pertofrane ♣)	*Adults:* 100-200 mg orally daily; may increase to 300 mg/day *Children (>12 years):* 25-50 mg orally daily; may increase to 100 mg/day over 1-2 weeks *Children (6-12 years):* 1-5 mg/kg orally every 8-12 hours
imipramine (Impril ♣, Norfranil, Novo Pramine ♣, Tofranil)	*Adults:* 25-50 mg orally every 6-8 hours; maximum dosage 300 mg/day; may give total dosage at bedtime *Children (>12 years):* 12.5-25 mg orally every 12 hours; maximum dosage 75 mg/day *Children (6-12 years):* 12.5 mg orally every 12 hours; maximum dosage 25 mg every 12 hours
nortriptyline (Aventyl, Pamelor)	*Adults:* 25 mg orally every 6-8 hours up to 150 mg/day
Serotonin and Norepinephrine Reuptake Inhibitors	
duloxetine (Cymbalta)	*Adults:* 20-30 mg orally every 12 hours
venlafaxine (Effexor)	*Adults:* 25 mg orally every 8-12 hours; maximum dosage 125 mg every 8 hours; extended release (XR)—75 mg once daily
Norepinephrine and Dopamine Reuptake Inhibitors	
buPROPion (Wellbutrin)	*Adults:* 100 mg orally twice daily; maximum dosage 450 mg or 150 mg every 8 hours
Combined Reuptake Inhibitors and Receptor Blockers	
mirtazapine (Remeron)	*Adults:* 15 mg orally daily in single bedtime dose; maximum dosage 45 mg/day
nefazodone (Serzone)	*Adults:* 100 mg orally twice daily; maximum dosage 600 mg/day or 300 mg every 12 hours
trazodone (Desyrel)	*Adults:* 50 mg orally 3 times a day; maximum dosage 200 mg every 8 hours

Intended Responses

- Depression is corrected.
- Symptoms of depressed mood are decreased.

Side Effects. SSRI drugs have many side effects. The most common side effects of SSRIs include drowsiness, dizziness, fatigue, insomnia, GI upset (e.g., nausea, diarrhea, dyspepsia, and flatulence), and impotence with decreased interest in sexual activity. Other side effect include apathy, anxiety, nervousness, confusion, headache, weakness, abdominal pain, anorexia, dry mouth, increased saliva, increased sweating, weight gain, and tremors. Venlafaxine (Effexor) can cause increased blood pressure.

Common side effects of TCAs include lethargy, sedation, drowsiness, fatigue, blurred vision, dry eyes, dry mouth, hypotension, and constipation.

Side effects occur more often in the first few days and often improve over time.

Adverse Effects. TCAs such as amitriptyline (Elavil), desipramine (Norpramin), imipramine (Tofranil), and nortriptyline (Aventyl) may cause serious adverse cardiac effects, including unstable ventricular dysrhythmias (abnormal heart rhythms) or asystole (absence of a heart rhythm).

Venlafaxine (Effexor), duloxetine (Cymbalta), and bupropion (Wellbutrin) may cause seizures. Mirtazapine (Remeron) can lead to neutropenia (decreased white blood cells [WBCs]), which increases the risk of infection. Nefazodone has been known to cause liver failure or liver toxicity.

Thoughts of suicide may increase in children, adolescents, and young adults when taking antidepressants; a warning appears on all labels for these drugs.

Signs of allergic reactions to antidepressants include chest pain, increased or irregular heart rhythm, shortness of breath, fever, hives, rash, itching, difficulty breathing or swallowing, swelling, decreased coordination, shaking hands (tremors), dizziness, light-headedness, and thoughts of hurting oneself.

Serotonin syndrome is a rare adverse effect that occurs when levels of serotonin are very high. Signs and symptoms of serotonin syndrome include anxiety, agitation, sweating, confusion, tremors, restlessness, lack of coordination, and rapid heart rate.

What To Do *Before* Giving Antidepressants

In addition to the general responsibilities related to drugs for psychiatric problems (p. 431), ask whether the patient has a family history of depression. Ask about usual bowel pattern, fluid intake, and diet. Notify the prescriber if the patient is taking the herbal preparation, St. John's wort.

If a patient is taking a TCA, ask about smoking because smoking cigarettes may decrease the effectiveness of these drugs.

Wellbutrin may be prescribed as Wellbutrin SR, the sustained-release form, which is administered in two doses at least 8 hours apart. Wellbutrin XL extended-release tablets should be taken once a day in the morning. Wellbutrin SR and XL tablets should be swallowed whole and never chewed, divided, or crushed.

What To Do *After* Giving Antidepressants

In addition to the general responsibilities related to drugs for psychiatric problems (p. 431), reassess the patient's mental status to determine his or her response to drugs. Monitor the patient for drug side effects, adverse effects, or allergic reactions and report them to the prescriber.

What To Teach Patients Taking Antidepressants

In addition to the general responsibilities related to teaching patients about drugs for psychiatric problems (p. 431), explain that their prescriber may start with a low drug dose and gradually increase it until therapeutic antidepressant effects are achieved.

Remind patients that antidepressants can control the symptoms of depression but will not cure depression. Teach them that it may take 1 to 8 weeks before symptoms of depression improve. Remind patients to take their antidepressant even when feeling well.

Explain that antidepressants may need to be discontinued gradually to avoid adverse effects.

Teach patients that Wellbutrin works by correcting the imbalance of the neurotransmitters dopamine and norepinephrine and that it may be prescribed as

Common Side Effects

Antidepressants

GI upset, Nausea, Diarrhea, Flatulence, Dyspepsia, Constipation

Dizziness

Drowsiness, Fatigue

Impotence, Decreased libido

Drug Alert!

Interaction Alert

Be sure to ask a patient about the use of St. John's wort, an herbal product used to treat depression. It should not be taken with antidepressant drugs.

QSEN: Safety

Drug Alert!

Interaction Alert

Ask patients taking a TCA drug about smoking because smoking cigarettes may decrease the effectiveness of these drugs.

QSEN: Safety

Drug Alert!

Teaching Alert

Be sure to teach patients who are taking an antidepressant that it may take 1 to 8 weeks before symptoms of depression improve.

QSEN: Safety

Clinical Pitfall

Instruct patients not to stop taking an antidepressant without first talking to their prescriber.

QSEN: Safety

Wellbutrin SR (sustained-release form, which is administered in two doses at least 8 hours apart) or Wellbutrin XL (extended-release tablets that should be taken once a day in the morning). Instruct patients that Wellbutrin SR and XL tablets should be swallowed whole and never chewed, divided, or crushed.

Tell patients that frequent mouth rinses and good oral hygiene can minimize the effects of dry mouth.

Instruct patients taking an SSRI to take the dose once a day in the morning or evening.

Caution patients taking a monoamine oxidase inhibitor (MAOI) and transitioning to an SSRI, TCA, or other antidepressant that these drugs should not be used for at least 14 days after discontinuing MAOI drugs because of a life-threatening drug interaction called *serotonin syndrome.* Teach that symptoms of this syndrome include confusion, agitation, restlessness, stomach disturbances, sudden elevated temperature, extremely high blood pressure, and severe seizures.

Life Span Considerations for Antidepressants

Pediatric Considerations. SSRIs, TCAs, and other antidepressant drugs should be used with caution in depressed children and adolescents because the risk for suicidal thoughts or actions may increase while taking these drugs. Fluoxetine (Prozac) may cause unusual excitement, restlessness, irritability, or trouble sleeping in children because they are more sensitive to the effects of this drug. Venlafaxine (Effexor) may slow growth and weight gain in children. A child's growth should be monitored carefully while taking this drug.

Considerations for Pregnancy and Lactation. SSRIs have a moderate likelihood of increasing the risk for birth defects or fetal harm. However, these drugs have not been tested during pregnancy. Paroxetine (Paxil) should be avoided in pregnancy. Some SSRIs pass through breast milk and may have unwanted effects such as drowsiness, decreased feeding, and weight loss in the breastfeeding infant. TCAs have a moderate to high likelihood of increasing the risk for birth defects or fetal harm.

Considerations for Older Adults. Older adults may require lower doses of SSRIs because of possible increased reaction to the effects and side effects of these drugs and slower metabolism of drugs such as escitalopram (Lexapro). Older patients with kidney disease or liver failure should be given lower doses of these drugs because they are metabolized by the liver and kidneys.

ANXIETY

Anxiety is a feeling of apprehension, fear, or worry. It can occur without a cause and may not be based on a real-life situation. Symptoms of anxiety vary with the form of anxiety disorder (Box 27-3).

Common anxiety disorders include panic disorder, generalized anxiety disorder, phobic disorder, obsessive-compulsive disorder, and posttraumatic stress disorder (PTSD).

Panic disorders are separate and intense periods of fear or feelings of doom that develop over a short period of time such as 10 minutes. A panic attack, the main symptom of panic disorder, is characterized by anxiety or terror and usually lasts between 15 and 30 minutes.

Generalized anxiety disorder (GAD) is when a person experiences excessive, almost daily anxiety and worry for more than 6 months. It affects about 3% of the population in the United States. Women are twice as likely as men to be affected. GAD most often begins during childhood or adolescence, but it may begin at any age.

Phobic disorders are intense, persistent, recurrent fears of certain objects (for example, snakes) or situations (for example, speaking in front of a group) that can cause a panic attack.

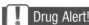
Clinical Pitfall

SSRIs, TCAs, and other antidepressant drugs should not be used for at least 14 days after discontinuing MAOI drugs because of the risk of the life-threatening drug interaction *serotonin syndrome.*

QSEN: Safety

Drug Alert!

Action/Intervention Alert

Monitor children and adolescents carefully because antidepressant drugs may increase the risk of suicidal thoughts or actions.

QSEN: Safety

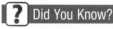
Did You Know?

Women are twice as likely as men to develop GAD.

Box 27-3	Symptoms of Anxiety

PANIC DISORDER
- Chest pain
- Chills or hot flashes
- Dizziness
- Feeling of being detached from the world (derealization)
- Fear of dying
- Nausea
- Numbness and tingling
- Palpitations
- Sense of choking
- Shortness of breath
- Sweating
- Trembling

GENERALIZED ANXIETY DISORDER
- Difficulty concentrating
- Easy fatigue
- Excessive, unrealistic worry
- Irritability
- Muscle tension
- Restlessness
- Sleep disturbance

PHOBIC DISORDER
- Intense, persistent, recurrent fear of certain objects (for example, snakes, spiders, blood)
- Intense, persistent, recurrent fear of certain situations (for example, heights, speaking in front of a group, public places)
- Panic attack possibly triggered by objects and situations

OBSESSIVE-COMPULSIVE DISORDER
- Obsessive thoughts such as:
  - Excessive focus on religious or moral ideas
  - Fear of being contaminated by germs or dirt or contaminating others
- Fear of causing harm to yourself or others
- Fear of losing or not having things you might need
- Intrusive sexually explicit or violent thoughts and images
- Order and symmetry—the idea that everything must line up "just right"
- Superstitions—excessive attention to something considered lucky or unlucky
- Compulsive behaviors such as:
  - Accumulating "junk" such as old newspapers, magazines, empty food containers, or other things for which you do not have a use
  - Counting, tapping, repeating certain words, or doing other senseless things to reduce anxiety
  - Excessively double checking things such as locks, appliances, and switches
  - Ordering or making groups of things even or arranging things "just so"
  - Praying excessively or engaging in rituals triggered by religious fear
  - Repeatedly checking in on loved ones to make sure they are safe
  - Spending a lot of time washing or cleaning

STRESS DISORDERS (POSTTRAUMATIC STRESS DISORDER)
- Avoiding activities, places, or people associated with the triggering event
- Being hypervigilant
- Difficulty concentrating
- Difficulty sleeping
- Feeling a general sense of doom and gloom along with decreased positive emotions and hopes for the future

Obsessive-compulsive disorder (OCD) is characterized by obsessive thoughts and compulsive actions. The person with OCD becomes trapped in a pattern of repetitive thoughts and behaviors that do not make sense and are distressing but are very difficult to overcome.

Posttraumatic stress disorder (PTSD) leads to anxiety and is caused by exposure to death or near-death experiences such as floods, fires, earthquakes, shootings, automobile accidents, or war. The traumatic experience recurs in thoughts and dreams.

Treatment of anxiety depends on the cause. Short-term anxiety attacks can be treated at home with interventions such as talking with a supportive person, meditating, taking a warm bath, resting in a dark room, or performing deep-breathing exercises. Strategies for coping with anxiety and stress include eating a well-balanced diet, getting enough sleep, exercising regularly, limiting caffeine and alcohol, avoiding nicotine and recreational drugs, using relaxation techniques, and balancing fun activities with responsibilities. Group therapy may be useful for anxieties such as fear of flying. Physical conditions may be treated with drugs or surgery. An example of a physical cause for anxiety is a tumor called a *pheochromocytoma*, which causes

 Memory Jogger

The common anxiety disorders include panic disorder, GAD, phobic disorder, OCD, and PTSD.

the adrenal glands to produce excessive amounts of adrenaline. Surgical removal of this tumor can resolve the symptom of anxiety. Symptoms of hyperthyroidism include anxiety. Careful diagnosis is essential because many of the symptoms of hyperthyroidism are also found in anxiety disorder. Hyperthyroidism and anxiety are often confused. Medical or surgical treatment of hyperthyroidism can also resolve the anxiety. Counseling or psychotherapy may also be helpful. Antianxiety drugs are often prescribed to control the symptoms of anxiety.

REVIEW OF RELATED PHYSIOLOGY AND PATHOPHYSIOLOGY

Anxiety that is perceived as out of proportion with what is normal or expected may escalate through a feedback circle (Figure 27-5). Physical symptoms may affect the heart (increased rate, pounding), lungs (increased rate and depth, shortness of breath), and nervous system (tremors, headaches). Emotional symptoms of anxiety include apprehension, dread, irritability, restlessness, and difficulty concentrating. Causes and factors associated with anxiety include mental conditions, physical conditions, the effects of drugs, or a combination of these causes. Box 27-4 summarizes the causes of the mental condition and the external factors associated with anxiety.

TYPES OF DRUGS FOR ANXIETY

ANTIANXIETY DRUGS

How Antianxiety Drugs Work

Mild anxiety is a common experience and usually requires no drug treatment. Moderate-to-severe anxiety is a symptom of psychiatric disorders such as phobia, panic disorder, OCD, and PTSD.

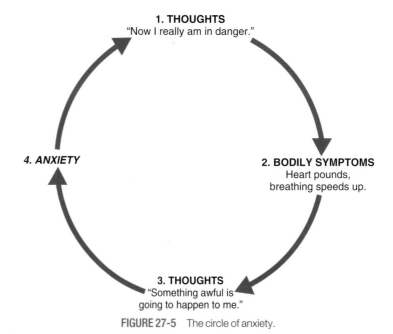

1. THOUGHTS
"Now I really am in danger."

2. BODILY SYMPTOMS
Heart pounds,
breathing speeds up.

3. THOUGHTS
"Something awful is
going to happen to me."

4. ANXIETY

FIGURE 27-5   The circle of anxiety.

Box 27-4	Causes and External Factors Associated with Anxiety

- Financial stress
- Lack of oxygen such as high-altitude sickness, emphysema, and pulmonary embolus
- Side effect of medication
- Stress at work
- Stress from a serious medical illness
- Stress from emotional trauma such as death of a loved one
- Stress from school
- Stress in personal relationships such as marriage
- Symptoms of a medical illness
- Use of illicit drugs such as cocaine

Chronic and severe anxiety are treated with **antianxiety drugs**, also called *anxiolytics* or *minor tranquilizers*. Most drugs used to treat anxiety also cause sedation or sleep and are likely to cause *dependence* (the psychologic craving for, or physiologic reliance on, a chemical substance) when taken for an extended period.

In the past **benzodiazepines** were the most commonly prescribed drugs for treatment of anxiety. When taken as directed, these drugs allow many patients with anxiety to lead nearly normal lives. Buspirone (BuSpar) and SSRIs such as sertraline (Zoloft), paroxetine (Paxil), fluoxetine (Prozac), and venlafaxine (Effexor) are now prescribed to treat anxiety more commonly than benzodiazepines because they have milder side effects and patients are less likely to become dependent on them. The major benefit of benzodiazepines is that they act within 30 minutes and may be given as needed, whereas it may take SSRIs 3 to 5 weeks to control anxiety. Benzodiazepines also decrease symptoms of alcohol withdrawal and prevent delirium tremens.

Benzodiazepines are CNS depressants that increase the inhibitory actions of gamma-aminobutyric acid (GABA) in the brain. GABA is a neurotransmitter that transmits messages from brain cell to brain cell. It sends a message to the brain neurons to slow down or stop firing. This quiets the brain and decreases anxiety.

SSRIs relieve anxiety by affecting the action of the neurotransmitter serotonin in the brain. Serotonin stays in the synaptic gap longer, and transmission of impulses is slowed. It is also theorized that these drugs may affect the limbic system, which is the part of the brain associated with emotions. They calm and relax people with anxiety; however, they may take several weeks to become effective.

Buspirone (BuSpar) binds the neuroreceptors for serotonin and dopamine in the brain and increases norepinephrine metabolism to relieve anxiety. Binding the neurotransmitters slows the transmission of impulses and quiets the brain to relieve anxiety.

Diazepam (Valium) has a longer half-life, which makes it a less attractive choice than other benzodiazepine drugs. Because benzodiazepine drugs are potentially addictive, they should not be prescribed for a patient with a substance abuse disorder.

Generic names, trade names, and dosages of drugs for anxiety are listed in the following table. Be sure to consult a drug handbook for information about any specific antianxiety drug.

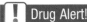

Drug Alert!

Action/Intervention Alert

Monitor patients taking antianxiety drugs for signs of dependence because most of these drugs are likely to cause dependence when taken for a long time.

QSEN: Safety

Drug Alert!

Teaching Alert

Teach patients that it may take SSRI drugs 3 to 5 weeks to control anxiety.

QSEN: Safety

Did You Know?

Beta blockers, which are usually prescribed for hypertension, are sometimes prescribed for patients facing anxiety-producing events such as performing on stage or making a speech.

Dosages for Common Antianxiety Drugs

Drug	Dosage
Benzodiazepines	
alprazolam (Apo-Alpraz ♣, Nu-Alpraz ♣, Xanax)	*Adults:* 0.25-0.5 mg orally every 8-12 hours; do not exceed 4 mg/day; extended release (XR)—1-10 mg once daily
clonazepam (Gen-Clonazepam ♣, Klonopin, Novo-Clonazepam ♣)	*Adults:* 0.125-0.25 mg orally every 12 hours
clorazepate (Novo-Clopate ♣, Tranxene)	*Adults:* 5 mg orally daily at bedtime; maximum dosage 60 mg/day
chlordiazepoxide (Librium, Novopoxide ♣)	*Adults:* Oral—7.5-10 mg as a single dose at bedtime or as 2-3 divided doses daily, maximum dose 60 mg daily; IM/IV—50-100 mg first dose, then 25-50 mg 3-4 times daily *Children (>6 years):* Oral—5 mg 2-4 times daily *Children (>12 years):* IM/IV—25-50 mg per dose
diazepam (Valium, Vivol ♣)	*Adults:* Oral—0.5-2.5 mg every 6 hours or 1-5 mg every 12 hours; IM/IV—2-10 mg, repeat every 3-4 hours as needed
lorazepam (Ativan, Nu-Loraz ♣)	*Adults:* 1-3 mg orally every 12 hours; maximum dosage 10 mg/day, or 5 mg every 12 hours
oxazepam (Novoxapam ♣, Serax)	*Adults:* 10-30 mg orally 3-4 times daily
Anxiolytics	
busPIRone (BuSpar)	*Adults:* 2.5-5 mg orally every 8 hours; maximum dosage 60 mg/day

Did You Know?

Librium (chlordiazepoxide) is named for *libré* (French for "free") and *liber* (Latin for "freedom") because it was the first benzodiazepine developed that freed patients from the symptoms of anxiety.

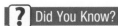 **Do Not Confuse**

Klonopin *with* Clonidine

An order for Klonopin may be confused with Clonidine. Klonopin (clonazepam) is a benzodiazepine drug use to treat anxiety and psychosis, whereas Clonidine is a central-acting adrenergic drug used to treat hypertension.

QSEN: Safety

Common Side Effects

Antianxiety Drugs

Dizziness,   Drowsiness,   Headache
Unsteadiness,   Fatigue
Ataxia

 Clinical Pitfall

Patients should not stop taking benzodiazepine drugs suddenly because of the risk for life-threatening withdrawal symptoms, including nervousness, restlessness, tremulousness, weakness, and seizures.

QSEN: Safety

⚠ Drug Alert!

Teaching Alert

Teach patients to avoid using alcohol, sleeping pills, or prescription pain drugs while taking antianxiety drugs.

QSEN: Safety

Intended Responses
- Anxiety is relieved without too much sedation.
- Symptoms of anxiety are decreased.
- Sense of well-being is improved.

Side Effects. The most common side effects of benzodiazepines are related to their CNS effects. They include drowsiness, dizziness, light-headedness, fatigue, ataxia, and unsteadiness. Other side effects include sleepiness, depression, lethargy, apathy, memory impairment, disorientation, amnesia, delirium, headache, slurred speech, behavioral changes, euphoria, dysarthria, and inability to perform complex mental functions. Additional common side effects include nervousness, irritability, difficulty concentrating, "glassy-eyed" appearance, changes in heart rate and blood pressure, changes in bowel function, and skin rashes. With chlordiazepoxide (Librium), there is pain at intramuscular sites after injection.

Common side effects of buspirone include dizziness and drowsiness. Others may include excitement, fatigue, headache, insomnia, nervousness, weakness, blurred vision, nasal congestion, sore throat, tinnitus, chest pain, palpitations, tachycardia, nausea, rash, myalgia, lack of coordination, numbness, paresthesia, clammy skin, and sweating.

Adverse Effects. Life-threatening adverse effects of benzodiazepines include seizures and coma. Buspirone can result in hallucinations and heart failure.

Suddenly stopping a benzodiazepine can cause a potentially life-threatening reaction of withdrawal symptoms, including nervousness, restlessness, tremulousness, weakness, and seizures. The patient may become dehydrated or delirious or may develop insomnia, confusion, and visual or auditory hallucinations.

Suicidal ideation (creating a plan to carry out suicide) may occur with patients taking clonazepam (Klonopin).

What To Do *Before* Giving Antianxiety Drugs
In addition to the general responsibilities related to drugs for psychiatric problems (p. 431), check for history of drug of substance dependencies.

What To Do *After* Giving Antianxiety Drugs
In addition to the general responsibilities related to drugs for psychiatric problems (p. 431), assess gait for steadiness. Continue to monitor level of anxiety to assess the effectiveness of the drug. Assess for and continue to monitor the patient for suicidal ideation.

Because of the tendency to become dependent on benzodiazepines, give these drugs only as prescribed. While patients are taking these drugs, observe for signs of dependency and report them to the prescriber.

What To Teach Patients Taking Antianxiety Drugs
In addition to the general responsibilities related to teaching patients about drugs for psychiatric problems (p. 431), instruct patients to take these drugs, especially benzodiazepines, exactly as prescribed to decrease the chance of dependence. Teach patients taking antianxiety drugs to avoid drinking alcohol, taking sleeping pills, or taking prescription pain drugs at the same time because of the danger of more severe CNS depression.

Tell patients that the prescriber may want to wean them off of these drugs gradually because stopping suddenly can cause withdrawal symptoms such as sweating, vomiting, muscle cramps, tremors, or seizures.

Teach patients about the signs of dependence and instruct them to report these signs immediately to their prescriber.

Teach patients to avoid alcohol and other CNS depressants while taking benzodiazepines because of the added sedative effects.

Instruct patients not to take benzodiazepines with antacids because antacids decrease their absorption. Tell them to take these drugs 1 hour before or 2 hours after an antacid.

Remind patients taking alprazolam (Xanax), diazepam (Valium), midazolam (Versed), triazolam (Halcion), or buspirone (BuSpar) to avoid drinking grapefruit juice while taking these drugs because grapefruit juice slows their metabolism and causes increased blood concentration.

Life Span Considerations for Antianxiety Drugs

Pediatric Considerations. Children are more sensitive to the effects of benzodiazepines and more likely to experience side effects. Using clonazepam (Klonopin) during childhood may cause decreased mental and physical growth. Clonazepam should not be used in children younger than 18 years with panic disorders because safety and effectiveness have not been established.

Considerations for Pregnancy and Lactation. Benzodiazepines have a high likelihood of increasing the risk for birth defects or fetal harm and should not be used during pregnancy. Chlordiazepoxide (Librium) and diazepam have caused birth defects when used during the first trimester of pregnancy. Use of benzodiazepines during pregnancy causes the fetus to become dependent on these drugs and can cause withdrawal symptoms after birth. These drugs should not be taken when a woman is breastfeeding because they can cause drowsiness, difficulty with feeding, and weight loss in the infant. Physical dependence and withdrawal symptoms may also occur in breastfed infants.

Considerations for Older Adults. Older adults are more sensitive to the effects of benzodiazepines and are more at risk for side effects. Older adults should be monitored for respiratory depression. Benzodiazepines may cause daytime drowsiness, falls, and injuries. Teach older adults to change positions slowly and to use handrails when going up or down stairs. Instruct family members to assess older adults who are taking benzodiazepines for changes in cognition or reduced mental alertness. Low doses of benzodiazepines should be used with these patients because they are more sensitive to the effects and side effects of these drugs. Drowsiness may be much more intense in older adults. Instruct them not to drive or use dangerous equipment until they know how the drug will affect them. Chlordiazepoxide and clorazepate (Tranxene) are not recommended for older adults because they have a long half-life. Buspirone should be started at 5 mg twice a day for these patients.

PSYCHOSIS

Psychosis is a loss of contact with reality that may be brief or long term. Common symptoms of psychosis include *delusions* (false ideas about what is occurring or personal identity), *illusions* (mistaken perceptions), and *hallucinations* (seeing or hearing things that are not there). Other symptoms of psychosis are listed in Box 27-5. An example of a delusion is when a person exaggerates his or her sense of self-importance and is convinced that he or she has special powers, talents, or abilities. The person may believe that he or she is a famous movie star or a saint. An example of an illusion is when a person thinks that he or she hears voices in the wind. The most common type of hallucination is hearing imaginary voices (*auditory*

Box 27-5 **Symptoms of Psychosis**

- Confusion
- Depression and sometimes suicidal thoughts
- Disorganized thoughts or speech
- Emotion exhibited in an abnormal manner
- Extreme excitement (mania)
- False beliefs (delusions)
- Loss of touch with reality
- Mistaken perceptions (illusions)
- Seeing, hearing, feeling, or perceiving things that are not there (hallucinations)
- Unfounded fears or suspicions

 Drug Alert!
Teaching Alert

Be sure to teach patients to take benzodiazepines exactly as prescribed to decrease the risk for developing dependence on these drugs.

QSEN: Safety

 Drug Alert!
Teaching Alert

Teach patients that the signs of dependence on benzodiazepines include:
- Strong desire or need to continue taking the drug
- Need to increase the dose to feel the effects of the drug
- Withdrawal effects after the drug is stopped (for example, irritability, nervousness, trouble sleeping, abdominal cramps, trembling, or shaking)

QSEN: Safety

 Drug Alert!
Teaching Alert

Teach patients taking a benzodiazepine to take the drug 1 hour before or 2 hours after an antacid.

QSEN: Safety

 Drug Alert!
Teaching Alert

Teach patients who take alprazolam, diazepam, midazolam, triazolam, or buspirone to avoid drinking grapefruit juice.

QSEN: Safety

Clinical Pitfall

Benzodiazepines should not be used during pregnancy because the fetus can become dependent on these drugs and experience withdrawal symptoms after birth.

QSEN: Safety

 Drug Alert!
Teaching Alert

Teach family members to watch for and report changes in cognition or decreased mental alertness in older adults taking antianxiety drugs.

QSEN: Safety

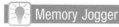 **Memory Jogger**

Psychotic disorders include delusions, illusions, and hallucinations.

hallucination) that give commands, make comments, or warn of impending danger. A visual hallucination occurs when a person sees something that is not there, such as a bright light, a shape, or a human figure. A person who is experiencing a psychotic episode may be unaware that anything is wrong and unable to ask for help.

Treatment of psychosis includes psychologic therapies such as counseling, guided discussion, and cognitive behavior therapy to help change or eliminate unwanted thoughts or beliefs. Antipsychotic drugs help to decrease auditory hallucinations and delusions and stabilize thinking and behavior. Hospital care may be needed to ensure a patient's safety because a person with psychosis may harm himself or herself or others. Many symptoms of psychosis can be controlled with long-term treatment.

REVIEW OF RELATED PHYSIOLOGY AND PATHOPHYSIOLOGY

The exact cause of psychotic disorders is not known. One theory is that these disorders develop because the brain overreacts to neurotransmitters (substances that carry messages between nerves) in the brain. Heredity may also play a part in the development of psychotic disorders such as schizophrenia, which tends to run in families. Psychosis may be caused by a variety of medical or psychiatric problems. Box 27-6 summarizes potential causes of psychosis.

TYPES OF DRUGS FOR PSYCHOSIS

ANTIPSYCHOTICS

How Antipsychotics Work

 Memory Jogger

Most antipsychotic drugs work by causing CNS depression.

Sometimes called neuroleptics or major tranquilizers, **antipsychotic drugs** are prescribed to treat and control the symptoms of psychosis such as hallucinations and delusions. These drugs produce a tranquillizing effect that helps to relax the CNS, allowing patients to function appropriately and effectively. They also control the symptoms of other psychiatric disorders that may lead to psychosis such as bipolar disorder.

All antipsychotic drugs tend to block dopamine receptors in the dopamine pathways in the brain. The normal effect of releasing the neurotransmitter dopamine is decreased. Transmission of impulses is decreased, which in turn decreases the symptoms of hallucinations, illusions, and delusions.

 Memory Jogger

Major tranquilizers are the drugs most commonly prescribed to treat psychosis.

Major tranquilizers are the most commonly prescribed drugs for psychosis. Other drugs used to treat psychosis include lithium carbonate (Lithonate) and thiothixene (Navane).

Antipsychotic drugs are occasionally used to treat acute delirium. The danger of using these drugs is prolonged or worsening agitation, especially when using older drugs such as haloperidol (Haldol). These drugs should no longer be prescribed for patients with dementia unless the patient is agitated, aggressive, or showing psychotic behavior that is distressing to patients or dangerous to others. Antipsychotic drugs should never be used at the whim of a caregiver for the sole purpose of restraining patients who wander, have insomnia, or do not cooperate.

Clinical Pitfall

Antipsychotic drugs should never be used to restrain patients who wander, have insomnia, or are uncooperative.

QSEN: Safety

Generic names, trade names, and doses of drugs for psychosis are listed in the following table. Be sure to consult a drug handbook for information about a specific antipsychotic drug.

Box 27-6 **Potential Causes of Psychosis**

- Alcohol and other drugs
- Bipolar disorders (manic depression)
- Brain tumors
- Dementia (Alzheimer's and other degenerative brain disorders)
- Epilepsy
- Psychotic depression
- Schizophrenia
- Stroke

Dosages for Common Drugs for Psychosis

Drug	Dosage
Antipsychotics	
aripiprazole (Abilify)	*Adults:* 10-15 mg orally daily *Adolescents:* 2 mg orally daily; gradually increase to 10 mg daily
chlorproMAZINE (Chlorpromanyl , Largactil , Thorazine)	*Adults:* Oral—10-25 mg 2-4 times daily, usual dosage 300 mg/day in divided doses; IM—25-50 mg, maximum dosage 400 mg every 3-12 hr as needed *Children:* Oral—0.55 mg/kg every 4-6 hr as needed; IM—0.55 mg/kg every 6-8 hr as needed
clozapine (Clozaril)	*Adults:* 25 mg orally 1-2 times daily; gradually increase to target dosage of 300-450 mg/day
olanzapine (Zyprexa)	*Adults:* 5-10 mg orally once daily; increase to 10-15 mg/day; maximum dosage 20 mg/day
prochlorperazine (Compazine, Prorazin , Stemetil)	*Adults/Children >12 years:* 5-10 mg orally 3-4 times daily up to 150 mg/day *Adults:* IM—10-20 mg every 2-6 hr up to 200 mg/day *Children 2-12 years:* IM—132 mcg/kg; not to exceed 10 mg per dose
quetiapine (Seroquel)	*Adults:* 25 mg orally twice daily; maximum dosage 800 mg/day
risperidone (Risperdal)	*Adults:* 1-3 mg orally twice daily; maximum dosage 6 mg/day
ziprasidone (Geodon)	*Adults:* 20 mg orally twice daily; maximum dosage 80 mg twice daily Intramuscular 10-20 mg; maximum dosage 40 mg/day *Children:* Safety and efficacy has not been established
Other Drugs	
lithium carbonate (Carbolith , Eskalith, Lithizine , Lithonate)	*Adults/Children >12 years:* 300-600 mg orally 3 times daily *Children <12 years:* 15-20 mg orally daily in 3-4 divided doses; maximum dose 2400 mg daily
thiothixene (Navane)	*Adults:* Oral—2 mg 3 times daily or 5 mg twice daily, maximum dosage 60 mg/day; IM—4 mg 2-4 times daily, maximum dosage 30 mg/day

Intended Responses

- Signs and symptoms of psychosis, including hallucinations and delusions, are decreased.
- Behavior is improved (or there is less antisocial behavior).
- Schizophrenic behavior is decreased.
- Suicidal behavior is decreased.

Side Effects. Early in treatment, common side effects of antipsychotic drugs related to CNS depression may include sedation and drowsiness, dizziness when changing positions, lethargy, restlessness, insomnia, and GI upset (e.g. nausea, vomiting, and diarrhea). Other side effects include agitation, headache, hypotension, tachycardia, muscle spasms, tremor, weakness, dry mouth, dry eyes, blurred vision, weight gain, photosensitivity, and constipation.

Do Not Confuse

chlorproMAZINE *with* chlorproPAMIDE

An order for chlorpromazine may be confused with chlorpropamide. Chlorpromazine is an antipsychotic drug used to treat psychosis, whereas chlorpropamide is a sulfonylurea used to treat type 2 diabetes.

QSEN: Safety

Do Not Confuse

Clozaril *with* Colazal

An order for Clozaril may be confused with Colazal. Clozaril is an antipsychotic drug used to treat psychotic disorders, whereas Colazal is a GI anti-inflammatory drug used to treat mild to moderate ulcerative colitis.

QSEN: Safety

Do Not Confuse

Zyprexa *with* Celexa or Zyrtec

An order for Zyprexa may be confused with Celexa or Zyrtec. Zyprexa is used to treat psychotic disorders, whereas Celexa is an SSRI drug used to treat depression. Zyrtec is an antihistamine used to treat allergies.

QSEN: Safety

Common Side Effects

Antipsychotics

Drowsiness, Insomnia, Lethargy

Dizziness

GI upset, Nausea, Vomiting, Diarrhea

Hand tremor (Lithium)

Adverse Effects. Several life-threatening adverse effects can occur with antipsychotic drugs. Tardive dyskinesia, a disorder characterized by involuntary movements (extrapyramidal symptoms) most often affecting the mouth, lips, and tongue and sometimes the trunk or other parts of the body such as arms and legs, can be caused by all antipsychotics. However, this adverse effect is much more common with first-generation drugs. Several drugs sometimes cause seizures, including clozapine, haloperidol, olanzapine, quetiapine, and lithium.

Neuroleptic malignant syndrome is a rare, potentially life-threatening disorder involving dysfunction of the autonomic nervous system. The autonomic nervous system is the branch of the nervous system responsible for regulating such involuntary actions as heart rate, blood pressure, digestion, and sweating. Muscle tone becomes rigid with tremors, body temperature and respiratory rate are markedly elevated, heart rate is tachycardic, blood pressure may be elevated or decreased, and consciousness is also severely affected. All antipsychotic drugs can cause this syndrome.

Neutropenia (decreased white blood cells) can result from taking clozapine or prochlorperazine. Clozapine can also cause myocarditis (inflammation of the heart muscle).

Quetiapine (Seroquel) and risperidone (Risperdal) cause increased risk of death in older adults with dementia.

What To Do *Before* Giving Antipsychotics

In addition to the general responsibilities related to drugs for psychiatric problems (p. 431), monitor fluid intake and urine output. Obtain a baseline weight.

Assess baseline level of psychosis. Check orientation, mood, and behavior. Be sure to observe that patients swallow these drugs. Ask about suicidal thoughts.

Ask patients about smoking because smoking may decrease the effectiveness of olanzapine and clozapine.

What To Do *After* Giving Antipsychotics

In addition to the general responsibilities related to drugs for psychiatric problems (p. 431), monitor intake and output and daily weight. Monitor bowel function. Report constipation to the prescriber and encourage the patient to drink extra fluids.

Reassess the patient's mental status, monitoring orientation, mood, and behavior for changes. Watch for sedation. Continue to monitor for suicidal thoughts.

Give antipsychotic drugs with food if the patient develops GI upset symptoms.

What To Teach Patients Taking Antipsychotics Drugs

In addition to the general responsibilities related to drugs for psychiatric problems (p. 431), teach patients that their prescriber may start with a low dose and gradually increase it to achieve therapeutic effects. Be sure to teach patients about the side effects and adverse effects of these drugs and to notify their prescriber if any of these symptoms occur. Tell them to immediately report sore throat, unusual bleeding or bruising, rash, or tremors.

Remind patients about the importance of psychotherapy to help keep psychosis under control.

Teach them to avoid alcohol and other CNS depressants while taking these drugs.

Tell patients to monitor bowel function and to increase activity, fluid intake, and fiber-containing foods to prevent constipation. Remind them to take these drugs and antacids at least 2 hours apart to prevent decreased absorption. Instruct patients to take these drugs with food if GI upset occurs.

Let patients know that some of these drugs may cause urine to be abnormally colored (for example, prochlorperazine may turn urine pink or reddish-brown).

Protective clothing, hats, and sunscreens should be used to protect against *photosensitivity* (sensitivity to light). Frequent mouth rinses and oral care can help minimize dry mouth.

Drug Alert!

Action/Intervention Alert

Before giving an antipsychotic, be sure to ask the patient about suicidal thoughts and initiate suicide precautions if needed.

QSEN: Safety

Drug Alert!

Action/Intervention Alert

Encourage patients taking antipsychotic drugs to drink extra fluids to prevent constipation.

QSEN: Safety

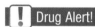

Drug Alert!

Action/Intervention Alert

Discuss with patients the importance of psychotherapy in addition to antipsychotic drug therapy to help keep their psychosis under control.

QSEN: Safety

Drug Alert!

Teaching Alert

Tell patients taking prochlorperazine (Compazine) that it may turn their urine pink or reddish-brown.

QSEN: Safety

Instruct patients taking quetiapine (Seroquel) to avoid temperature extremes because this drug impairs body temperature regulation.

Teach patients taking quetiapine (Seroquel) or olanzapine (Zyprexa) to avoid grapefruit and grapefruit juice during therapy. Grapefruit can interfere with metabolism of the drug, causing increased blood levels and increased risk for side effects or adverse effects.

Life Span Considerations for Antipsychotics

Pediatric Considerations. Side effects and adverse effects are more likely in children because they are more sensitive to the effects of these drugs.

Considerations for Pregnancy and Lactation. Drugs for psychosis have a moderate risk of increased likelihood for birth defects or fetal harm and should be avoided during pregnancy. These drugs may cross the placenta and cause unwanted side effects such as involuntary movements on the newborn infant. These drugs should not be taken during breastfeeding. Lithium has a high risk of increased likelihood for birth defects or fetal harm and should be avoided during pregnancy and breastfeeding.

Considerations for Older Adults. Side effects and adverse effects are more likely in older adults because they are more sensitive to the effects of these drugs. They should start with lower doses of all antipsychotic drugs. Older adults with renal insufficiency should also be started with lower doses.

Most of the antipsychotic drugs, especially chlorpromazine (Thorazine) can cause a rapid fall in blood pressure when changing from a sitting to a standing position (orthostatic hypotension). Teach older adults to change positions slowly and to sit on the edge of the bed for a few moments before standing. Remind them to always use handrails when going up or down stairs.

Lithium can cause excessive urination and quickly lead to dehydration, especially in older adults. Remind older adults to drink daily about the same amount of fluid they lose in urination. Also remind them to notify the prescriber if they are too nauseated and cannot take in as much fluid as they should.

 Drug Alert!

Teaching Alert

Instruct patients taking quetiapine (Seroquel) to avoid temperature extremes because this drug impairs body temperature regulation.

QSEN: Safety

 Drug Alert!

Teaching Alert

To prevent falls, teach older adults to change positions slowly while taking chlorpromazine (Thorazine) because it can cause a rapid drop in blood pressure.

QSEN: Safety

Get Ready for Practice!

Key Points

- Mental illness can be caused by biologic or psychologic factors.
- Women are twice as likely as men to develop depression, but men are less likely to seek treatment for depression.
- Depression can be mistaken as part of the aging process, and many older adults go undiagnosed and untreated.
- Many people with depression do not seek treatment because they do not recognize that it is a treatable illness.
- Anxiety may occur without a cause or may be based on a real-life situation.
- Physical reactions such as increased heart rate, sweating, trembling, fatigue, and weakness often occur with anxiety.
- A person experiencing a psychotic disorder may be unaware that anything is wrong and unable to ask for help.
- Treatment for depression, anxiety, and psychosis includes psychotherapy, counseling, and medications.

- It may take up to 8 weeks for improvement of depression symptoms after an antidepressant drug is prescribed.
- Be sure to ask a patient with a mental disorder about suicidal thoughts.
- Instruct patients not to stop taking these drugs without talking with their prescriber.
- Assess a patient with an anxiety disorder for physical signs such as changes in blood pressure, heart rate, and respiratory rate.
- Teach patients taking benzodiazepines to take the drugs exactly as prescribed to decrease the risk of developing drug dependence.

Additional Learning Resources

evolve Be sure to visit your Evolve website (http:// evolve.elsevier.com/Workman/pharmacology/) for additional online resources.

SG Go to your Study Guide for additional learning activities to help you master this chapter content.

Review Questions

See the Answer Keys—In-text Review Questions for answers to these questions.

Test Yourself on the Basics

1. How do tricyclic antidepressants (TCAs) work in the treatment of depression?
   A. TCA drugs inhibit the reuptake of neurotransmitters.
   B. TCA drugs decrease the amount of serotonin in the brain.
   C. TCA drugs lower the levels of neurotransmitters.
   D. TCA drugs work very slowly to correct chemical imbalances in the brain.

2. Why are SSRI drugs prescribed more often than TCA drugs for the treatment of depression?
   A. TCA drugs are more likely to lead to dependence.
   B. SSRI drugs have fewer side effects than TCA drugs.
   C. TCA drugs lead to more adverse effects.
   D. SSRI drugs work more rapidly than TCA drugs.

3. Which class of drugs is most likely to lead to dependence when prescribed?
   A. TCAs
   B. SSRIs
   C. Benzodiazepines
   D. Antipsychotic drugs

4. A patient is prescribed olanzapine (Zyprexa) for treatment of psychosis. What information from the patient must you report to the prescriber?
   A. The patient tells you that he uses St. John's wort.
   B. The patient tells you that he exercises every day.
   C. The patient tells you that he eats a lot of fast foods.
   D. The patient tells you that he smokes cigarettes.

5. The patient prescribed a benzodiazepine drug tells you that he is considering suicide. What must you do? (Select all that apply.)
   A. Notify the prescriber.
   B. Hold the benzodiazepine drug.
   C. Ask for an order for leather restraints.
   D. Initiate suicide precautions.
   E. Ask the patient if he or she has a suicide plan.

Test Yourself on Advanced Concepts

6. How do selective serotonin reuptake inhibitors (SSRIs) work to treat depression?
   A. By inhibiting the reuptake of the neurotransmitters norepinephrine, dopamine, or serotonin by nerve cells
   B. By inhibiting the actions of gamma-aminobutyric acid (GABA) in the brain
   C. By increasing the amount of the neurotransmitter serotonin in the brain
   D. By inhibiting the activity of monoamine oxidase preventing the breakdown of monoamine neurotransmitters

7. A patient who has been taking amitriptyline (Elavil) to treat depression has developed dizziness with a blood pressure of 94/60. The patient tells the unlicensed assistive personnel (UAP) that he needs to get up to use the bathroom. What are your best instructions for the UAP?
   A. Keep the patient on bedrest and offer him a bedpan.
   B. Have the patient take slow deep breaths and keep the head of his bed in a supine position.
   C. Have the patient get up slowly and sit on the side of the bed before standing.
   D. Keep the patient in bed until we can get an order for a bedside commode.

8. A patient prescribed the SSRI paroxetine (Paxil) 4 weeks ago tells you that it is not working and asks if she can have diazepam (Valium) instead? What is your best response?
   A. "Paroxetine has fewer side effects than diazepam."
   B. "Paroxetine is less likely to cause dependence than diazepam."
   C. "Paroxetine can take from 1 to 8 weeks for symptoms of depression to improve."
   D. "Diazepam interacts with other drugs and food, whereas paroxetine can be taken without regard to other drugs or food."

9. Which antidepressant drug may cause unusual excitement, irritability, and trouble sleeping when prescribed for children?
   A. fluoxetine (Prozac)
   B. sertraline (Zoloft)
   C. venlafaxine (Effexor)
   D. duloxetine (Cymbalta)

10. The patient prescribed chlorpromazine (Thorazine) is at risk for constipation. What is your best action?
    A. Call the prescriber and ask for an order for stool softeners.
    B. Instruct the patient to drink extra fluids every day.
    C. Teach the patient about foods that are low in fiber.
    D. Tell the patient about the importance of exercise in preventing constipation.

11. After giving a patient risperidone (Risperdal) she tells you that she feels nauseated. What is your best action?
    A. Notify the prescriber immediately.
    B. Check the patient of signs of an allergic reaction.
    C. Give the drug on an empty stomach.
    D. Provide the patient with food when giving this drug.

12. The patient prescribed chlorpromazine (Thorazine) tells you that that he is very active and spends a lot of time outdoors. What best advice do you teach this patient?
    A. "Be sure to wear protective clothing when you are outside."
    B. "There is no need to change the amount of time you spend outside."
    C. "You may need to get a membership to a gym and stay indoors."
    D. "Be sure to drink more fluids whenever you spend time outdoors."

13. What precautions will you teach an older adult who is prescribed chlorpromazine (Thorazine)?
    A. Chlorpromazine can cause an increase in thirst, so the older adult should drink more fluids.
    B. Chlorpromazine can cause excessive urination, which can lead to dehydration, so drink more fluids.
    C. Chlorpromazine can cause dizziness, so be sure to change positions slowly.
    D. Chlorpromazine can cause kidney function to decrease, so a diuretic drug may also be prescribed.

14. The prescriber orders imipramine (Tofranil) 300 mg orally in three divided doses. Imipramine comes in scored 50-mg tablets.
    A. How many mg do you give for each dose? _____ mg
    B. How many tablets would you give for each dose? _____ tablet(s)

15. The prescriber's order for a patient with generalized anxiety disorder is for lorazepam (Ativan) 0.02 mg/kg every 3 hours IV as needed. The patient's weight is 55 kg. Lorazepam is available as 2 mg/mL.
    A. How many mg do you give for each dose? _____ mg
    B. How many milliliters do you give for each dose? _____ mL

Critical Thinking Activities

See the Answer Keys—Critical Thinking Activities for answers to these activities.

Mrs. Woolsey is a 48-year-old housewife whose husband works full time and whose children are grown. She tells you that her life doesn't seem to have any purpose and that she often spends the day in her robe. She states that her only friend died 6 months ago from pancreatic cancer.
1. What is Mrs. Woolsey's likely diagnosis?
2. Which class of drugs is the prescriber most likely to try for this patient?
3. Why are these drugs the best choice for Mrs. Woolsey?
4. What are key points that you would include when teaching the patient about these drugs?

Objectives

After studying this chapter you should be able to:

1. List the names, actions, usual adult dosages, possible side effects, and adverse effects of drugs for sleep.
2. Explain what to do before and after giving a drug for sleep.
3. Explain what to teach patients taking drugs for sleep, including what to do, what not to do, and when to call the prescriber or pharmacist.
4. Describe life span considerations related to drugs for sleep.

Key Terms

barbiturates (bär-BĬ-chŭrets) (p. 451) A class of drugs formed from barbituric acid that induce a general depression over all central nervous system functions and induce sedation.

benzodiazepine receptor agonists (bĕn-zō-dī-ĂZ-ĕ-pēnz rē SĔP-tŭrz) (p. 451) A class of non-benzodiazepine sedative-hypnotics that interact with the same receptor site that benzodiazepine drugs do, turning on the receptors to induce sleep.

benzodiazepines (bĕn-zō-dī-ĂZ-ĕ-pēnz) (p. 451) A class of drugs that depress the central nervous system by binding to gamma aminobutyric acid receptors, resulting in hypnotic and sedating effects. They are used mainly to control symptoms of anxiety or stress.

sedatives (SĔD-ĕ-tĭvz) (p. 451) Drugs that promote sleep by targeting signals in the brain to produce calm and ease agitation.

INSOMNIA

REVIEW OF RELATED PHYSIOLOGY AND PATHOPHYSIOLOGY

Sleep is a natural and necessary periodic state of rest for the mind and body. When we sleep, our bodies rest and restore energy levels. Sleep helps a person recover from illness, cope with stress, and solve problems. During sleep, consciousness is partially or completely lost, the eyes close, body movements decrease, metabolism slows, and responsiveness to external stimuli declines.

Insomnia is the inability to go to sleep or remain asleep throughout the night. It is the most common sleep problem. Most people experience acute, short-term insomnia at some time during their lives. People of any age may have insomnia. Symptoms include difficulty falling asleep, waking often during the night or early morning, and not feeling rested after sleep.

Failing to get enough sleep because of insomnia causes *sleep deprivation*, which is a shortage of quality, undisturbed sleep that reduces physical and mental well-being. Coordination, judgment, reaction time, and social function are all impaired by lack of sleep. Drowsiness interferes with the ability of the brain to concentrate, learn, and remember. Simple tasks seem more difficult to perform, and complex tasks may seem impossible to complete. People become anxious, moody, and impatient and have increased difficulty interacting with others.

Signs of sleep deprivation include falling asleep at the wheel while driving, watching television, or reading a book; sleeping for extra-long periods; difficulty awaking in the morning; irritability during the day; and falling asleep during quiet times of the day. Sleep deprivation may be short term or long term.

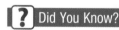 Did You Know?

Sleep deprivation decreases immune function and increases the risk for infection.

DRUGS FOR INSOMNIA

The most commonly prescribed sleep drugs are **sedatives**, a broad group of drugs that promote sleep by acting on signals in the central nervous system (CNS) to produce calm and ease agitation. Sedatives include benzodiazepine receptor agonists, benzodiazepines, antihistamines, sedating antidepressants, and skeletal muscle relaxants.

Benzodiazepine receptor agonists, also called non-benzodiazepine sedative-hypnotics, are a class of drugs that interact with the same receptor site that benzodiazepine drugs do, turning on the receptors to induce sleep. Drugs from this class are now the first-line sleep aids to treat insomnia. They are less likely to be addictive but must be carefully monitored by the prescriber because of the possibility of misuse. **Benzodiazepines** are drugs that depress the central nervous system (CNS) by binding to gamma aminobutyric acid (GABA) receptors, resulting in hypnotic and sedating effects. GABA is an inhibitory rather than excitatory neurotransmitter in the brain. When increased amounts of GABA are present or GABA receptors are stimulated, CNS activity is reduced. Although benzodiazepines are mainly used to treat anxiety or stress, a few are used as a short-term treatment of insomnia. They can be habit forming when used for prolonged periods of time (more than 2 to 4 weeks) and are no longer the first-line drugs for insomnia.

Older drugs sometimes still used to treat insomnia for short time periods are the barbiturate-based drugs. **Barbiturates** are drugs formed from barbituric acid that induce a general depression over all CNS functions along with inducing sedation. Both motor and sensory functions are inhibited, and the seizure threshold is elevated. Although rarely used for general insomnia, the barbiturates may be prescribed short-term when other drugs for insomnia have not been successful. Most barbiturates, including those used for sleep, are categorized as Schedule II controlled substances with a high potential for abuse and dependence. In addition, because all CNS functions are depressed, overdoses with the barbiturates are serious and can lead to death. These drugs are more commonly used to induce sedation and reduce anxiety before surgery. Some are used as part of seizure control management with epilepsy.

Antihistamines are drugs used to treat allergies and allergic reactions. Some, such as diphenhydramine (Allerdryl ♣, Benadryl) and dimenhydrinate (Dramamine, Gravol ♣), have sedating effects and are available over the counter. See Chapter 6 for a complete discussion of the actions and uses of antihistamine drugs as well as the responsibilities.

Sedating antidepressants also have some effect for insomnia, especially trazodone, amitriptyline, and doxepin. See Chapter 27 for a complete discussion of the action and uses of antidepressants as well as the responsibilities. Generic names, brand names, and dosages of the most commonly prescribed drugs for insomnia are listed in the following table. Be sure to consult a drug reference textbook for information about specific drugs used to treat insomnia.

Skeletal muscle relaxants are another group of drugs that are used at times for insomnia. The most common ones used for this purpose are the carbamates and the cyclobenzaprines. Both of these drug groups work by depressing the CNS and produce significant sedation. A more complete discussion of the actions, dosages, responsibilities, and side effects of these drugs is presented in Chapter 30.

 Clinical Pitfall

The barbiturate drugs (pentobarbital and secobarbital) are rarely used for insomnia because they are classified as Schedule II controlled substances with a high potential for abuse and addiction.

QSEN: Safety

Dosages for Common Drugs for Insomnia

Drug	Dosage
Benzodiazepine Receptor Agonists	
eszopiclone (Lunesta)	*Adults:* 2-3 mg orally at bedtime
zolpidem (Ambien)	*Adults:* 10 mg orally at bedtime; extended release—12.5 mg at bedtime

Continued

Dosages for Common Drugs for Insomnia—cont'd

Drug	Dosage
zaleplon (Sonata)	*Adults:* 10 mg orally at bedtime (dosage range is 5-20 mg)
Benzodiazepines	
flurazepam (Dalmane, Novoflupam ✿, Somnol ✿)	*Adults:* 15-30 mg orally at bedtime
quazepam (Doral)	*Adults:* 7.5-15 mg orally at bedtime
triazolam (Gen-Triazolam ✿, Halcion, Novotriolam ✿)	*Adults:* 0.125-0.25 mg orally at bedtime (maximum dose 0.5 mg)
estazolam (ProSom)	*Adults:* 1-2 mg orally at bedtime
temazepam (Restoril)	*Adults:* 7.5-30 mg orally at bedtime
Barbiturates	
pentobarbital (Nembutal)	*Adults:* 100-200 mg orally at bedtime *Children:* 2-6 mg/kg orally at bedtime
secobarbital (Seconal)	*Adults:* 100 mg orally at bedtime
Miscellaneous Sedative-Hypnotic	
chloral hydrate (Aquachloral, Somnote)	*Adults:* 0.5 to 1 g orally or rectally at bedtime *Children:* 50 mg/kg orally up to 1 g at bedtime

How Drugs for Insomnia Work

Benzodiazepines such as temazepam (Restoril) and benzodiazepine receptor agonists such as zaleplon (Sonata) relieve insomnia by either stimulating an increase in the inhibitory neurotransmitter GABA (gamma aminobutyric acid) in the brain or acting as an agonist at the GABA receptor in the brain. These actions cause depression of selected areas of the CNS. Antihistamines such as diphenhydramine (Benadryl) and sedating antidepressants such as trazodone (Desyrel) produce drowsiness and mild sedation, which enhances sleep.

Common Side Effects

Drugs for Insomnia

Drowsiness   Dizziness   Dry mouth

Headache   GI discomfort

Intended Responses
- Insomnia is relieved, and sleep is improved.
- Person is sedated, and sleep is induced.
- Length of time to fall asleep is decreased.
- Sleep duration is increased.

Side Effects. Benzodiazepine receptor agonists can cause amnesia, daytime drowsiness, dizziness, and a feeling of "being drugged." Additional side effects of zaleplon (Sonata) include hallucinations, impaired memory, and impaired psychomotor functions for a brief period of time after the drug dose.

Benzodiazepines may cause confusion, daytime drowsiness, decreased ability to concentrate, dizziness, headache, and lethargy. These drugs can also cause blurred vision, constipation, diarrhea, nausea, and vomiting.

Adverse Effects. Drugs for insomnia are metabolized by the liver and excreted by the kidney. When liver or kidney function is reduced, drug levels can become very high, with more side effects and adverse effects. A very concerning side effect of the benzodiazepine receptor agonists is *somnambulism*, sleepwalking. Some people taking these have had episodes of sleep-eating and sleep-driving without any recollection of these actions. It is not known how common the problem of somnambulism is among patients prescribed benzodiazepine receptor agonists.

Benzodiazepines are potentially addictive. Psychologic and physical dependence can develop within a few weeks or months of regular or repeated use. In addition,

Clinical Pitfall

A concerning side effect of the benzodiazepine receptor agonists is the possibility of sleepwalking, sleep-eating, and sleep-driving with the patient having no recollection of these actions.

QSEN: Safety

overdose is possible. The reversal agent for a benzodiazepine overdose is flumazenil (Romazicon). When given intravenously, it can reverse the sedation effects of a benzodiazepine overdose. Its duration of action is not as long as any of the benzodiazepines. This means that more than one dose may be needed. It does not reverse the depressed respiratory functions associated with benzodiazepine overdose, and the patient may still need mechanical ventilation. Flumazenil can lower the seizure threshold, especially in a person who has used benzodiazepines for a long time.

What To Do *Before* Giving Drugs for Insomnia

In addition to the general actions to take listed in Chapter 2 before giving any drug for insomnia to a patient for the first time, ask the patient about usual sleep patterns and his or her specific difficulty with sleeping. In addition, ask about a history of depression, confusion, falls, and pain. Assess the patient's current mental status.

What To Do *After* Giving Drugs for Insomnia

For patients in an acute care or residential setting who are taking a drug for insomnia for the first time, check the patient's vital signs and assess the level of consciousness. Watch for changes in heart rate, blood pressure, and level of consciousness. Check for orthostatic hypotension, excessive sedation, or confusion, especially in older adults.

Instruct the patient to call for help when getting out of bed and ensure that the call light is within easy reach because these drugs can cause drowsiness and dizziness. Remind the patient to get up or change positions slowly.

What To Teach Patients Taking Drugs for Insomnia

Tell patients to take these drugs exactly as directed by the prescriber and remind them of the importance of follow-up appointments to monitor the progress of treatment. Remind patients never to take a double dose of these drugs. Tell them to report side effects to the prescriber.

Teach patients taking benzodiazepines about the possibility of becoming dependent on these drugs when they are taken for extended periods of time. Remind them that drugs for insomnia should be taken only for a short period of time (2 to 4 weeks) and only when needed.

Tell patients that drugs for insomnia should not be taken unless there is adequate time to sleep (4 to 8 hours, depending on the sleep drug). Suggest to patients taking any of the benzodiazepine receptor agonists to have another person with them for the first night they take the drug to determine whether somnambulism will be a problem. Instruct patients taking any sedative drug to go to bed immediately after taking the drug because of its rapid onset of action. Remind them that the amnesia side effect can be reduced or avoided if they are able to get 4 or more hours of sleep after taking the drug. Warn patients not to take these drugs on overnight airplane flights of less than 7 to 8 hours because they may experience transient memory loss called *traveler's amnesia*.

Because drugs for insomnia can cause drowsiness and blurred vision, caution patients to avoid driving, operating heavy or complicated equipment, or performing any activities that require alertness. Also stress the importance of not drinking alcohol while taking these drugs to avoid potentiating the sedating effects.

Life Span Considerations for Drugs for Insomnia

Pediatric Considerations. Watch children receiving any sedating drug for unusual or paradoxical responses. A paradoxical response is one that is opposite of what is expected.

Considerations for Pregnancy and Lactation. Benzodiazepines have a high likelihood of increasing the risk for birth defects or fetal harm and should not be taken during pregnancy. Most benzodiazepine receptor agonists have a moderate likelihood of increasing the risk for birth defects or fetal harm and are generally

Clinical Pitfall

Do not give flumazenil (Romazicon) to anyone who has a seizure disorder.

QSEN: Safety

Drug Alert!

Action/Intervention Alert

To better monitor for side effects, assess the level of consciousness before giving a drug for insomnia.

QSEN: Safety

Drug Alert!

Teaching Alert

Teach patients taking benzodiazepine receptor agonists to go to bed immediately after taking a dose of these drugs.

QSEN: Safety

Drug Alert!

Teaching Alert

Teach patients to be sure that there is adequate time (4 to 8 hours) for sleep before taking a drug for insomnia.

QSEN: Safety

Drug Alert!

Teaching Alert

Teach patients taking an insomnia drug to avoid alcohol and other CNS-depressing substances because of the risk for oversedation.

QSEN: Safety

Clinical Pitfall

Most drugs for insomnia should not be taken during pregnancy or breastfeeding.

QSEN: Safety

considered safe for use during pregnancy, but only if the benefits outweigh the possible side effects. Most drugs for insomnia cross the placenta and enter breast milk and can have sedating effects on the fetus or infant.

Considerations for Older Adults. Older adults should be given lower doses of drugs for insomnia because they are more sensitive to the effects of these drugs and more likely to experience side effects. In addition, older adults are at increased risk for falls while taking these drugs.

Get Ready for Practice!

Key Points

- All drugs to relieve insomnia cause some degree of central nervous system depression.
- Psychologic and physical dependence can develop within a few weeks or months of regular or repeated use of many drugs for insomnia.
- The barbiturate drugs (pentobarbital and secobarbital) are rarely used for insomnia because they are classified as Schedule II controlled substances with a high potential for abuse and addiction.
- To better monitor for effectiveness and for side effects, assess the level of consciousness before giving a drug for insomnia.
- Teach patients taking drugs for insomnia to be sure that there is adequate time for sleep (4 to 8 hours) before taking these drugs.
- A concerning side effect of the benzodiazepine receptor agonists is the possibility of sleepwalking, sleep-eating, and sleep-driving with the patient having no recollection of these actions.
- A family member should be taught to watch the patient taking a benzodiazepine receptor agonist for sleepwalking.
- Warn patients to avoid operating any heavy equipment, driving a car, or making critical decisions while under the influence of any CNS depressant drug.

Additional Learning Resources

evolve Be sure to visit your Evolve website (http://evolve.elsevier.com/Workman/pharmacology/) for additional online resources.

SG Go to your Study Guide for additional learning activities to help you master this chapter content.

Review Questions

See the Answer Keys—In-text Review Questions for answers to these questions.

Test Yourself on the Basics

1. With which drug for insomnia should you warn the patient about the side effect of sleepwalking, sleep-eating, or sleep-driving?
   A. eszopiclone (Lunesta)
   B. flurazepam (Dalmane)
   C. cyclobenzaprine (Flexeril)
   D. chloral hydrate (Aquachloral)

2. What should you instruct the patient to do immediately after taking a benzodiazepine receptor agonist?
   A. Drink at least 8 oz of water with the tablet or capsule.
   B. Go to bed within 5 to 10 minutes after taking the drug.
   C. Check your pulse for 1 full minute after taking the drug.
   D. Listen to soft and relaxing music to ensure adequate sleep.

3. Which drugs belong to the benzodiazepine receptor agonist class? (Select all that apply.)
   A. chloral hydrate (Somnote)
   B. estazolam (ProSom)
   C. eszopiclone (Lunesta)
   D. flurazepam (Dalmane)
   E. secobarbital (Seconal)
   F. triazolam (Halcion)
   G. zaleplon (Sonata)
   H. zolpidem (Ambien)

4. Which drug for insomnia is rarely used now because it is a Schedule II drug with a high potential for abuse and dependence?
   A. chloral hydrate (Aquachloral)
   B. flurazepam (Dalmane)
   C. pentobarbital (Nembutal)
   D. zolpidem (Ambien)

Test Yourself on Advanced Concepts

5. Why should a patient taking a CNS depressant avoid drinking alcohol?
   A. Alcohol can potentiate the sedating effect of these drugs.
   B. Alcohol reduces the pupil size increasing the risk for falls.
   C. Drinking alcohol with a CNS depressant lowers blood glucose levels.
   D. Combining a CNS depressant with alcohol increases the risk for urinary retention.

6. What is the reversal agent for a benzodiazepine overdose?
   A. caffeine
   B. naloxone (Narcan)
   C. protamine sulfate
   D. flumazenil (Romazicon)

7. Which statement made by a person prescribed to take zolpidem (Ambien) indicates a need for more teaching?
   A. "I always go to bed as soon as I take this drug."
   B. "I am so glad that this drug is so safe and has no potential for dependence."
   C. "I will be sure to take this drug only when I have time to sleep for at least 4 hours."
   D. "I will not drink alcoholic beverages or take any other sleep aid when I am taking this drug."

8. A 40-year-old man is prescribed 600 mg of chloral hydrate orally. The liquid chloral hydrate you have on hand is 250 mg/5 mL. How many mL is the correct dose for this patient? _____ mL

Critical Thinking Activities

See the Answer Keys—Critical Thinking Activities for answers to these activities.

A 48-year-old woman comes to the office and asks for some secobarbital (Seconal). She reports that her husband died in a car crash 2 weeks ago and that she has not slept more than 1 hour a day since the accident. She remembered that her mother used to take Seconal occasionally years ago for insomnia. She also takes ibuprofen daily for mild arthritis.

1. What type of drug is secobarbital?
2. What type of drug is ibuprofen?
3. Is there any reason these two drugs cannot be taken at the same time?
4. Are there any dangers associated with secobarbital use for this woman?
5. Is there another drug or drug class that would be better for this woman?

Objectives

After studying this chapter you should be able to:

1. Describe the proper technique to administer eye drops and eye ointments.
2. List the names, actions, usual adult dosages, possible side effects, and adverse effects of drugs for glaucoma.
3. Describe what to do before and after giving drugs for glaucoma.
4. Explain what to teach patients taking drugs for glaucoma, including what to do, what not to do, and when to call the prescriber.
5. Describe life span considerations for drugs for glaucoma.

Key Terms

alpha-adrenergic agonists (ăd-rĕn-ĔRJ-ĭk ĂG-ō-nĭsts) (p. 464) Drugs that bind to receptor sites in the eye that bind to naturally occurring adrenalin, which "turns on" the receptor and reduces the amount of aqueous humor produced.

beta-adrenergic blocking agents (BĔ-tă ăd-rĕn-ĔRJ-ĭk blŏk-ēng Ă-jĕntz) (p. 462) Drugs that bind to adrenergic receptor sites and act as antagonists, which prevents naturally occurring adrenalin from binding to the receptors.

carbonic anhydrase inhibitors (CAIs) (kăr-BŎN-ĭk ăn-HĪ-drăz ĭn-HĬB-ĭ-tŏrz) (p. 466) A type of diuretic that also can lower intraocular pressure by reducing production of aqueous humor by as much as 60%.

cholinergic agents (kō-lĭn-ĔRJ-ĭk Ă-jĕntz) (p. 465) Drugs that increase the response that occurs when the naturally produced substance (acetylcholine) binds to its receptor

and activates it. In the eye, less aqueous humor is produced, and its flow is improved.

glaucoma (glŏ-KŌ-mă) (p. 458) A condition in which the aqueous humor does not drain normally out of the eye, causing a rise in intraocular pressure to levels that may damage the optic nerve.

intraocular pressure (IOP) (ĭn-trŭ-ŎK-yū-lŭr PRĔSH-ŭr) (p. 457) The fluid pressure inside the eyeball that helps to maintain the correct shape of the eye. The normal range for intraocular pressure is 10 to 20 mm Hg.

prostaglandin agonists (prŏ-stă-GLĂN-dĭn ĂG-ō-nĭsts) (p. 461) Drugs that bind to prostaglandin receptor sites in the eye and cause eye blood vessel smooth muscles to relax, which allows these blood vessels to dilate and drain more aqueous humor.

OVERVIEW

The eye, along with the brain, is the organ that allows sight (vision). The most common problems affecting the eye that can be treated or controlled by drug therapy are inflammation, infection, and glaucoma. These disorders are most often treated with drugs delivered as eye drops and eye ointments. General issues for ophthalmic therapy are discussed on pp. 458-461 in this chapter. Chapter 6 discusses various types of anti-inflammatory drugs, nearly all of which have an ophthalmic form. Chapters 8, 9, and 10 discuss the drug therapy for bacterial infections, viral infections, and fungal infections. Many anti-infective drugs have an ophthalmic form. This chapter focuses on drug therapy to manage glaucoma, which can be controlled if found and treated early, allowing the patient to continue to have effective vision.

REVIEW OF RELATED PHYSIOLOGY AND PATHOPHYSIOLOGY

PHYSIOLOGY

The eyes are able to change light into nerve impulses that are sent to the brain, where images are "seen." Figure 29-1 shows the features of the eye from the front (looking at a person directly in the face). The eye is a hollow ball made up of several layers. At the front of the eye is the *cornea*, the clear portion of the sclera that covers the

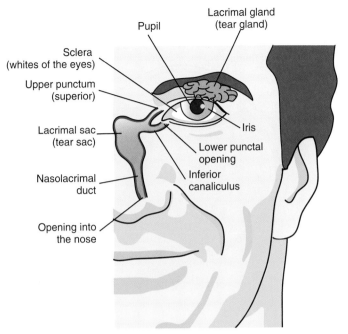

Pupil

Lacrimal gland
(tear gland)

Sclera
(whites of the eyes)

Upper punctum
(superior)

Lacrimal sac
(tear sac)

Iris

Lower punctal
opening

Inferior
canaliculus

Nasolacrimal
duct

Opening into
the nose

FIGURE 29-1   Features of the external eye (front view) along with the tear gland and duct system.

front section over the eye and allows light to enter. The *iris* is the ring of color that surrounds the pupil. The *pupil* is a round opening in the center of the iris that lets light into the eye. It dilates to increase in size, letting more light into the eye, and constricts to decrease in size, letting less light into the eye. *Miosis* is constriction of the pupil, making the opening smaller and letting less light into the eye. *Mydriasis* is dilation of the pupil, making the opening larger and letting more light into the eye (Figure 29-2).

The hollow eyeball is filled with clear substances that allow light to bend and penetrate all the way from the front of the eye to the back wall of the eye to the retina. The *retina* is the lining of the back part of the eye, opposite the pupil, that contains light-sensitive photoreceptors. *Photoreceptors,* the true sense organs for vision, are special smaller nerve endings of the large optic nerve. Photoreceptors react to light and change it into electrical impulses that are transmitted to the brain, where they are perceived as images. Figure 29-3 shows a cutaway side view of the eye. The optic nerve connects the photoreceptors in the retina to the brain and sends impulses that are changed to images in the brain.

The eye is divided into two segments, the posterior segment and the anterior segment (see Figure 29-3). The *posterior segment* is the entire back part of the eye from the lens to the area of the sclera where the optic nerve leaves the eye. It contains the *vitreous body (vitreous humor),* which is the gel-like filling of the eye. The *anterior segment* is the front of the eye that extends from the lens to the cornea and contains both the anterior and posterior chambers. It is filled with a small amount of clear fluid known as *aqueous humor.* Because the eye is hollow and needs to retain a ball-shape for vision, the gel in the posterior segment (vitreous body) and the fluid in the anterior segment (aqueous humor) must be present in set amounts that apply pressure inside the eye to keep it round. This pressure is known as **intraocular pressure (IOP)**, and it has to be just right. If the pressure is too low, the eyeball is soft and collapses, preventing light from striking the photoreceptors in the back of the eye. If the pressure is too high, it compresses blood vessels in the eye, reducing blood flow and oxygen delivery to the photoreceptors. Without enough oxygen, the photoreceptors and the optic nerve die, and sight is lost permanently.

Aqueous humor is the clear fluid made continuously by the ciliary body. This fluid circulates from the posterior chamber through the pupil and into the anterior chamber,

Memory Jogger

Constriction of the pupil is miosis (small word, small pupil size). Dilation of the pupil is mydriasis (larger word, larger pupil size).

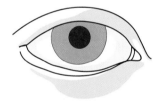

A   Normal pupil slightly dilated for moderate light.

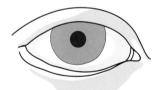

B   Miosis—pupil constricted when exposed to increased light or close work, such as reading. (Smaller word, smaller opening.)

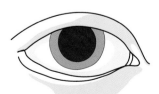

C   Mydriasis—pupil dilated when exposed to reduced light or when looking at a distance. (Larger word, larger opening.)

FIGURE 29-2   Miosis and mydriasis.

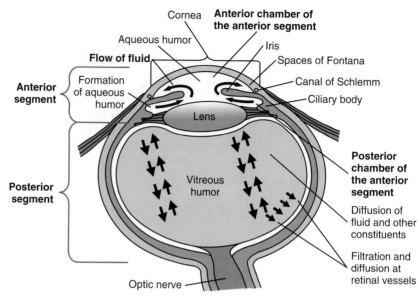

Cornea   **Anterior chamber of the anterior segment**

Aqueous humor

Iris

Flow of fluid

Spaces of Fontana

Anterior segment   Formation of aqueous humor

Canal of Schlemm

Ciliary body

Lens

Posterior chamber of the anterior segment

Posterior segment

Vitreous humor

Diffusion of fluid and other constituents

Filtration and diffusion at retinal vessels

Optic nerve

FIGURE 29-3   Side view (cutaway) of the internal features of the eye and flow of aqueous humor.

where it drains (see Figure 29-3). At the outer edges of the iris, beneath the cornea, there are blood vessels (the *trabecular network*) that collect this fluid and drain it through the canal of Schlemm, returning it to the blood. About 1 mL of aqueous humor is always present in each eye, but it is continuously made and reabsorbed. When fluid is made at the same rate that it is reabsorbed, the pressure inside the eye remains within the normal range (10 to 20 mm Hg). When fluid is reabsorbed too slowly, the amount in the eye increases, and so does the IOP.

PATHOPHYSIOLOGY

Glaucoma is a condition of increased IOP caused by an increase in the amount of aqueous humor. Both eyes can have the problem, or it may affect only one eye. There are many types and causes of glaucoma. The most common type is a chronic condition related to aging called *primary open-angle glaucoma (POAG),* which affects both eyes. Although we usually think of glaucoma as a disorder of older adults, children can also have it. In children the problem most often is caused by eye trauma that blocks the canal of Schlemm and usually only affects one eye.

POAG occurs when aqueous humor is made at the normal rate but reabsorption is reduced, leading to an increase in the amount of fluid and pressure inside the eye. This type of glaucoma is painless and has no early symptoms. The damage occurs so slowly that the patient may not even be aware that sight is being lost. Usually side vision (also known as *peripheral vision*) is lost first. Once photoreceptors die, they cannot be replaced. Without treatment, glaucoma leads to blindness.

GENERAL ISSUES FOR LOCAL EYE DRUG THERAPY

Drugs placed directly into the eye are *local* eye drug therapy. Eye drops are thin, sterile, liquid drugs that are squeezed as a small drop or drops from a small container. Eye ointments are thick, greasy drugs that stay in contact with the eye surface longer than drops. They can deliver a high concentration of drug and blur vision for minutes to hours after instillation.

Although drugs for eye problems can be taken orally or by another systemic method, they most often are administered as eye drops or eye ointments. Other routes include eye injections and placing drug disks on or in the eye. The following section discusses information about the correct use of eye drops and eye ointments, regardless of their specific actions or why they are prescribed.

Memory Jogger

Keeping the IOP within the normal range (10 to 20 mm Hg) is important to maintain vision.

Memory Jogger

Drug therapy for glaucoma does not cure the problem; it only controls it.

Many different drug types can be delivered as eye drops or eye ointments. Each type has different actions and effects, along with some common actions and effects. General responsibilities for the common effects of eye drops and eye ointments are listed in the following paragraphs. Any specific responsibilities are listed with each individual drug class.

The intended responses for all drug therapies for glaucoma are:
* IOP is reduced to the normal range.
* There is no further loss of sight.

What To Do *Before* Giving Eye Drugs

Check the order to see which eye is to receive the drug. A problem may affect only one eye, and the drug should be applied only to that eye. To avoid confusion, issues related to the right eye are indicated by writing "right eye" rather than using the Latin abbreviation "OD" *(oculus dexter)*. Issues related to the left eye are indicated as "left eye" rather than "OS" *(oculus sinister)*. Issues related to both eyes are indicated as either "both eyes" or "left and right eyes" rather than "OU" *(oculus uterque)*. When eye drugs are prescribed, the prescriber should indicate which eye or eyes are to be treated, and the pharmacist or pharmacy technician indicates this information on the drug bottles. If the eye drop bottle or eye ointment tube is not labeled with this information, the health care professional labels it to correspond to the eye or eyes being treated.

Always wash your hands. Although the eye is not sterile, aseptic technique is used when touching the eye or placing drugs into the eye because it is not well protected by the immune system and can be infected easily.

Many eye drugs come in different strengths. Always check the strength prescribed with that of the drug you have on hand to be sure that you are giving the correct dose.

Check to be sure that a tube of ointment is for ophthalmic (eye) use. Some drugs for the eye are also available as regular topical ointments, but these contain larger particles that should not be placed in the eye.

Check to see whether any other eye drops are to be administered. If so, wait at least 10 minutes after instilling the first set and before instilling the second set of eye drops. If more than two drugs are to be instilled, wait at least 10 minutes between each set.

If a patient wears contact lenses, ask him or her to remove them before instilling the drop into the eye. For some drugs, the contact lens can be replaced 15 minutes after the drug is instilled. For other drugs, especially ointments, contact lenses should not be worn until drug therapy is complete. Inspect the eye for redness, drainage, or open areas. If open areas are present, check to determine whether the drug can be instilled. Some drugs should not be instilled into an eye with open areas because the drug is rapidly absorbed into systemic circulation when applied to an open area, and the side effects are widespread. For other drugs, this is not a problem.

For ointments, after removing the cap from the ointment tube, squeeze a small amount out onto a tissue (without touching the tip of the tube or letting it come into contact with the tissue) and discard this ointment. This action reduces the chance of instilling contaminated ointment into the patient's eye.

Follow the steps in Box 29-1 for placing eye drops or ointments into another person's eye. Figure 29-4 shows a common technique for instilling eye drops or ointments.

What To Do *After* Giving Eye Drugs

For any eye drop that can have systemic side effects, apply gentle pressure to the punctum in the corner of the eye nearest the nose for about 1 minute (Figure 29-5). The *punctum* is the opening of the tube at the inner corner of the eye that drains tears into the nose and mouth (see Figure 29-1). This area is also called the *inner canthus*

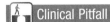

Clinical Pitfall

Avoid the use of the Latin terms for right eye (OD), left eye (OS), and both eyes (OU).

QSEN: Safety

Interaction Alert

Always wait at least 10 minutes between instilling different eye drops to prevent a drug interaction or dilution of drug concentration.

QSEN: Safety

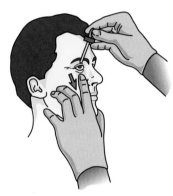

FIGURE 29-4   Correct technique for instilling eye drops.

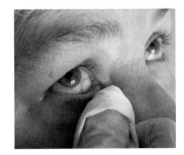

FIGURE 29-5   Applying punctal occlusion to prevent systemic absorption.

| Box 29-1 | How to Instill Eye Drops or Ointments |

SELF-ADMINISTRATION

1. Check the name, strength, expiration date, color, and clarity of the eye drops to be instilled. If the drug is an ointment, be sure that it is an ophthalmic (eye) preparation and not a general topical ointment.
2. Check to see whether only one eye is to have the drug or if both eyes are to receive the drug.
3. If both eyes are to receive the same drug and one eye is infected, use two separate bottles or tubes and carefully label each with "right" or "left" for the correct eye.
4. Wash your hands.
5. Remove the cap from the bottle or tube, keeping the cap upright to prevent contaminating it.
6. Tilt your head backward, open your eyes, and look up at the ceiling.
7. Using your nondominant hand, gently pull the lower lid down against your cheek, forming a small pocket.
8. Hold the eye drop bottle or ointment tube (with the cap off) like a pencil with the tip pointing down with your dominant hand.
9. For ointment, squeeze a small amount out onto a tissue (without touching the tip to the tissue) and discard this ointment.
10. Rest the wrist that is holding the bottle or tube against your mouth or upper lip.
11. For eye drops, gently squeeze the bottle and release the prescribed number of drops into the pocket that you have made with your lower lid. Do not touch any part of the eye or lid with the tip of the bottle. For ointment, gently squeeze the tube and release a small amount of ointment into the pocket that you have made with your lower lid. Do not touch any part of the eye or lid with the tip of the tube.
12. Gently release the lower lid.
13. Close the eye gently (without squeezing the lids tightly) and roll your eye under the lid to spread the drug across the eye.

14. For eye drops, gently press and hold the corner of the eye nearest the nose to close off the punctum and prevent the drug from being absorbed systemically.
15. Without pressing on the lid, gently blot or wipe away any excess drug or tears with a tissue.
16. Gently release the lower lid.
17. Keep the eye closed for about 1 minute.
18. Place the cap back on the bottle or tube.
19. Wash your hands again.
20. Do not drive or operate heavy machinery while your vision is blurry.

ADMINISTERING DRUGS TO ANOTHER PERSON

1. Follow self-administration steps 1 through 5.
2. Put on gloves if secretions are present in or around the eye.
3. Explain the procedure to the patient.
4. Have the patient sit in a chair and the person applying the drug stand behind the patient (or alternatively stand in front of the patient who is sitting in a chair or over the patient who is lying in bed).
5. Ask the patient to tilt the head backward, with the back of the head resting against the body of the person applying the drug (or against the back of the chair) and looking up at the ceiling.
6. Gently pull the lower lid down against the patient's cheek, forming a small pocket.
7. Hold the eye-drop bottle or ointment tube (with the cap off) like a pencil, with the tip pointing down.
8. For ointment, squeeze out and discard a small amount of ointment as described in step
9. Follow steps 11 through 16.
10. Tell the patient to keep his or her eyes closed for a minute.
11. Remove your gloves.
12. Place the cap back on the bottle or tube.
13. Wash your hands again.
14. Remind the patient not to drive or operate heavy machinery while his or her vision is blurry.

| (!) Drug Alert! |

Teaching Alert

Teach patients the steps in Box 29-1 for correctly instilling drops into one or both eyes. Using saline eye drops for practice, demonstrate the steps to patients and have patients demonstrate them back to you. If a patient has physical problems or is confused and cannot instill the eye drops, teach a family member, friend, or neighbor how to do this correctly.

Teach patients how to use punctal occlusion by applying pressure over the punctum immediately after instilling the drops. This action keeps the drug on the eye longer and helps to prevent systemic effects.

QSEN: Safety

and can be blocked by lightly pressing on it. Applying pressure to this area immediately after drops are instilled lets the drug coat the entire eye before any of it leaves the area. This action is called *punctal occlusion* and reduces systemic absorption of the drug.

Instruct patients to keep the eye closed for about 1 minute after instilling the drug to ensure that it spreads evenly across the eye.

What To *Teach* Patients Taking Eye Drugs

Teach patients to use eye drugs exactly as prescribed. Some people, especially older adults, may not consider eye drops to be a true drug. They also may believe that "if 1 drop is good, 10 drops will be better." Explain that using more drops than prescribed increases the chance that the drug will be absorbed into the blood and result in systemic effects. In addition, the effect of the drug on the eye may be too strong when extra drug is applied.

Administering eye drugs to an infant or child can be difficult. Sudden head movement can cause the tip of the bottle or tube to scratch the eye.

Older adults may have more difficulty self-administering eye drops because of physical limitations. Adaptive devices are available that hold the bottle of eye drops and help keep the eyelids open. When the device is placed around the eye, the tip of the bottle lines up directly over the center of the eye (Figure 29-6). The patient then only has to trigger the right number of drops. Although this method does not place the drops in a lid pocket, it is acceptable.

Instruct patients not to share the eye ointment with anyone else to prevent spreading eye infections from one person to another.

Remind patients not to drive or use heavy equipment while the drug is in their eye and vision is blurred.

Remind patients to report any new symptoms (general or specific to the eye) to their prescriber as soon as possible. Stress that they should call their prescriber or go to the emergency department immediately if they have a sudden loss or reduction of vision.

Life Span Considerations for Drugs Used to Treat Glaucoma

Pediatric Considerations. The safety and effectiveness of these drugs have not been established in children. However, glaucoma can occur in children and must be treated to preserve sight. Teaching the child, the parent, or any other caregiver how to instill eye drops safely is critical (see Box 29-1). It is also important to stress that if only one eye is affected, which is common when glaucoma is the result of trauma, the drugs must only be placed in the affected eye.

Considerations for Pregnancy and Lactation. Most drugs for glaucoma therapy have a moderate likelihood of increasing the risk for birth defects or fetal harm. Unless the risk for sight loss is severe, these drugs should be avoided during the first trimester of pregnancy and used with caution during the later 6 months of pregnancy. Breastfeeding is not recommended during glaucoma therapy.

Considerations for Older Adults. Focus on correct technique for administering eye drops. Teach older adults with physical limitations how to use adaptive devices for eye-drop administration.

TYPES OF DRUGS FOR GLAUCOMA

Drugs for glaucoma improve the reabsorption of aqueous humor and/or reduce the amount that is made. These actions restore good blood flow inside the eye and keep the remaining photoreceptors of the optic nerve healthy. Most glaucoma drugs are administered as eye drops. For sudden-onset glaucoma (acute closed-angle glaucoma), systemic drugs may be used.

PROSTAGLANDIN AGONISTS

How Prostaglandin Agonists Work

Prostaglandins agonists bind to prostaglandin receptor sites in the eye and relax eye blood vessel smooth muscles, which allows these blood vessels to dilate and drain more aqueous humor. This allows the fluid to leave the eye more quickly and lowers the IOP. The prostaglandin agonists are very effective, are used only once a day, and seem to have fewer systemic side effects than other drugs. Generic names, trade names, and usual dosages of these drugs are listed in the following table. Be sure to consult a drug reference book for specific information about glaucoma drugs.

Drug Alert!

Teaching Alert

Ensure that the patient understands the importance of taking only the correct dose of the drug and occluding the punctum immediately after placing the drops in his or her eye.

QSEN: Safety

Drug Alert!

Teaching Alert

If infants or young children need eye drugs, demonstrate drug instillation to the parent or guardian and teach them to obtain the assistance of another adult.

QSEN: Safety

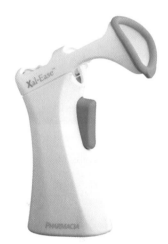

FIGURE 29-6 The Xal-Ease adaptive device for self-administering eye drops. (From Pfizer, Inc., New York.)

Drug Alert!

Teaching Alert

Teach patients using eye drugs for any eye problem to immediately call their prescriber or go to the emergency department if a sudden reduction or loss of vision occurs.

QSEN: Safety

Memory Jogger

The five classes of drugs to treat glaucoma are:

- Prostaglandin agonists
- Beta blockers
- Alpha-adrenergic agonists
- Cholinergic drugs
- Carbonic anhydrase inhibitors

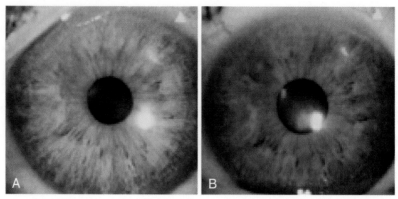

FIGURE 29-7 Changes in iris color associated with prostaglandin agonist drug therapy for glaucoma. **A,** Before treatment. **B,** After treatment. (From Yanoff, M., & Duker, J. (2009). *Ophthalmology* (3rd ed.). St. Louis: Mosby.)

Dosages for Common Prostaglandin Agonists

Drug	Dosage (Adults and Children)
bimatoprost (Lumigan)	1 drop of a 0.01% solution or a 0.03% solution in affected eye or eyes daily in the evening
latanoprost (Xalatan)	1 drop (1.5 mcg) in affected eye or eyes daily in the evening
travoprost (Travatan)	1 drop (0.004% solution) in affected eye or eyes daily in the evening

Common Side Effects

Prostaglandin Agonists

Itchiness, Redness

(!) Drug Alert!

Administration Alert

Do not instill prostaglandin agonists into an eye that does not have an intact surface.

QSEN: Safety

(!) Drug Alert!

Teaching Alert

Remind patients using a prostaglandin agonist for glaucoma in only one eye not to place the drops in the unaffected eye even though their eye colors may now be different.

QSEN: Safety

Side Effects. The most common side effects of prostaglandin agonists are eye itching, eye redness, a permanent change in the iris color from lighter colors to brown (Figure 29-7), thickening and lengthening of the eyelashes, and darkening of the skin on the eyelids.

Adverse Effects. Adverse effects related to systemic absorption of prostaglandin agonists are rare. These include muscle weakness, hypotension, elevated liver enzymes, and an increase in body hair.

What To Do *Before* and *After* Giving Prostaglandins Agonists

In addition to the general responsibilities related to eye drug therapy (pp. 458-461), inspect the eye for any corneal abrasions or other signs of trauma. These drugs should not be used if the surface of the eye is not intact.

What To *Teach* Patients Taking Prostaglandins Agonists

In addition to teaching the patient about the general care needs and precautions related to eye drugs (pp. 460-461), remind patients that using higher doses than prescribed can reduce the effectiveness of the drug in controlling glaucoma.

Tell patients that eye and eyelid color can change over time and that the lashes can become thicker and longer. If only one eye has glaucoma, the color and lash changes will occur only in that eye. Stress that the drug should *not* be used in the eye that does not have glaucoma.

BETA-ADRENERGIC BLOCKING AGENTS

How Beta-Adrenergic Blocking Agents Work

Beta-adrenergic blocking agents are drugs that bind to adrenergic receptor sites and act as antagonists in the ciliary body, which prevents naturally occurring adrenalin from binding to the receptors. This response in the eye causes less aqueous humor to be produced and also causes the fluid to be absorbed slightly. Generic names, trade names, and common dosages of these drugs are listed in the following table. Be sure to consult a drug reference for specific information about glaucoma drugs.

Dosages for Common Beta-Adrenergic Blocking Drugs

Drug	Dosage (Adults)
betaxolol hydrochloride (Betoptic, Kerlone)	1-2 drops (0.5% solution) in affected eye every 12 hr
carteolol (Cartrol, Ocupress)	1 drop (1% solution) in affected eye every 12 hr
levobetaxolol (Betaxon)	1 drop (0.5% ophthalmic suspension) in affected eye every 12 hr
levobunolol (AK-Beta, Betagan)	1-2 drops (0.25% solution) in affected eye every 12 hr; 1-2 drops (0.5% solution) in affected eye once daily
metipranolol (OptiPranolol)	1 drop (0.3% solution) in affected eye every 12 hr
timolol ❶ (Betimol, Istalol, Timoptic)	1 drop (0.25% solution or 0.5% solution) in affected eye once or twice daily
timolol GFS ❶ (gel-forming solution) (Timoptic-XE, timolol-GFS)	1 drop (0.25% solution or 0.5% solution) in affected eye once or twice daily

❶ High-alert drug.

Side Effects. Common side effects for beta blockers used in the eye include tearing, blurred vision, and a mild burning sensation within the first few minutes after the drug is instilled. Later tear production is reduced; and the eyes are dry, itchy, and red. The pupil is constricted *(miosis)*. The eyelids can become inflamed and crusty.

Adverse Effects. Long-term use of beta blockers can increase the risk for cataracts. The most serious adverse effects occur when these drugs are absorbed systemically. They can block beta receptors in the heart, slowing the heart rate, and may even lead to heart failure. In the lungs beta blockers can make the airways narrower, making asthma and bronchitis worse.

What To Do *Before* Giving Beta-Adrenergic Blocking Agents
In addition to the general responsibilities related to eye drug therapy (pp. 458-461), check the patient's vital signs (especially blood pressure, heart rate, respiratory rate, and pulse oximetry). Use these data as a baseline to determine whether an adverse reaction occurs.

Check to see whether the patient is also taking an oral beta blocker for control of blood pressure or heart rhythm problems. An oral drug taken along with beta-blocking eye drops could make the adverse effects more severe.

Check the patient's record to determine whether the patient has asthma, chronic obstructive pulmonary disease (COPD), or heart failure. Beta blockers should be used cautiously in patients with any of these problems.

What To Do *After* Giving Beta-Adrenergic Blocking Agents
In addition to the general responsibilities related to eye drug therapy (pp. 460-461), tell the patient to call you immediately if wheezing develops or dizziness is present. Check his or her blood pressure, heart rate, respiratory rate, and pulse oximetry at least every 4 hours for the presence of an adverse effect. Notify the prescriber if the heart rate drops below 60 beats per minute, wheezes develop, or the pulse oximetry reading drops below 92%.

What To *Teach* Patients Taking Beta-Adrenergic Blocking Agents
In addition to teaching the patient about the general care needs and precautions related to eye drugs, remind patients that excessive use of these drugs increase the risk for heart and breathing problems.

Tell patients to use good light when reading and to be careful in darker rooms. The pupil of the eye will not open further to let in more light, and it may be harder to see objects in dim light. This problem can increase the risk for falls.

Remind patients with diabetes that drugs from this class can mask the symptoms of hypoglycemia if the drug is absorbed systemically.

Common Side Effects

Beta-Adrenergic Blocking Agents

Miosis, Itchiness, Redness

 Memory Jogger

When beta-blocking eye drops are absorbed systemically, they can worsen asthma and heart failure.

 Drug Alert!

Action/Intervention Alert

Notify the prescriber immediately if heart rate drops or difficulty breathing develops after a beta blocker has been instilled in the eye.

QSEN: Safety

Life Span Considerations for Beta-Adrenergic Blocking Agents

Considerations for Older Adults. Focus on preventing severe systemic side effects. With high doses, systemic absorption is possible, and the effects on the cardiac and respiratory systems can be severe. Heart failure and bronchospasms can become worse. The risk for hypoglycemia increases among patients with diabetes. Thus these drugs should either not be used or used cautiously in older adults who have heart failure, asthma, COPD, other respiratory problems, or diabetes. If they are used, stress the importance of using the right dose and the need to occlude the punctum after administration.

ALPHA-ADRENERGIC AGONISTS

How Alpha-Adrenergic Agonists Work

Alpha-adrenergic agonists are drugs that bind to alpha-adrenergic receptor sites that bind to naturally occurring adrenalin, which "turns on" the receptor and reduces the amount of aqueous humor produced in the eye. They also dilate the pupil and improve fluid flow through it. These actions reduce the amount of fluid in the eye, lowering the IOP.

When used as eye drops, the effects of these drugs should be present only in the eye. They are normally used for short-term therapy to prevent or reduce pressure after eye surgery. Generic names, trade names, and common dosages of these drugs are listed in the following table. Be sure to consult a drug reference for specific information about glaucoma drugs.

Dosages for Common Alpha-Adrenergic Agonists

Drug	Dosage
apraclonidine (Iopidine)	1-2 drops (0.5% solution) in affected eye every 8 hr
dipivefrin hydrochloride (AK-Pro, Propine)	1 drop (0.1% solution) in affected eye every 12 hr

Common Side Effects

Alpha-Adrenergic Agonists

Tearing, Blurred vision, Itchiness, Redness

Side Effects. Common side effects are tearing and blurred vision for a few minutes after instilling the drug. The pupil dilates (*mydriasis*) and remains dilated, even when there is plenty of light. The sclera may also be red and itchy. Less common side effects include eyelid crusting, eye discharge, and nasal dryness.

Adverse Effects. If the drug is absorbed systemically, the patient may become drowsy. Blood pressure can decrease, and the heart rate can become slow and irregular. Usually these symptoms occur only when the drug is overused.

What To Do *Before* Giving Alpha-Adrenergic Agonists

In addition to the general responsibilities related to eye drug therapy (pp. 458-461), check the patient's vital signs, especially blood pressure and heart rate. Use this information as a baseline to determine whether an adverse reaction is occurring.

Check to see whether the patient also takes a monoamine oxidase (MAO) inhibitor drug. Alpha-adrenergic agonists are contraindicated for use in these patients.

! Drug Alert!

Interaction Alert

Alpha-adrenergic agonist eye drops for glaucoma should not be administered to anyone who is taking a monoamine oxidase inhibitor or who has taken a drug from this class within the past 14 days.

QSEN: Safety

What To Do *After* Giving Alpha-Adrenergic Agonists

In addition to the general responsibilities related to eye drug therapy (pp. 459-460), check the patient's vital signs at least once per shift to determine whether the drug is having an effect on blood pressure or heart rate.

Most alpha-adrenergic agonists should be protected from light and heat. The container is a solid color that does not allow light to enter. Refrigerate these drugs, but do not allow them to freeze.

What To *Teach* Patients Taking Alpha-Adrenergic Agonists

In addition to teaching the patient about the general care needs and precautions related to eye drugs, teach patients to store the drug properly and protect it from light.

Because the pupil is dilated, patients have increased sensitivity to light. Teach them to wear sunglasses when in the sunlight or other bright light conditions.

! Drug Alert!

Teaching Alert

Remind patients using alpha-adrenergic agonists to wear sunglasses when in bright light conditions.

QSEN: Safety

If the patient has been prescribed to use the drug for a limited time such as 1 week, remind him or her not to continue the drug beyond that time period. These drugs not only lower elevated IOP, they can also lower normal IOP, which can cause problems.

CHOLINERGIC DRUGS

How Cholinergic Agents Work

Cholinergic agents increase the response that occurs when the naturally produced substance (acetylcholine) binds to its receptor and activates it. One type of cholinergic drug is an acetylcholine agonist and acts just like acetylcholine. The other type of cholinergic drug works on the enzyme that destroys acetylcholine. The result of this action is that there is more natural acetylcholine around to bind to the acetylcholine receptor.

By either acting like acetylcholine or allowing it to remain in higher concentrations, the cholinergic drugs lower IOP by decreasing the amount of aqueous humor produced and improving its flow. These drugs make the pupil smaller (miosis) but at the same time make more room between the iris and the lens, allowing the fluid to flow better through the pupil even though it is smaller. Generic names, trade names, and common dosages of these drugs are listed in the following table. Be sure to consult a drug reference for specific information about glaucoma drugs.

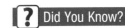 **Did You Know?**

Cholinergic drugs are named after acetylcholine.

Dosages for Common Cholinergic Drugs

Drug	Dosage
carbachol (Carboptic, Carbastat, Isopto Carbachol)	2 drops (1.5% solution or 3% solution) in affected eye every 8 hr
echothiophate (Phospholine Iodide)	1 drop (0.125% solution) in affected eye once or twice daily
pilocarpine (Adsorbocarpine, Akarpine, Isopto Carpine, Ocu-Carpine, Ocusert, Piloptic, Pilopine, Pilostat)	1-2 drops (1% solution or 2% solution) in affected eye every 6 to 8 hr, depending on strength of solution and patient response to the drug

Side Effects. The local side effects of cholinergic drugs for the eye include miosis, tearing, a mild burning sensation, blurred vision, and eye redness. These drugs are absorbed easily through the mucous membranes of the eyelids and can cause systemic effects such as headache, flushing, increased saliva, and sweating.

Adverse Effects. When larger amounts of the drug are absorbed into the blood, systemic adverse effects are possible. These include hypotension, heart rhythm problems, diarrhea, and urinary incontinence.

What To Do *Before* and *After* Giving Cholinergic Drugs

In addition to the general responsibilities related to eye drug therapy, check the patient's vital signs, especially blood pressure, heart rate, respiratory rate, and pulse oximetry. Use these data as a baseline to determine whether an adverse reaction is occurring.

Check to see whether the patient is also taking an oral cholinergic drug for other health problems (such as urinary retention or myasthenia gravis). An oral drug taken along with the eye-drop form of a cholinergic drug could make adverse effects more severe.

Check the patient's record to determine whether he or she has asthma, COPD, or heart failure. Cholinergic drugs should be used cautiously in patients with any of these problems because the drugs can make them worse.

If excess drug is present on the patient's skin, wipe it off immediately to prevent systemic side effects (these drugs can be absorbed through the skin).

Common Side Effects

Cholinergic Drugs

Miosis, Tearing, Itchiness, Redness

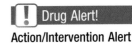 **Drug Alert!**

Action/Intervention Alert

Wipe any excess drug from the patient's skin to prevent systemic side effects.

QSEN: Safety

Drug Alert!

Action/Intervention Alert

Notify the prescriber immediately if the heart rate drops below 60 or if breathing problems develop after a cholinergic drug has been administered.

QSEN: Safety

Check the patient's blood pressure, heart rate, respiratory rate, and pulse oximetry at least every 4 hours for the presence of an adverse effect. Notify the prescriber if the heart rate drops below 60 beats per minute, wheezes develop, or the pulse oximetry reading drops below 92%.

Tell the patient to call you immediately if he or she develops wheezing or notes an increase in drooling or sweating or if dizziness is present.

Remind the patient that the pupils will not open as wide when light is low. He or she may need more light to read and see easily.

What To *Teach* Patients Taking Cholinergic Drugs

In addition to teaching patients about the general care needs and precautions related to eye drugs, tell patients to use good light when reading and be careful in darker rooms. The pupil of the eye will not open wider to let in more light, and it may be harder to see objects in dim light. This problem can increase the risk for falls.

Tell patients to report an increase in drooling or sweating to their prescriber immediately because these are often the symptoms of drug overdose.

 Do Not Confuse

acetaZOLAMIDE *with* acetoHEXAMIDE

An order for acetaZOLAMIDE can be confused with acetoHEX-AMIDE. AcetaZOLAMIDE is a drug to treat glaucoma, whereas aceto-HEXAMIDE is a drug for type 2 diabetes.

QSEN: Safety

CARBONIC ANHYDRASE INHIBITORS

How Carbonic Anhydrase Inhibitors Work

Carbonic anhydrase inhibitors (CAIs) are a type of diuretic that also can lower IOP by reducing production of aqueous humor by as much as 60%. They can be taken orally and as eye drops to control glaucoma. Generic names, trade names, and common dosages of these drugs are listed in the following table. Be sure to consult a drug reference for specific information about glaucoma drugs.

Dosages for Common Carbonic Anhydrase Inhibitors

Drug	Dosage (Adults)
acetaZOLAMIDE (Diamox)	250 mg orally 1 to 4 times daily (sustained-release capsules) 500 mg IV over 1 min; may repeat the dose in 2-4 hr
brinzolamide (Azopt)	1 drop (1% solution) in affected eye every 8 hr
dorzolamide (Trusopt)	1 drop (2% solution) in affected eye every 8 hr
methazolamide (Neptazane)	50-100 mg orally every 8 to 12 hr

 Do Not Confuse

Diamox *with* Diabinese

An order for Diamox can be confused with Diabinese. Diamox is a diuretic drug to treat glaucoma, whereas Diabinese is an older drug used for type 2 diabetes.

QSEN: Safety

Common Side Effects

Carbonic Anhydrase Inhibitors

Blurred vision, Itchiness, Redness

Side Effects. When carbonic anhydrase inhibitors are used as eye drops, the most common side effect is blurred vision briefly after instilling the drug. The sclera may also become red and itchy.

When these drugs are given systemically, there are many more side effects such as changes in blood glucose levels (up or down), headache, fever, nausea, vomiting, and diarrhea.

Adverse Effects. Carbonic anhydrase inhibitors are related to the sulfonamide antibacterial drugs ("sulfa" drugs). If a patient has an allergy to sulfonamides, he or she may also have an allergy to carbonic anhydrase inhibitors, even when they are used as eye drops.

When taken systemically, these drugs can cause acidosis; severe skin reactions; electrolyte imbalances; dizziness; confusion; and numbness of the hands, feet, and face. Carbonic anhydrase inhibitors also interact with many drugs. Be sure to check a drug handbook or the package insert before administering any of these drugs by mouth or as an injection.

What To Do *Before* Giving Carbonic Anhydrase Inhibitors

In addition to the general responsibilities related to eye drug therapy, ask the patient whether he or she is allergic to sulfonamide antibacterial drugs. Because carbonic anhydrase inhibitors are a type of sulfonamide, the patient may also have an allergy to these drugs. If he or she has a known allergy to sulfonamides, report this to the prescriber before administering the eye drops.

What To Do *After* Giving Carbonic Anhydrase Inhibitors

In addition to the general responsibilities related to eye drug therapy (pp. 459-460), after giving the first dose of a drug from this class, check the patient's vital signs every hour for the first 2 hours. Also ask the patient whether any shortness of breath, dizziness, or general skin itchiness is occurring. These are all symptoms of an allergic reaction.

Life Span Considerations for Carbonic Anhydrase Inhibitors

Pediatric Considerations. Carbonic anhydrase inhibitors are not used in children with glaucoma because these drugs slow growth when used long term.

Considerations for Pregnancy and Lactation. Carbonic anhydrase inhibitors are known to cause birth defects in animals. Unless the risk for sight loss is severe, these drugs should be avoided during pregnancy. Carbonic anhydrase inhibitors are not recommended during breastfeeding.

Considerations for Older Adults. The use of carbonic anhydrase inhibitors can increase the risk for acidosis. The risk for acidosis is low when the patient is taking the drug in eye-drop form. However, misuse or overuse of the drug can lead to acidosis and other systemic problems.

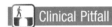

Drug Alert!

Administration Alert

Do not administer a carbonic anhydrase inhibitor to a patient who has a "sulfa drug" allergy.

QSEN: Safety

Clinical Pitfall

Do not give carbonic anhydrase inhibitors to children or women who are pregnant or breastfeeding.

QSEN: Safety

Get Ready for Practice!

Key Points

- Use aseptic technique when instilling eye drugs because the eye can easily become infected.
- Apply only ointments that are labeled "for ophthalmic use" in the eye.
- Place eye drops or eye ointments only in the affected eye.
- If both eyes are to be treated and one eye is infected, use a separate bottle or tube for each eye.
- Place the drops or ointment into a pocket created by gently pulling the lower lid downward.
- Never touch any part of the patient's eye with the tip of the bottle or tube.
- Drugs administered as eye drops can enter the blood and cause systemic effects.
- When instilling eye drops that can have systemic effects, apply gentle pressure to the corner of the eye nearest the nose (the inner canthus where the drainage ducts are located) for 1 to 2 minutes after instilling the drops.
- Teach the patient to use eye drops or ointments exactly as directed and never to use more drug than prescribed.
- Glaucoma can occur at any age and can affect one or both eyes.
- Untreated glaucoma leads to blindness.
- The goal of glaucoma therapy is to keep the IOP within normal range and prevent loss of photoreceptors.
- Most drugs for glaucoma come in different strengths; be sure to check the strength of the drug that you have on

hand with that of the prescription to prevent overdosing or underdosing.
- Adrenergic agonists cause the pupils to dilate and the eye to be more sensitive to light. Urge patients to wear dark glasses or a hat with a brim in bright conditions.
- Beta blockers and cholinergic drugs make the pupil smaller even in low-light conditions. Teach patients to be more cautious in dim lighting to avoid falls and to use more light to read or do close work.
- Beta blockers and cholinergic drugs, if absorbed systemically, can slow the heart rate, lower blood pressure, and cause asthma. Be sure to warn patients about these side effects and tell them to notify their prescriber if symptoms appear or worsen.
- Warn patients with diabetes that beta blockers can mask the symptoms of hypoglycemia. Blood glucose levels may need to be checked more often.
- Over time the prostaglandin agonist eye drops change the color of the iris to brown, darken the eyelids, and increase the number and length of eyelashes.

Additional Learning Resources

evolve Be sure to visit your Evolve website (http://evolve.elsevier.com/Workman/pharmacology/) for additional online resources.

SG Go to your Study Guide for additional learning activities to help you master this chapter content.

Review Questions

See the Answer Keys—In-text Review Questions for answers to these questions.

Test Yourself on the Basics

1. Which brand name drugs belong to the prostaglandin agonist class? Select all that apply.
   A. Betaxon
   B. Iopidine
   C. Lumigan
   D. Ocupress
   E. Piloptic
   F. Travatan
   G. Trusopt
   H. Xalatan

2. Which adverse effect can occur as a result of excessive use of prostaglandin agonists?
   A. Asthma
   B. Hypertension
   C. Urinary retention
   D. Increased body hair

3. For which eye-drop-delivered drug is it most important that the corneal surface be intact?
   A. dorzolamide (Trusopt)
   B. metipranolol (OptiPranolol)
   C. pilocarpine (Akarpine)
   D. travoprost (Travatan)

4. Which eye drops for glaucoma are most likely to cause miosis? Select all that apply.
   A. brimonidine (Alphagan)
   B. brinzolamide (Azopt)
   C. carbachol (Isopto)
   D. dipivefrin (AK-Pro)
   E. echothiophate (Phospholine Iodide)
   F. latanoprost (Xalatan)
   G. methazolamide (Neptazane)
   H. timolol (Timoptic)

5. Which patient problem is a contraindication for use of the beta-adrenergic antagonist drugs?
   A. Asthma
   B. Blurred vision
   C. Constipation
   D. Diabetes type 1

Test Yourself on Advanced Concepts

6. Which drug for glaucoma must be avoided for patients who have an allergy to sulfa drugs?
   A. carteolol (Ocupress)
   B. dorzolamide (Trusopt)
   C. levobunolol (Betagan)
   D. dipivefrin hydrochloride (Propine)

7. You are teaching a family member to apply eye drops before a patient's surgery. Into which exact area do you instruct the drops to be instilled?
   A. The corner of the eye nearest the nose
   B. The corner of the eye nearest the side of the head
   C. The center of the eye where the pupil is located
   D. The pocket created by pulling down the lower lid

8. Which patient response is most important to check after administering an adrenergic agonist for control of glaucoma?
   A. Heart rate and rhythm
   B. 24-hour urine output
   C. Level of consciousness
   D. Pupil size and shape

9. A patient is prescribed to receive acetazolamide (Diamox) 250 mg orally immediately for an increased intraocular pressure. The drug you have on hand is acetazolamide 125 mg/tablet. How many tablets will you give for the 250-mg dose? _____tablets

10. A patient is prescribed latanoprost (Xalatan), 1 drop per eye twice each day (every 12 hours) for control of glaucoma. The bottle contains 4 mL of drug, and 16 drops = 1 mL. How many days will the bottle of eye drops last if the patient uses the drug exactly as prescribed? _____ days

Critical Thinking Activities

See the Answer Keys—Critical Thinking Activities for answers to these activities.

Mr. Green is a 79-year-old widower who has just been diagnosed with glaucoma and has been prescribed latanoprost (Xalatan) 1 drop (1.5 mcg) in both eyes once daily. He is fiercely independent and lives alone in a small apartment. His daughter, who is a nurse, lives about 30 minutes away and visits him twice a week. In addition to glaucoma, he has mild heart failure for which he takes furosemide (Lasix) 40 mg once daily and carvedilol (Coreg) 12.5 mg twice daily. He also has a "frozen shoulder" on the right side (his dominant side) from a previous injury. As a result, he cannot bring his right hand up to his face. He is concerned that he won't be able to instill his own eye drops. You are concerned that he may only use the drops twice weekly when his daughter visits.

1. What type of drug is latanoprost, and what are the side effects?
2. Considering his other health problems, is this a good drug for him? Why or why not?
3. What problems can occur if he only receives the eye drops twice weekly?
4. How can you work with the patient to help him remain independent and use his glaucoma medication correctly?

Drug Therapy for Osteoporosis, Arthritis, and Skeletal Muscle Relaxation

http://evolve.elsevier.com/Workman/pharmacology/

Objectives

After studying this chapter you should be able to:

1. List the names, actions, usual adult dosages, possible side effects, and adverse effects of drugs for osteoporosis and arthritis.
2. Explain what to teach patients about drugs for osteoporosis and arthritis.
3. List the names, actions, usual adult dosages, possible side effects, and adverse effects of drugs for skeletal muscle relaxation.
4. Explain what to do before and after giving a drug for skeletal muscle relaxation.
5. Explain what to teach patients about drugs for skeletal muscle relaxation.

Key Terms

benzodiazepines (běn-zō-dī-ĂZ-ě-pēnz) (p. 476) A class of psychotropic drugs with hypnotic and sedative effects used to control symptoms of anxiety or stress and as sleeping aids for insomnia (see Chapters 27 and 28).

bisphosphonates (BĪ-ō-FŎS-fō-nātz) (p. 472) A class of drugs known as calcium-modifying drugs that both prevent bones from losing calcium and increase bone density.

carbamates (KĂR-bă-mātz) (p. 477) A class of drugs that act centrally to depress most central nervous system activity and reduce motor neuron depolarization, leading to skeletal muscle relaxation.

cyclobenzaprines (sī-klō-BĚN-ză-prēnz) (p. 477) A class of drugs similar in structure to the tricyclic antidepressants that change the influence of serotonin in the spinal cord, which reduces nerve impulse transmission and leads to skeletal muscle relaxation.

estrogen agonists/antagonists (ĔS-trō-jěn ĂG-ŏ-nĭsts/ăn-TĂG-ŏ-nĭsts) (p. 472) Hormone receptor drugs that selectively bind to and activate estrogen receptors in some tissues and bind to and block estrogen receptors in other tissues.

osteoclast monoclonal antibodies (ŏs-tē-ō-KLĂST mŏ-nō-KLŌ-năl ăn-tĭ-BŎD-ēz) (p. 472) Drugs composed of antibodies directed against immature osteoclasts.

skeletal muscle relaxants (SKĔL-ĭ-tăl MŬS-ăl rē-LĂK-sănts) (p. 476) A class of drugs that act by depressing the central nervous system, resulting in a reduction of skeletal muscle spasms, increased sedation, reduction of pain perception, and increased mobility of affected skeletal muscles.

uric acid synthesis inhibitors (Ū-rĭk ĂS-ĭd SĬN-thě-sĭs ĭn-HĬB-ĭ-tŏrz) (p. 475) Drugs that prevent the formation of uric acid resulting in lower blood levels of uric acid and prevention of hyperuricemia.

THE MUSCULOSKELETAL SYSTEM

The musculoskeletal system is composed of bones and muscles. Bones form the framework for the body and support the positions of other organs and tissues. Some bones are organized to work with other bones to allow body movement or locomotion. The organized connections of bones for the purpose of movement are the joints. However, bones alone cannot move the body. Skeletal muscles and their associated structures (tendons and ligaments) are attached to bones for the main purpose of movement. Muscles are attached as opposing groups around joints in a way that when one muscle group contracts (shortens), the joint flexes so that the two connecting bones move toward each other by pulling motions (Figure 30-1, *A*). To straighten the bones around a joint, the flexor muscles relax (stretch) and the opposing muscles (extensors) contract so that the bones are pulled back into their original positions (Figure 30-1, *B*). Skeletal muscles do not normally

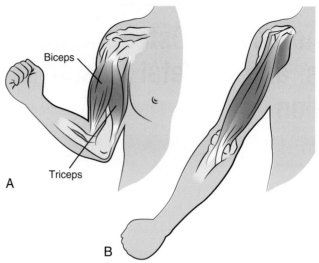

FIGURE 30-1 **A,** Biceps contracted, bending the elbow and moving forearm up toward the shoulder. **B,** Triceps contracted, pulling the forearm down, straightening the elbow.

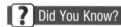

Did You Know?

Muscles move bones around joints by pulling the bones, never by pushing the bones.

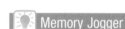

Memory Jogger

Osteoclastic activity reduces bone density and strength whereas osteoblastic activity improves bone density and strength.

contract on their own. They require stimulation from the nervous system. Thus smooth, coordinated motion requires the input of the nervous system to alternately stimulate the opposing muscle groups that cause joints to bend and then straighten. The major problems that can occur with the musculoskeletal system that can be managed with drug therapy are osteoporosis, arthritis, and skeletal muscle spasms.

OSTEOPOROSIS

REVIEW OF RELATED PHYSIOLOGY AND PATHOPHYSIOLOGY

For bones to be strong enough to provide continuing support throughout the life span, they must stay firm and dense. Bone formation with the removal of old bone cells (*osteocytes*) and replacement with new bone cells occurs throughout life. The process of old bone cell removal is known as *osteoclastic activity*. Osteoclastic activity also causes bones to lose minerals, especially calcium, a process known as *bone resorption of calcium*. Replacement with new bone cells is known as *osteoblastic activity*.

In infancy, childhood, and adolescence, osteoblastic activity occurs at a faster rate than osteoclastic activity. This results in bones becoming longer as the individual grows taller, and becoming more dense to support body structures as the individual grows heavier. In addition to bone cells, minerals such as calcium and phosphorus deposit and form a matrix within the bone to add density and strength. Osteoblastic activity and hormones contribute to the deposition and retention of these minerals, as does weight-bearing. (The more weight-bearing, the more signals are sent to the bones indicating that remaining strong and dense is important.)

In adulthood, the osteoblastic activity and osteoclastic activity should be balanced so that bone does not become longer or thicker but does maintain its density. The desired actions are that as older cells are removed, they are replaced with an equal number of new cells and that minerals are retained in the matrix for bone strength.

As a person ages, osteoblastic activity can slow down. If osteoclastic activity then continues at a normal or faster rate, bone formation becomes unbalanced with bone cell removal occurring faster than bone cell replacement. This results in thinner, more fragile bones that can break easily. When osteoclastic activity outstrips osteoblastic activity, bone mineral loss also reduces bone density.

The problem of imbalanced bone metabolism is known as *osteoporosis*. It is likely that all older people have some degree of osteoporosis as a result of normal aging. However, some conditions and factors speed up this process. Osteoporosis occurs to a greater degree and at earlier ages among people who are smaller statured (women more than men), those who have a strong family history of the problem, those who smoke, those who are taking corticosteroids on a daily basis, those who have lower levels of androgens (men) or lower levels of estrogen (women), and those who do not participate in sufficient weight-bearing activity. (Weight-bearing activity includes walking, dancing, running, and performing resistance exercises. Swimming, cycling, and most upper body exercises are *not* considered sufficiently weight-bearing to prevent or delay osteoporosis.)

Many health problems are associated with osteoporosis. Foremost is the greatly increased risk for bone fractures and the resulting mobility limitations. However, other problems can occur as bone density decreases unevenly. Posture changes, and the person loses height as the spine bends forward, outward, or inward (Figure 30-2). These changes can limit lung expansion and lead to pulmonary problems.

TYPES OF DRUGS TO MANAGE OR SLOW OSTEOPOROSIS

A variety of different types of drugs and supplements are used to manage or slow the progression of osteoporosis. These include the categories of nutritional supplements (vitamins and minerals), bisphosphonates, estrogen agonists/antagonists, and osteoclast monoclonal antibodies.

Nutritional Supplements

Bone density and strength depend on an adequate supply of the mineral calcium. Calcium in the diet is absorbed in the small intestine in the presence of activated vitamin D. Without adequate amounts of activated vitamin D, little if any dietary calcium is absorbed. This is why some sources of calcium, such as milk, are fortified by having vitamin D added to them. Anyone at risk for developing osteoporosis or who actually has osteoporosis is recommended to supplement the diet with additional calcium and vitamin D. Issues related to the nutritional supplementation with these substances and other substances are presented in Chapter 24.

 Memory Jogger

Osteoporosis occurs with aging, but the rate of progression varies as a result of many individual patient factors.

 Memory Jogger

The drugs used to manage or prevent osteoporosis include:
- Nutritional supplements (calcium and activated vitamin D)
- Bisphosphonates
- Estrogen agonists/antagonists
- Osteoclastic monoclonal antibodies.

 Did You Know?

Your intestinal tract cannot absorb dietary calcium without sufficient amounts of activated vitamin D.

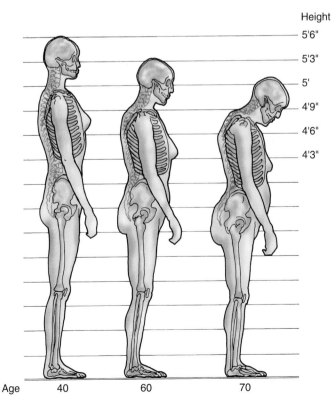

FIGURE 30-2   A normal spine at age 40 years and osteoporotic changes at ages 60 and 70 years. (From Ignatavicius, D. D., & Workman, M. L. (2016). *Medical-surgical nursing: Patient-centered collaborative care* (8th ed.). St. Louis: Saunders.)

Memory Jogger

The generic names of the bisphosphonates all have the syllable "dron" in the middle.

Memory Jogger

Remember that agonists activate the receptor site of a cell and mimic the actions of naturally occurring body substances or hormones, whereas antagonists block the receptor site of a cell and prevent the actions of naturally occurring body substances or hormones.

Do Not Confuse

Fosamax *with* Flomax

An order for Fosamax can be confused with Flomax. Fosamax is a drug to manage or prevent osteoporosis and Flomax is a drug to improve urine flow for men with an enlarged prostate gland.

QSEN: Safety

Do Not Confuse

Actonel *with* Actos

An order for Actonel (risedronate) can be confused with Actos. Actonel is a bisphosphonate drug to manage or prevent osteoporosis. Actos is an antidiabetes drug to control blood glucose levels.

QSEN: Safety

Bisphosphonates

Bisphosphonates are a type of calcium-modifying drug that both prevents bones from losing calcium and increases bone density, rather than just maintaining bone density. The major use for these drugs is the prevention and management of osteoporosis with reduction of the risk for bone fractures, especially in women. They are less effective in preventing and managing osteoporosis in men. Other approved uses for these drugs include the prevention of skeletal fractures in patients with bone metastases and multiple myeloma, Paget's disease, and for the treatment of hypercalcemia associated with cancer.

Currently prescribed bisphosphonates are second- and third-generation drugs that contain nitrogen and are much more effective than the first-generation drugs. These drugs are only effective in people who have an adequate intake of both calcium and vitamin D. For this reason, some formulations of the bisphosphonates also contain calcium and vitamin D. Bisphosphonates as therapy for osteoporosis are not indicated for children.

Estrogen Agonists/Antagonists

Estrogen agonists/antagonists are hormone receptor drugs that selectively bind to and activate estrogen receptors in some tissues and bind to and block estrogen receptors in other tissues. For many years, it has been known that osteoporosis developed and progressed more rapidly after menopause, when a woman's estrogen production was very low. Estrogen and estrogen agonists have a protective influence in preventing bone density loss. Initially, postmenopausal women were give estrogen agonists for this action. However, the estrogen agonists activated estrogen receptors in all tissues, causing many problems. These problems included enhanced growth of breast and uterine tumors, formation of blood clots, and thickened uterine lining tissues leading to excessive dysfunctional uterine bleeding. Because the estrogen agonists/antagonists are selective in which estrogen receptors they activate and which ones they block, some of the problems associated with estrogen use after menopause to prevent or manage osteoporosis are reduced.

Osteoclast Monoclonal Antibodies

Osteoclast monoclonal antibodies are drugs composed of antibodies directed against immature osteoclasts. Binding of these antibodies to immature osteoclasts prevents their maturation and reduces their actions of reducing bone density and strength. Just like any other drug composed of antibodies, severe allergic reactions are possible. For this reason, this drug should be prescribed only to treat severe osteoporosis in patients for whom other treatments have not been effective.

Dosages for Common Drugs to Prevent or Manage Osteoporosis

Drug	Dosage
Bisphosphonates	
alendronate (Fosamax)	*Adults:* 10 mg orally daily
ibandronate (Boniva)	*Adults:* 2.5 mg orally daily, *or* 150 mg orally once per month, *or* 3 mg IV bolus, once every 3 months
risedronate (Actonel, Atelvia)	*Adults:* 5 mg orally daily, *or* 35 mg orally once weekly, *or* 75 mg orally twice per month, *or* 150 mg orally once per month
zoledronic acid (Reclast)	*Adults:* 5 mg IV infusion over 15 to 30 minutes once yearly
Estrogen Agonists/Antagonists	
estrogen/bazedoxifene (Duavee)	*Adults:* 1 tablet orally daily (contains 0.45 mg of conjugated estrogen and 20 mg of bazedoxifene)
raloxifene (Evista)	*Adults:* 60 mg orally once daily
Monoclonal Antibodies	
denosumab (Prolia)	*Adults:* 60 mg subcutaneously once every 6 months

How Drugs for Osteoporosis Work

Bisphosphonates all work by moving blood calcium into the bone, binding to calcium in the bone, and preventing osteoclasts from destroying bone cells and resorbing calcium. It also inhibits the activity of tumor necrosis factor (TNF) within bone, preventing certain white blood cells from damaging or destroying bone. It is not known exactly how the bisphosphonates increase bone production.

Estrogen agonists/antagonists work by agonizing (activating) estrogen receptors in the bone, which leads to reduced calcium resorption and increased bone density. At the same time, the estrogen antagonist portion of the drug blocks estrogen receptors in breast tissue and uterine tissue. This prevents excessive growth of breast tissue (that may promote breast cancer cell growth) and overgrowth of uterine endometrial tissues that can lead to excessive uterine bleeding.

Osteoclast monoclonal antibodies work by binding to a receptor on immature osteoclasts and on certain white blood cells, preventing them from becoming mature. It is only the mature osteoclasts and white blood cells that either directly attack bone cells and bone matrix or produce substances that degrade bone cells and bone matrix. The effects of osteoclast monoclonal antibodies result in decreased bone loss and increased bone density and strength.

Intended Responses
- Bones maintain density and strength.
- Blood calcium levels remain normal.
- Bone fractures do not occur.

Side Effects. The most common side effects of the *bisphosphonates* are abdominal pain, headache, esophageal reflux, and nausea. The most common side effects of the *estrogen agonist/antagonists* are muscle spasms, nausea, and indigestion. The most common side effects of *osteoclast monoclonal antibodies* are skin rashes and musculoskeletal pain.

Adverse Effects. The most serious adverse effect of the *bisphosphonates* is the development of jawbone necrosis (osteonecrosis), especially with tooth extraction or other invasive dental procedures involving the jawbone in which the bone is damaged. The exact mechanism through which these drugs cause osteonecrosis is not known but it is thought to occur because the drugs interfere with bone healing. It is more common in patients taking higher doses and with intravenous administration of the drug. Jaw osteonecrosis also is an adverse effect of *osteoclast monoclonal antibodies*.

The most common adverse effect of the *estrogen agonists/antagonists* is the increased risk for thrombotic events, which include deep vein thrombosis, stroke, myocardial infarction, and pulmonary embolism. Because of this risk, these drugs should not be used by anyone who has had a previous thrombotic event or who smokes.

The major adverse effect of *osteoclast monoclonal antibodies* is severe allergic reactions and possible anaphylaxis. The risk for severe allergic reaction increases with repeated dosage of the drug.

What To *Teach* People Taking Drug Therapy for Osteoporosis

Teach patients taking oral *bisphosphonates* to take the drug early in the morning, right after breakfast, and to drink a full glass of water. To prevent esophageal reflux and irritation, teach patients to remain in the upright position (sitting, standing, or walking) for at least 30 minutes after taking an oral bisphosphonate. Stress to patients the need to inform their dentists or oral surgeons that they are taking a *bisphosphonate* or an *osteoclast monoclonal antibody* before any tooth extraction or invasive dental procedure involving the jawbone.

Common Side Effects of Drugs for Osteoporosis

Bisphosphonates

Abdominal pain, Nausea, Esophageal reflux   Headache

⚠ Drug Alert!

Administration Alert

Assess the patient for an allergic reaction during and after subcutaneous injection of denosumab (Prolia). Keep emergency equipment in the room with the patient.

QSEN: Safety

ARTHRITIS

REVIEW OF RELATED PHYSIOLOGY AND PATHOPHYSIOLOGY

Arthritis is a progressive degeneration of bones and cartilage at joints. As the degeneration progresses, the surrounding joint tendons, ligaments and fibrous capsule are all affected. This results in greatly reduced joint function, reduced mobility, and pain.

There are different types of arthritis, which are based on the major causes of the disorder. Drug management of arthritis is determined by the specific cause and type of the arthritis, as well as the degree of damage and joint function loss.

Osteoarthritis is the most common form and usually occurs as a "wear-and-tear" disorder in weight-bearing joints as a result of chronic use. It is more common in people who are overweight and in those who have engaged in activities that chronically stress, abuse, or excessively use specific joints (such as repetitive motions). Although the disorder is affected by lifestyle, familial, and genetic factors also affect personal susceptibility to the problem. Osteoarthritis is not caused by autoimmune or inflammatory disorders, but joint inflammation can result from the damage and contributes to the pain and disability.

A variety of other types of arthritis have inflammation as part of the cause. *Rheumatoid arthritis* is an autoimmune disease in which the immune system cells fail to recognize cartilage and other joint tissues to be normal body tissue and start immunologic attacks targeting them. One body chemical in particular is involved in the attack, tumor necrosis factor (TNF). The result is severe inflammation that leads to progressive destruction of all joint tissues. Loss of joint function can occur early and progresses with pain and tissue loss.

Psoriatic arthritis is another type of autoimmune disorder that occurs in some patients who also have the skin manifestations of psoriasis, which is actually a systemic disease, not just a skin problem. Some of the same immune system cells and cell products that attacked the connective tissues of the skin also attack and destroy the connective tissues of joints. Psoriatic arthritis has inflammation as a cause of tissue destruction rather than as a result of tissue damage. It can affect any joint but is most common in the feet, hips, and lower spine.

Gouty arthritis or *gout* is a joint problem that stems from excessive uric acid crystals in the blood (hyperuricemia) precipitating into joints and starting an inflammatory process that then leads to progressive damage. For most people with this type of arthritis, the episodes of pain, swelling, and inflammation occur intermittently with periods of no symptoms in between. The problem can occur either when the person ingests excessive amounts of foods, especially proteins, that are first converted into purines and then converted into uric acid or when the person has a metabolic problem that reduces the elimination of uric acid by the kidneys. So with excessive ingestion of uric acid–forming foods, the cause is lifestyle-related (about 10% of all cases). In reduced elimination or uric acid (about 90% of all cases), the basic problem is a metabolic one in which not enough enzymes that help eliminate uric acid are present, especially when greater amounts of uric acid–producing foods are ingested. This problem can be familial.

TYPES OF DRUGS TO MANAGE ARTHRITIS

DRUGS FOR PAIN CONTROL

Drugs for pain are used for any type of arthritis when an acute episode causes pain. These drugs do not reduce the existing tissue damage or prevent progression of the disease; they merely modify the person's perception of the pain severity. Chapter 7 provides a detailed discussion of the actions, side effects, adverse effects, and other specific issues for the various types of drugs used in pain control.

ANTI-INFLAMMATORY DRUGS

A wide variety of anti-inflammatory drugs are used to manage all types of arthritis. For those types that have an immunologic basis (such as rheumatoid arthritis,

Memory Jogger

About 10% of cases of gouty arthritis result from lifestyle choices and 90% result from metabolic problems.

psoriatic arthritis, and gouty arthritis), the anti-inflammatory drugs can reduce or slow the tissue damage as well as reduce the symptoms of arthritis. Common drugs for this purpose are the nonsteroidal anti-inflammatory drugs (NSAIDs), corticosteroids, and disease-modifying anti-rheumatic drugs (DMARDs). Chapter 6 provides a detailed discussion of the actions, side effects, adverse effects, and other specific issues for the various types of anti-inflammatory drugs.

DRUGS FOR HYPERURICEMIA AND GOUT

Although pain-control drugs and anti-inflammatory drugs are used to control symptoms of gouty arthritis and gout, they do not address the actual cause, hyperuricemia. Drugs that reduce blood uric acid levels are divided into **uric acid synthesis inhibitors** that prevent the formation of uric acid and an enzyme that increases uric acid excretion. Rasburicase is the drug that increases uric acid excretion. It is only used for gout when uric acid levels are extremely high and must be brought down quickly. It is not approved for use to prevent gouty arthritis. Its most common usage is to reduce hyperuricemia related to cancer therapy (tumor lysis syndrome).

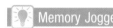
Memory Jogger

The three classes of drugs used to manage arthritis are:
- Drugs for pain control
- Anti-inflammatory drugs
- Drugs for hyperuricemia

Dosages to Manage Hyperuricemia and Gout

Drugs	Dosages
Uric Acid Synthesis Inhibitors	
allopurinol (Aloprim, Zyloprim)	*Adults:* initially 100 mg orally daily. Increased by 100 mg weekly until serum uric acid levels are reduced to 6 mg/dL or lower. Maximum dose is 800 mg orally daily *Children:* Safety and efficacy have not been established
febuxostat (Uloric)	*Adults:* 40-80 mg orally once daily *Children:* Safety and efficacy have not been established
Enzyme	
rasburicase (Elitek)	*Adults:* 0.2 mg/kg/IV over 30 minutes once daily for 5 days *Children:* Safety and efficacy have not been established

How Drugs for Gout Work

The uric acid synthesis inhibitors each reduce an enzyme important in the conversion of purines (mostly derived from dietary proteins) into uric acid. As a result, uric acid levels can be lowered to a normal level that does not precipitate in joints.

Rasburicase breaks down existing uric acid crystals in the blood and converts them to allantoin. This product is inactive and easily excreted. As a result, blood uric acid levels are rapidly reduced.

Intended Responses
- Pain, swelling, and redness are reduced.
- Physical function is increased.
- Progression of joint damage is slowed or prevented.

Side Effects. The most common side effects of the uric acid synthesis inhibitors are headache, rash, and slight nausea. The most common side effects of rasburicase are rash, abdominal pain, mucositis, and nausea.

Common Side Effects
Uric Acid Synthesis Inhibitors

Headache   Rash   Nausea

Adverse Effects. Neither allopurinol nor febuxostat have common adverse effects. There does appear to be a slightly increased risk for myocardial infarction, heart failure, and stroke when taking these drugs long term. However, these events are rare.

Administration Alert

Assess the patient for an allergic reaction throughout the infusion of rasburicase and for 2 hours after the infusion. Keep emergency equipment in the room with the patient.

QSEN: Safety

Rasburicase is associated with extreme hypersensitivity reactions and anaphylaxis. This drug also can cause hematologic problems when given to a person who has a deficiency of the enzyme glucose-6-phosphate dehydrogenase (G6PD). This health problem is most common among black individuals, and rasburicase is contraindicated for black people.

What To Teach Patients Taking a Uric Acid Synthesis Inhibitor
Remind patients taking allopurinol to take it after a full meal. For both types of uric acid synthesis inhibitors, teach the patient the importance of maintaining a good fluid intake, especially of water throughout the day.

Life Span Considerations for Drugs to Manage Hyperuricemia and Gout
Considerations for Pregnancy and Lactation. The uric acid synthesis inhibitors and rasburicase have a moderate likelihood of increasing the risk for birth defects or fetal harm. They have caused problems in pregnant laboratory animals and should not be used in pregnancy unless the benefits to the mother outweigh the risks to the fetus. Breastfeeding is not recommended while taking any of these drugs.

MUSCLE SPASMS

REVIEW OF RELATED PHYSIOLOGY AND PATHOPHYSIOLOGY

Skeletal muscles are voluntary muscles with excitable membranes that require stimulation by motor nerves (another type of excitable tissue) to depolarize and contract. For example, when you want to scratch your nose, you first consciously think about scratching your nose. The motor area of the brain triggers the nerves that specifically control the muscles of one arm and hand so that only those muscles are depolarized and you just scratch your nose without having a whole body muscle response. If, for some reason, the nerves connecting your brain to your arm and hand's skeletal muscles are not working, the muscles will not contract and no movement occurs.

A *skeletal muscle spasm* is the involuntary contraction of a single muscle, group of related muscles, or just a part of a muscle. This most often occurs when a nerve or nerves controlling contraction to that muscle depolarizes spontaneously and inappropriately. Common causes of inappropriate nerve depolarization include pressure on the nerve, swelling along the nerve path, and electrolyte imbalances, especially low blood calcium and magnesium levels. Spasms can also occur when a muscle is irritated or damaged. When a large muscle has a spasm, rather than just an isolated twitch, intense pain from a lack of oxygen getting to the muscle can result. (Think about how it feels to have a "Charlie horse" in your calf muscle.) In some instances, skeletal muscle spasms are repeated muscle twitches that are less painful but very annoying. In either case, muscle function is reduced during spasms and twitches.

SKELETAL MUSCLE RELAXANTS
Skeletal muscle relaxants are drugs that act by depressing the central nervous system (CNS), which reduces motor nerve depolarization and results in a reduction of skeletal muscle spasms and increased mobility of affected skeletal muscles. They are used for pain and insomnia when excessive skeletal muscle contractions or spasms contribute to these problems. The most commonly used skeletal muscle relaxants are the carbamates, the cyclobenzaprines, and the **benzodiazepines** (which are discussed in Chapter 28).

Generic names, brand names, and dosages of the most commonly prescribed skeletal muscle relaxants for muscle spasms are listed in the following table. Be sure to consult a drug reference book for information about specific skeletal muscle relaxant drugs.

 Memory Jogger

The three classes of skeletal muscle relaxants are:
- Carbamates
- Cyclobenzaprine
- Benzodiazepines

Dosages for Common Skeletal Muscle Relaxant Drugs

Drug	Dosage
Carbamates	
methocarbamol (Robaxin)	*Adults:* Initially 1.5-2 g orally every 6 hr for 2-3 days; maintenance—4-4.5 g total daily, orally given in 3-6 divided doses 1-2 g intravenously at a rate of 300 mg/minute *Children:* Safety and efficacy have not been established
carisoprodol (Soma, Soprodol 350, Vanadom)	*Adults and Adolescents:* 250-350 mg orally 3 times daily and at bedtime *Children:* Safety and efficacy have not been established
cyclobenzaprine (Flexeril, Amrix)	*Adults:* 5-10 mg orally 3 times daily *Children:* Safety and efficacy have not been established

How Skeletal Muscle Relaxants Work

The exact mechanism of action for the carbamates is unknown but these drugs work in the CNS rather than directly on muscle tissue. The drugs depress most CNS activity, leading to skeletal muscle relaxation.

The chemical structure of cyclobenzaprine is very similar to the tricyclic antidepressants. This drug is thought to cause muscle relaxation by its actions in the CNS rather than directly on muscle tissue. The drug changes the influence of serotonin in the spinal cord, leading to reduced motor nerve impulse transmission and skeletal muscle relaxation.

Intended Responses
- Skeletal muscle relaxation
- Reduced muscle spasms
- Sedation
- Pain relief
- Increased mobility of affected muscles

Side Effects. The most common side effects of the carbamates are flushing, hypotension, bradycardia, and fainting. The most common side effects of cyclobenzaprine are dizziness, headache, and the anticholinergic effects of dry mouth, blurred vision, and urinary retention.

Adverse Effects. The most common adverse effects of the carbamates are amnesia, and angioedema. The drug should be used cautiously, if at all, in patients who have a seizure disorder because it can lower the seizure threshold. When methocarbamol is given intravenously and infiltration or extravasation (leakage of fluid into the tissues) occurs, pain, phlebitis, and sloughing at the injection site may occur.

The most common adverse effects of cyclobenzaprine are cardiac dysrhythmias and prolonged cardiac conduction. This drug is not to be used in a patient who is recovering from a myocardial infarction or who has any preexisting, persistent heart rhythm problem. In addition, cyclobenzaprine should never be prescribed for a patient who is taking a monoamine oxidase inhibitor (MAOI) drug because of the risk for severe hypertension and serotonin syndrome (see Chapter 27). Cyclobenzaprine also lowers the seizure threshold and should never be used for patients who have a seizure disorder.

What To Do *Before* Giving Skeletal Muscle Relaxants

In addition to the general actions to take listed in Chapter 2 before giving any drug to a patient for the first time, assess the level of consciousness, cognition, and skeletal muscle reactivity. Also asked whether he or she has a seizure disorder or has ever had a seizure in the past because these drugs lower the seizure threshold.

Common Side Effects
Carbamates

Flushing

Hypotension

Bradycardia

Fainting

Common Side Effects
Cyclobenzaprine

Dizziness

Urinary retention

Blurred vision

⚠️ Drug Alert!
Administration Alert

The carbamates and cyclobenzaprine should not be given to anyone who has a seizure disorder because these drugs lower the seizure threshold.

QSEN: Safety

Before giving the first dose of cyclobenzaprine, assess the patient's blood pressure and radial and apical pulses for any skipped beats, extra beats, or any other type of irregular heart beat. If you find any persistent heart beat irregularity, notify the prescriber before administering the drug.

What To Do *After* Giving Skeletal Muscle Relaxants

Assess for level of consciousness and degree of skeletal muscle relaxation or muscle weakness after giving any class of skeletal muscle relaxants. Patients may become very drowsy and are at risk for falling. Raise the side rails and remind them to call for help to get out of bed for any reason.

Muscle relaxants can cause a sudden lowering of blood pressure, especially when the patient changes position *(orthostatic hypotension).* Help the patient change position slowly. When getting out of bed, he or she should sit for a few minutes on the side of the bed before attempting to get up. Help him or her during walking to prevent falling.

Both classes of drugs can cause urinary retention. If a patient receiving one of these drugs has an enlarged prostate gland, assess for symptoms of urine retention.

For patients receiving intravenous dosages (by bolus or continuous infusion) of a carbamate, assess the site immediately after giving a bolus dose or every 2 hours during a continuous infusion. Assess for pain, redness, swelling, or a cord-like feel over the vein. If any signs of infiltration are present, stop the infusion, remove the IV, and notify the prescriber.

After giving the first dose of cyclobenzaprine, assess the patient's radial and apical pulses hourly for any skipped beats, extra beats or any other type of irregular heartbeat. If you find persistent irregularity, notify the prescriber. Also assess the patient's blood pressure for sudden-onset hypertension.

What To *Teach* Patients Taking Skeletal Muscle Relaxants

For any type of skeletal muscle relaxant, remind patients that these drugs are to be taken only on a short-term basis. Usually the drugs are prescribed for 2 to 3 weeks because of their potential for abuse.

Just like for any drug that causes sedation, warn patients to avoid operating any dangerous equipment, driving a car, or making critical decisions while under the influence of these drugs. Also remind the patient to avoid alcohol because the sedation effect of these drugs is potentiated by alcohol.

Teach patients taking cyclobenzaprine to take their pulse daily and to report new-onset, persistent irregularities to the prescriber. Instruct them to go to the nearest emergency department or call 911 if they develop shortness of breath or chest pain.

Because cyclobenzaprine increases sun sensitivity and can lead to severe sunburn, remind patients to use sunscreen, hats, and protective clothing during sun exposure.

Life Span Considerations for Skeletal Muscle Relaxants

Considerations for Pregnancy and Lactation. The carbamates and cyclobenzaprine have a low to moderate likelihood of increasing the risk for birth defects or fetal harm. They can be used during pregnancy; however, it is recommended that the drugs be used only if clearly needed. The carbamates appear to be excreted in breast milk and should be used cautiously with breastfeeding. The infant should be monitored closely, especially for drowsiness and gastrointestinal problems. It is not known whether cyclobenzaprine enters breast milk.

Considerations for Older Adults. The carbamates are not recommended for older adults because of the sedation and anticholinergic effects. The muscle relaxant effect also causes muscle weakness and increased the risk for falls. Cyclobenzaprine is used with caution in older adults and only when clearly needed, because the muscle weakness and anticholinergic effects are similar to the carbamates.

Drug Alert!

Action/intervention Alert

When administering an intravenous dose of a carbamate, assess for pain, redness, swelling, or a cord-like feel over the vein that indicate an infiltration or extravasation.

QSEN: Safety

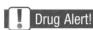

Drug Alert!

Teaching Alert

Warn patients to avoid operative any heavy equipment, driving a car, or making critical decisions while under the influence of any drug for pain or sleep that causes CNS depression.

QSEN: Safety

Get Ready for Practice!

Key Points

- Osteoclastic activity reduces bone density and strength, whereas osteoblastic activity increases bone density and strength.
- Osteoporosis occurs with aging, but the rate of progression varies as a result of many individual patient factors.
- The drugs used to manage or prevent osteoporosis include nutritional supplements (calcium and activated vitamin D), bisphosphonates, estrogen agonists/antagonists, and osteoclastic monoclonal antibodies.
- Your intestinal tract cannot absorb dietary calcium without sufficient amounts of activated vitamin D.
- Patients taking oral bisphosphonates must remain in the upright position for at least 30 minutes after taking the drug to prevent esophageal reflux and irritation.
- The generic names of the bisphosphonates have the syllable "dron" in the middle.
- Remind patients taking estrogen agonists/antagonists not to use tobacco or nicotine to reduce the risk for thrombotic events.
- Osteoclast monoclonal antibodies have a greater incidence of severe hypersensitivity reactions than any other drug class for osteoporosis.
- The enzyme rasburicase has a high risk for severe hypersensitivity reactions.
- About 10% of cases of gouty arthritis result from lifestyle choices, and 90% result from metabolic problems.
- The three classes of drugs used to manage arthritis are drugs for pain control, anti-inflammatory drugs, and dugs for hyperuricemia.
- The three classes of skeletal muscle relaxants are carbamates, cyclobenzaprines, and benzodiazepines.
- When administering an intravenous dose of a carbamate, assess for pain, redness, swelling, or a cord-like feel over the vein that indicate an infiltration or extravasation.
- Warn patients to avoid operative any heavy equipment, driving a car, or making critical decisions while under the influence of any CNS depressant drug.

Additional Learning Resources

evolve Be sure to visit your Evolve website (http://evolve.elsevier.com/Workman/pharmacology/) for additional online resources.

SG Go to your Study Guide for additional learning activities to help you master this chapter content.

Review Questions

See the Answer Keys—In-text Review Questions for answers to these questions.

Test Yourself on the Basics

1. Which drugs belong to the bisphosphonate class? Select all that apply.
   A. alendronate (Fosamax)
   B. denosumab (Prolia)
   C. estrogen/bazedoxifene (Duavee)
   D. ibandronate (Boniva)
   E. raloxifene (Evista)
   F. risedronate (Actonel)
   G. zoledronic acid (Reclast)
2. Which class of drugs to treat osteoporosis is most likely to cause a severe allergic or hypersensitivity reaction?
   A. bisphosphonates
   B. estrogen agonists/antagonists
   C. monoclonal antibodies
   D. nutritional supplements
3. Why is activated vitamin D often prescribed to be taken with calcium supplements for management of osteoporosis?
   A. Vitamin D is the activated form of the mineral calcium.
   B. Intestinal absorption of dietary calcium requires the presence of activated vitamin D.
   C. Calcium and vitamin D together form a hard substance that increases bone density and strength.
   D. Most drugs for osteoporosis are more effective when blood levels of calcium and vitamin D are at least normal.
4. Which class of drugs is most effective at reducing episodes of gouty arthritis?
   A. Anti-inflammatories
   B. Opioids or narcotics
   C. Uric acid synthesis inhibitors
   D. Disease-modifying antirheumatic drugs
5. For which condition or health problem is a contraindication for the use of rasburicase (Elitek)?
   A. Osteoporosis
   B. G6PD deficiency
   C. Diabetes mellitus
   D. Previous thrombotic event
6. For which patient is methocarbamol (Robaxin) contraindicated?
   A. 27-year-old patient who is 6 months pregnant
   B. 35-year-old woman who takes oral contraceptives
   C. 55-year-old man with diabetes and peripheral neuropathy
   D. 75-year-old man who had cataract surgery 1 week ago

Test Yourself on Advanced Content

7. A woman taking a bisphosphonate sees all of these medical professionals annually. Which professional is it most important that she report her use of bisphosphonates?
   A. Ophthalmologist
   B. Endocrinologist
   C. Gynecologist
   D. Dentist

8. Which activity should you tell a patient prescribed to take raloxifene (Evista) to avoid?
   A. Drinking a glass of wine daily
   B. Drinking caffeinated beverages
   C. Walking and running
   D. Smoking cigarettes

9. Which drug class reduces skeletal muscle spasms by changing the influence of serotonin in the spinal cord?
   A. Carbamates
   B. Cyclobenzaprines
   C. Anti-inflammatories
   D. Monoclonal antibodies

10. What are the most common adverse effects of the carbamates?
    A. Amnesia and angioedema
    B. Phlebitis and skin sloughing
    C. Slow and irregular pulse
    D. Muscle spasms and twitches

11. Which instruction is most important to teach a patient prescribed to take alendronate (Fosamax), 10 mg daily?
    A. "Be sure to rotate injection sites every week."
    B. "Be sure to take the drug 1 hour before or at least 2 hours after a meal."
    C. "Report any headaches you experience to your prescribed immediately."
    D. "Remain in the upright position for at least 30 minutes after taking the drug."

12. What is the main reason drugs for osteoporosis are prescribed only for adults?
    A. Children absorb dietary calcium much better than adults do.
    B. Osteoporosis seldom occurs in people less than 40 years old.
    C. Most of these drugs interfere with the lengthening of bones.
    D. When given to people who are growing, bones become too dense.

13. A patient with gouty arthritis is now prescribed to take 500 mg of allopurinol (Aloprim) orally once daily. The tablets available are 100 mg and 300 mg. What combination of these tablets would be the prescribed dose? _____-mg tablets, _____300-mg tablets

14. A patient is prescribed to receive 3 mg of ibandronate (Boniva) by IV bolus. The drug on hand is a solution with a concentration of 1 mg/mL. How many milliliters is the prescribed dose? ___ mL

Critical Thinking Activities

See the Answer Keys—Critical Thinking Activities for answers to these activities.

Mrs. Short is a 62-year-old woman who finished menopause 5 years ago. At her annual physical examination this year, she was discovered to be 1.5 inches shorter than 5 years ago, and tests revealed significant bone density loss. Her primary care provider has prescribed ibandronate (Boniva) 2.5 mg orally daily for this problem.

1. What class of drug is ibandronate, and how does it work?
2. Mrs. Short asks whether she should take calcium supplements. What is your response? Provide a rationale for your response.
3. What instructions should you provide to this patient for how and when to take this drug?
4. What drug-associated problems should you teach her to report to the prescriber?

chapter

Drug Therapy for Male Reproductive Problems

31

Objectives

After studying this chapter you should be able to:

1. List the common names, actions, usual adult dosages, possible side effects, and adverse effects of drugs for benign prostatic hyperplasia.
2. Describe what to do before and after giving drugs for benign prostatic hyperplasia.
3. Explain what to teach patients taking drugs for benign prostatic hyperplasia, including what to do, what not to do, and when to call the prescriber or pharmacist.
4. Describe life span considerations for drugs for benign prostatic hyperplasia.

5. List the common names, actions, usual adult dosages, possible side effects, and adverse effects of drugs for male hormone replacement therapy and erectile dysfunction.
6. Describe what to do before and after giving drugs for male hormone replacement therapy and erectile dysfunction.
7. Explain what to teach patients taking drugs for male hormone replacement therapy and erectile dysfunction, including what to do, what not to do, and when to call the prescriber or pharmacist.
8. Describe life span considerations for drugs for male hormone replacement therapy and erectile dysfunction.

Key Terms

androgens (ĂN-drō-jĕnz) (p. 481) The group of male sex hormones that includes testosterone.

benign prostatic hyperplasia (BPH) (bĕ-NĪN prō-STĂT-ĭk hī-pŭr-PLĀ-zhĕ) (p. 481) Enlargement of the prostate gland caused by an increased number of cells in the gland. Formerly known as benign prostatic hypertrophy.

erectile dysfunction (ĕ-RĔK-tĭl dĭs-FŬNK-shŭn) (p. 488) The inability to achieve or maintain an erection for sexual intercourse.

prostate gland (PRŎS-tāt GLĂND) (p. 481) A walnut-size male sex gland that surrounds the upper part of the urethra and secretes substances into seminal fluid.

testosterone (tĕs-TŎS-tĕ-rōn) (p. 485) A hormone (sex hormone) produced in the testes that encourages development and maintenance of male sexual characteristics.

BENIGN PROSTATIC HYPERPLASIA

REVIEW OF RELATED PHYSIOLOGY AND PATHOPHYSIOLOGY

Located between the bladder and the penis, the **prostate gland** is a walnut-sized male sex gland that surrounds the upper part of the urethra and secretes a milky white mix of simple sugars, enzymes, and alkaline chemicals into seminal fluid (Figure 31-1). These secretions improve the chance of pregnancy with intercourse by increasing the amount of seminal fluid, improving sperm movement, and reducing acidity in the vagina. The activity and size of the prostate gland depend on the presence of testosterone, the main androgen secreted by the testes and adrenal glands. (**Androgens** are a group of male sex hormones that includes testosterone, dihydrotestosterone [DHT], and androstenedione.) The prostate gland has testosterone receptors in the nucleus of each cell that bind circulating testosterone. When bound, these receptors trigger the genes for prostate cell growth and activity.

Many men over age 50 have **benign prostatic hyperplasia (BPH)**, an enlargement of the prostate gland as a result of increased numbers of cells in the gland. Although the amount of circulating testosterone decreases with age, the number of testosterone

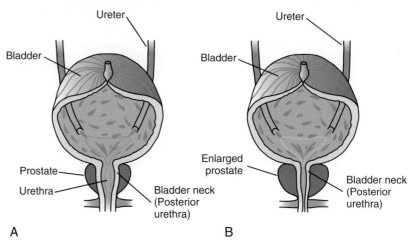

FIGURE 31-1   **A,** Normal prostate gland. **B,** Enlarged prostate gland showing the narrowing of the urethra, decreasing urine flow.

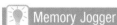

Memory Jogger

As men age, testosterone levels decrease but the number of testosterone receptors in the prostate increases.

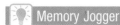

Memory Jogger

Because the signs and symptoms of BPH and prostate cancer are the same, urge any man with symptoms of BPH to be seen by his physician to rule out prostate cancer.

QSEN: Safety

Memory Jogger

The two main groups of drugs used to treat BPH are DHT inhibitors and selective alpha-1 blockers.

receptors in the prostate gland *increases*. Because of this, even small amounts of testosterone, especially DHT, are more likely to bind with receptors and eventually cause the prostate gland to enlarge.

Because of its location, when the prostate enlarges, it squeezes the urethra, narrowing it and decreasing urine flow from the bladder (see Figure 31-1).

Symptoms of BPH are:
- Increased frequency of urination
- *Nocturia* (increased urination at night)
- Difficulty in starting (hesitancy) and continuing urination
- Reduced force and size of the urine stream
- The feeling of incomplete bladder emptying
- Dribbling after urinating

Signs and symptoms of BPH are the same as for prostate cancer. Any man with symptoms of BPH should be seen by his physician to rule out prostate cancer.

The symptoms of prostate enlargement are uncomfortable and can interfere with adequate sleep and rest. Often urine stays in the bladder much longer than normal, leading to urinary tract infection. With rapid or severe enlargement, the bladder can become completely blocked, with urine backing up into the ureters and kidneys, leading to kidney damage or failure. With severe blockage, surgery is needed. When symptoms are mild to moderate, drug therapy can reduce prostate pressure and improve urine flow.

TYPES OF DRUGS FOR BENIGN PROSTATIC HYPERPLASIA

DHT INHIBITORS AND SELECTIVE ALPHA-1 BLOCKERS

Selective alpha-1 blockers and DHT inhibitors are the two main categories of drugs used to treat prostate enlargement. Because the actions of these two drug types differ, they can be used alone or together to improve urine flow.

How Drugs for Benign Prostatic Hyperplasia Work. Selective alpha-1 blockers act to relax smooth muscle tissue in the prostate gland, the neck of the bladder, and the urethra. These smooth muscles contain alpha-1 adrenergic receptors. When the receptors are activated, the smooth muscle constricts, tightening the prostate, which increases the pressure and squeezes the urethra. Smooth muscle in the bladder neck and urethra also contract and make the urethra narrower. When these receptors are bound with selective alpha-1 blockers, the smooth muscle relaxes, placing less pressure on the urethra and improving urine flow.

DHT inhibitors work directly on the prostate gland. They are a "counterfeit" drug that looks like testosterone and binds to the enzyme that normally converts testosterone to DHT, its most powerful form. This counterfeit drug cannot be converted to DHT, and although it is bound to the enzyme, the enzyme is not available to convert the real testosterone to DHT. With much less DHT in the prostate, the cells in the prostate gland do not receive the signal to grow. As a result, the gland shrinks and puts less pressure on the urethra, allowing better urine flow.

Dosages for Common Drugs for BPH

Drug	Dosage (Adult Men Only)
DHT Inhibitors	
dutasteride (Avodart)	0.5 mg orally once daily
finasteride (Proscar)	5 mg orally once daily
Selective Alpha-1 Blockers	
alfuzosin (UroXatral, Xatral 🍁)	10 mg orally once daily
doxazosin (Cardura)	1 mg orally once daily at bedtime
silodosin (Rapaflo)	8 mg orally once daily
tamsulosin (Flomax, Novo-Tamsulosin 🍁)	0.4-0.8 mg orally once daily 30 minutes after a meal
terazosin (Hytrin)	1 mg orally once daily at bedtime

Intended Responses
- Pressure on the urethra is decreased.
- Urine flow from the bladder through the urethra is improved.
- BPH symptoms (frequency, difficulty starting or stopping the urine stream, dribbling, excessive nighttime urination, feeling of incomplete bladder emptying) are decreased.

Side Effects. The most common side effect of drugs for BPH is a decreased interest in sexual activity (decreased libido).

Side effects for DHT inhibitors also include erectile dysfunction, decreased seminal fluid, and reduced fertility. Other side effects for some men are a slowing of hair loss from the scalp and, in some cases, scalp hair regrowth.

Selective alpha-1 blockers may lower blood pressure, especially when changing positions (orthostatic hypotension), causing dizziness or light-headedness. Other side effects may include back pain and runny or stuffy nose.

Adverse Effects. Drugs for BPH are metabolized by the liver. If the patient's liver is impaired, the drug is excreted more slowly, and higher blood levels could result. Higher blood levels lead to more severe side effects. Patients with liver impairment should be prescribed lower dosages of these drugs.

DHT inhibitors can adversely affect other hormone or sex tissues. Breast changes such as enlargement, lumps, pain, or fluids leaking from the nipple can occur. Any of these changes or pain in the testicles is a reason to consult a physician, who will likely stop the drug.

DHT inhibitors can cause birth defects when taken or handled by a pregnant woman. Women who are pregnant or who may become pregnant should avoid handling the tablets or capsules, especially if they are crushed or broken. Because these drugs enter the seminal fluid of men who take them, men should wear a condom when having sex with a woman who is pregnant or may become pregnant.

Alpha-1 blockers are excreted by the kidneys. Patients who have renal impairment retain the drug longer and have more severe hypotension. Although these drugs are not toxic to the kidney (*nephrotoxic*), they should not be taken by patients who have severe renal impairment or kidney failure.

Tamsulosin is made from a sulfonamide and may cause an allergic reaction in patients who are allergic to sulfa drugs.

Common Side Effects

Drugs for BPH

Decreased libido

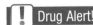 **Drug Alert!**

Interaction Alert

The patient who has an allergy to sulfa drugs may also have an allergy to tamsulosin.

QSEN: Safety

All of the alpha-1 blockers can interact with many other drugs and herbal supplements, especially antihypertensives, cardiac drugs, and drugs for erectile dysfunction. The interactions can be complex and serious.

Alpha-1 blockers have been associated with a problem called *floppy iris syndrome* during cataract surgery. With this problem, the iris does not respond as expected to drugs that dilate or constrict it and can collapse toward the surgical site. Although this is not a reason to stop the drug, the surgeon performing cataract surgery must take special steps to prevent a floppy iris from causing complications.

What To Do *Before* Giving Drugs for BPH

The signs and symptoms of BPH are the same as for prostate cancer. Before a drug for BPH is taken, the patient should have a digital rectal examination by his prescriber and have his blood tested for prostate-specific antigen (PSA) levels to rule out prostate cancer.

Because liver impairment can increase the blood level of the drugs for BPH, make sure that the patient does not have a liver problem before starting these drugs. Check the patient's most recent laboratory values for liver problems (elevated liver enzymes). (See Table 1-3 for a listing of normal values.)

Because alpha-1 blockers may cause orthostatic hypotension, take the patient's blood pressure in the lying, sitting, and standing positions.

If a patient will be taking tamsulosin, ask whether he has ever had an allergic reaction to sulfa drugs. If he has had such a reaction, report this to the prescriber.

What To Do *After* Giving Drugs for BPH

Assess the patient for orthostatic (postural) hypotension and related problems (dizziness, light-headedness), especially after the first dose. Remind the patient to call for assistance when getting out of bed.

What To *Teach* Patients Taking Drugs for BPH

Remind patients to continue their annual prevention and early detection practices for prostate cancer. These include a digital rectal examination and blood PSA levels.

Caution men taking DHT inhibitors to make sure that women who are or may become pregnant do not come into contact with the drug or handle it. Methods for men to reduce exposure to women include:

- Wearing a condom during sexual intercourse
- Not donating blood (which could be given to a pregnant woman)

Some common herbal preparations have an action similar to that of DHT inhibitors. They include saw palmetto (*Serenoa repens*) and soy isoflavones. If a man takes a DHT inhibitor with one of these substances, it is possible that it could increase the intended responses of the drug, including side effects.

Teach patients taking alpha-1 blockers to change positions slowly, especially when rising to a standing position, because a rapid drop in blood pressure can cause dizziness. Although this problem is more likely to occur when a patient first takes an alpha-1 blocker, it can occur at any time, especially if he is dehydrated or taking drugs for hypertension, erectile dysfunction drugs, or cardiac drugs such as beta blockers or calcium channel blockers. Warn patients to avoid driving or operating dangerous equipment until they know how the drugs will affect them.

Warn patients taking alpha-1 blockers to tell all other health care providers that they are taking this drug because of the potential for drug interactions. Also warn them not to take over-the-counter drugs without checking with their prescriber.

Remind patients taking an alpha-1 blocker to inform their surgeon that they are taking this drug when cataract surgery is being planned.

Life Span Considerations for Drugs for BPH

Pediatric Considerations. DHT inhibitors and selective alpha-1 blockers should not be administered to children or adolescents.

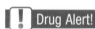

Drug Alert!

Interaction Alert

Alpha-1 blockers interact with many drugs and herbal supplements. Before giving an alpha-1 blocker, ask the patient about all other drugs or supplements he takes and then check with the pharmacist to avoid a possible drug interaction.

QSEN: Safety

Drug Alert!

Teaching Alert

Remind men taking DHT inhibitors that it may take 3 to 6 months of therapy before the prostate shrinks and symptoms improve.

QSEN: Safety

Drug Alert!

Teaching Alert

Instruct patients who take a DHT inhibitor with saw palmetto (*Serenoa repens*) or soy isoflavones to notify the prescriber if any unusual side effects occur.

QSEN: Safety

Considerations for Pregnancy and Lactation. DHT inhibitors have a very high likelihood of increasing the risk for birth defects or fetal harm. They are teratogens and can cause birth defects, especially in male fetuses. Women who are pregnant, may become pregnant, or are breastfeeding should not take these drugs or handle them if the tablet or capsule is crushed or broken. Although selective alpha-1 blockers have a low likelihood of increasing the risk for birth defects or fetal harm, they are used *only* to treat BPH in men and are not indicated for women, regardless of pregnancy or breastfeeding status.

Considerations for Older Adults. Drugs for BPH are more commonly prescribed for older men. Prostate cancer is much more common in this age group. Ensure that older men taking drugs for BPH understand the need to have annual prostate cancer screening.

The risk for orthostatic (postural) hypotension is higher in older patients taking alpha-1 blockers than in younger adults, especially with the first dose. Monitor older adults carefully for severe hypotension.

MALE HORMONE REPLACEMENT THERAPY

REVIEW OF RELATED PHYSIOLOGY AND PATHOPHYSIOLOGY

Testosterone is a hormone (sex hormone), produced in the testes, that helps with development and maintenance of male sex characteristics. It is also important for maintaining muscle mass, adequate levels of red blood cells (RBCs), bone density, sense of well-being, and sexual and reproduction functions. As men age, the level of testosterone in their bodies decreases. This is a natural phenomenon that begins around age 30 and continues through the remainder of life. Low blood testosterone level, also called hypogonadism, occurs in many men over age 45. There are also several other potential causes of low testosterone (Box 31-1).

Symptoms of insufficient testosterone include (Figure 31-2):

- Decreased interest in sex
- Decreased sense of well-being
- Depression, irritability
- Difficulty concentrating and remembering
- Erectile dysfunction
- Decreased muscle and increased body fat
- Anemia (fatigue, decreased energy)
- Decreased bone density
- Decreased body hair

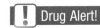

Drug Alert!

Teaching Alert

Teach patients prescribed drugs for BPH to schedule annual prostate cancer screening.

QSEN: Safety

Memory Jogger

Testosterone levels begin to decrease around age 30 and continue to decrease for the rest of a man's life.

Box 31-1	**Causes of Low Testosterone Levels**

- Injury, infection, or loss of the testicles
- Chemotherapy or radiation treatment for cancer
- Genetic abnormalities such as Klinefelter's syndrome (extra X chromosome)
- Hemochromatosis (too much iron in the body)
- Dysfunction of the pituitary gland (a gland in the brain that produces many important hormones)
- Inflammatory diseases such as sarcoidosis (a condition that causes inflammation of the lungs)
- Medications, especially hormones used to treat prostate cancer and corticosteroid drugs
- Chronic illness
- Chronic kidney failure
- Liver cirrhosis
- Stress
- Alcoholism
- Obesity (especially abdominal)

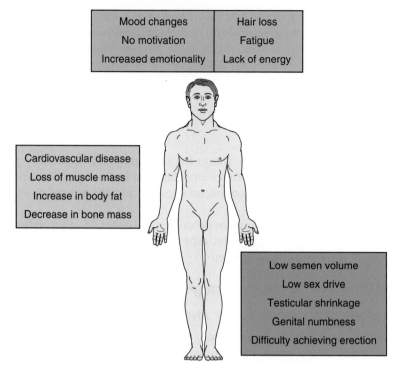

FIGURE 31-2 Signs of low testosterone.

Box 31-2 | **Methods of Testosterone Replacement**

- Intramuscular injections, given anywhere from 2 to 10 weeks apart
- Testosterone patch worn either on the body or on the scrotum (the sac that contains the testicles)
- Testosterone gel applied to the skin or inside the nose
- Mucoadhesive material applied above the teeth twice a day
- Oral tablets
- Long-acting subcutaneous implant
- Testosterone stick (apply like underarm deodorant)

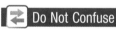 **Do Not Confuse**

Testosterone *with* Testolactone

An order for testosterone can be mistaken for testolactone. Testosterone is used for hormone replacement. Testolactone is used to treat advanced stage breast cancer.

QSEN: Safety

How Drugs for Testosterone Replacement Work

Testosterone replacement therapy drugs promote growth and development of men's sexual organs, as well as help maintain secondary sexual characteristics. Box 31-2 lists methods of testosterone replacement. Testosterone is a schedule III drug (with moderate to low potential for physical and psychological dependence). Oral testosterone tablets are available but are generally not used because of the danger of liver damage. Be sure to consult a drug handbook for additional information on testosterone drugs.

Dosages for Common Testosterone Drugs

Drug	Dosage
testosterone (Cypionate, Andriol ♦)	IM: 50-400 mg every 2-4 weeks
testosterone patch (Androderm)	Transdermal patch: 4 mg/day patch applied to arm or upper body once daily at night
testosterone gel (AndroGel, Testim)	50 mg applied to skin on abdomen, shoulders, or upper arms once daily
testosterone mouth patch (Striant)	30 mg applied to upper gums near two front teeth every 12 hr
testosterone pellets (Testopel)	SC: 150-450 mg every 3 to 6 months

Intended Responses
- *Anabolic effects* (e.g., increased muscle mass and bone density)
- *Androgenic effects* (e.g., maturation of sex organs, development of secondary sex characteristics such as deepened voice and growth of pubic and axillary hair)
- Relief of symptoms
- Increased interest in sex

Side Effects. Side effects of testosterone are uncommon. Some side effects include acne or oily skin, mild fluid retention, increased size of prostate with difficulty urinating, breast enlargement, sleep apnea, and decreased testicle size. Pain or inflammation may occur at intramuscular (IM) injections sites, and pruritus (itching), erythema (redness), or skin irritation may occur with transdermal patches.

Adverse Effects. Liver damage, including peliosis hepatitis, neoplasms, and hepatocellular carcinoma, are adverse effects of these drugs. Increases in the incidence of heart attacks and strokes have been reported and are a major concern.

What To Do *Before* Giving Testosterone Replacement Drugs
Ask men about a history of prostate or breast cancer because if this is present, they should not receive testosterone replacement therapy. Before this therapy, all men should have prostate cancer screening including a rectal exam and PSA blood test.

Also check for history of diabetes, kidney, liver, or cardiovascular disease. Testosterone can cause decreased blood glucose levels.

Get a baseline weight and blood pressure. Check lab tests including complete blood count (CBC with Hgb/Hct), liver function tests, electrolytes, and cholesterol.

What To Do *After* Giving Testosterone Replacement Drugs
Check weight every day to assess for fluid retention, and report weight gain of 5 or more pounds to the prescriber. Assess blood pressure at least twice a day. Monitor lab tests including electrolytes, liver function tests, hemoglobin/hematocrit, and cholesterol.

Assess injection sites for redness, swelling, or pain. Ask the patient about his sleep pattern. In collaboration with nutrition services, ensure that the patient's diet contains adequate protein and calories

What To *Teach* Patients Taking Testosterone Replacement Drugs
Teach patients to check weight daily (same time, scale, and amount of clothes) and report a weight gain of 5 pounds or more per week to the prescriber. Tell them to report frequent erections, difficulty with urination, or breast enlargement to the prescriber.

Tell patients to include high protein sources in their diet. If a patient experiences gastrointestinal discomfort, teach them to eat small frequent meals.

Instruct patients to consult with the prescriber before taking any other drugs while receiving testosterone replacement therapy. Also tell them that regular follow-up visits with the prescriber as well as laboratory tests are necessary.

For patients prescribed testosterone gels or patches, teach families to avoid touching patient skin, linen, or clothing that has been in contact with the drug.

Life Span Considerations for Testosterone Replacement Drugs
Pediatric Considerations. Safe use has not been established. Testosterone replacement must be used with caution in children.

Considerations for Pregnancy and Lactation. Testosterone has a very high likelihood of increasing the risk for birth defects or fetal harm and should not be used during pregnancy or breastfeeding.

Common Side Effects

Testosterone Drugs

Itching (pruritus)   Difficulty urinating   Sleep apnea

Male breast enlargement

! Drug Alert!

Action/Intervention Alert

Be sure that patients receive prostate cancer screening before beginning testosterone replacement therapy.

QSEN: Safety

! Drug Alert!

Action Alert

Report a weight gain of 5 pounds in a week to the prescriber because this indicates fluid retention that can occur with testosterone therapy replacement.

QSEN: Safety

 Clinical Pitfall (Black Box Alert)

Testosterone can cause virilization in children and women after secondary exposure. Warn them to avoid touching skin, clothing, or linens that have come into contact with testosterone preparations.

QSEN: Safety

Considerations for Older Adults. Older adults are at increased risk of prostate hyperplasia, or growth stimulation of occult prostate carcinoma.

ERECTILE DYSFUNCTION

REVIEW OF RELATED PHYSIOLOGY AND PATHOPHYSIOLOGY

Penile erections occur as a result of a complex process involving the central nervous, peripheral nervous, hormonal, and vascular systems. An abnormality occurring in any of these systems can interfere with the ability to develop and sustain an erection, or ejaculate and experience an orgasm.

Erectile dysfunction (ED) is the inability of a man to achieve or maintain an erection sufficient for satisfying sexual activity. For more than 20 years, ED (also called *impotence*) has been recognized as a common problem as men age. Many men are affected by age 40, and the incidence continues to increase as men age.

Organic risk factors for ED include cardiovascular disease (e.g., hypertension, atherosclerosis, hyperlipidemia), diabetes, drug side effects (e.g., antihypertensives), alcohol use, smoking, pelvic surgery or trauma, neurological disease, obesity, and radiation to the pelvis. Hormone deficiency or hypogonadism (reduction or absence of hormone secretion or other physiological activity of the gonads [testes]) can also cause ED. Functional (psychological) ED may be caused by depression, anxiety, or stress.

ED is diagnosed by a thorough history and a complete physical examination. Signs and symptoms of ED include:
- Difficulty getting an erection
- Difficulty keeping an erection
- Decreased sexual desire

Treatment may include penile pumps, implants, surgery, psychological counseling, or drugs. Phosphodiesterace-5 (PDE-5) inhibitor drugs have been very successful in treating ED in many men.

How Drugs for Erectile Dysfunction Work

When a man develops an erection, blood fills tissue in the penis, which causes it to become enlarged and stiff. Phosphodiesterase-5 inhibitor drugs (PDE-5) relax smooth muscle and allow the penis to fill with blood (Figure 31-3). Each of these drugs requires sexual stimulation to cause an erection. They begin working within 20 or 30 minutes to an hour. The effects of sildenafil and vardenafil last for up to 4 hours, whereas the effects of tadalafil can last up to 36 hours.

In addition to treating ED, some of these drugs are prescribed to increase blood flow in the lungs of people who have pulmonary vascular problems such as pulmonary arterial hypertension and some forms of pulmonary fibrosis (see Chapter 21). Be sure to consult a drug handbook for additional information about a specific ED drug.

Dosages for Common Drugs for Erectile Dysfunction

Drug	Dosage (Adult Men Only)
sildenafil (Viagra)	50 mg orally once daily, 30 min to 1 hr before sexual activity
tadalafil (Cialis)	2.5 mg orally once daily, 30 min to 1 hr before sexual activity
vardenafil (Levitra)	10 mg orally once daily, 1 hr before sexual activity

Intended Responses
- Ability to have an erection
- Ability to maintain an erection
- Increased interest in sexual intercourse

Memory Jogger

ED may be caused by organic or functional factors.

Memory Jogger

Drugs for erectile dysfunction require sexual stimulation to cause an erection.

Do Not Confuse

Sildenafil *with* Tadalafil or Vardenafil

An order for sildenafil can be mistaken for tadalafil or vardenafil. All three drugs are used to treat ED. Be sure you administer the prescribed drug.

QSEN: Safety

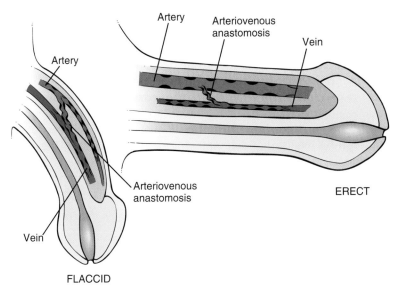

FIGURE 31-3   The normal erection process. (From Swartz, M. (2015). *Textbook of physical diagnoses: History and examination.* St. Louis: Saunders.)

Side Effects. Common side effects of PDE-5 drugs include acid reflux, heartburn, indigestion, diarrhea, nasal congestion, flushing of skin, bloody nose, headache, and muscle aches. Patients may experience changes in vision, hearing, or postural hypotension, but these are not common.

Adverse Effects. PDE-5 drugs may cause prolonged erections lasting more than 4 hours. *Priapism* (painful erections lasting more than 6 hours) can occur but are rare. Tadalafil may cause nephrotoxicity, neurotoxicity, or pleural effusions. If these drugs are taken with nitrate drugs, angina (chest pain) or heart attack (MI) can occur.

What To Do *Before* Giving Drugs for Erectile Dysfunction
Ask patients about cardiovascular problems, including angina, and about benign prostatic hyperplasia (BPH). Check laboratory test results for kidney and liver function. Contact the prescriber if the patient is taking a nitrate drug because giving the two drugs together may result in severe hypotension.

Check baseline heart rate, blood pressure, and oxygen saturation. Assess cardiovascular status. Ask about current medications (these drugs are contraindicated for patients using any form of nitrate drug because extreme low blood pressure can occur) and herbal preparation use (St. John's wort may decrease concentration of the drugs). Patients taking alpha-adrenergic blockers with these drugs may also experience hypotension.

What To Do *After* Giving Drugs for Erectile Dysfunction
Continue to monitor patients' heart rate, blood pressure, and oxygen saturation. Ask patients about any vision or hearing changes. Assess patients for intended or side effects such as headache, flushing, and gastrointestinal upset. Instruct them to report prolonged or painful erections.

Give acetaminophen (if ordered) for headache relief.

What To *Teach* Patients Taking Drugs for Erectile Dysfunction
Teach patients that these drugs have no effect without sexual stimulation. Instruct patients to notify the prescriber immediately for an erection that lasts longer than 4 hours or if they experience priapism (prolonged painful erections). Also teach patients to report any sudden loss of vision or hearing to the prescriber.

Common Side Effects

Erectile Dysfunction Drugs

GI discomfort   Headache   Muscle aches

Nasal congestion

⚠ Drug Alert!

Administration Alert

PDE-5 drugs for ED should not be taken at the same time as nitrate drugs because of the danger of extremely low blood pressure. Angina (chest pain) or heart attack (myocardial infarction) can occur.

QSEN: Safety

⚠ Drug Alert!

Administration Alert

Patients prescribed a drug for erectile dysfunction should not take the herbal preparation St. John's wort because it can decrease the concentration and effect of these drugs.

QSEN: Safety

⚠ Drug Alert!

Teaching Alert

Teach patients to report prolonged or painful erections to the prescriber.

QSEN: Safety

Drug Alert!

Teaching Alert

Tell patients to take drugs for erectile dysfunction 30 minutes to an hour before anticipated sexual activity.

QSEN: Safety

Drug Alert!

Teaching Alert

Teach patients not to take drugs for erectile dysfunction with prescribed nitrate drugs because they may cause severe hypotension.

QSEN: Safety

Tell patients to take the drugs 30 minutes to an hour before anticipated sexual activity. Teach that the action of sildenafil and tadalafil lasts 4 hours, and vardenafil lasts up to 36 hours.

Instruct patients to avoid the use of nitrate drugs while taking these drugs. Teach patients how to monitor blood pressure and heart rate.

Tell patients to avoid alcohol while taking these drugs because it increases the risk of orthostatic hypotension. Also teach patients to avoid grapefruit and grapefruit juice because it may increase the concentration of the drugs and cause toxicity. Tell patients that high-fat meals may delay maximum effectiveness of these drugs.

Remind patients to get up slowly when rising from a lying or sitting position because of side effects such as dizziness, light-headedness, or hypotension.

Get Ready for Practice!

Key Points

- An enlarged prostate squeezes the urethra, narrowing it and decreasing urine flow from the bladder.
- Because BPH and prostate cancer have similar symptoms, all men being treated for BPH should be screened for prostate cancer annually.
- Women who are pregnant, may become pregnant, or are breastfeeding should neither take DHT inhibitors nor handle these drugs if the tablet or capsule is crushed or broken.
- Orthostatic hypotension may occur with selective alpha-1 blocker therapy, especially with the first dose.
- As men age, the testosterone levels in their bodies decrease.
- Testosterone replacement methods include IM, subcutaneous, patch, and gel.
- Men with a history of prostate or breast cancer should not receive testosterone replacement therapy.
- Report weight gain of 5 pounds or more in a week with testosterone replacement because this indicates fluid retention.
- Family members should avoid touching skin, clothing, or linens that have been in contact with testosterone preparations.
- Erectile dysfunction can be caused by organic or functional factors.
- Drugs for erectile dysfunction require sexual stimulation to work.
- Report any prolonged or painful erections to the prescriber immediately.
- Drugs for erectile dysfunction should not be taken with nitrate drugs or alcohol because of the increased risk for severe hypotension.
- Drugs for erectile dysfunction also may be used to treat pulmonary artery hypertension and some forms of pulmonary fibrosis.
- Teach patients to take drugs for erectile dysfunction 30 minutes to an hour before anticipated sexual activity, and teach them that achieving an erection requires sexual stimulation.

- Teach patients to report erections that last longer than 4 hours or are painful.

Additional Learning Resources

evolve Be sure to visit your Evolve website (http://evolve.elsevier.com/Workman/pharmacology/) for additional online resources.

SG Go to your Study Guide for additional learning activities to help you master this chapter content.

Review Questions

See the Answer Keys—In-text Review Questions for answers to these questions.

Test Yourself on the Basics

1. Which are the two main groups of drugs used to treat BPH?
   A. Phosphodiesterace-5 inhibitors
   B. DHT inhibitors
   C. Testosterone replacement drugs
   D. Selective alpha-1 blockers
   E. Non-selective alpha-1 blockers
2. Which patient should not receive testosterone replacement?
   A. Older male with history of tuberculosis
   B. Younger male with history of 20% body surface burns
   C. Middle-aged male with history of prostate cancer
   D. Older male with history of gastroesophageal reflux disease
3. A 50-year-old man is prescribed sildenafil (Viagra) for erectile dysfunction. For which herbal preparation in use by the patient will you need to notify the prescriber or pharmacist?
   A. Black cohosh
   B. Echinacea

C. Feverfew

D. St. John's wort

4. What is the most common side effect of drugs prescribed to treat BPH?

A. Decreased libido

B. Hypotension

C. Angina

D. Hair loss

5. Which class of drugs would you instruct a patient taking an ED drug to avoid?

A. Calcium channel blockers

B. Nitrates

C. Angiotensin-converting enzyme inhibitors

D. Beta blockers

Test Yourself on Advanced Concepts

6. The patient prescribed tamsulosin (Flomax) asks you how this drug will help his benign prostate hyperplasia (BPH). What is your best response?

A. "It works directly on the prostate gland to shrink it."

B. "It works with testosterone by converting it to its most powerful form."

C. "It relaxes smooth muscle tissue in the prostate, neck of the bladder, and urethra."

D. "It increases pressure inside the bladder to help increase the urine stream."

7. Which action is most important before administering tamsulosin (Flomax) to a patient?

A. Check the patient's blood pressure lying, sitting, and standing.

B. Elevate the head of the bed to at least 45 degrees.

C. Check the patient's baseline weight and height.

D. Warn the patient that side effects may include hair loss from the scalp.

8. Which precaution is most important to teach a patient prescribed tamsulosin (Flomax) for treatment of BPH?

A. Avoid donating blood.

B. Be sure to have annual prostate cancer screenings.

C. Do not take this drug if you are allergic to "sulfa" drugs.

D. Do not drink alcoholic beverages while taking this drug.

9. An older adult male is prescribed finasteride (Proscar) for BPH. Which age-related teaching point will you be sure to include during discharge teaching?

A. Take acetaminophen if you experience a headache.

B. Be sure to have your annual screening for prostate cancer.

C. You may experience an increase in urine output.

D. You may experience a rash, but it will improve over a couple of weeks.

10. The patient is prescribed tadalafil (Cialis) for erectile dysfunction. For which adverse effect should you monitor after administering this drug?

A. Flushing of the skin

B. Nasal congestion with itching

C. Indigestion with acid reflux

D. Prolonged painful erection

11. A patient prescribed sildenafil (Viagra) for erectile dysfunction is also prescribed isosorbide dinitrate. What is your best action?

A. Administer the drugs if blood pressure is within normal range.

B. Contact the prescriber.

C. Hold both drugs if the heart rate is high.

D. Administer the sildenafil at night and isosorbide in the morning.

12. A 52-year-old man is prescribed testosterone gel (AndroGel) for low serum testosterone. What must you teach his wife about this drug?

A. "Be sure to provide your husband with high carbohydrate meals."

B. "Avoid touching linen or clothing that has been in contact with the drug."

C. "Your husband may experience impotence as a result of this drug."

D. "If your husband experiences hair loss, be sure to contact the prescriber."

13. An older adult male receives IM testosterone every 2 weeks at the prescriber's office. For which condition(s) is this patient at increased risk to develop? (Select all that apply.)

A. Prostate hyperplasia

B. Hypertension

C. Type 2 diabetes mellitus

D. Prostate cancer

E. Priapism

F. Enlargement of breast tissue

14. A patient with BPH is prescribed 0.8 mg of tamsulosin (Flomax) daily. The drug comes in 0.4 mg capsules. How many capsules will you teach the patient to take? _____ capsule(s)

15. A patient with low serum testosterone is prescribed testosterone (Cypionate) 150 mg IM every 2 weeks. Testosterone comes as 100 mg/mL. How many milliliters will you give with each dose? _____ mL

Critical Thinking Activities

See the Answer Keys—Critical Thinking Activities for answers to these activities.

Mr. Miles, a 65-year-old man, is visiting his health care provider for an annual checkup. He tells you that he has been experiencing difficulty with urination, including increased frequency, urinating more at night, difficulty starting his urine stream, and dribbling after urination. He states that after urination, he feels like his bladder is not emptied.

1. What diagnosis is suggested by Mr. Miles's symptoms?

2. What classes of drugs do you expect will be prescribed for Mr. Miles, and how will these drugs work?

3. What important teaching points will you include regarding the diagnosis and its treatment?

Drug Therapy for Female Reproductive Issues

Objectives

After studying this chapter you should be able to:

1. List the names, actions, usual dosages, possible side effects, and adverse effects of drugs for perimenopausal hormone replacement.
2. Explain what patients taking perimenopausal hormone replacement drugs need to know, including what to do, what not to do, and when to call the prescriber or pharmacist.
3. List the names, actions, possible side effects, and adverse effects of hormonal drugs for contraception.
4. Explain what patients taking hormonal drugs for contraception need to know, including what to do, what not to do, and when to call the prescriber or pharmacist.
5. Describe life span considerations for drugs for perimenopausal hormone replacement drugs and for hormonal drugs for contraception.

Key Terms

estrogen (ĔS-trō-jĕn) (p. 492) The main female sex hormone secreted by the ovaries and adrenal glands.

follicle-stimulating hormone (FŎL-ĭ-kŭl STĬM-yū-lā-tĭng HŌR-mŏn) (p. 492) Hormone secreted by the pituitary gland that causes the ovary to secrete estrogen and allows one ovum each month to complete maturation.

hormonal contraception (hŏr-MŌN-ŭl kŏn-tră-SĔP-shŭn) (p. 496) The use of hormone-based drugs that suppress ovulation and prevent pregnancy.

progesterone (prō-JĔS-tŭr-ōn) (p. 493) The female hormone that supports pregnancy by maintaining the thickened uterine lining.

REVIEW OF RELATED PHYSIOLOGY AND PATHOPHYSIOLOGY

The cyclic hormone changes that occur during adolescence and continue throughout a woman's menstruating years promote conception and pregnancy. Conception occurs when a mature egg (*ovum*) is released from a woman's ovary and is fertilized by a sperm (*spermatozoon*) during sexual intercourse. When the fertilized egg then successfully implants in the uterus, the condition of pregnancy results, and an infant may be born 9 months later. The maturation of an egg and proper preparation of the uterine lining to support pregnancy depend on the presence and timing of specific hormones.

Menstruation is the periodic shedding of the uterine lining that occurs as a result of the cyclic changes of hormone levels in females. *Menarche* is the beginning of the years of menstruation in an adolescent female. It occurs as a result of the secretion of *gonadotropin-releasing hormone (GnRH)* in the brain. This hormone starts to be secreted in both females and males at the beginning of puberty so that sex hormone secretion can occur and cause the physical changes leading to interest in sexual activity (*libido*) and the ability to perform sexual intercourse. **Estrogen** is the main female sex hormone secreted by the ovaries and adrenal glands.

In females the secretion of GnRH stimulates the release of two hormones from the pituitary gland: follicle-stimulating hormone (FSH) and luteinizing hormone (Figure 32-1). **Follicle-stimulating hormone** causes the ovary to secrete estrogen and allows one ovum in the ovary to complete maturation each month. As estrogen levels rise in the blood, the lining of the uterus grows and thickens (see Figure 32-1). After about

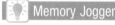
Memory Jogger

GnRH is secreted by the hypothalamus of both males and females to start the hormone changes needed for puberty.

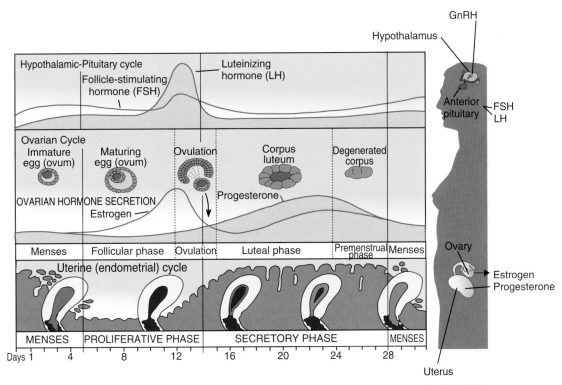

FIGURE 32-1 Hormone interactions for ovulation and menstruation. *GnRH*, Gonadotropin-releasing hormone.

14 days of lining growth, it is thick enough to support the implantation of a fertilized egg. At this optimal midcycle time, GnRH triggers the pituitary gland to release *luteinizing hormone,* which causes secretion of progesterone by the ovary and allows the release of a mature ovum. This process is known as *ovulation.* The outer covering *(corpus luteum)* from the released ovum also secretes progesterone.

Progesterone supports any pregnancy that occurs by maintaining the thickened uterine lining and allowing it to secrete nutrients needed by the early embryo. If fertilization and pregnancy do not occur, the outer covering from the released ovum degenerates in about 12 days, and circulating levels of estrogen and progesterone drop. The loss of these hormones allows the lining of the uterus to stop growing and to shed as menstruation. Figure 32-2 shows the feedback loops controlling the secretion of estrogen and progesterone.

When the mature ovum is fertilized by a sperm, the outer covering from the released ovum continues to grow and secrete both estrogen and progesterone. Together these hormones keep the uterine lining thickened and secreting nutrients to support a pregnancy until the placenta develops enough to take over these functions for the rest of the pregnancy. So pregnancy depends first on *conception* in which a mature ovum is released from the ovary and fertilized by a sperm. Then, within 5 to 8 days, the fertilized ovum must implant itself into the prepared uterine lining.

 Memory Jogger

Estrogen causes the uterine lining to thicken during the first half of the menstrual cycle. Progesterone maintains the lining and causes it to secrete nutrients during the second half of the cycle. The drop in the level of these hormones allows menstruation to occur.

MENOPAUSE

Menopause is the cessation of menstrual periods and ovulation. Natural menopause occurs as a result of age-related changes in the ovary in which glandular cells shrink and become nonfunctional, a process called *involution.* The ovaries become smaller and no longer respond to the brain hormones by secreting estrogen and releasing mature eggs. Natural menopause occurs gradually, over months to years. (Menopause caused by surgery or drug therapy can be sudden.)

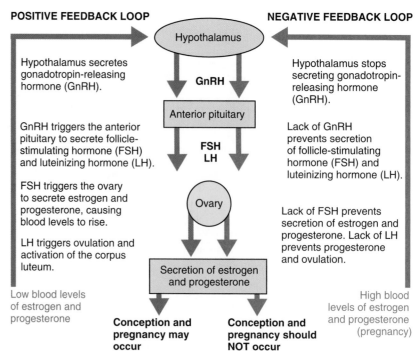

POSITIVE FEEDBACK LOOP   **NEGATIVE FEEDBACK LOOP**

Hypothalamus secretes gonadotropin-releasing hormone (GnRH).

GnRH triggers the anterior pituitary to secrete follicle-stimulating hormone (FSH) and luteinizing hormone (LH).

FSH triggers the ovary to secrete estrogen and progesterone, causing blood levels to rise.

LH triggers ovulation and activation of the corpus luteum.

Low blood levels of estrogen and progesterone

Hypothalamus stops secreting gonadotropin-releasing hormone (GnRH).

Lack of GnRH prevents secretion of follicle-stimulating hormone (FSH) and luteinizing hormone (LH).

Lack of FSH prevents secretion of estrogen and progesterone. Lack of LH prevents progesterone and ovulation.

High blood levels of estrogen and progesterone (pregnancy)

Conception and pregnancy may occur

Conception and pregnancy should NOT occur

FIGURE 32-2 Positive and negative feedback control over estrogen and progesterone secretion.

Perimenopause is the transition in a woman from having regular hormone cycles with menstrual periods to the time when menstrual periods have stopped for a full year. During this time, hormone levels change, causing the woman to have a variety of uncomfortable but usually minor symptoms.

When the glandular cells of the ovary shrink, they no longer produce normal levels of estrogen. The decreased blood levels of estrogen trigger the brain to secrete GnRH, which then triggers the pituitary gland to secrete FSH (see Figure 32-2). Before menopause the FSH acts on the ovary and causes ovarian cells to secret estrogen, which then inhibits the pathway through negative feedback. With nonfunctional ovarian cells unable to respond to FSH by increasing estrogen secretion, this pathway is disrupted for a time. The continued low blood levels of estrogen constantly stimulate the brain to secret GnRH in large amounts, resulting in the secretion of very large amounts of FSH (Figure 32-3). This extra FSH is useless because the ovary cannot respond to it, and it has effects on other body tissues. Box 32-1 lists the symptoms associated with decreased estrogen levels and increased FSH levels.

High levels of FSH act on blood vessels, making them dilate suddenly, resulting in the woman experiencing sudden whole-body flushes and radiant heat. These are commonly called *hot flashes* or *hot flushes*. At night these flushes are often followed by excessive sweating that leaves nightclothes and bedding wet.

Memory Jogger

Menopause symptoms are caused by low levels of estrogen and high levels of FSH.

Do Not Confuse

Premphase *with* **Prempro**

An order for Premphase can be confused with Prempro. Although both drugs are used for perimenopausal hormone replacement therapy, the dosages of the combined hormones are different, and the drugs should not be interchanged.

QSEN: Safety

TYPES OF PERIMENOPAUSAL HORMONE REPLACEMENT DRUGS

CONJUGATED ESTROGENS

How Perimenopausal Hormone Replacement Therapy Works

Hormone replacement therapy (HRT) is the replacement of naturally secreted estrogen and progesterone with exogenous hormones during the perimenopausal period. Providing low doses of estrogen increases blood estrogen levels, which helps with perimenopausal symptoms in two ways. First it relieves the direct problems from low estrogen levels (see Box 32-1). Second, it also inhibits the feedback system and lowers the levels of FSH. This reduces the side effects of high FSH levels (see Box 32-1).

Positive but ineffective feedback loop

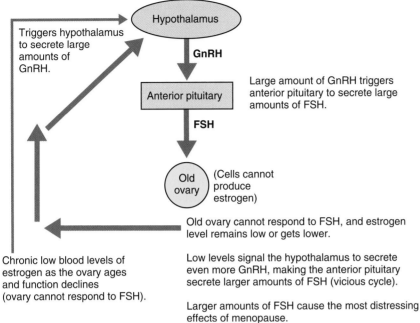

Triggers hypothalamus to secrete large amounts of GnRH.

Large amount of GnRH triggers anterior pituitary to secrete large amounts of FSH.

(Cells cannot produce estrogen)

Old ovary cannot respond to FSH, and estrogen level remains low or gets lower.

Low levels signal the hypothalamus to secrete even more GnRH, making the anterior pituitary secrete larger amounts of FSH (vicious cycle).

Chronic low blood levels of estrogen as the ovary ages and function declines (ovary cannot respond to FSH).

Larger amounts of FSH cause the most distressing effects of menopause.

FIGURE 32-3 Mechanism for hot flushes and night sweats associated with menopause. *FSH*, Follicle-stimulating hormone; *GnRH*, gonadotropin-releasing hormone.

Box 32-1   **Common Perimenopausal Symptoms**

SYMPTOMS RELATED TO REDUCED ESTROGEN LEVELS
- Atrophy of vaginal tissue
- Dry skin
- Increased rate of osteoporosis
- Painful intercourse
- Reduced cervical mucus

SYMPTOMS RELATED TO HIGH FOLLICLE-STIMULATING HORMONE LEVELS
- Decreased mental concentration
- Hot flushes
- Night sweats
- Sleep difficulties

Dosages for Common Perimenopausal Hormone Replacement Therapy Drugs

Drug	Dosage (Adults Only)
conjugated estrogens (Cenestin, C.E.S. ♣, Enjuvia, Premarin)	0.3 mg, 0.45 mg, or 0.625 mg orally once daily, given cyclically or continuously, alone in women without a uterus, in combination with a progestin in women with a uterus
conjugated estrogens; medroxyPROGESTERone	
(Premphase)	0.625 mg of conjugated estrogens orally once daily on days 1-14, then 1 light-blue tablet (0.625 mg conjugated estrogens and 5 mg medroxyPROGESTERone acetate) orally once daily on days 15-28
(Prempro)	0.3 mg or 0.45 mg along with medroxyPROGESTERone acetate 1.5 mg/day, or 0.625 mg along with medroxyPROGESTERone 2.5 mg, and then 0.625 mg along with 5 mg medroxyPROGESTERone for those not responding to lower doses

Common Side Effects

Perimenopausal Hormone
Replacement Therapy

Acne

👤 Clinical Pitfall

Patients taking perimenopausal
HRT should not smoke because of
the increased risk for blood clot
formation.

QSEN: Safety

💡 Memory Jogger

Taking perimenopausal HRT drugs
more often than prescribed or not
following instructions for timing
increases the risk for excessive
uterine bleeding.

Intended Responses
- The number and severity of hot flushes and night sweats are reduced.
- Vaginal dryness is reduced.

Side Effects.   Common side effects of perimenopausal HRT include breast tenderness, breakthrough bleeding, fluid retention, weight gain, and acne. These occur with conjugated estrogen alone and when combined with progesterone.

Adverse Effects.   Recent studies indicate that women taking estrogen-based HRT have a slightly higher incidence of myocardial infarction (heart attack). For this reason, estrogen-based HRT is not recommended for long-term therapy.

Drugs for perimenopausal HRT increase blood clotting, placing the patient at risk for thrombosis and emboli. Cigarette smoking worsens this risk. Results of increased clot formation include increased risks for heart attack, stroke, pulmonary embolism, and deep vein thrombosis.

In women who have a uterus and who take perimenopausal HRT, the uterine lining can become excessively thick, increasing the risk for excessive uterine bleeding.

The hormones in perimenopausal HRT can increase the growth of cancers that are hormone sensitive such as cervical, breast, ovarian, and uterine cancers. These drugs should not be used in women who have a history of these types of cancer. These hormones also increase the risk for liver impairment, gallbladder disease, and pancreatitis.

What To *Teach* Patients Taking Perimenopausal Hormone Replacement Therapy

Teach women to take drugs for perimenopausal HRT exactly as prescribed with regard to dosage and timing.

Urge patients who smoke to either quit or reduce smoking during the time that they take these drugs.

Teach patients to check the color of the roof of the mouth and the whites of the eyes weekly for the presence of a yellow tinge. Tell them to report jaundice, a sign of liver toxicity, to their prescriber as soon as possible.

Teach patients to seek medical attention immediately if they have chest pain or difficulty breathing, swelling in one leg, or symptoms of stroke.

CONTRACEPTION

In the United States, the age when females begin menarche (start menstruating) and can become pregnant may be as young as 9 years. Although sexual maturity is often early, social maturity is considerably later. Many people prefer to prevent pregnancy at least temporarily while still engaging in sexual intercourse.

Contraception is the intentional prevention of pregnancy. Many methods are used to prevent pregnancy. The most reliable method is completely abstaining from sexual intercourse, which may not be a reasonable choice for many people. Other forms of contraception include surgery, barrier methods, spermicidal foams and gels, and intrauterine devices. Specific drugs can be highly effective at preventing conception and pregnancy.

TYPES OF DRUGS FOR HORMONAL CONTRACEPTION

Hormonal contraception is the use of hormones that suppress ovulation and prevent pregnancy. It is highly effective when used appropriately. The hormones that prevent conception and pregnancy can be taken orally; used as topical applications in the form of transdermal patches, uterine rings, and released by a device directly in the uterus; implanted under the skin; and injected parenterally as a slow-absorbing drug form (Table 32-1). The most commonly used form of hormonal contraception is the

Table 32-1	Common Hormonal Contraceptives
GENERIC NAMES	**TRADE NAMES**
Combination Oral Contraceptives	
drospirenone; ethinyl estradiol	Yasmin
ethinyl estradiol; desogestrel	Apri, Azurette, CAZIANT, Cyclessa, Desogen, Kariva, Mircette, Ortho-Cept, Pimtrea, Reclipsen, Solia, Velivet
ethinyl estradiol; ethynodiol diacetate	Demulen, Kelnor, Zovia
ethinyl estradiol; levonorgestrel	Aviane, Enpresse, Jolessa, Lessina, Levlen, Levlite, Levora, Lutera, Portia, Quasense, Seasonale, Seasonique, Sronyx, Tri-Levlen, Triphasil, Trivora
ethinyl estradiol; norethindrone	Aranelle, Balziva, Brevicon, Femcon, Genora, Jenest, Leena, Modicon, Necon, Norinyl, Nortrel, Ortho-Novum, Ovcon, Tri-Norinyl, Zenchent
ethinyl estradiol; norethindrone acetate	Estrostep, Femhrt, Junel, Loestrin, Microgestin, Primella, Tilia, Tri-Legest
ethinyl estradiol; norgestimate	MonoNessa, Ortho Tri-Cyclen, Previfem, Sprintec-28, Tri-Previfem, Tri-Sprintec, TriNessa
ethinyl estradiol; norgestrel	Cryselle, Low-Ogestrel, Ogestrel, Ovral
mestranol; norethindrone	Genora, Necon, Necon, Norinyl, Ortho-Novum
Combination Topical Contraceptives	
Vaginal Rings	
ethinyl estradiol; etonogestrel	NuvaRing
Patches	
ethinyl estradiol; norelgestromin	Ortho Evra
Progestin-Only Oral Contraceptives	
norethindrone	Aygestin, Camila, Errin, Jolivette, Nor-QD, Nora-BE, Ortho Micronor
norgestrel	Ovrette
Intrauterine Contraceptives (Progestin Only)	
levonorgestrel	Mirena
Subcutaneous Implants (Progestin Only)	
etonogestrel	Implanon
levonorgestrel	Norplant

oral contraceptive. *Oral contraceptives* (OC) (often called birth control pills or BCPs) are hormone-based drugs taken orally that are generally effective in prevention of pregnancy. Regardless of the form of hormonal contraception used, the mechanism of action and side effects are the same.

How Hormonal Contraceptives Work

As described earlier in the chapter, the control of natural estrogen and progesterone secretion is through a "feedback" system of the hormone pathway that includes the hypothalamus, the pituitary gland, and the ovary (see Figure 32-2). Oral contraceptives interfere with the body's natural production of estrogen and progesterone by *turning off* the tissues in the pathway through *negative feedback* (see Figure 32-2). The most effective oral contraceptives contain two types of hormones, a synthetic estrogen and a synthetic type of progesterone known as a progestin. When a woman consistently takes this hormone combination, the blood levels of estrogen and progesterone are high, which sends signals to the hypothalamus that secretion of these hormones is not needed. Thus, GnRH secretion is inhibited. Without GnRH, the anterior pituitary does not secrete FSH and LH. As a result, the ovary does not produce more estrogen or progesterone. Without this influence, ovulation does not occur, and the lining of the uterus stays thin, unable to support a pregnancy. In a sense, oral contraceptives fool the endocrine system by mimicking pregnancy hormones. This "feeds back" to the hypothalamus, signaling that further hormone production is not needed.

 Memory Jogger

Hormonal contraceptives are more convenient and less disruptive to sexual spontaneity than are barrier methods.

 Memory Jogger

Hormonal contraceptives fool the endocrine system into not secreting estrogen and progesterone by mimicking pregnancy hormones.

Some oral contraceptives contain only progestin rather than a combination of estrogen and progestin. These are known as "mini-pills" and raise blood levels of progesterone, causing the hormone pathway to be turned off through negative feedback. The exact mechanism by which the surge of LH and ovulation are prevented is not known. However, in addition to suppressing ovulation, other changes occur that prevent pregnancy. These changes include thickening of the cervical mucus, which prevents movement of sperm into the uterus, and changing of the endometrium so that a pregnancy is not supported. These progestin-only oral contraceptives are usually taken daily continuously. The specific drugs in combination and their dosages vary, as does the dosing schedule. Be sure to consult a drug handbook for specific dosages and scheduling.

Intended Responses
- Suppression of ovum maturation
- Suppression of ovulation
- No conception and pregnancy

Side Effects. Common side effects of oral contraceptives include breast enlargement and tenderness, nausea, fluid retention, weight gain, and breakthrough bleeding. The severity of side effects is related to the dosage of the specific hormones used for contraception. Some women have more acne while taking oral contraceptives and others have less acne.

Adverse Effects. Oral contraceptives increase the risk for blood clots that can cause deep vein thrombosis, pulmonary embolism, myocardial infection, and stroke, especially among women who smoke and in those older than 35 years.

Most oral contraceptives (and other hormonal contraceptives) cause some degree of fluid and sodium retention, leading to hypertension. Women with moderate to severe hypertension should not use hormonal contraceptives.

Estrogen and progestin are metabolized by the liver and can cause liver toxicity. The patient with liver toxicity has elevated liver enzymes, yellowing of the skin and whites of the eyes, tiredness, dark urine, pale or clay-colored stools, and nausea. The woman with known liver problems should not use hormonal contraceptives.

The synthetic hormones in oral contraceptives and other hormonal contraceptives can increase the growth rate of cancer cells sensitive to the presence of hormones. Such cancers include cervical cancer and breast cancer. Hormonal contraceptives should not be used by women who have or who have had breast cancer or cervical cancer.

The oral contraceptives that use drospirenone as the progestin (Ocella, Yasmin, YAZ28) can increase the serum potassium level (normal levels 3.5 to 5.0 mEq/L or mmol/L), leading to *hyperkalemia*. When severe, it can cause complete heart block and other life-threatening irregular heart rhythms. This drug combination should be avoided in women who have kidney, liver, or adrenal disease and in those who are taking other drugs that increase potassium levels (e.g., angiotensin-converting enzyme (ACE) inhibitors for hypertension, potassium-sparing diuretics).

What To *Teach* Women Taking Hormonal Contraceptives
Oral contraceptives require a full cycle before they are effective. Teach the woman to use an additional method of contraception during the first cycle.

Check the recommended scheduling of the specific contraceptive prescribed. The scheduling is important for best effectiveness. Remind the woman to take the drug as recommended or an unplanned pregnancy may result.

Instruct the woman to take the oral contraceptive with food once daily. She should take the drug at the same time each day for best effect and to remember to take it. Remind her not to take more than one dose per day.

A major adverse effect of hormonal contraceptives is the increased risk for developing blood clots, especially among women who smoke. Stress the importance of not smoking or using nicotine in any form.

Common Side Effects
Perimenopausal Hormone Replacement Therapy

Nausea, weight gain   Breast tenderness

 Memory Jogger

The most serious adverse effect of hormonal contraceptives is the formation of blood clots that could lead to deep vein thrombosis, myocardial infarction, pulmonary embolism, and stroke.

 Drug Alert!

Interaction Alert

Oral contraceptives interact with many drugs and herbal supplements. Ask the patient about *all* other drugs, including over the counter, or supplements she takes, then check with the pharmacist to avoid a possible drug interaction.

QSEN: Safety

 Drug Alert!

Teaching Alert

Remind women that oral contraceptives are only effective at preventing pregnancy when taken exactly as prescribed.

QSEN: Safety

If one dose is missed within the cycle, the drug should still be effective in preventing pregnancy. However, if more than one dose is missed within a cycle, especially if two doses in a row are missed, tell the woman to continue to use it for the rest of the cycle but also to use another method of contraception for the rest of the cycle.

Warn women using hormonal contraceptives to be sure and tell any other health care provider that they are taking this drug because of the potential for drug interactions. Also, warn women not to take any over-the-counter drug without checking with the health care provider who prescribed the contraceptive.

Tell the woman to notify the prescriber if she develops yellowing of the skin or eyes, darkening of the urine, or lightening of the stools. These problems are signs of liver toxicity, a serious adverse effect of hormonal contraceptives.

Remind women that although hormonal contraceptives protect against pregnancy, they provide no protection against HIV and other sexually transmitted diseases. Condom use is needed to protect against contracting these infections.

Life Span Considerations for Perimenopausal Hormone Replacement Therapy and for Hormonal Contraception

Pediatric Considerations. Hormone replacement drugs and hormonal contraception are not approved for children of either gender before puberty. Early chronic exposure can cause growth of the long bones to stop.

Considerations for Pregnancy and Lactation. Hormone replacement therapy drugs and hormonal contraceptives should not be taken during pregnancy. Women should be tested for pregnancy or know for certain that they are not pregnant before starting these drugs. If a woman suspects that she has become pregnant while using hormone replacement therapy or a hormonal contraceptive, she should see her prescriber immediately.

Breastfeeding while using hormonal contraceptives is not recommended. These drugs interfere with lactation. They are also present in breast milk and may have adverse effects on the infant.

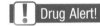 **Drug Alert!**

Teaching Alert

Remind women that hormonal contraceptives provide no protection against HIV or any other sexually transmitted disease.

QSEN: Safety

Get Ready for Practice!

Key Points

- Drugs for perimenopausal hormone replacement should be taken only short term to reduce the symptoms of menopause.
- Drugs for perimenopausal HRT increase blood clot formation, increasing the risks for heart attack, stroke, pulmonary embolism, and deep vein thrombosis.
- Women on perimenopausal hormone replacement therapy should not smoke.
- Hormonal contraception is a reversible form of birth control.
- Whether taken orally or applied as a patch, vaginal ring, intrauterine device, or implanted into subcutaneous tissue, hormonal contraceptives have the same mechanism of action and side effects.
- The estrogen and progesterone in hormonal contraceptives disrupt the female hormone pathway by using negative feedback and mimicking pregnancy hormones.
- The severity of side effects and the incidence of adverse effects are related to the dosage of the specific hormones used for contraception.

- Hormonal contraception should not be used by women who smoke; have a personal history of breast, uterine, ovarian, or cervical cancer; have moderate to severe hypertension; or have other significant risk factors for stroke or myocardial infarction.
- Teach women to seek medical help immediately for any symptom associated with deep vein thrombosis, myocardial infarction, stroke, or pulmonary embolism.
- Hormonal contraceptives do not protect against sexually transmitted diseases

Additional Learning Resources

evolve Be sure to visit your Evolve website (http://evolve.elsevier.com/Workman/pharmacology/) for additional online resources.

SG Go to your Study Guide for additional learning activities to help you master this chapter content.

Review Questions

See the Answer Keys—In-text Review Questions for answers to these questions.

Test Yourself on the Basics

1. Which activity must you advise the patient to avoid while taking perimenopausal hormone replacement therapy?
   A. Smoking cigarettes
   B. Having sexual intercourse
   C. Drinking alcoholic beverages
   D. Engaging in moderate-to-heavy exercise

2. Which side effects are most commonly associated with perimenopausal hormone replacement therapy? (Select all that apply.)
   A. Acne
   B. Breast tenderness
   C. Fluid retention
   D. Hair thinning
   E. Increased risk for urinary tract infection
   F. Night sweats
   G. Vaginal dryness
   H. Weight gain

3. For women who have a uterus and who are taking perimenopausal hormone replacement therapy, which adverse effect of the therapy is possible?
   A. Unplanned pregnancy
   B. Excessive uterine bleeding
   C. Increased risk for miscarriage
   D. Delayed ovulation suppressing fertility

4. Which hormone-based drug for birth control is delivered as an intrauterine contraceptive?
   A. etonogestrel (Implanon)
   B. ethinylestradiol, norethindrone (Brevicon)
   C. levonorgestrel (Mirena)
   D. norethindrone (Jolivette)

5. Which electrolyte should be closely monitored in any patient using an oral contraceptive that contains drospirenone?
   A. Sodium
   B. Potassium
   C. Calcium
   D. Magnesium

Test Yourself on Advanced Concepts

6. For which woman is the use of perimenopausal hormone replacement therapy contraindicated?
   A. 50-year-old who had her gall bladder removed 10 years ago
   B. 55-year-old who had a hysterectomy 15 years ago
   C. 45-year-old who was treated for breast cancer 5 years ago
   D. 48-year-old who used oral contraceptives for 20 years

7. How do hormonal contraceptives that contain only progestin (progesterone) prevent pregnancy?
   A. Inhibiting a woman's libido.
   B. Keeping the uterine lining too thick to allow fertilization.
   C. Thickening the cervical mucus and preventing sperm movement.
   D. Tightening the opening of the cervix, preventing sperm from entering.

8. A woman who wants to use hormonal contraception has all these health problems. Which one makes the use of this type of birth control a poor choice for her?
   A. She has hepatitis C.
   B. She is 20 lb overweight.
   C. Her mother died of ovarian cancer.
   D. Her menstrual periods are irregular.

9. A woman who has used hormonal contraception for 3 years calls and tells you that she has had pain in her right groin for 2 days and now her right leg is swollen. What is your best action?
   A. Reassure her that this is an expected side effect of hormonal contraception.
   B. Tell her that this means the contraception has failed and she is pregnant.
   C. Suggest that she elevate her legs and apply a heating pad.
   D. Tell her to notify the prescriber immediately.

10. Why should hormonal contraception be discontinued if pregnancy occurs?
    A. The hormonal contraceptives are expensive and no longer needed when pregnancy occurs.
    B. The risk for birth defects is increased with the use of hormonal contraceptives during pregnancy.
    C. The hormones in the contraceptive compete with natural hormones of pregnancy and increase the risk for miscarriage.
    D. Taking hormonal contraceptives during pregnancy greatly increases the risk for development of excessive uterine bleeding at delivery.

Critical Thinking Activities

See the Answer Keys—Critical Thinking Activities for answers to these activities.

A 28-year-old mother of two calls and tells you that she "had the stomach flu" last week and could not hold down any food for 3 days. She tells you that she usually takes Norinyl and not only did not take it while she was sick, she also forgot to take it for the next 4 days. She is concerned about an unplanned pregnancy.

1. What type of drug is Norinyl?
2. What are the side effects of this drug?
3. Is she correct in worry about an unplanned pregnancy as a result of forgetting to take this drug for 7 days? Why or why not?
4. What should you tell her about contraception?

Medication Administration Skills*

Skill 1 Performing Hand Hygiene with Soap and Water

ACTION (RATIONALE)

1. Inspect hands, observing for visible soiling, breaks, or cuts in the skin and cuticles. (*Poor personal hygiene and an open area of the skin provide areas in which microorganisms are able to grow.*)
2. Determine amount of contaminant on hands. (*Determines the type of hand hygiene needed.*)
3. Assess areas around the skin that are contaminated. (*Prevents contamination of hands during and after hand hygiene procedure.*)
4. Adjust the water to appropriate temperature and force. (*Water that is too hot can chap skin, and too much force causes splashing and may spread microorganisms to other areas, especially your clothing.*)
5. Wet hands and wrists under the running water, always keeping hands lower than elbows. (*Hands are the most contaminated part of the upper extremities; water should flow from the wrists [least contaminated area] over the hands, and then down the drain.*)
6. Lather hands with liquid soap (about 1 teaspoon). (*Soap lather emulsifies fat and aids in cleansing.*)
7. Wash hands thoroughly with a firm, circular motion and friction on back of hands, palms, and wrists. Wash each finger individually, paying special attention to areas between fingers and knuckles by interlacing fingers and thumbs and moving hands back and forth, causing friction. (*Helps to loosen soil and microorganisms, both resident [normally present] and transient [acquired from contamination].*)

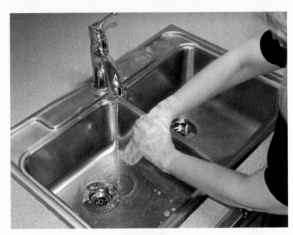

Step **7**

8. Wash for 15 to 30 seconds. (*The greater the contamination, the more need for longer washing.*)
9. Rinse wrists and hands completely, again keeping hands lower than elbows. (*Water should run from cleaner area [the wrists] over the hands, and then down the drain, rinsing the dirt and microorganisms away.*)

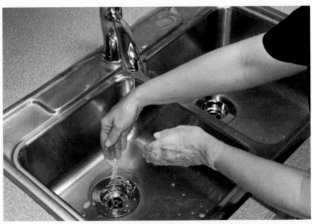

Step **9**

Continued

---

*Skills from Cooper, K., & Kelly, G. (2015). *Foundations of nursing*, ed 7, St. Louis, Mosby.

Skill 1   Performing Hand Hygiene with Soap and Water—cont'd

10. Dry hands thoroughly with paper towels. Start by patting at fingertips, then hands, and then wrists and forearms. *(Prevents chapping. Drying should progress from clean to less clean, and the cleanest areas are now your fingers and hands.)*

11. If it is necessary to turn off faucets manually, use a dry paper towel. *(Keeps clean hands from touching contaminated handles.)*

12. Use hospital-approved hand lotion if desired. *(Keeps skin soft and lubricated so it does not crack easily.)*

13. Inspect hands and nails for cleanliness. *(Ensures cleanliness of hands and nails.)*

14. If hands are not visibly soiled, use an alcohol-based waterless antiseptic for routine decontamination of hands in all clinical situations, unless you are caring for a patient with *Clostridium difficile* or *Candida* infection. The spores are unaffected by alcohol, so soap and water must be used in this instance.

15. Provide patient teaching.

16. Explain to the patient the importance of hand hygiene. *(Helps the patient understand that hand hygiene slows down the spread of infection.)*

17. If contamination occurs, it is necessary to reassess technique.

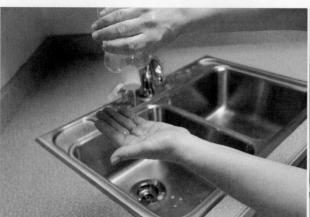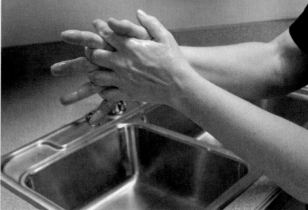

Step **14**

Skill 2   Gloving

ACTION (RATIONALE)

Donning Gloves

1. Remove gloves from dispenser. *(Keeps gloves handy and ready for use.)*

2. Inspect gloves for perforations. *(Prevents pathogenic microorganisms from entering through perforation in gloves.)*

3. Don gloves when ready to begin patient care. Wearing gloves with a gown does not necessitate any special technique for putting them on; wear them pulled over cuffs of gown. *(Ensures full coverage of your wrists.)*

4. Change gloves after direct handling of infectious material such as wound drainage. *(Prevents cross contamination.)*

Skill 2   Gloving—cont'd

5. Do not touch side rails, tables, or bed stands with contaminated gloves. *(Prevents spread of microorganisms throughout environment.)*

Removing Gloves

6. Remove first glove by grasping outer surface at palm with other gloved hand and pulling glove inside out and off. Place this glove in the hand that is still gloved. *(Prevents you from touching your own skin with contaminated glove.)*

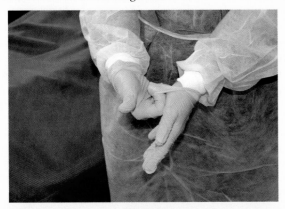

Step **6**

7. Remove second glove by placing finger under cuff and turning glove inside out and over other glove. Drop gloves into waste container. *(Prevents you from touching contaminated glove. Wraps contamination inside gloves to help protect others.)*

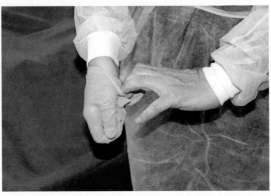

Step **7**

8. Perform hand hygiene. *(Helps prevent cross contamination.)*
9. Provide patient teaching.
10. If contamination occurs, it is necessary to reassess technique.

Skill 3   Administering Tablets, Pills, and Capsules

ACTION (RATIONALE)

1. Follow the eight "rights" of medication administration. *(Prevents medication errors.)*
2. Perform the three label checks. *(Prevents medication errors.)*
3. Follow Standard Precautions. *(Prevents spread of microorganisms.)*
4. Perform hand hygiene. *(Prevents spread of microorganisms.)*
5. If using a unit-dose package, place unopened medication package in medicine cup. *(Prevents medication errors.)*

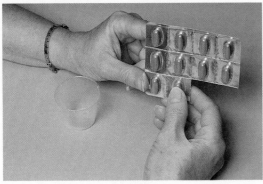

Step **5**

6. If using a multidose bottle, pour tablet, without touching it, into cap of bottle. *(Prevents contamination.)*
7. Pour tablet from cap into medicine cup.
8. If pouring from multidose bottle and patient is to receive several tablets, use a separate cup for medications such as digitalis, and label this cup with the name of the medication. If the patient's pulse is less than 60 bpm, withhold the medication and report this action to the RN and the health care provider. *(By placing digitalis in a separate cup marked with the medication's name, it will be identified easily.)*
9. If a tablet needs to be broken in half to administer half the dose, use gloved hands or a cutting device. Break the tablet along the scored line located along the center of the tablet. The nurse may be required to dispose of the remainder of the tablet or save it in its original container, depending on the health care facility's policy.
10. If a patient has difficulty swallowing, the nurse may need to use a mortar and pestle or other pill-crushing device. The crushed medication is often mixed with applesauce, yogurt, or some other soft food item. The nurse should ask the patient his or her preference regarding what to place the

Continued

Skill 3   Administering Tablets, Pills, and Capsules—cont'd

medication in. It is important for the nurse to remember that is not appropriate to crush drugs that are capsules, enteric-coated, long acting, or slow release. These types of drugs are developed to prevent stomach irritation, or the medication may be destroyed by gastric acids. Some medications are not meant to be crushed because crushing increases the absorption rate and the medication is meant to be released and absorbed slowly. If the medication label specifies "extended release," "sustained release," "XL," "SR," or "CD," then the medication should not be crushed.

11. Any medications dropped in the course of the medication pass must be disposed of according to facility policy. *(Prevents contaminated medications from being administered to patient.)*

12. Transport medication to patient's room.
13. Identify patient by checking identification bracelet and per facility policy. *(Prevents medication errors.)*
14. Explain procedure to patient.
15. Document administration of medication on medication administration record (MAR) with time, date, and name or with computerized documentation.
16. Return at an appropriate time to assess patient's response to medication. *(Enables you to determine effectiveness of medication and any occurrence of adverse reactions. Some medication routes act more quickly than other routes.)*
17. Document side effects and therapeutic responses per facility policy.

Step 5 figure from Potter, P. A., Perry, A.G., Stockert, P., et al. (2013). *Fundamentals of nursing* (8th ed.). St. Louis: Mosby.

Skill 4   Administering Liquid Medications

ACTION (RATIONALE)

1. Follow the eight "rights" of medication administration. *(Prevents medication errors.)*
2. Perform the three label checks. *(Prevents medication errors.)*
3. Follow Standard Precautions. *(Prevents spread of microorganisms.)*
4. Perform hand hygiene. *(Prevents spread of microorganisms.)*
5. Remove liquid preparation from patient's drug box, bin, medication cabinet, or computerized medication dispenser.
6. Check dose/milliliter and total volume of medication in container.
7. Calculate dosage; if the dose ordered is different from the dose/milliliter stated on the label, calculate correct dose; if ordered medication is labeled according to a different measurement system, convert by using appropriate equivalent. Work calculation on paper.
8. Check calculations with another nurse. *(Helps prevent errors.)*
9. Obtain medicine cup that is graduated (has markings indicating marked amount; total volume of cup is 30 mL, or 1 oz) or appropriate graduated syringe. *(For accuracy.)*
10. Face label of bottle toward palm of hand *(to avoid soiling label)*; if label becomes soiled, return the

bottle to the pharmacy. Do not give medication if label is unreadable. *(Maintains accuracy and prevents errors.)*

11. Place medicine cup on flat surface to pour while you watch at eye level, or hold medication cup up at eye level while you pour. *(Maintains accuracy.)*
12. Place cap of bottle with inner rim up to prevent contaminating inside of cap. *(To prevent contaminating remaining contents of bottle.)*
13. Read dosage amount at lowest level of meniscus (curve formed by liquid's upper surface). *(For accuracy.)*

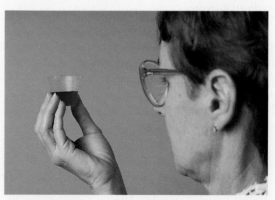

Step **13**

Skill 4   Administering Liquid Medications—cont'd

14. Transport medication to patient's room.
15. Identify patient by checking identification bracelet and per facility policy. (*Prevents medication errors.*)
16. Explain procedure to patient.
17. Document administration on medication administration record, whether on paper copy or

with computer. Note time, date, and medication name.
18. Return at appropriate time to assess patient's response to medication. (*Enables you to determine effectiveness of medication and any occurrence of adverse reactions.*)
19. Document assessment findings in progress notes.

Step 13 figure from Potter, P. A., & Perry, A. G. (2009). *Fundamentals of nursing: Concepts, process, and practice* (7th ed.). St. Louis: Mosby.

Skill 5   Administering Sublingual Medications

ACTION (RATIONALE)

1. Follow the eight "rights" of medication administration. (*Prevents medication errors.*)
2. Perform the three label checks. (*Prevents medication errors.*)
3. Follow Standard Precautions. (*Prevents spread of microorganisms.*)
4. Perform hand hygiene. (*Prevents spread of microorganisms.*)
5. Transport drug to patient's room and identify patient by checking identification bracelet and per facility policy. (*Prevents medication errors.*)
6. Don gloves and place tablet under patient's tongue. (*Reduces spread of microorganisms and prevents absorption of medication into your skin.*)

7. Do not give patient water immediately afterwards. (*Water reduces absorption of medication.*)
8. Instruct patient not to swallow tablet but to let it dissolve. (*Swallowing reduces absorption of medication.*)
9. Teach patient how to place medication under tongue when self-administering. Instruct patient to let it dissolve.
10. Remove gloves and wash hands. (*Reduces spread of microorganisms.*)
11. Record sublingual administration of medications per facility policy.
12. Return to assess patient's response to medication. (*Enables you to determine effectiveness of medication and any occurrence of adverse reactions.*)
13. Document assessment findings in progress notes.

Skill 6   Administering Buccal Medications

ACTION (RATIONALE)

1. Follow the eight "rights" of medication administration. (*Prevents medication errors.*)
2. Perform the three label checks. (*Prevents medication errors.*)
3. Follow Standard Precautions. (*Prevents spread of microorganisms.*)
4. Perform hand hygiene. (*Prevents spread of microorganisms.*)
5. Transport drug to patient's room and identify patient by checking identification bracelet and per facility policy. (*Prevents medication errors.*)
6. Don gloves and place medication between patient's cheek and gum. (*Prevents spread of microorganisms.*)

7. Do not give patient water immediately afterwards. (*Reduces absorption of medication.*)
8. Instruct patient not to swallow tablet but to let it dissolve.
9. Teach patient how to place medication between gum and cheek when self-administering.
10. Remove gloves and wash hands. (*Reduces spread of microorganisms.*)
11. Record buccal administration of medications per facility policy.
12. Return to assess patient's response to medication. (*Enables you to determine effectiveness of medication and any occurrence of adverse reactions.*)
13. Document assessment findings in progress notes.

Skill 7   Administering Eyedrops and Eye Ointments

ACTION (RATIONALE)

1. Follow the eight "rights" of medication administration. (*Prevents medication errors.*)
2. Perform the three label checks. (*Prevents medication errors.*)
3. Follow Standard Precautions. (*Prevents spread of microorganisms.*)
4. Gather equipment. (*Organizes procedure.*)
   - Eyedrops
   - Gloves
   - Cotton ball or tissue
   - Sterile saline
5. Perform hand hygiene. (*Prevents spread of microorganisms.*)
6. Confirm medication is ophthalmic preparation. Transport medication to patient's room.
7. Identify patient by checking identification bracelet and asking patient's name and birth date. (*Prevents medication errors.*)
8. Introduce yourself; explain procedure. (*Establishes trust.*)
9. Provide privacy; position back of patient's head on pillow; direct patient's face upward toward ceiling.
10. Determine which eye is to receive the medication or whether both eyes should.
11. Don gloves. (*Reduces spread of microorganisms.*)
12. Remove exudate; clean eye as needed with sterile solution of saline or water; use cotton balls to wipe away exudate; use one cotton ball per stroke, wiping from inner canthus outward. (*Cleansing eye from inner to outer canthus avoids introducing microorganisms into lacrimal ducts. Soaking allows easy removal of dried exudate that harbors microorganisms.*)
13. To apply drops:
    a. Expose lower conjunctival sac by having patient look upward while gentle traction is applied to lower eyelid.

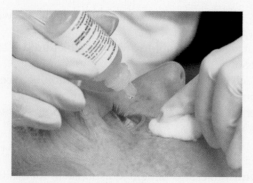

Step **13a**

b. Put prescribed number of drops into conjunctival sac, not onto eyeball. (*Therapeutic effect of drug is obtained only when drops enter sac.*)
c. Conjunctival sac normally holds one or two drops. (*Applying drops to conjunctival sac provides even distribution of medicine across eye.*)
d. Use tissue to apply gentle pressure above bone at inner corner of eyelid for 1 to 2 minutes. (*Minimizes absorption into circulatory system.*)
e. Apply sterile dressing, if it is ordered.

14. To apply ointment:
    a. Expose lower conjunctival sac by having patient look upward while gentle traction is applied to lower eyelid.

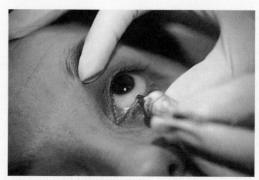

Step **14a**

b. Squeeze ointment into lower conjunctival sac.
c. Ask patient to close eye and move it around in circular motion. (*Spreads medication evenly.*)
d. Apply sterile dressing, if it is ordered.

15. After applying drops or ointment to an eye, leave patient in comfortable position; clean up the work area.
16. Remove gloves and wash hands. (*Reduces spread of microorganisms.*)
17. Answer patient's questions and, if appropriate, teach patient to perform self-care.
18. Record administration of medications per facility policy.
19. Return to assess patient's response to medication. (*Enables you to determine effectiveness of medication and any occurrence of adverse reactions.*)
20. Document assessment findings in progress notes.

Steps 13a and 14a figures from Potter, P. A., Perry, A.G., Stockert, P., et al. (2013). *Fundamentals of nursing* (8th ed.). St. Louis: Mosby.

Skill 8   Administering Eardrops

ACTION (RATIONALE)

1. Follow the eight "rights" of medication administration. *(Prevents medication errors.)*
2. Perform the three label checks. *(Prevents medication errors.)*
3. Follow Standard Precautions. *(Prevents spread of microorganisms.)*
4. Gather equipment. *(Organizes procedure.)*
   - Eardrops
   - Gloves
   - Cotton ball
5. Perform hand hygiene. *(Prevents spread of microorganisms.)*
6. Confirm medication is otic preparation. Transport medication to patient's room.
7. Identify patient by checking identification bracelet and per facility policy. *(Prevents medication errors.)*
8. Introduce yourself; explain procedure. *(Establishes trust.)*
9. Provide privacy.
10. Determine which ear is to receive the medication; position patient with affected ear upward.
11. Don gloves. *(Reduces spread of microorganisms.)*
12. Remove external exudate from ear; it is necessary to obtain an order for irrigating the ear. *(Drainage harbors microorganisms and sometimes impedes distribution of medication into the canal.)*
13. Draw medication into dropper.
14. Instill drops:
    a. *For adults and for children older than 3 years:* Turn head with affected side up; pull earlobe upward and back to straighten external auditory canal; instill drops without touching ear with dropper. *(Straightening of ear canal provides direct access to deeper external structures.)*

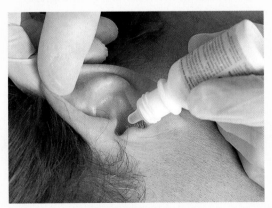

Step **14a**

b. *For children younger than 3 years:* Turn head with affected side up; pull earlobe downward and back; instill drops without touching ear with dropper. *(Straightening of ear canal provides direct access to deeper external structures.)*

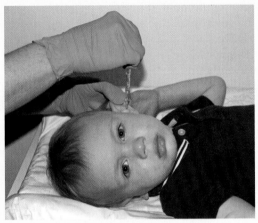

Step **14b**

15. Tell patient to remain in same position for 5 to 10 minutes to allow medication to drain into ear by gravity. *(To promote distribution of drops in ear canal.)*
16. Place a cotton ball loosely into ear as needed. *(Prevents escape of medication when patient sits or stands.)*
17. Remove gloves.
18. Leave patient in comfortable position; clean work area.
19. Answer patient's questions and, if appropriate, teach patient self-care.
20. Perform hand hygiene. *(Reduces spread of microorganisms.)*
21. Record administration of medications per facility policy.
22. Return to assess patient's response to medication. *(Enables you to determine effectiveness of medication and any occurrence of adverse reactions.)*
23. Document assessment findings in progress notes.

Skill 9   Administering Nose Drops

ACTION (RATIONALE)

1. Follow the eight "rights" of medication administration. (*Prevents medication errors.*)
2. Perform the three label checks. (*Prevents medication errors.*)
3. Follow Standard Precautions. (*Prevents spread of microorganisms.*)
4. Gather equipment. (*Organizes procedure.*)
   - Nose drops
   - Gloves
   - Tissues
5. Perform hand hygiene. (*Prevents spread of microorganisms.*)
6. Confirm medication is nasal preparation. Transport medication to patient's room.
7. Identify patient by checking identification bracelet and per facility policy. (*Prevents medication errors.*)
8. Introduce yourself; explain procedure. (*Establishes trust.*)
9. Provide privacy.
10. Don gloves. (Reduces spread of microorganisms.)
11. If patient is an adult or older child, ask patient to clear nose of accumulations by blowing gently into tissue. (*Allows absorption of medication.*)
12. Determine which nostril is to receive the medication or whether both nostrils should.
13. Position patient:
    a. *Adult or older child:* Have patient lie down, hanging head backward over edge of bed (if condition permits) or with pillow under shoulders to hyperextend the neck if patient can tolerate it. (*Promotes absorption of medication.*)
    b. *Younger child:* Position child on bed with head backward and downward. (*Promotes absorption of medication.*)
    c. *Infant:* Hold infant with head backward and downward. (*Promotes absorption of medication.*)
14. After drawing medication into dropper, instill medication while holding dropper above (not touching) nostril being treated.

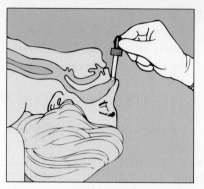

Step **14**

15. If orders specify treatment in both nostrils, repeat procedure to instill drops in other nostril.
16. Tell patient to hold position for a few minutes. (*Allows medication to remain in place.*)
17. Remove gloves.
18. Tell patient to refrain from blowing nose immediately after instillation. (*Prevents removal of medication.*)
19. Offer tissues for later use.
20. Leave patient in comfortable position; clean work area.
21. Answer patient's questions and, if appropriate, teach patient self-care.
22. Perform hand hygiene. (*Reduces spread of microorganisms.*)
23. Record administration of medications per facility policy.
24. Return to assess patient's response to medication. (*Enables you to determine effectiveness of medication and any occurrence of adverse reactions.*)
25. Document assessment findings in progress notes.

Step 14 figure from Clayton, B.D., Stock, Y. N. (2007). *Basic pharmacology for nurses* (14th ed.). St. Louis: Mosby.

Skill 10 Administering Nasal Sprays

ACTION (RATIONALE)

1. Follow the eight "rights" of medication administration. (*Prevents medication errors.*)
2. Perform the three label checks. (*Prevents medication errors.*)
3. Follow Standard Precautions. (*Prevents spread of microorganisms.*)
4. Gather equipment. (*Organizes procedure.*)
   - Nasal spray
   - Gloves
   - Tissues
5. Perform hand hygiene. (*Prevents spread of microorganisms.*)
6. Confirm medication is nasal preparation. Transport medication to patient.
7. Determine which nostril is to receive the medication or whether both should.
8. Identify patient by checking identification bracelet and per facility policy. (*Prevents medication errors.*)
9. Introduce yourself; explain procedure. (*Establishes trust.*)
10. Provide privacy; position patient upright.
11. Don gloves. (*Reduces spread of microorganisms.*)
12. Have patient gently blow nose, if capable, to clear nasal passages of accumulations. (*Promotes absorption of medication.*)
13. Compress one nostril.
14. Shake bottle while holding it upright. (*To mix solution.*)
15. Insert tip of spray bottle into patient's patent nostril.
16. Instruct patient to inhale through the nose; while patient inhales, squeeze bottle.
17. If orders specify treatment in both nostrils, repeat procedure for other nostril.
18. Tell patient to refrain from blowing nose for a few minutes; offer tissues for later use. (*Promotes absorption of medication.*)
19. Answer patient's questions and, if appropriate, teach self-administration.
20. Remove gloves and wash hands. (*Reduces spread of microorganisms.*)
21. Record administration of medications per facility policy.
22. Return to assess patient's response to medication. (*Enables you to determine effectiveness of medication and any occurrence of adverse reactions.*)
23. Document assessment findings in progress notes.

Skill 11 Administering a Metered-Dose Inhaler

ACTION (RATIONALE)

1. Follow the eight "rights" of medication administration. (*Prevents medication errors.*)
2. Perform the three label checks. (*Prevents medication errors.*)
3. Follow Standard Precautions. (*Prevents spread of microorganisms.*)
4. Gather equipment. (*Organizes procedure.*)
   - Gloves
   - Inhaler
   - Canister
   - Spacer device
5. Perform hand hygiene. (*Prevents spread of microorganisms.*)
6. Transport medications to patient's room.
7. Identify patient by checking identification bracelet and per facility policy. (*Prevents medication errors.*)
8. Introduce yourself; explain procedure. (*Establishes trust.*)
9. Provide privacy.
10. Don gloves. (*Reduces spread of microorganisms.*)
11. Allow patient opportunity to manipulate inhaler, canister, and spacer device (e.g., AeroChamber). Explain and demonstrate how canister fits into inhaler. (*Patient needs to be familiar with how to assemble and use equipment.*)
12. Explain what metered dose is and warn patient about overuse of inhaler, including drug side effects. (*Patient needs to know the dangers of excessive inhalations because of risk of serious side effects. If drug is received in recommended doses, side effects are minimal.*)

Continued

Skill 11   Administering a Metered-Dose Inhaler—cont'd

13. Remove mouthpiece cover from inhaler. Shake inhaler well. *(Ensures mixing of medication in canister.)*
14. Position inhaler:
    a. *Without AeroChamber (spacer):* Have patient open lips and place inhaler ½ to 1 inch (1 to 2 cm) from mouth with opening toward back of pharynx. Lips will not touch inhaler. *(Prevents rapid influx of inhaled medication and subsequent airway irritation. Positioning the mouthpiece 1 to 2 cm from the mouth is considered the best way to deliver the medication without a spacer.)*

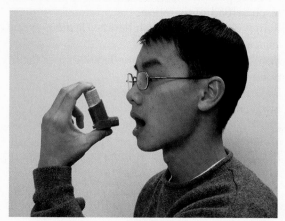

Step **14a**

    b. *With AeroChamber (spacer):* Have patient exhale fully and then grasp mouthpiece with teeth and lips while holding inhaler with thumb at the mouthpiece and fingers at the top. *(Spacers are recommended because the device allows particles of the medication to "ride" the breath into the airways rather than hit the back of the pharynx.)*

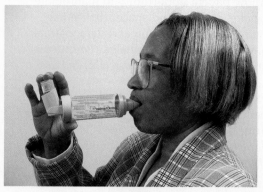

Step **14b**

15. Instruct patient to press down on inhaler to release medication while inhaling slowly and deeply through mouth.
16. Instruct patient to breathe in slowly for 2 to 3 seconds and to hold breath for approximately 10 seconds. *(Holding breath allows tiny drops of aerosol spray to reach deeper branches of airway.)*
17. Instruct patient to exhale through pursed lips.
18. Instruct patient to wait 2 to 5 minutes between puffs. More than one puff is usually prescribed. *(First inhalation opens airways and reduces inflammation. Second or third inhalation penetrates more deeply into airways.)*
19. If more than one type of inhaled medication is prescribed, wait 5 to 10 minutes between inhalations or as ordered by health care provider. *(Drug administration is prescribed at intervals during day to promote bronchodilation and keep side effects to a minimum.)*
20. Explain that patient will sometimes feel gagging sensation in throat caused by droplets of medication on pharynx or tongue.
21. Instruct patient in removing medication canister and cleaning inhaler in warm water. *(To remove residue that can interfere with proper distribution of medication.)*
22. Instruct patient to rinse mouth with water and spit.
23. *Evidence-based practice for patient to determine when the metered-dose inhaler (MDI) is empty:* In the past, patients were taught to determine the remainder of medication in the canister of their MDI by floating it in water. This method was found to be very inaccurate because of the variety of canister sizes and designs. Patients used different methods to try to determine whether a canister was empty and tended to use the medication canister much longer than its intended duration. When MDIs do not have built-in dose counters, instruct the patient in how to count doses still available in the canister by calculating the number of puffs used per day to calculate the number of days to expect the inhaler to last.

Steps 14a and 14b figures from Potter, P. A., Perry, A.G., Stockert, P., et al. (2013). *Fundamentals of nursing* (8th ed.). St. Louis: Mosby.

Skill 12   Applying Topical Agents

ACTION (RATIONALE)

1. Follow the eight "rights" of medication administration. (*Prevents medication errors.*)
2. Perform the three label checks. (*Prevents medication errors.*)
3. Follow Standard Precautions. (*Reduces spread of microorganisms.*)
4. Gather equipment. (*Organizes procedure.*)
   - Gloves
   - Medication
   - Washing materials
5. Perform hand hygiene. (*Reduces spread of microorganisms.*)
6. Transport medication to patient's room.
7. Identify patient by checking identification bracelet and per facility policy. (*Prevents medication errors.*)
8. Introduce yourself; explain procedure to patient. (*Establishes trust.*)
9. Provide privacy; place patient in comfortable position that allows exposure of selected site.
10. Don gloves. (*Reduces spread of microorganisms and prevents absorption of topical agent into your skin.*)
11. Read prescription instructions carefully. (*For accuracy.*)
12. Prepare medicinal agent (ointments, creams, and lotions sometimes have to be squeezed or removed with a tongue blade, depending on preparation used).
13. Wash affected area, removing debris, encrustations, and previous medications. (*Removal of debris enhances penetration of topical drug through skin. Cleansing removes microorganisms resident in remaining debris.*) Area should be allowed to dry. (*Allows for better adherence to the skin.*)
14. With gloves on, apply medication lotion, ointment, or cream via paper, or apply medication patch directly to skin. When using medication patches, be certain to remove plastic from disk before applying to skin. (*Essential for absorption of medication. Do not massage medication into skin; this can cause a bolus of medication to be administered.*)
15. Remove gloves.
16. Leave patient in comfortable position.
17. Answer patient's questions, and teach patient to perform self-applications if appropriate.
18. Clean work area.
19. Wash hands. (*Reduces spread of microorganisms.*)
20. Document administration per facility policy on paper copy of medication administration record or with computerized documentation system.
21. Return to assess patient's response to medication. (*Enables you to determine effectiveness of medication and any occurrence of adverse reactions.*)
22. Document assessment findings in progress notes.

Skill 13   Administering Rectal Suppositories

ACTION (RATIONALE)

1. Follow the eight "rights" of medication administration. (*Prevents medication errors.*)
2. Perform the three label checks. (*Prevents medication errors.*) Ensure that the patient does not have any contraindications for giving the type of medication in a suppository form.
3. Follow Standard Precautions. (*Prevents spread of microorganisms.*)
4. Gather equipment. (*Organizes procedure.*)
   - Gloves
   - Lubricant
   - Suppository
   - Souffle cup
5. Perform hand hygiene. (*Prevents spread of microorganisms.*)
6. Obtain suppository from refrigerator or from patient's medication bin.
7. Place unopened suppository into medicine cup or souffle cup (ungraduated disposable paper cup).
8. Introduce yourself; explain procedure to patient. (*Enlists patient's cooperation and establishes trust.*)
9. Identify patient by checking identification bracelet and per facility policy. (*Prevents medication errors.*)
10. Provide privacy.
11. Don clean gloves. (*Protects you from fecal material and reduces the spread of microorganisms.*)

Continued

Skill 13   Administering Rectal Suppositories—cont'd

12. Position patient in Sims' position (on left side with upper leg flexed at knee). (*Position exposes anus and helps patient to relax external anal sphincter. Left-side positioning lessens the likelihood that the suppository or feces will be expelled.*)
13. Unwrap suppository.
14. Maintain privacy; expose patient's buttocks.
15. Assess anus externally and gently palpate rectal vault as needed. (*Enables you to determine presence of active rectal bleeding, as well as to note whether rectum contains feces, which potentially cause problems with suppository placement.*) Do not palpate a patient's rectum after rectal surgery. If a patient has hemorrhoids, always use a generous amount of a lubricating gel and gently manipulate the tissues to visualize the anus for insertion of the suppository.
16. Apply water-soluble lubricant to tapered end of suppository. (*Lubrication reduces friction as suppository enters rectal area.*)
17. Ask patient to take deep breath; insert tapered end of suppository beyond internal anal sphincter. Insert suppository as patient exhales to relax anal

sphincter. (*Forcing suppository through constricted sphincter causes discomfort.*)
18. Ask patient to retain suppository as long as possible. (*This allows the medication to completely dissolve and absorb through mucous membranes of rectum into capillaries of systemic circulatory system.*) Hold the patient's buttocks together to help patient retain suppository. (*Provides sufficient time for the effects of the suppository to reach the maximum effectiveness.*)
19. Discard gloves.
20. Perform hand hygiene. (*Reduces spread of microorganisms.*)
21. Help patient assume a comfortable position.
22. Document administration of suppository per facility policy.
23. Return to assess patient's response to medication. (*Enables you to determine effectiveness of medication and any occurrence of adverse reactions.*)
24. Document assessment findings in progress notes.

Bibliography

Abate, K., & Buttaro, T. (2015). Safe and effective NSAID use. *The Nurse Practitioner, 40*(6), 18–22.

Adams, B., & Fergusin, K. (2014). Pharmacologic management of pulmonary arterial hypertension. *AACN Advanced Critical Care, 25*(4), 309–316.

Alexander-Magalee, M. A. (2013). Addressing pharmacology challenges in older adults. *Nursing, 43*(10), 58–60.

Anderson, P., & Townsend, T. (2015). Preventing high-alert medication errors in hospital patients. *American Nurse Today, 10*(5), 18–22.

Aschenbrenner, D. (2012). Statins receive key labeling revisions. *American Journal of Nursing, 112*(8), 21–23.

Aschenbrenner, D. (2013). Drug watch. *American Journal of Nursing, 113*(2), 23–24. *113*(3), 22–23; *113*(4), 28–29; *113*(8), 23–24; *113*(9), 26–27; *113*(10), 22–23; *113*(11), 22–23.

Aschenbrenner, D. (2014). Drug watch. *American Journal of Nursing, 114*(1), 24–25. *114*(2), 24–25; *114*(3), 22–23; *114*(4), 24–25; *114*(5), 24–25; *114*(6), 20–21; *114*(8), 21–22; *114*(9), 24–25; *114*(10), 22–23; *114*(11), 23–24.

Aschenbrenner, D. (2015). Drug watch. *American Journal of Nursing, 115*(1), 22–23. *115*(2), 20–21; *115*(5), 23–24.

Baldwin, K., & Walsh, V. (2014). Independent double-checks for high-alert medications: Essential practice. *Nursing, 44*(4), 65–67.

Barnsteiner, J. H. *Medication reconciliation.* (2008). Retrieved from <http://www.ncbi.nlm.nih.gov/books/NBK2648/>.

Bartlett, D. (2011). Drug therapy gets personal with genetic profiling. *American Nurse Today, 6*(5), 23–27.

Beery, T. A., & Workman, M. L. (2012). *Genetics and genomics in nursing and health care.* Philadelphia: F.A. Davis.

Berryman, S., Jennings, J., Ragsdale, S., Lofton, T., Huff, D., & Rooker, J. (2012). Beers criteria for potentially inappropriate medication use in older adults. *Medsurg Nursing, 21*(3), 129–132.

Blake, T. (2012). Three medication pathways for bipolar disorder. *Nursing, 42*(5), 28–35.

Boyce, B., & Yee, B. (2012). Incidence and severity of phlebitis in patients receiving peripherally infused amiodarone. *Critical Care Nurse, 32*(4), 27–34, 71.

Brandmeyer, E., & Thimmesch, A. (2014). Using coenzyme Q10 in clinical practice. *Nursing, 44*(3), 63–66.

Buonocore, D., & Wallace, E. (2014). Comprehensive guideline for care of patients with heart failure. *AACN Advanced Critical Care, 25*(2), 151–162.

Cheek, D. (2013). What you need to know about pharmacogenomics. *Nursing, 43*(3), 44–48.

Clinical Pharmacology. Retrieved from <http://www.clinicalpharmacology.com/default.aspx>.

Cookson, K. (2013). Dimensional analysis: Calculate dosages the easy way. *Nursing, 43*(6), 57–62.

Cooper, B., & Sejnowski, C. (2013). Serotonin syndrome: Recognition and treatment. *AACN Advanced Critical Care, 24*(1), 15–20.

Cranwell-Bruce, L. (2011). Biological disease modifying antirheumatic drugs. *Medsurg Nursing, 20*(3), 147–149.

Crawford, C., & Johnson, J. (2012). To aspirate or not: An integrative review of the evidence. *Nursing, 42*(3), 20–25.

Daniels, G., & Schmelzer, M. (2013). Giving laxatives safely and effectively. *Medsurg Nursing, 22*(5), 290–296, 302.

Darcy, D. (2014). What's new in anticoagulation for patients with atrial fibrillation? *American Nurse Today, 9*(11), 7–10.

Duncan, J., & Corcoran, J. (2007). *Pediatric high-alert medications: Evidence-based safe practices for nursing professionals.* Marblehead, MA: HCPro.

Felicilda-Reynaldo, R. (2013). A review of anticholinergic medications for overactive bladder symptoms. *Medsurg Nursing, 22*(2), 119–123.

Felicilda-Reynaldo, R. (2013). Circulation savers: Thrombolytic therapy. *Medsurg Nursing, 22*(6), 393–397.

Felicilda-Reynaldo, R., & Kenneally, M. (2015). A review of antihypertensive medication, Part I. *Medsurg Nursing, 24*(3), 177–181.

Frith, K. (2013). Medication errors in the intensive care unit. *AACN Advanced Critical Care, 24*(4), 389–404.

Gann, M. (2015). How informatics nurses use bar code technology to reduce medication errors. *Nursing, 45*(3), 60–66.

Gibson, J., & Raphael, B. (2014). Understanding beta-blockers. *Nursing, 44*(6), 55–59.

Glowacki, D. (2015). Effective pain management and improvements in patients' outcomes and satisfaction. *Critical Care Nurse, 35*(3), 33–43.

Guenter, P., & Boullata, J. (2013). Drug administration by enteral feeding tube. *Nursing, 43*(12), 26–33.

Hussar, D. A. (2012). New drugs 2012, part 1. *Nursing, 42*(3), 38–45.

Hussar, D. A. (2012). New drugs 2012, part 2. *Nursing, 42*(7), 38–44.

Hussar, D. A. (2013). New drugs 2013, part 1. *Nursing, 43*(2), 36–46.

Hussar, D. A. (2013). New drugs 2013, part 2. *Nursing, 43*(7), 42–49.

Hussar, D. A. (2014). New drugs 2014, part 1. *Nursing, 44*(2), 44–54.

Hussar, D. A. (2014). New drugs 2014, part 2. *Nursing, 44*(7), 26–33.

Hussar, D. A. (2014). New drugs 2014, part 3. *Nursing, 44*(10), 28–34.

Hussar, D. A. (2015). New drugs 2015, part 1. *Nursing, 45*(4), 40–48.

Institute for Safe Medication Practices. *ISMP's list of error-prone abbreviations, symbols, and drug designations.* (2013). Retrieved from <http://www.ismp.org/Tools/errorproneabbreviations.pdf>.

Institute for Safe Medication Practices. *ISMP's list of confused drug names.* (2015). Retrieved from <http://www.ismp.org/Tools/Confused-Drug-Names.aspx>.

Institute for Safe Medication Practices. *ISMP's list of high-alert medications.* (2015). Retrieved from <http://www.ismp.org/Tools/HighAlertMedicationList.asp>.

Jalkut, M. (2014). Ketorolac as an analgesic agent for infants and children after cardiac surgery. *AACN Advanced Critical Care, 25*(1), 23–30.

Jones, J. (2014). Misread labels as a cause of medication errors. *American Journal of Nursing, 114*(3), 11.

Kuebler, K. (2014). Using morphine in end-of-life care. *Nursing, 44*(4), 60.

Lampe, J. (2014). Beware of oversimplifying mealtime insulin dosing for hospital patients. *American Nurse Today, 9*(9), 9–12.

Leung, J., Nelson, S., & Leloux, M. (2014). Pharmacotherapy during the end of life: Caring for the actively dying patient. *AACN Advanced Critical Care, 25*(2), 79–88.

Macedo, M. (2015). The effects on growth of inhaled corticosteroids in children with persistent asthma. *American Journal of Nursing, 115*(6), 21.

Mandrack, M., Cohen, M., Featherling, J., Gellner, L., Judd, K., Kienle, P., et al. (2012). Nursing best practices using automated dispensing cabinets: Nurses' key role in improving medication safety. *Medsurg Nursing, 21*(3), 134–139.

Matzo, M., & Dawson, K. (2013). Opioid-induced neurotoxicity. *American Journal of Nursing, 113*(10), 51–56.

Merchant, N., & Waldrop, J. (2012). The safety and advantages of pentavalent vaccines. *The Nurse Practitioner, 37*(4), 48–53.

National Coordination Council for Medication Error Reporting and Prevention. *Medication error index report.* (2015). Retrieved from <http://www.nccmerp.org/home>.

Polizzi, M. (2015). Drug therapy 101. *Nursing, 45*(1), 44–46.

Porter, R. (2014). Medication errors in the intensive care unit: Ethical considerations. *AACN Advanced Critical Care, 25*(1), 56–62.

Rosini, J., & Dogra, P. (2015). Pharmacology for insomnia: Consider the options. *Nursing, 45*(3), 38–45.

Ruggiero, J., Smith, J., Copeland, J., & Boxer, B. (2015). Discharge time out: An innovative nurse-driven protocol for medication reconciliation. *Medsurg Nursing, 24*(3), 165–172.

Scordo, K., & Pickett, K. (2015). Managing hypertension: Piecing together the guidelines. *Nursing, 45*(1), 28–33.

Sculli, G., & Sine, D. (2011). *Soaring to success: Taking crew resource management from the cockpit to the nursing unit.* Danvers, MA: HCPro.

Shaffer, C., & Aymong, L. (2014). Administering vaccines. *Nursing, 44*(10), 46–50.

Shanks, L. (2011). Medication calculation competency. *American Journal of Nursing, 111*(10), 67–69.

Sherrod, M., Sherrod, N., & Cheek, D. (2015). Following the guideline for reducing cardiovascular risk with statins. *Nursing, 45*(6), 41–46.

Smith, G., Wagner, J., & Edwards, J. (2015). Epilepsy update part 1: Refining our understanding of a complex disease. *American Journal of Nursing, 115*(5), 40–47.

Smith, G., Wagner, J., & Edwards, J. (2015). Epilepsy update part 2: Nursing care and evidence-based treatment. *American Journal of Nursing, 115*(6), 34–44.

Spivak, I. (2015). Oral anticoagulants and atrial fibrillation: An update for the clinical nurse. *Medsurg Nursing, 24*(2), 95–100.

Thompson, N. (2013). Chemotherapy and biotherapy drugs for autoimmune diseases. *American Nurse Today, 8*(9), 22–26.

Tzeng, H., Yin, C., & Schneider, T. (2013). Medication error-related issues in nursing practice. *Medsurg Nursing, 22*(1), 13–16, 50.

U.S. Food and Drug Administration. (2014). Content and format of labeling for human prescription drugs and biologics: Requirements for pregnancy and lactation labeling. *Federal Register, 79*(233), Part II. Retrieved from <http://www.gpo.gov/fdsys/pkg/FR-2014-12-04/pdf/214-28241.pdf>.

Vitale, S. (2012). What your patient needs to know about CAM. *Nursing, 42*(8), 59–61.

Wallis, L. (2014). A combination drug for HIV prevention in high-risk groups. *American Journal of Nursing, 114*(8), 15.

Wallis, L. (2014). Milliliter-only instructions could reduce parents' dosing errors. *American Journal of Nursing, 114*(10), 16.

Williams, T., King, M., Thompson, J., & Champagne, M. (2014). Implementing evidence-based medication safety interventions on a progressive care unit. *American Journal of Nursing, 114*(11), 53–62.

Wilson, K. (2013). Choosing the right line for the right time. *Nursing, 43*(12), 66–68.

Zurawski, R. (2014). Carbapenem-resistant Enterobacteriaceae: Occult threat in the intensive care unit. *Critical Care Nurse, 34*(5), 44–52.

Index

Page numbers followed by "*f*" indicate
figures, "*t*" indicate tables, and "*b*" indicate
boxes.